P9-DVV-075

EAT RIGHT

4

YOUR TYPE

Complete
Blood Type Encyclopedia

Most Riverhead Books are available at special quantity discounts for bulk purchases for sales promotions, premiums, fund-raising, or educational use. Special books, or book excerpts, can also be created to fit specific needs.

For details, write: Special Markets, The Berkley Publishing Group, 375 Hudson Street, New York, New York 10014.

EAT RIGHT 4 YOUR TYPE

Complete
Blood Type Encyclopedia

**The A–Z Reference Guide for the Blood Type Connection to
Symptoms, Disease, Conditions, Vitamins, Supplements, Herbs and Food**

Dr. Peter J. D'Adamo
with Catherine Whitney

RIVERHEAD BOOKS
New York

Riverhead Books
Published by The Berkley Publishing Group
A division of Penguin Putnam Inc.
375 Hudson Street
New York, New York 10014

Every effort has been made to ensure that the information contained in this book is
complete and accurate. However, neither the publisher nor the authors are engaged in
rendering professional advice or services to the individual reader. The ideas, procedures,
and suggestions contained in this book are not intended as a substitute for consulting with
your physician. All matters regarding your health require medical supervision. Neither
the authors nor the publisher shall be liable or responsible for any loss, injury, or damage
allegedly arising from any information or suggestion in this book. The opinions expressed
in this book represent the personal views of the authors and not of the publisher.

Copyright © 2002 by Hoop-A-Joop, LLC
Book design by Tiffany Kukec
Cover design by Thomas Tofuri

All rights reserved. This book, or parts thereof, may not be reproduced
in any form without permission.

Published simultaneously in Canada.

First Riverhead trade paperback edition: January 2002

Visit our website at www.penguinputnam.com

Library of Congress Cataloging-in-Publication Data

D'Adamo, Peter
Eat right for your type complete blood type encyclopedia / Peter D'Adamo, with
Catherine Whitney
p.   cm.
ISBN 1-57322-920-2
1. Blood groups.   2. Health.   3. Medicine, Popular.   I. Whitney, Catherine.   II. Title

QP98.D3335 2002
612.1'1825—dc21
2001048776

PRINTED IN THE UNITED STATES OF AMERICA

10   9   8   7   6   5   4   3   2

For Teresa and Mary—and a sunny day

Contents

PART ONE
The Basics of the ABO Blood Groups

PART TWO
A–Z Blood Group Guide to Health and Medical Conditions

Contents

Contents

Contents

PART THREE
Blood Group Protocols

ACKNOWLEDGMENTS

The *Eat Right 4 Your Type Complete Blood Type Encyclopedia* represents the most comprehensive database of blood type–related scientific and medical information available in one volume.

Since the publication of *Eat Right 4 Your Type* in late 1996, we have seen the blood type diet introduced to millions of readers and translated into more than forty languages. The foundation created by this first bestselling title has since been strengthened with the addition of *Cook Right 4 Your Type*, in 1999, and *Live Right 4 Your Type*, in 2001. We have made full use of Internet technology to offer support and education and enable important feedback from thousands of readers around the world, through our website, www.dadamo.com.

The development of this encyclopedia has relied on the talents and dedication of many professionals. I want to express my deep thanks to those who have been most instrumental in its creation:

Martha Mosko D'Adamo, my wife and partner, who provided support, feedback and inspiration throughout the entire creative process.

My literary agent, Janis Vallely, who has been a treasured colleague and friend, as well as a wonderful advocate.

Amy Hertz, my editor at Riverhead/Putnam, who has nurtured my work with patience and skill. Her unflagging enthusiasm and steady hand have been invaluable.

Catherine Whitney, my writer, and her partner, Paul Krafin, who have transformed incredibly complex science into lively prose and easy-to-understand guidelines. Their agent, Jane Dystel, continues to provide advice and encouragement.

I would also like to acknowledge others who have made significant contributions to this encyclopedia: my colleague Bronner Handwerger, N.D., whose medical insights and research abilities enabled us to create a comprehensive and cutting-edge encyclopedia; Heidi Merritt, whose reliable instincts and attention to detail were essential to this complex effort; and our fine illustrators, Deborah Schuler and Paul Whitney.

Special thanks to the wonderful staffs at Riverhead Books and Putnam, whose tireless efforts, under the direction of Susan Petersen, have produced such great success.

This encyclopedia would not be possible were it not for the work of countless scientists and researchers, whose pioneering work throughout the twentieth century has enhanced our understanding of the evolution, biology and genetics of blood type. In particular, I am indebted to my father, James D'Adamo, N.D., who has given me a wonderful scientific legacy.

USERS GUIDE

The following explanations and guidelines will help you navigate this encyclopedia, and make the most of its contents.

Scientific References

There are hundreds of scientific study references throughout the encyclopedia, appearing at the end of each section. Most of the articles cited may be accessed through Medscape's MEDLINE service (www.medscape.com).

Blood Type Databases

If you would like to pursue a more advanced understanding and application of the blood type science, Dr. D'Adamo's website (www.dadamo.com) contains the following databases:

Diet and Nutrition

TYPEbase®, a searchable food value database by blood group

NUTRIbase®, a searchable food nutrient database

RECIbase®, a searchable recipe database by blood group

SUPPbase®, a searchable database of nutritional supplements

PHYTObase®, a searchable database of medicinal herbs

FRANKENbase®, a searchable database of genetically engineered foods

Immunology

ALLERbase®, a searchable protein allergen database with links to external accessions

Outcomes

RESULTbase®, a searchable database of self-reported outcomes by individuals following the blood type diet

Lectins

LECster®, a searchable lectin characterization database, with references

Genetics

GENEBase®, a searchable genomic database

In addition, it is recommended that newcomers to this science read Dr. D'Adamo's foundational books, *Eat Right 4 Your Type: The Individualized Diet Solution to Staying Healthy, Living Longer & Achieving Your Ideal Weight* and *Live Right 4 Your Type: The Individualized Prescription for Maximizing Health, Metabolism, and Vitality in Every Stage of Your Life.*

A Word About Terminology

Although we often use the colloquial term "blood type" in everyday language, scientists normally employ the more precise term "ABO blood groups" to distinguish the ABO blood-typing system from the many other minor blood-typing systems. To remain consistent with the scientific data, the term "blood group" will be used in the medical text of this book.

PART I

Anthropological, Biological and Genetic Basis

This section contains the most current information available on the anthropology, biology and genetics of the ABO blood groups. It is the textual point of reference for health and medical information and recommendations.

PART II

Medical Conditions

The A–Z Blood Group Guide to Health and Medical Conditions contains blood group–specific information and recommendations for more than 250 medical conditions. We have taken care to cover only those conditions for which some blood group association exists. In some cases, that association has been validated in multiple studies and reflects a conclusion that is generally accepted in medical science.

Example: Blood group A's greater susceptibility to most cancers, and blood group O's higher than average risk of ulcers.

In other cases, where fewer studies have been conducted, the associations are less clear, and the data should be used judiciously.

Example: The association between blood group O and fibromyalgia.

If you do not find the condition you're concerned about in this encyclopedia, a blood group association has not yet been determined by laboratory research or clinical studies. However, you can gain some helpful general information by referring to the medical category of the condition—for example, IMMUNITY or AUTOIMMUNE DISEASES. You may also refer to Dr. D'Adamo's website (www.dadamo.com) for outcome reports by individuals, and for bulletin board discussions, where thousands of individuals have shared their results anecdotally.

Risk Charts

At the top of each medical condition is a risk chart, graphically representing what is known about blood group–specific risks for that condition. These charts serve only as a starting point for an investigation of risks. The association between blood groups and disease is not a simple matter of cause and effect. When we talk about blood type–related risk factors, we are not saying that being a particular blood type *in itself* creates a higher risk factor for certain diseases. Only that, in combination with other factors, such as family history, diet, lifestyle and environmental conditions, there may be an increased risk for developing a certain disease. In immeasurable increments, this risk factor may increase a lot, or it may increase a little. When we apply the blood type connection to the physiology of a particular disease, we can examine risk factors in a new context, calculate the variations in human physiology, and formulate treatments that go right to the heart of the susceptibility.

The values on the risk charts indicate the following:

LOW: Blood group provides some degree of protection.

AVERAGE: Blood group provides no known protection or risk.

HIGH: Blood group is a significant risk factor.

Therapies

Recommended therapies utilize the primary tool of blood group–specific protocols. These protocols (see part 3) are formulated according to the optimal food-supplement-behavioral formulas for each blood group. Additional highly specific recommendations are noted where appropriate.

Medical Condition Links

In order to provide the broadest possible range of information for each medical condition, there are two methods of linking them with other topics. The first is the use of SMALL CAPS in the text to indicate an item that is covered independently. In addition, each condition includes a list of related topics.

PART III

Blood Group–Specific Protocols

These 30 blood group-specific protocols are the functional health strategies to be used in addition to diet, exercise and general medical recommendations. These are the protocols that are recommended in the Therapies portion of the A–Z Blood Group Guide to Health and Medical Conditions (part 2).

In addition, the protocols are designed in a

modular format, making them available for use as needed for your general health and well-being. For example, you may wish to adhere to the Anti-stress Protocol for your blood group during a time of particularly high stress; the Surgery Recovery Protocol if you have had surgery; or the Antiviral Protocol if you are suffering from a viral infection, such as influenza.

Supplement names that appear in quotation marks—i.e., "ARAG"—are available through North American Pharmacal (see last page of text).

Note: These protocols are not meant as substitutes for the medical advice of physicians and other health-care professionals. Rather, they are intended to enhance medical treatments and provide overall health benefits.

Blood Group Food Base

This is the most detailed blood group–related food analysis to date. It not only provides values for ABO blood groups, non-secretors and minor blood groups, but also offers an explanation for why each food is considered beneficial, neutral or to be avoided, depending on your blood group.

Note: The basic values for each blood group are for secretors. Non-secretor variants are listed where appropriate.

Blood Group Supplement Base

The supplement database is a cross-reference for the blood group protocols, and also supplies additional information about the specific supplements recommended in each protocol. Listed here are the individualized blood group–specific beneficial effects of each supplement. This list is not intended as a comprehensive description of all supplements and their benefits, but as a targeted reference to help each blood group gain maximum health benefits.

PART ONE

The Basics of the ABO Blood Groups

1. THE ANTHROPOLOGY OF BLOOD GROUPS

2. A CENTURY OF BLOOD GROUP SCIENCE

3. BIOLOGICAL SIGNIFICANCE OF THE ABO BLOOD GROUPS

4. 9q34: THE ABO GENE

ONE

The Anthropology of Blood Groups

There is a vast span of human existence of which little is known. Archeological ruins from the beginnings of civilization have been unearthed, and there have been occasional discoveries of a more prehistoric nature, but not much else. The impermanency of our physical existence is responsible for this void; our flesh and body fluids rapidly decompose after death. Unless preserved by extraordinary means, even skeletal remains eventually crumble and disappear. Early peoples did not practice ceremonial burial. Left to the elements, bodies soon completely decomposed: "Dust to dust" was not a mere poetic metaphor. It was a recorded observation of our transient natures.

Only in the last century have scientists and anthropologists begun using biological markers such as the blood groups in the search for humanity's imprint on our distant past. These studies have allowed a greater understanding of the movements and groupings of early peoples as they adapted to changing climates, mutating germs, and uncertain food supplies. Recent analyses, using sophisticated genetic measures, have produced the most accurate picture to date of human evolution.

The variations, strengths, and weaknesses of each blood group can be seen as part of humanity's continual process of acclimating to different environmental challenges. Most of these challenges have involved the digestive and immune systems. It is no surprise, then, that many of the distinctions between the blood groups involve basic functions of our digestive and immune systems.

Evolution is usually considered in the context of millions of years, which is the time frame needed to explain the many differences between animals or other species. Yet humanity's own life span provides ample time for many small day-to-day refinements, representing the constant struggle between inherited traits and environmental challenges.

And although evidence indicates that the individual genetic mutations responsible for producing the ABO genes are quite ancient[1], this is of trivial importance to the actual demographics of the individual ABO blood groups in ancient populations. In genetics it is not the actual age of the gene that matters, but rather its frequency or drift. This is computed by geneticists using a formula called the Hardy-Weinberg equation. Hardy-Weinberg posits that if the only evolutionary force acting on the population is random mating, the gene frequencies remain unchanged and constant. For example, if you start off with a small number of a particular gene in a larger gene pool (such as the gene for blood group B in the gene pool for ABO blood type) and nothing other than random mating occurs, at the end of a period of time, you would still have a small number of B genes in the ABO gene pool.

So something other than random mating is responsible for the present-day differences in frequency between the ABO blood groups. There has to be another explanation for why there are such large populations of blood group O (40% to 45%) and A (35% to 40%) and much lower rates of groups B (4% to 11%) and AB (0 to 2%).

One explanation might be that perhaps the mutation that produced the B gene was just not as common an occurrence as the mutation that produced the A gene. Yet, if they occurred at the same time, why would this be? Also, if the mutations are of such paramount importance, why is the distribution of the B gene so geographically limited to an area of high concentration stretching as a belt of territory from the Himalayas to the Urals?

The answer lies not in the ancient nature of the mutations that produced the A and B genes, but rather in the interactions that occurred between early humans and their environment that were influenced by their ABO blood groups. These included the various areas and climates people chose to inhabit, each with their unique populations of microbes and foods that humans chose to catch or cultivate.

As humans migrated and were forced to adapt their diets to local conditions, the new diets provoked changes in their digestive tracts and immune systems, necessary for them to first survive and later thrive in their new habitats. Different foods metabolized in a unique manner by each ABO blood group probably resulted in that blood group achieving a certain level of susceptibility (good or bad) to the endemic bacteria, viruses, and parasites of the area. This probably more than any other factor was what has influenced the modern-day distribution of our blood group. It is fascinating to note that virtually all the major infectious diseases that ran so rampant throughout our preantibiotic history have ABO blood group preferences of one group or another[2].

This results from the fact that many microbes possess ABO "blood types" of their own. It is perhaps useful to understand that the ABO blood group antigens are not unique to humans, although humans are the only species with all four variants. They are relatively simple sugars that are abundantly found in nature. For example, a bacterium with an antigen on its surface that mimicked the blood group A antigen would have a much easier time infecting a person who was group A, since that bacteria would more likely be considered "self" to the immune system of a blood group A person. Also, microbes may adhere to the tissues of one ABO group in preference to another, by possessing specialized adhesion molecules for that particular blood group[3].

The horrors of the Black Plague, which ran unchecked throughout Europe in the thirteenth and fourteenth centuries, is a perfect example. The plague was a disease caused by bacterial infection and was almost certainly fatal to those who contracted it in the early years of its initial spread. By the fifteenth century, however, fatalities were rare, although many people continued to contract the infection. In just two generations, traits were developed in the survivors that protected them from fatal infections. Since these traits were necessary to survival, they were then passed on and retained as a form of genetic memory.

The Black Plague is especially interesting from the perspective of ABO blood groups, since *Yersinia pestis*, the source of the plague, is a bacterium that prefers individuals of a specific ABO group, in this case, group O[4,5].

The effects of ABO blood group on survival against most forms of epidemic illness is so distinct that a modern-day map of the ABO blood group distribution in Europe closely parallels the locations of major epidemics, with higher densities of blood group A and lower frequencies of blood group O in areas historically known to have had long histories of repeated pandemics.

On the other hand, in pre-urbanization days blood group O would have had the survival advantage against the flukes and worms that routinely infected early humans, probably because it is the only blood group with antibodies against two other antigens, A and B. These changes are reflected in the local success or failure of each of the blood groups, which appear to have each had a moment of preeminence at a critical juncture in our history: the ascent of humans to the top of the food chain (the early advantage of blood group O), the change from hunting and gathering to a highly concentrated, urban environment and agriculturally based diet (the ascent of blood group A), and the mingling and migration of the races from the African homeland to Europe and Asia (the opportunity for blood groups B and AB).

The Ancestral Foundation

Chemical analysis of the group O antigen reveals that, from a structural perspective, it is the simplest blood group and serves as the backbone for the synthesis of increasingly complex A, B and AB antigens. These later blood groups evolved by adding other sugars onto the basic O sugar, much as a modern city might be built upon the foundations of an ancient one. Thus, if the mutations that produced the A and B antigens are ancient, the gene for blood group O is infinitely older.

Another dimension testifying to the great antiquity of group O comes from the science of physical anthropology and suggests that a greater part of humanity's existence has been lived exclusively as group O.

New studies on mitochondrial DNA (mtDNA) support the theory that *Homo sapiens* emerged in Africa and only later infiltrated other regions. Unlike DNA, which is inherited from both parents and changes minutely with each generation, mtDNA is passed directly from mother to child. It is contained in eggs but not in sperm. Since only random mutations alter its sequence, it is a more accurate measure of the trajectory of human evolution. Extensive mtDNA studies demonstrate that humans evolved from a common ancestor. These studies also confirm the theory that the blood groups evolved as migratory mutations.

The extraordinarily high percentage of blood group O in "ancient" or otherwise isolated populations also testifies to its great age[6]. Even though the early migrations dispersed the gene for group O blood throughout the world, there are some extraordinary examples of "old" populations existing in our world today. Because of their geographic locations, these societies have remained isolated from interaction with other populations. If A, B and O had developed simultaneously, the isolated population groups would have had all of them. But these "old societies" are group O because genes for the later blood groups never had the opportunity to enter into their populations. They have remained unchanged.

The Basques are an ancient people whose origins are still a mystery. The Basque language, the only western European language not connected by Indo-European roots, appears to be related to several dialects found in small isolated populations in the valleys of the Caucasus Mountains. Although they look much like their French and Spanish neighbors, Basques possess the lowest frequency of blood group B—originally having no group B at all—and the highest frequencies of blood group O in Europe. Cattle, abundant on the European plains, and freshwater fish seem to have been the staples of their early existence, as evidenced by the extraordinary renderings of the famous cave paintings found in the Basque country.

More than 50% of the Basque population is Rh-negative, as opposed to 16% for the rest of Europe. Like the gene for group O, the genetic mechanism for the Rh-negative blood type is simpler, hence undoubtedly older, than the gene for Rh-positive.

Native Americans are another example of the "old peoples" existing in our world today. It has often been asserted that all full-blooded American Indians are group O, and recent studies on largely intermingled Amerindian populations show a very high (67% to 80%) predominance of O, indicating that their migration from Asia to Alaska was probably much earlier than previously believed[7,8]. Their high rate of blood group O suggests that the Amerindians and Eskimos are directly descended from Cro-Magnon ancestors, probably Mongolians, who migrated around 15,000 B.C. to the Americas. In contrast to the Basques, however, the Asian Amerindians must have mingled extensively with other Asian populations, picking up along the way the gene for Rh-positive blood.

As with the Basques, few Native Americans are group B, so they must have migrated to the Americas late enough to pick up the Rh-positive gene, but too early to pick up the gene for B[9]. This migration probably took place across the land bridge that at one time connected Siberia to Alaska. As the last Ice Age ebbed and the lands warmed and glaciers receded, the rising water levels eliminated the land bridge between Asia and America, bottling up the Native Americans and a high-O enclave and preventing for another 10,000 years any communication between the continents. Forensic studies support this theory: in Chile no B or AB blood groups have been noted either in pre-Columbian or Colonial mummies[10].

Another theory for the extremely high incidence of blood group O in Native Americans is that O individuals seem relatively resistant to syphilis and smallpox, having developed antibodies to the infections that were major killers of Native Americans when they were introduced into the Old World by Columbus[11].

Agricultural advances in the Americas were late in coming, because the new American homeland was abundantly populated with game and fish, which discouraged agriculture. Even corn, which was the staple grain, didn't appear to be domesticated until 4500 B.C., and common beans appear to be an even more recent addition, first being cultivated around 2200 B.C. So, as with the Basques, meats and not grains were the primary staple of the Native American diet.

In England, Wales, and Scotland, there is a strong association between ABO blood group and geographical differences in the death rate[12]. Studies of blood group distribution in the British Isles show a general increase of group O frequency from relatively low numbers in southern England to increasingly higher ones in northern England, Wales, Scotland, and Ireland[13]. This suggests that the Anglo-Saxons had relatively high A levels, and that O increased as the proportion of Celtic ancestry increased, although the origin of the high incidence of blood group O in the Irish may represent the remnants of Mesolithic peoples[14]. This is also the case with continental Europe, where the percentage of group O increases in northern Germans and Danes. It is also known that the Icelanders had high O frequencies, close to the frequencies found in the populations of Scotland and Ireland.

Among the Nomads of the Arabian Peninsula and the Berbers of the Atlas Mountains, two old populations, the frequency of the blood group O gene is high. Africans, on average, have more O genes and less A genes than do Europeans. So it can be seen that the gene carried by people who are blood group O is ancient by evolutionary standards.

The Age of the Hunter-Gatherers

Our first human ancestors likely emerged in sub-Saharan Africa between 170,000 and 50,000 years ago. These ancestors probably ate a rather crude, omnivorous diet of plants, grubs, and the scavenged leftovers of other, more successful predatory animals. Since humans have neither the sharp teeth nor claws of a true predator, one could speculate that these people were perhaps as much prey as predator. Yet within these early humans lay the greatest predatory tool yet devised: the human brain.

In a study published in the journal *Science*, anthropologists reported that tests made on the carbon content of teeth of *Australopithecus africanus*, a pre-human species, indicate that they ate large quantities of foods rich in carbon 13—such as grasses and sedges—or animals that ate these plants, or both. The research indicated that the australopithecines, which walked upright but also climbed trees, were already venturing out of their usual forest habitat to forage in open grasslands. It also suggested that hominids were consuming high-protein animal foods before the development of stone tools for butchering. They noted that many theories of human origins invoke a switch to a meat-rich diet to explain the sudden expansion of brain size with the first *Homo* species. If they were eating meat, it probably came from small animals that could be caught without tools or the scavenged remains of meals left by large predators[15].

Big game hunting by humans started in Africa about half a million years ago, although the full force of armed human bands may not have been felt much before 100,000 B.C.

Early humans' relationship to their environment changed dramatically with the appearance of our first direct ancestors, the Cro-Magnons, around 40,000 B.C. Named for a site in France where remains were first identified and studied, Cro-Magnons developed the beginnings of communication and tool working, and were also superb hunters. Using simple signals and gestures, they began to hunt in organized packs, wielding bone or simple stone weapons. This major advance catapulted what had been one of the less successful primates all the way to the top of the food chain. As skillful and formidable hunters, Cro-Magnons soon had little to fear from any animal rival.

Cro-Magnons possessed such modern human features as a higher, vertical forehead, a reduced brow ridge, a smaller face and teeth, and a chin. Their skeletons indicate great muscularity, suggesting they were employed in much more strenuous activities than are most modern peoples.

By the time of the Cro-Magnons, hunting and the consumption of a mostly carnivorous diet had become a way of life. It was in the midst of this carnivorous frenzy that the digestive attributes of blood group O reached their full expression, with the highly efficient acid and pepsin production of the stomach geared for the digestion of meat. With no natural predators (other than themselves) and an assured supply of game, the population of wily, physically agile Cro-Magnon hunters must have flourished.

Once early humans had gained ascendancy, it took a surprisingly short time for them to deplete the numbers of major game animals. By 50,000 B.C., most large game herds were already extinct in Africa. The scarcity of a primary food source led to widespread migration in search of new and fertile hunting grounds. The feast had come to an end. It had been a fairly routine task to feed a small hunting group on the kill of a single enormous animal carcass for a week or more. Now, having to hunt and kill a sufficient number of small game, most of whom proved fast and elusive, made survival much more difficult. Hunger began to take its toll on the previously successful tribes of hunters. The young, old, and weak fell by the wayside, succumbing to disease and starvation. Bands of hunters began warring with each other for the limited food supply.

This depletion of the large game in Africa, coupled with climatic changes and possibly population pressures, encouraged early humans to begin moving out of Africa. The more barren northern areas, previously covered with ice, had started to warm, while a shift in the trade winds began to parch and desiccate what had once been fertile land in the African Sahara.

All of these factors joined together into what was quite possibly the greatest series of migrations in human history. These migrations seeded the planet with a base population of blood group O, helping to make it the widespread and ubiquitous blood group it continues to be to this day.

The Wanderings

By 30,000 B.C., bands of Cro-Magnons were migrating eastward and northward in search of new hunting lands. By 20,000 B.C., migration into Europe and Asia was so significant that large game herds began disappearing from those areas as well.

Other food sources had to be discovered, and the search was a desperate one. Under these pressures, our ancestors may have become omnivorous again, feeding on a broader menu of new plant and animal species. In particular, the food re-

sources of the shore and the sea were systematically exploited for the first time.

Cro-Magnons were getting smarter and more creative, developing more sophisticated housing and clothing. These alterations allowed bands of hunters to search for new game herds in northern grasslands and forests. By 10,000 B.C., human hunting groups occupied all the main land masses of the earth, except for Antarctica. Hunting bands found their way to Australia between 40,000 and 30,000 years ago. Some 5,000 to 15,000 years later, other bands managed to cross the Bering Strait from Asia and entered the Americas. In these later, relatively more sophisticated hunting societies, the extermination of large game accelerated. Cro-Magnon hunting methods were becoming increasingly efficient, as evidenced by the vast number of animal bones piled up at some of the recently unearthed archeological sites. At Solutre, France for example, the remains of more than 10,000 horses have been found. At Dolni Vestonice in the Czech Republic, a large number of bones from extinct mammoths litter the site. Some archeologists estimate that from the time human migration to the Americas began about 15,000 years ago, it took less than one thousand years to exterminate most of the large game in North and South America. The reason that the Aztec civilization was so easily toppled by the Spanish Conquistadors was the sheer terror that the horse-mounted warriors brought to the relatively primitive Aztec foot soldiers. Horses were previously unknown to the Aztecs—in earlier migrations from north to central America, their ancestors had exterminated the wild horses of the American plains, slaughtering them for food.

They had no idea that horses could be used for far greater purposes than as a food source.

The expansion of Cro-Magnon hunting bands across the earth was a period of unalloyed success for humankind. The effect of a carnivorous diet on human growth was profound. The movement of the early humans to more temperate climates stimulated genetic responses. They developed lighter skins, less massive bone structures, and straighter hair. The skeleton, especially in Caucasians, matures slowly, and their lighter skin is better protected than darker skin against frostbite. Lighter skin is also better able to metabolize vitamin D, vital to survival in a land of shorter days and longer nights.

The dominance of the Cro-Magnons eventually brought about their own downfall. They suffered greatly from their own success. Overpopulation soon led to the exhaustion of available hunting grounds. Before long, most of the large game herds in the populated regions were destroyed by overhunting. This led to increased competition for a limited food supply. Competition led to war, and war to further migration.

The Agricultural Dawning

The Neolithic period, or "New Stone Age," followed the Paleolithic period or "Old Stone Age" of the Cro-Magnon hunters, beginning around 30,000 B.C. Agriculture and animal domestication are generally recognized as the hallmarks of its culture. The ability to cultivate grains and livestock allowed these early people to forgo the hand-to-mouth existence of their nomadic ancestors, and settle down in cities, allowing for substantial population concentrations. The British prehistorian V. Gordon Childe coined the term "Neolithic Revolution" to describe the change from a hunting and gathering society to one based on food production, and he considered it the greatest advance in human history after the marshaling of fire.

The Neolithic Period was also an important watershed in the distribution of the ABO blood groups. This new, relatively sedentary, agrarian lifestyle and the major change in diet resulted in a new mutation in the digestive tracts and immune systems of these early people. Many of them became carriers of group A blood. The blood group A variant allowed humans to tolerate and better assimilate grains and other agricultural products. Blood group A initially appeared in significant numbers in the early Caucasian peoples, sometime between 25,000 and 15,000 B.C., somewhere in western Asia or the Middle East. The gene for group A was carried into western Europe and Asia during the movement of these Neolithic societies, especially a branch termed the Indo-Europeans, where it penetrated extensively into the pre-Neolithic type O populations.

The Indo-Europeans appeared originally in South Central Russia, and between 3500 and 2000 B.C. spread southward into Southwestern Asia, especially to Iran and Afghanistan. At some point after this, they began to spread again, this time further westward, into Europe. Not only did their migration serve to transport the gene for group A to pre-Neolithic hunter-gatherers, but it also served as a major catalyst in stimulating the adoption of Neolithic developments, such as agriculture. Almost all modern Europeans share a common ancestry with the Indo-European peoples.

The invasion of the Neolithic Indo-Europeans was scattershot and incomplete. In some areas, pre-Neolithic societies were obliterated through warfare and intermingling, while leaving others, such as the Basques of Spain, relatively alone and intact.

The Neolithic Revolution was the original "diet revolution," as it introduced new foods and lifestyle habits into the simpler immune systems and digestive tracts of the early hunter-gatherers, and produced the environmental stress necessary to spark the development of a new blood group variation, A. As the digestive tract of this new blood group gradually lost its ability to digest the carnivorous diet of the hunter-gatherers, the simpler, pre-agricultural diet dependent largely on hunting and gathering disappeared.

The Emergence of the Collective

Settling into permanent communities presented new developmental challenges; the individualistic tendencies of the hunter-gatherer now gave way to a more structured society. Skill specialization can only evolve as part of a larger whole; the basket weaver is dependent on the farmer, the farmer on the toolmaker. One no longer thought of food only when hungry; fields needed to be sown and cultivated in anticipation of future reward.

The cultivation of wheat and barley, coupled with the domestication of food animals such as sheep, goats, pigs, chickens, and later cattle, first occurred between 9000 and 5000 B.C. in southwestern Asia, a fertile mixing ground in which all three major races commingled.

The new farming economies spread slowly from southeast Europe to the north and west. The permanent settlements that developed as a result of the new agrarian society gave rise to the early cities.

Neolithic sites in southeast Europe date from before 6000 B.C. and are located in areas with the most workable soils and temperate climate. Cattle, sheep, or pigs, in addition to wheat, barley, peas, beans, and flax, were raised. By 4000 B.C., a series of settlements were established on the lakeshores of Switzerland, and agriculture was adapted to the Alpine environment, with emphasis on cattle, legumes, and fruit, in addition to wheat.

Cereal crops and cattle were introduced to western France by 4000 B.C. and were in use in southern Scandinavia, the British Isles, and the northern European plains by about 3500 B.C., pushing the remaining hunter-gatherer peoples farther north into the wilderness, or influencing them to adopt the new, settled mode of life. 4000 B.C. marked the beginning of the Neolithic period in Britain and Ireland, and is denoted by an extensive clearing of the forests at that time for agriculture, burial rituals, and the building of "megalithic" structures such as Stonehenge in England.

There is good evidence to support the link between the ascendancy of blood group A and the development of the urban society. As discussed, many areas of the world that have long histories of urbanization and frequent outbreaks of plague, cholera, and smallpox show a predominance of group A over group O. This statistic clearly proved that group A was more resistant to and able to survive the infections common to densely populated areas. One might well wonder how blood group O survived at all—much less how it has remained to this day the most prevalent blood group on the planet. One reason might be the sheer amount of the group O gene in the gene pool; it is recessive in A and B and thus remains self-replicating.

Blood group A is found in the highest concentrations among western Europeans. Unlike blood groups B and O, there are many varieties of group A. The major grouping, A1, accounts for about 95% of all A blood. The largest subgroup, A2, is found principally in Northern Caucasians. A2 is found in very high concentration in Iceland and Scandinavia, particularly among the Lapps, ancient settlers of the area. They are almost unique in their high frequency of A, and have the highest frequency of A2, registering 42% in one group. The A2 gene is almost entirely confined to Caucasian populations. The European frequency of group A decreases as we head eastward.

Over much of Europe the frequency of the A gene is greater than 25%. It is also found in considerable numbers around the entire Mediterranean Sea, particularly in Corsica, Sardinia, Spain, Turkey, and the Balkans. It is clear that humankind most often laid down permanent settlements in those areas where conditions offered them the best chance of survival.

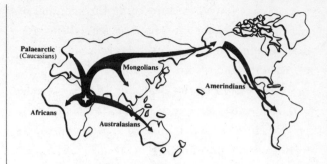

From their base in the ancestral homeland of Africa, early blood group O hunter-gatherers wandered throughout Africa and into Europe and Asia in search of new supplies of large game. As they encountered changing environmental conditions, they began to develop modern racial characteristics.

The Nomadic Mutation

The gene for blood group B first appeared in significant numbers somewhere around 10 to 15,000 B.C., the tail end of the Neolithic period, in the area of the Himalayan highlands now part of present-day Pakistan and India. As with the environmental conditions that spawned the advent of group A, the development of blood group B was in large part a response to changes in the environment. But unlike group A, which began to supplant group O as a response to new types of infections, then thrived as a result of the new dietary changes, group B appears to have been more of a response to climatic changes, followed by a different set of dietary adaptations. Life in the tropical flat savannahs of eastern Africa gave way to a harsher existence as the Cro-Magnon hunters migrated to the colder, drier, mountainous areas of the subcontinent and the barren endless plains of the central Asian steppes.

It is possible that blood group B may have been the only blood group with the capabilities to survive in such a harsh environment. There is some science behind this theory: For example, variability in levels of the hormones testosterone and estradiol and somatotropic hormones in mountaineers of the Pamirs and Kirghizes was examined in relation to their place of residence in terms of elevation above sea level. At high altitudes, blood O group had lower concentrations of estradiol and testosterone, while blood group B had the highest concentration[16]—making B better able to pass on its genes.

Under times of famine, two biological functions diminish: the ability to fend off infection and the ability to reproduce. Essentially omnivores, members of blood group B may have been the only blood group whose immune systems were capable of functioning with a diet described by one Roman historian as "soured milk and mare's blood." In addition to having the ability to survive pestilence, blood group B women may be more fertile than their group A and group O counterparts[17] and may begin to menstruate earlier[18].

Higher concentrations of the group B gene exist in direct relationship with the demographics of the preexisting caste system. Since the caste system was the direct result of consecutive layers of foreign conquest, it appears that the group B gene may have been introduced into the Indian subcontinent via conquest[19]. In a study among fourteen Hindu caste groups, besides Christian and Muslim populations of the West Godavari District, Andhra Pradesh, India, all the Hindu castes except Brahmin, Kshatriya, and Reddy exhibited relatively higher frequency of group B

over group A[20]. In a study of ABO distribution along the Silk Route of northwestern China, a distinct increase in blood group B was seen, especially when those subjects of Mongolian extraction were compared to Caucasians[21].

An almost continuous belt of mountainous terrain extends from the Urals in Russia to the Caucasus in Asia, and then to the Pyrenees of southern France. This barrier split the migrations of the blood groups into two basic routes: a northern stream and a southern one. The invaders taking the southern approach became the ancestors of the Mediterranean people and western Europeans, and carried with them the gene for blood group A. The Ural Mountains prevented a large migration westward from Asia, although small numbers of Caucasians entered eastern Europe, carrying with them the gene for blood group B, which they picked up by intermingling with the Asian Mongolians. This barrier served to divide blood groups into a western group, A, and an eastern group, B.

Blood group B Mongolians continued to travel northward, toward present-day Siberia. At various times the Mongolians penetrated large swaths of Eastern Europe, at one time reaching as far as the gates of Vienna, Austria. The Mongolians were certainly responsible for introducing the gene for blood group B into the eastern European populations. They developed a different culture, dependent on herding and emphasizing the use of cultured dairy products. These nomadic people were expert equestrians and wandered extensively over the Siberian flatlands, the great steppes. These nomads must have been compact, tightly knit, and genetically homogenous. A recent study using sophisticated polymerase chain reaction (PCR) technology determined the ABO groupings of the dried remains of nine human mummies that had been discovered in the Taklamakan desert in 1912. Of the nine, eight were group B[22].

Two basic blood group B population patterns emerged out of the Neolithic revolution in Asia: an agrarian, relatively sedentary population located in the south and east, and the wandering nomadic societies of the north and west. This schism stands as an important cultural remnant in Southern Asian cuisine—the use of dairy products remains practically nonexistent. To the Asian culture, dairy products are considered the food of the barbarian.

In the Middle East it appears that tribes of Semitic group B nomads may have infiltrated into preexisting Neolithic cultures, both passively and aggressively. Semitic peoples called the Hyksos were foreign rulers of Egypt during the Second Intermediate Period. Exactly who those foreign rulers were is not known, but it is assumed they were Asiatics. The Egyptian term for Hyksos merely means "rulers of foreign lands." It was once thought that foreign rule in Egypt would have necessarily entailed a violent overthrow, but instead there is the appearance of a peaceful takeover. More likely, the numbers of these foreigners slowly increased in the delta region until they became a powerful political force. Under the rule of the Hyksos, the continuity of Egyptian culture and ritual was preserved, indicating that these foreign kings had become fully Egyptianized. Persian suzerainty may have also added large amounts of the group B gene to the upper-class Egyptian gene pool; a third-century-B.C. Egyptian mummy, "Iset

Iri Hetes," was recently typed and found to be group B[23]. Interestingly, Africa in general (independent of any racial categorization) has a higher incidence of group B than Europe or the Middle East. Whether this is the result of intermingling or the original group B gene pool is unknown; however, it does imply that the links between ancient Egypt and sub-Saharan Africa are deeper and older than generally recognized.

The blood group characteristics of the various Jewish populations have long been of interest to anthropologists. As a general rule, regardless of their nationality or race, there is a trend toward higher-than-average rates of blood group B. The Ashkenazim of Eastern Europe and the Sephardim of the Middle East and Africa, the two major sects, share high rates of blood group B and bear no discernible differences. Babylonian Jews differ considerably from the predominantly group O present-day Arab population of Iraq in that they have a high frequency overall of blood group A and an even higher frequency of blood group B. The Jews of the Tafilalet Oasis in Morocco—an ancient community, now dispersed—also had a high frequency of the gene for blood group B, around 29% of the total society.

The Karaites, who have an extraordinarily high rate of blood group B, are members of a Jewish sect founded in Babylonia in the eighth century A.D. A singular community of Karaites continues to exist in Lithuania, and they were known to have migrated as a body from the Crimea. The Karaites consider themselves Jews by religion only, not by race. This claim of racial separation was accepted by the Nazi authorities, who controlled Lithuania during World War II. Because of this, the Karaites were spared the horrors of the Holocaust[24].

To modern-day anthropologists, blood group B continues to be an "Eastern" blood group. It is found in high numbers among Asians such as the Chinese, Indians, and Siberians. In Europe, blood group B is more frequently found in Hungarians, Russians, Poles, and other Eastern Europeans. It is not found in large numbers among Western Europeans. Among pre-Neolithic people, such as the Basques and Amerindians, group B is practically nonexistent.

Of all the ABO blood groups, group B shows the most clearly defined geographic distribution. Stretching as a great belt across the Eurasian plains and down to the Indian subcontinent, blood group B is found in increased numbers from Japan, Mongolia, China, and India up to the Ural Mountains. From there westward, the percentages fall until a low is reached at the extreme western end of Europe.

Blood group B is a distinctly non-Indo-European blood type. In Europe, only two areas with a high rate of blood group B appear: one among the group of non-Indo-European peoples known as the Finno-Ugrics (such as the Hungarians and the Finns), the other among the central Slavic peoples (Czechs, Southern Poles, and Northern Serbs). The Viking invaders may have also had a relatively high percentage of the B gene, since many of the towns of Britain and Western Europe that are linked to the coast by internal lines of communication such as large rivers have a disproportional amount of blood group B when compared to the surrounding territory.

The small numbers of blood group B in old and Western Europeans represents western migration by Asian nomadic peoples. This is most clearly seen in the easternmost Western Europeans, the Germans and Austrians, who have an unexpectedly high incidence of blood group B blood compared to their western neighbors. The highest frequency of blood group B in Germans occurs in the area around the upper and middle Elbe River, an important natural boundary between "civilization" and "barbarism" in ancient and medieval times.

Modern subcontinental Indians, a Caucasian people, have some of the highest frequencies of blood group B in the world. Interestingly, among the Asiatics, the Indians and the Japanese are the only groups that show high frequencies of blood group A as well. The northern Chinese and Koreans have high rates of blood group B, and lower rates of blood group A.

Nowadays, blood group B accounts for about 10% of the world's population.

Interminglings

Blood group AB is found in less than 5% of the population. It is certainly the most recent blood group. Unlike the other ABO blood groups, group AB resulted from the intermingling of group A Caucasian people and group B Mongolian people. Some of this may have been peaceful, but some must have been part of the violent turmoil that marked the great "Migration of Peoples" at the end of the Ancient Period (300 A.D. to 800 A.D.)

This time period was characterized by the collapse of the ancient civilizations, brought on by the influx of various wandering hordes of predominantly Eastern origin. The incidence of blood group B was probably very high in these steppe dwellers, so the appearance of group AB in Europe is probably the result of the intermingling of these Eastern invaders with their European hosts. In Europe, the distribution of this blood group parallels group B, with a low incidence in Western Europeans. There is a very high incidence of AB blood in subcontinental Indians, again probably the result of migration, conquest, caste distinctions, and intermingling.

Little evidence for the occurrence of group AB extends beyond 900 to 1,000 years ago, when a large western migration of Eastern peoples took place. Blood group AB is rarely found in European graves prior to 900 A.D. Studies of prehistoric grave exhumations in Hungary indicate a distinct lack of this blood group into the Langobard age (fifth to seventh century A.D.). This would seem to indicate that, up until that point in time, European populations of blood groups A and B did not come into common contact. If they did, they neither mingled nor intermarried.

Blood group AB may be a purely human invention. This blood group takes the concept of tolerance to the extreme, as it sees all things A-like or B-like as self, and manufactures no opposing blood group antibodies. As early as the 1940s it was noticed that blood group AB had a higher incidence of cancer than the other blood groups. On the plus side, group AB's tolerance perhaps minimizes the chances of allergies and other autoimmune diseases, such as arthritis and inflammation.

There may be a similar survival benefit with regard to possession of a B antigen that is shared between groups B and AB. For example, it has been noted that group B individuals are on average a bit taller than their A and O counterparts[25], and that group AB women are generally a bit heavier than those in the other ABO groups[26].

Something about AB "works" in a modern sense, because these people inherit the tolerance of both A and B. Perhaps this serves to enhance the AB immune system's abilities to manufacture more specific antibodies to microbial invaders, as it possesses neither anti-A or anti-B antibodies.

Blood Group Distribution Today

Our blood groups are not a hit-or-miss act of random genetics without any real purpose. Rather, the ABO blood groups are a set of differing solutions to a host of environmental variables, such as diet and infection, that insured the survival of the human race. The blood group adaptations were a change in "human antigenicity"—a biological desire to identify with the prevailing currents of the environment.

By looking at the distribution of blood groups today, we can see the threads of our evolutionary history. In the United States, O is the most prevalent blood group and A is second, followed by B, and finally AB. The breakdown in Great Britain is very similar to the U.S. percentages. In Germany there are slightly more A than O; B and AB remain almost the same as U.S. percentages. In Japan and China, A, O, and B are fairly evenly split, and the AB percentage increases over that found in European populations.

Until the end of World War II, physical anthropology usually meant the comparison of various physical characteristics of the body between different human populations and individuals. This usually included measurements of the body and its parts, especially the skull. However, probably as a result of the intensive use of blood transfusions during the war, the blood groups have come to provide an alternative to the often highly subjective methods of body measurement. Here was a definitive biological marker that could be used to map migrations and classify human groupings. Physical anthropology had its first scientific tool.

"History is bunk," wrote industrialist Henry Ford. It is a quote with the ring of truth in it. We are destined to interpret past events through the eyes of those who left the records (usually the victors), using our own modern-day thoughts and rationales. Losers rarely write history, and it is impossible for us to fully inhabit the minds and experiences of our predecessors. Yet there is something very intellectually and emotionally riveting about understanding the ebb and flow of our human experience. Not only is it fascinating from an intellectual standpoint, but we also can see, feel and touch the modern-day physical ramifications of these long-ago events.

In that sense, we are all survivors.

REFERENCES

1. O'hUigin C, Sato A, Klein J. Evidence for convergent evolution of A and B blood group antigens in primates. *Hum Genet.* 1997;101:141–148.

2. Garratty G. Blood group antigens as tumor markers, parasitic/bacterial/viral receptors, and their association with immunologically important proteins. *Immunol Invest.* 1995;24:213–232.

3. Jorgensen G. Human genetics and infectious diseases. *MMW Munch Med Wochenschr.* 1981;123:1447–1452.

4. Pestana de Castro AF, Perreau P, Rodrigues AC, Simoes M. Haemagglutinating properties of Pasteurella multocida type A strains isolated from rabbits and poultry. *Ann Microbiol (Paris).* 1980;131:255–263.

5. Doughty BR. The changes in ABO blood group frequency within a mediaeval English population. *Med Lab Sci.* 1977; 34:351–354.

6. Mourant AE. *Blood Relations: Blood Groups and Anthropology.* Oxford, NY: Oxford University Press; 1983.

7. Harb Z, Llop E, Moreno R, Quiroz D. Coastal Chilean populations: genetic markers in four locations. *Rev Med Chil.* 1998;126:753–760.

8. Gorodezky C, Castro-Escobar LE, Escobar-Gutierrez A. The HLA system in the prevalent Mexican Indian group: the Nahuas. *Tissue Antigens.* 1985;25:38–46.

9. Solovenchuk LL. [Genetic structure of the populations of native inhabitants in the northeastern USSR. III. Asiatic Eskimo and the coast and reindeer Chukchi]. *Genetika.* 1984;20:1902–1909.

10. Mitchell JR. An association between ABO blood-group distribution and geographical differences in death-rates. *Lancet.* 1977;1:295–297.

11. Cavalli-Sforza LL, Menozzi P, Piazza A. *The History and Geography of Human Genes.* Princeton: Princeton University Press, 1994.

12. Allison MJ, Hossaini AA, Munizaga J, Fung R. ABO blood groups in Chilean and Peruvian mummies. II. Results of agglutination-inhibition technique. *Am J Phys Anthropol.* 1978;49:139–142.

13. Mascie-Taylor CG, Lasker GW. Migration and changes in ABO and Rh blood group clines in Britain. *Hum Biol.* 1987;59:337–344.

14. Tills D, Teesdale P, Mourant AE. Blood groups of the Irish. *Ann Hum Biol.* 1977;4:23–24.

15. Wilford JN. Study of prehumans' teeth suggests that they

dined on meat. *The New York Times International.* January 15, 1999.

16. Spitsyn VA, Bets LV, Anikeeva AV, Spitsyna NK. Influence of environmental and genetic factors on levels of testosterone, estradiol and somatotropic hormones in mountaineers of the Pamir. *Vestn Ross Akad Med Nauk.* 1997;7:46–51.

17. Kelso AJ, Siffert T, Thieman A. Do type B women have more offspring?: an instance of asymmetrical selection at the ABO blood group locus. *Am J Human Biol.* 1995;41–44.

18. Balgir RS. Menarcheal age in relation to ABO blood group phenotypes and haemoglobin-E genotypes. *J Assoc Physicians India.* 1993;41:210–211.

19. Sengupta S, Dutta MN. Genetic investigations among the Ahom of Assam. *J Indian Med Assoc.* 1991;89:13–15.

20. Vijayalakshmi M, Naidu JM, Suryanarayana B. Blood groups, ABH saliva secretion and colour vision deficiency in Hindu castes and religious groups of West Godavari, Andhra Pradesh, India. *Anthropol Anz.* 1994;52:305–313.

21. Iwasaki M, Kobayashi K, Suzuki H, et al. Polymorphism of the ABO blood group genes in Han, Kazak and Uygur populations in the Silk Route of northwestern China. *Tissue Antigens.* 2000;56:136–142.

22. Lin Z, Kondo T, Minamino T, Sun E, Liu G, Ohshima T. Genotyping of ABO blood group system by PCR and RFLP on mummies discovered at Taklamakan desert in 1912. *Nippon Hoigaku Zasshi.* 1996;50:336–342.

23. Klys M, Opolska-Bogusz B, Prochnicka B. A serological and histological study of the Egyptian mummy 'Iset Iri Hetes' from the Ptolemaic period III-IB. C. *Forensic Sci Int.* 1999; 99:229–233.

24. Mourant AE. *Blood Relations: Blood Groups and Anthropology.* Oxford, NY: Oxford University Press: 1983.

25. Borecki IB, Elston RC, Rosenbaum PA, Srinivasan SR, Berenson GS. ABO associations with blood pressure, serum lipids and lipoproteins, and anthropometric measures. *Hum Hered.* 1985;35:161–170.

26. Kelso AJ, Maggi W, Beals KL. Body weight and ABO blood types: Are AB females heavier? *Amer J Hum Biol.* 1994; (6):385–387.

TWO

A Century of Blood Group
Science

Since their discovery at the beginning of the twentieth century, the ABO blood groups have emerged as the most reliable measure of human individuality and diversity. Their influence spans the entire spectrum of the physiological, psychological, and social orders.

Knowledge of their significance bridges many of the chasms in our understanding of human life—from how we have survived to the way we interact with our environment. The blood groups allow us to follow humanity's many migrations across this ancient planet.

As we look at the unraveling of the mysteries of the blood groups during the past century, we can see the patchwork of human identity come together, piece by piece, confirming the interre-

latedness of biology and destiny. It has been a fascinating and provocative journey.

The Discovery of ABO Blood Groups

The idea that blood circulated throughout the body was first proposed in 1628 by Englishman William Harvey, who published his theories in his famous book *On the Motion of the Heart and Blood in Animals*. Harvey was a student of Hieronymus Fabricius, an esteemed scientist and surgeon at the University of Padua in Italy. Fabricius, an ardent anatomist, had observed the one-way valves in veins, but had not figured out exactly what their role was. The popular belief of the day held that blood was circulated by a sort of pulsing action of the arteries.

From knowledge gained on the battlefield, early physicians knew that an extreme loss of blood produced shock and death. By the sixteenth century, physicians were attempting to replace blood lost in surgery or battle with the blood of a healthy donor. However, it was immediately recognized that success or failure was wildly unpredictable; some of these early attempts at transfusion succeeded in spectacular fashion, while others only seemed to hasten the demise of the patient. In their attempts to find a predictable way to exchange blood, physicians even tried using the blood of other animals, such as lambs, dogs and rabbits. Even milk and salt water were used. Unfortunately, most of the time these variations were terrible failures. Until the twentieth century, loss of blood was the most frequent cause of death in childbirth and on the battlefield.

Then, in 1888, at the University of Dorpat (now Tartu) in Estonia, a researcher doing work on his doctoral thesis made a discovery that would provide a vital clue to the mystery. While studying the toxicity of castor oil on laboratory animals, Herman Stillmark was shaken by the extreme suffering the animals endured. He decided to attempt his experiments on cell cultures instead of live animals. When Stillmark mixed an extract of castor seeds with blood, he made a startling observation: the red blood cells were agglutinated— that is, they clumped together, "like in clotting"[1]. Stillmark discovered that the agglutination by castor bean seeds occurred in some animal species but not in others and that castor seeds could also agglutinate liver cells, skin cells and white blood cells of some species as well. What Stillmark had discovered was for many years termed a "toxic principle" in the plant, and it was more than a half century before the protein responsible for these toxic effects was effectively isolated and given the name *ricin*, from the Latin name for castor beans (*Ricinus communis*). The discovery of agglutination was an important medical breakthrough. For the first time, a direct reaction between other substances and blood had been demonstrated.

Stillmark's work started a series of theses and papers at the University that investigated other agglutinating toxins. In 1891 it was discovered that the jequirty plant (*Abrus precatorius*) also possessed agglutinating properties. Croton, a third toxin isolated from the seeds of the "Physic-nut," *Croton tiglium*, was also shown to have differences in behavior toward different animal blood cells. Some red blood cells were simply destroyed (rabbit, crow), some strongly agglutinated (ox, pig, sheep, pike, perch, and frog), some moderately agglutinated (cat), and some very slightly agglutinated (human).

These early papers on agglutination by plant toxins had a stimulating effect on the burgeoning science of immunology and correlated with other earlier findings that described other agglutinating proteins from animal origin, such as many snake venoms.

This immediately caught the attention of German bacteriologist Paul Erlich, who recognized that he could investigate certain immunologic problems using plant agglutinins rather than relying on bacterial toxins, such as diphtheria. Using abrin and ricin, Ehrlich carried out a number

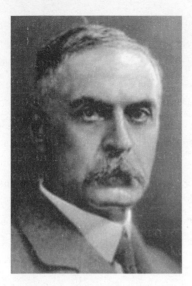

Dr. Karl Landsteiner received the Noble Prize in 1930 for his discovery of ABO blood group antigens and antibodies.

of experiments that established some of the fundamental concepts of immunology. For example, rabbits fed small amounts of jequirty seeds developed a certain degree of immunity against the abrin, and injecting abrin intravenously could increase their immunity. By this experiment Ehrlich was able to demonstrate the specificity of serum proteins (later known as antibodies) found in the serum of animals after the administration of abrin and ricin. For example, anti-abrin could neutralize the activity of abrin, but not that of ricin, and vice versa. The specificity of the basic antibody molecule and the induction of tolerance remain to this day the basic cornerstones of immunology.

Erhlich's findings concerning the specificity of most antibody molecules also paved the way for the discovery of the ABO blood groups twelve years later, by establishing the dynamics of what would become known as antigen-antibody reaction. In 1900, Dr. Karl Landsteiner, an Austrian-American physician and scientist, observed that when blood from different individuals was mixed, agglutination of the red cells took place—in some cases, but not in others. From these diverse reactions, it was possible to distinguish three distinct blood groups, O, A, and B. A fourth group, AB, would soon be added. For the first time, transfusions could occur in a safe and predictable manner. Considering the sheer number of human lives saved by Landsteiner's discovery, it ranks as one of the greatest medical breakthroughs of all time—one for which Landsteiner would receive the Nobel Prize in 1930. With Philip Levine and Alexander Weiner, he would go on to discover the Rh blood system in 1946, thus resolving another puzzling complication of maternal-fetal reactions.

Independently of Landsteiner, Jan Jansky, a Czech doctor of medicine and professor at Charles University in Prague, was simultaneously reaching similar conclusions at the beginning of the century. Jansky, a specialist in the field of neurology and psychiatry, was analyzing the blood of more than 3,000 subjects to learn whether he could detect coagulation differences in the blood of schizophrenics and other psychotics. In the process of his investigation, Jansky noted four distinct blood groupings, and published his work on groups O, A, B, and AB in 1907.

More Than Just Transfusions

While the implications of these discoveries for safe blood transfusions was clear, Landsteiner's curiosity about blood group reactions took him into wider territories. Blending Stillmark's research on agglutination and Ehrlich's research on immunology with his own findings on blood group reactions, he began experimenting with different substances and their impact on red blood cells. In 1908, he showed that small amounts of an agglutinin from the common lentil bean would clump the red blood cells of a rabbit, but even high amounts had no effect on the red blood cells of pigeons. He was also able to demonstrate that plant agglutinins attached to red blood cells could be liberated by raising the temperature to 50°C or by treating the agglutinated cells with pig gut mucus (providentially enough, a rich source of the blood group A antigen). Landsteiner was prepared to publish his findings showing the link between plant substances and blood groups in 1914, but war intervened and his work would not see print until 1933.

Although he appeared to have recognized the reactivity between certain plant toxins and red blood cells, Lansteiner apparently did not seem to search for any relationship that would have made them applicable as blood typing tools. In the four decades following his discovery, little new research was conducted, although a few new sources of agglutinins were discovered, including soy beans, lima beans, and peanuts.

However, in 1945 William Clouser Boyd, Ph.D., working at Boston University's School of Medicine, discovered that some agglutinins can be blood group specific, being able to clump the blood of one type but not of another. The agglutinin found in lima beans clumped only type A red blood cells, but not those of type O or B. Boyd

coined the term *lectin* to mean any agglutinin capable of clumping cells by linking up their surface sugars. *Lectin* is derived from the Latin word *legere,* which means "to pick or choose." Lectins have very specific tastes when it comes to agglutination, only working on very specific combinations of sugars, much like a lock and its particular key.

As Boyd himself described in a 1970 issue of the *Annals of the NY Academy of Science,* his discovery of blood group–specific lectins came as he studied a table Landsteiner had used to summarize his animal data.

AGGLUTININ FROM	TITER OF BLOOD FOR		AGGLUTININ FROM	TITER OF BLOOD FOR	
	Rabbit	Pigeon		Horse	Pigeon
Beans	125	2000	*Abrus precatorius*	128	256
Lentils	160	0	Castor bean	4	512

TABLE I. Titers of different plant agglutinins for the red cells of different species

"One day toward the end of 1945, looking at this table in the second English edition of Landsteiner's book, I was seized with the idea that if such extracts could show species specificity, they might even show individual specificity; that is, they might possibly affect the red cells of some individuals of a species and not affect others of the same species. Therefore, I asked one of my assistants to go out to the corner grocery store and buy some dried lima beans. Why I said lima beans instead of the more common pea beans or kidney beans I shall never know. But if we had bought practically any other bean we would not have discovered anything new.

"The lima beans were ground and extracted with

salt solution. The resulting extract agglutinated erythrocytes of some human individuals, but those of others only weakly, if at all. It was immediately evident that the differences were correlated with blood groups.

"The ease with which this discovery was made misled me, and aside from a rather oblique reference to it in the second edition of my *Fundamentals of Immunology*, which I was working on at the time, I did not publish this observation until 1949, when I reported on an investigation of 262 varieties of plants belonging to 63 families and 186 genera.

"I proposed that these blood-antigen-specific plant agglutinins (which are also specific precipitins) be called "lectins"—from the Latin *legere*, to pick out or choose—intending thus to call attention to their specificity without begging the question as to their nature."

Blood Groups and Their Human Distributions

The first scientific study of blood group distribution was first attempted by Ludwik and Hanka Hirschfeld, a Polish husband-wife team of immunologists, during World War I[2]. Working among the ethnically diverse Allied forces stationed at Salonika, Greece, the Hirschfelds used the new knowledge of blood groups to study racial and nationality characteristics. They systematically analyzed the blood groups of several different ethnic continents among soldiers in the English and French colonial armies, including Vietnamese, Senegalese, Indian, and various other war prisoners. Each group contained over 500 or

more subjects. They found, for example, that the rate of blood group B ranged from a low of 7.2% of the population of English subjects to a high of 41.2% in Indians, and that Western Europeans in general had a lower incidence of blood group B than Balkan Slavs, who had a lower incidence than Russians, Turks, and Jews, who again had a lower occurrence than Vietnamese and Indians. The distribution of blood group AB essentially followed the same pattern, with a low of 3% to 5% in Western Europeans and a high of 8.5% in Indians.

Blood groups A and O were essentially the reverse of groups B and AB. The percentage of group A remained fairly consistent at 40% among Europeans, Balkan Slavs, and Arabs, while being quite low among West Africans, Vietnamese, and Indians. Forty-six percent of the English population tested were group O, which accounted for only 31.3% of the Indians tested.

Modern analysis, largely derived from blood bank records, probably contains the blood groups of more than 20 million individuals from around the world. Yet these large numbers can do no more than confirm the original observations of the Hirschfelds. Interestingly, at the time no scientific publication felt compelled to publish their material, which for a while languished in an obscure anthropology journal.

In the 1920s several anthropologists first attempted racial classification based on blood groups. Based on earlier work, in 1929 Laurance Snyder published a book called *Blood Grouping in Relationship to Clinical and Legal Medicine*[3] in which he proposed a comprehensive classification system based on blood group. This book was especially interesting because it largely focused on the distribution of the ABO groups, the only tool to be had at the time. The Rh and MN groups had yet to be discovered.

Perhaps because of the chaotic aftermath of World War I and the Depression, the subsequent three decades saw little interest or activity in using the blood groups as an anthropological tool.

In 1950, William Boyd, who was proving himself to be a man of diverse interests and abilities, used his prior work with blood groups to combat racist notions that predominated in America. Collaborating with noted science fiction writer Isaac Asimov, Ph.D., he published *Races and People*[4], a seminal work on the subject. Boyd contended that blood groups served as a far more reliable determination of race than other measures, such as skin color and national origin. He cited four reasons for this conclusion, all of which resonated for the times. First, blood group was a hidden characteristic. One couldn't determine a person's blood group by merely looking at him. It prevented judgments made on superficial and prejudicial bases. Second, unlike other physical characteristics, blood groups were inherited in precise ways. Third, blood groups remained intact from the moment of fertilization until death. They were permanent. Finally, blood groups served as conclusive evidence of the ways humans mixed with one another throughout history. There was no such thing as "purity" of race. The various blood groups were found all over the world. The only factor that changed was the frequency of their occurrence.

Earlier, Boyd analyzed the ABO blood group system, along with two minor systems, MN and Rh, that had been subsequently identified[5]. (See

chapter 3.) From his analysis he isolated six "genetic races," following patterns of immigration that would have been impossible to track by using skin color or other obvious characteristics:

CLASSIFICATION	ABO BLOOD GROUP	MN BLOOD GROUP	RH BLOOD GROUP
Early European	High O; no B	Higher than average N	High Rh
European (Caucasoid)	High A_2; moderate representation of all	Normal frequencies of M	Higher than average Rh
African (Negroid)	High B; relatively high A_2		Higher than average Rh; very high representation of rare Rh genes
Asiatic (Mongolian)	High B; little A_2		Little Rh
American Indian	Very high O; little if any A or B		No Rh
Australoid	High A_1; no A_2	High N	No Rh

TABLE II. Boyd's Classifications

Early European group: Possessing the highest incidence (over 30%) of the Rh-negative gene, probably no group B, and a relatively high incidence of group O. The gene for blood group N was possibly somewhat higher than in present-day Europeans. This group is represented today by its modern descendants, the Basques.

European (Caucasoid) group: Possessing the next highest incidence of the Rh-negative gene and a relatively high incidence of group A_2, with moderate frequencies of other blood group genes. Normal frequencies of the gene for blood group M.

African (Negroid) group: Possessing a tremendously high incidence of a rare type of Rh positive gene, Rh0, and a moderate frequency of Rh negative; relatively high incidence of group A_2 and the rare intermediate types of group A, and a rather high incidence of group B.

Asiatic (Mongolian) group: Possessing high frequencies of group B, and little if any of the genes for group A_2 and Rh-negative.

American Indian group: Possessing little or no group A and probably no B or Rh-negative. Very high rates of group O.

Australoid group: Possessing high incidence of group A_1, but not A_2 or Rh-negative; high incidence of the group N gene.

Boyd's classification made more sense than the earlier classification systems because it also fit the geographic distributions of the individual races more accurately.

In the 1950s, as emphasis shifted to genetic characteristics, scientific interest increased in the blood groups and other markers that have known genetic bases. In the 1960s, a brilliant Italian population geneticist named Luigi Luca Cavalli-Sforza produced a "tree" of human evolution, based largely on genetic evidence collected over the decades, primarily blood group studies. Cavalli-Sforza collected blood group data in the villages and mountain communities around Parma, Italy. Using the well-established network of Catholic parishes, he solicited the support of parish priests in blood-typing parishioners—often in sacristies after Sunday Mass. The branches of Cavalli-Sforza's tree spread from a common ancestor in Africa to Asia, Australia, and North America. Other branches from Africa spread to the European areas, replacing Neanderthals as the

original population source. Cavalli-Sforza's research added to the evidence that, contrary to popular belief, races were not genetically distinct, but rather a mix with only superficial distinctions. He would later write that Europeans, drawing from both African and Asian ancestry, were the most genetically mixed-up race on earth.

He used this fact to make a pointed dig at Arthur de Gobineau, a 19th-century French author whose work had influenced German racism. De Goubineau "would die of rage and shame at this suggestion," he wrote gleefully, "since he believed that Europeans . . . were the most genetically pure race, most intellectually gifted and the least weakened by racial mixing."

Frank Livingstone, one of the premier blood group paleoserologists, even rejected the concept of race altogether[6,7]. Livingstone theorized that although biological variability existed between the populations of organisms comprising a species, this variability did not conform to the discrete packages we call races. Rather, these distinctions were "clines"—gradients of physiological change in a group of related organisms, usually along a line of environmental transition.

In tracking the course of humanity using blood groups, the early paleoserologists were able to draw significant conclusions about how the human race survived. A. E. Mourant, a physician and anthropologist who published two key works, *Blood Groups and Disease*[8] and *Blood Relations: Blood Groups and Anthropology*[9], collected much of the available material on the subject. There is good evidence for considerable effects of selection on blood group distribution. Infection undoubtedly accounted for the majority of natural selection in prehistoric populations. This can be explained by the phenomenon of *horror autotoxicus*—that is, the body's inherent aversion to producing antibodies to self antigens.

Mourant was the first to hypothesize that the relatively high distribution of group A in areas with historically high incidence of plague (Turkey, Greece, Italy) would point to selective disadvantage for group O, proven immunochemically by blood group studies on various *Yersinia* species. Antigenic similarity exists between the blood groups and a great variety of bacterial, rickettsial, and helminthic species, including typhoid, streptococci (group A), staphylococci (group O), *Shigella*, and *Proteus*. Strong proof for the theory that blood group was a critical influence on the survival of early humanity is the fact that virtually every infectious disease known to influence population demographics (malaria, cholera, typhus, smallpox, influenza, and tuberculosis) has had a "preferred" blood group that is especially susceptible and an opposing blood group that is resistant. Many experts have made strong arguments that the pressure applied by infectious diseases along blood group lines has been one of the factors, if not the primary factor, influencing natural selection and blood group distributions.

Blood Groups and Personality: The Science and the Pseudoscience

While physical anthropologists were tracing the evolution of the human race using blood groups, others were exploring the influence of blood groups from another perspective. The twen-tieth century had also seen the flowering of a new kind of science—one that sought to explain the mysteries of the mind in addition to the mysteries of the body. Inevitably, blood groups emerged as a subject of investigation. In the 1920s, Takeji Furukawa, a Japanese psychology professor, studied relations between blood group and character[10]. Furukawa proposed a theory on the relation between blood groups and temperament. He majored in experimental education in college, and upon his employment at a women's high school he worked in its administration office. He came to believe that the temperamental differences of applicants were responsible for the inability to predict school performance from the results of their entrance examinations. He was from a family of many doctors, and was familiar with blood groups, the newest physiological discovery of the day. Furukawa published some of his work in the German *Journal of Applied Psychology* in 1931 and so influenced several European psychologists to begin to examine the concept in greater detail. German psychologist Karl H. Gobber took Furukawa's work to deeper levels. In Switzerland, Dr. K. Fritz Schaer used the students of the Swiss Military Academy as test subjects in researching blood groups and personality. However, considering the fascist tidal wave that was washing over Germany and was soon to engulf Europe and the world in its brutal grip, Furukawa's work became essentially lost in the maelstrom for a couple of decades.

Two major figures in psychology, Raymond Cattell[11,12] and Hans Eysenck[13], would later study blood groups peripherally in the course of their work on personality. Both were interested in studying personality as an organic, biochemical function rather than as a product of socialization and upbringing.

Cattell made several significant contributions to the development of research tools and techniques that tracked the individual differences in cognitive abilities, personality, and motivation. He developed the 16 Personality Factor (16PF) personality assessment device, designed to evaluate the personality patterns of a "normal" adult, which is still in wide use today.

In 1964 and again in 1980, Cattell studied blood groups using his 16PF system. A sample of 323 Caucasian Australians was characterized with respect to 17 genetic systems (including 7 blood groups) and 21 psychological variables. His results showed that:

1. Blood group AB individuals were significantly more self-sufficient and group-independent than types O, A or B.

2. Blood group A individuals were more prone to severe anxiety than blood group O individuals.

Using Cattell's 16PF tool, another researcher studied the relationship between ABO blood group and personality factors in 547 south Mississippi schoolchildren. It was found that the mean scores for each personality factored differed by ABO blood type. Blood group O students were found to be more tense than blood group A or blood group B students. On the other hand, blood group AB students were the most tense of all[14].

Psychologist Hans Eysenck, who was born in Berlin, studied in France and at London University, and was professor of psychology at London University from 1955 to 1983, similarly pioneered the idea that genetic factors play a large part in determining the psychological differences between people. Eysenck's major contribution to psychology was his theory of personality, sometimes called the PEN System (Psychoticism, Extroversion, and Neuroticism). According to Eysenck, these variables were the result of physiological and chemical preferences; for example, introverts have higher levels of activity in the corticoreticular loop of the brain, and thus are chronically more cortically aroused, than extroverts.

Eysenck looked at differences between nationalities in their occurrences of particular personality characteristics as a reflection of the rates of certain ABO blood groups in their populations. He used earlier studies that showed significant differences in the frequency of the ABO blood groups among European introverts and extroverts, and between highly emotional and relaxed people. These results showed that emotionality was significantly more common in blood group B individuals than in blood group A individuals, and that introversion was more common in blood group AB than the other blood groups.

In one study, Eysenck looked at two population samples, one British, the other Japanese. Since previous studies had shown that Japanese samples were more naturally introverted and more neurotic than British samples, he predicted that the Japanese, as compared to the British, would have a higher proportion of blood group AB and a lower ratio of blood group A to blood group B.

This was confirmed by looking at the established blood group frequencies for the two countries.

Taken as a whole, these investigations into blood groups and personality caused barely a ripple in the growing field of psychology. Popular interest in the subject did not occur until 1971, when Masahiko Nomi, a Japanese journalist, wrote a series of popular books on the subject of personality and blood type. Nomi's work is typically uncontrolled and largely anecdotal; one never gets a clear idea of exactly how he arrived at his conclusions. Because of this he has been heavily assailed by the Japanese psychological community, although his books are phenomenally popular[15].

Although the effects of blood groups on such a complicated aspect of expression as personality continue to remain unclear and contradictory, they may be just the tip of a much bigger iceberg—the relationship that occurs between ABO blood group and stress at the genetic level. Here observations achieved some credibility in recent years, when a moderate number of studies linked ABO blood groups to a diverse series of mental disorders, including associations between blood group O and bipolar disorder[16–19] and blood group A and obsessive-compulsive disorder[20–21]. Other studies implied that the genetics of ABO blood groups might influence the amount and kind of neurochemicals and hormones secreted in conditions of stress. For example, blood group O individuals are known to respond to stress by secreting large amounts of catecholamines, such as adrenaline. In addition, there is evidence that they tend to eliminate adrenaline less efficiently under stress than their A, B, and AB counterparts. Because of

high circulating levels of adrenaline, it would not be surprising to find that the incidence of "type A behavior" is actually higher in blood group O, a fact that has been shown for young men recovering from acute heart attacks[22].

Blood group A and B individuals were shown to manufacture higher levels of the adrenal stress hormone cortisol when under stress, and blood group A individuals were least effective at removing excess cortisol over time when compared with the other blood groups. High levels of cortisol have been linked with obsessive-like thought patterns, a higher incidence of heart disease, metabolic inefficiency, and lower immune function[23,24]. In addition, the blood of group A individuals has been shown to become more viscous when under stress when compared to the other ABO blood groups[25]. Perhaps this is the result in part of a known association between group A and a tendency toward higher levels of various clotting factors[26].

First Links Between Blood Groups and Biological Function

As early as 1921, a study in the British *Journal of Experimental Pathology*[27] examined blood group frequencies in patients suffering from various types of carcinoma and concluded individuals of group AB were more prone to cancer in general, a finding echoed by two later studies, done in the 1930s[28–29]. This was the beginning of a growing body of raw data showing blood group–specific propensities for disease, but these studies were fraught with difficulty, largely due to confounding factors such as ethnic or geographic factors. In addition, many times a negative result was reached that was later shown to be the result of faulty statistical analysis. For example, stimulated by the first cancer study, a larger study done at the Mayo Clinic in the 1920s analyzed the blood groups of 2,446 patients and concluded that there was no association between blood group and cancer as previously reported, and in fact no association between blood group and disease at all[30]. Among the diseases examined and included in the negative results were several, such as pernicious anemia and stomach ulcers, for which there is no longer any doubt about a strong link with blood group. Had the Mayo investigators used more reliable statistical tools, the blood group associations would have been discovered. Unfortunately, the Mayo Clinic report sidetracked interest in the study of blood groups and disease for a considerable period of time.

The first strong link between ABO blood groups and a non-blood-related disease was reported in 1936 by Luigi Ugelli, an Italian physiologist. Ugelli found the incidence of bleeding ulcers highest in men who were blood group O, an association that has now been confirmed with extensive studies[31].

After a hiatus during World War II, interest again developed in looking at the link between blood groups and disease. In 1953, when researchers demonstrated an association between group A and higher incidences of stomach carcinoma[32], there was a resurgence of clinical interest in blood group disease studies, which skyrocketed during the late 1950s and 1960s. The use of newer, more powerful analytic tools to study large populations

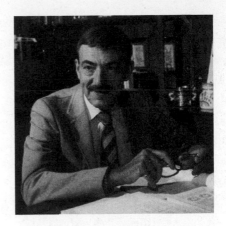

James D'Adamo, N.D.

for the first time provided the mathematical basis for accurate research. In a paper published in 1960[33], researchers demonstrated a "strikingly high" increase of group O among ulcer sufferers compared to controls, with a correspondingly lower incidence of the other blood groups, a finding corroborated by numerous other researchers[34]. In addition to these links with diseases of the digestive tract, researchers also began to find associations between blood groups and physiological functions. Blood group O was shown to have higher levels of stomach hydrochloric acid[34-36], pepsinogen[37], and gastrin—all important digestive factors necessary for proper protein digestion and the intestinal enzyme alkaline phosphatase[38], an important digestive enzyme necessary for fat absorption. Blood group A was shown to have higher levels of blood clotting factors and a greater incidence of heart disease and elevated cholesterol[39].

My father, James D'Adamo, N.D., was the first to advance the theory that the ABO blood groups could be employed as a method of optimizing diet. During the 1960s he noticed that although many patients did well on strict vegetarian and low-fat diets, a certain number did not appear to improve, and several did poorly or even worsened. A sensitive man with keen powers of deduction and insight, he reasoned that there should be some sort of "key" that he could use to determine differences in the dietary needs of his patients. He rationalized that since blood was the great source of nourishment to the body, perhaps some aspect of the blood could help to identify these differences.

Through the years and with countless patients, a pattern emerged. Patients who were blood group A seemed to do poorly on high-protein diets consisting of large amounts of meat, but did well on vegetable proteins such as soy and tofu. When group A patients ate large amounts of dairy, it tended to produce copious amounts of mucous discharge in their sinuses and respiratory passages. When they increased their level of physical activity and exercise, group As tended to feel less well than when they did lighter forms of exercise, such as Hatha yoga.

On the other hand, group O patients tended to thrive on high-protein diets, and they often stated that high-intensity activities, such as jogging and aerobics, energized them and improved their moods. In 1980, my father condensed his observations and dietary recommendations into a book titled *One Man's Food*, inspired by the saying "One man's food may be another man's poison."

At the time of the publication of my father's book, I was in my third year of naturopathic studies at Seattle's John Bastyr College. In 1982, for a Clinical Rounds requirement in my senior year, I scanned the medical literature to see if there was a correlation between ABO blood group and a predilection for certain diseases, and whether any of this supported my father's diet theory. As I knew that his book was based on his own subjective impressions of the blood types, and not on any objective methods of evaluation, I wasn't sure what I would find.

After an extensive literature search at the University of Washington's Health Sciences Library, I collected a large amount of seemingly unrelated information about certain rare diseases that were associated with blood type, and several common diseases that apparently were not. I also found a large number of digestive diseases and functions linked to blood type—information I had not learned in medical school. These were the first revelations that suggested a scientific basis for my father's empirical observations.

As I continued my investigation, I found other key correlations and I published my data in 1982 in a paper titled "Diet, Disease and the ABO Blood Groups: A Review of the Literature."

I spent the next twenty years continuing my research, in particular advancing the study of blood group–specific lectins and their effects on digestion and immunity. In the clinical setting of my practice, I used this increasingly viable science to successfully treat thousands of patients. In late 1996, I published *Eat Right 4 Your Type: The Individualized Diet Solution to Staying Healthy, Living Longer and Achieving Your Ideal Weight* (Putnam).

By that point, there were more than a thousand published studies on the associations of blood groups and disease. It was difficult to argue with the general pattern that emerged from the large body of statistical data on malignancy, coagulation, and infection. Discoveries in membrane chemistry, tumor immunology, and infectious disease (especially relating to bacterial receptors) added a scientific rationale and bolstered the credibility of earlier statistical studies. Some of the more recent findings on parasitic/bacterial/viral receptors, the hematological abnormalities seen when high frequency blood group antigens are missing, and the association with immunologically important proteins were most convincing in demonstrating a blood group association.

Yet, even as the body of research continued to expand, linking blood group individuality to diet and disease, the mainstream medical community largely remained unaware of the breakthroughs. In most medical schools, the study of ABO blood groups was still limited to its role as a complicating factor in transfusions—a limitation Landsteiner, Boyd, and others transcended almost a century ago.

By 2000, using the tools of the Internet, I had compiled a Blood Type Outcome Registry, consisting of nearly 4,000 reports from individuals of every blood type, based on the level of improvements they experienced in diseases and chronic conditions after using the blood type diet plans (see part 3). Many of these results were fortified by "hard" data, including blood tests and physician reports. The level of overall satisfaction reported was quite astounding: Regardless of blood group, a consistent 90% to 93% rate of overall satisfaction with the results of the diet was reported, with improvements in digestion, overall sense of energy and well-being, and weight loss being the most common results reported. The sig-

nificance of these findings goes beyond a simple degree of satisfaction or a beneficial health improvement. It scientifically challenges the validity of any "one size fits all" diet philosophy. Nine out of 10 blood group O individuals report beneficial results from a high-protein diet, while 9 out of 10 blood group A individuals report a similar rate of success with a predominantly low-protein diet.

One person's food is indeed someone else's poison.

The development of the nonprofit Institute for Human Individuality (IfHI) now promises to take the research even further. In alliance with the Southwest College of Naturopathic Medicine, IfHI will do the large-scale clinical studies needed to evaluate the efficacy of the Blood Type Diet with regard to a variety of common chronic diseases, including rheumatoid arthritis and several cancers.

Future History

As a new century dawns, it appears that widespread acceptance of blood group science will ultimately rely on the explosive discoveries being forged in DNA research and biotechnology. In essence, medical science may finally be catching up with the non-transfusion significance of the ABO blood groups. This is especially to be seen in the field of molecular oncology, the study of cancer on a molecular level. Here the ABO blood groups are assuming a greater role with the release of each scientific journal. For example, the finding that many tissues first signal their conversion into cancer cells by losing the ability to synthesize ABO antigens[40,41] has furthered our understanding of the early, premalignant changes that cells undergo before they become deadly and begin to spread (metastasize).

Nanorobotics: The Future of Blood Groups?

Today we are witnessing even more remarkable possibilities for blood groups to play a role in every aspect of human health and healing. An exciting new technology called nanotechnology, which employs knowledge of the blood groups as one of its key determining factors, is about to make an enormous impact on how medicine will be practiced in the near future. Nanotechnology is the process of creating microscopic machines that will enter our bodies to perform specific tasks. They will intervene with disease and heal heretofore unreachable mechanisms deep within us—even the narrowest veins and tiniest cells will be open to this new medical miracle. Nano (meaning "incredibly small") technology will be created by controlling the manufacture of individual atoms.

These manipulated biomolecules will become known as *nanobots*—robots of microscopic proportions. Researchers are currently working on the means to tailor devices and materials on the scale of billionths of a meter. They will eventually acquire the ability to engineer living structures, biological machines no larger than molecules such as DNA. In a time reminiscent of the film *Fantastic Voyage,* many medical futurists foresee tiny robotic biomolecules that will be placed into the body, perhaps engineered to destroy specific cancer cells or repair damaged DNA material. These nanobots will be programmed to identify specific ABO antigens as measures of identity, so they can instantly spot the mutations that cause disease.

The scattershot days of contemporary medical intervention may soon be considered as antique as the Model T Ford. Physicians may soon be able to design tiny tools to safely and effectively repair the damaged nanoscopic machinery of a diseased body, just as a mechanic works on a car's engine today using tools that are on the same scale as the engine. It sounds like science fiction—and until recently it was—but it's reaching the verge of possibility because teams of doctors and scientists are combining advances from biology and chemistry with the synthesis and fabrication of tools from chemical engineering and the microchip industry.

Robert A. Freitas is considered the father of nanomedicine, and he's quite interested in using blood groups as determinants of individuality in the new field. As Freitas writes in his book *Nanomedicine:* "A nanorobot, searching for a particular set of approximately 30 blood group antigens, would require about three thousandths (3/1000) of a second to make the self/non-self determination for a particular red cell membrane it encountered. A nanorobot seeking to determine the complete blood group type of the membrane, and must in the worst case search all 254 known blood antigen types, would require at most 2 seconds to make these determinations"[42]. Perhaps in the near future, a biological microrobot may reassemble damaged genetic material, or destroy killer microbial invaders, reading blood group antigens to accomplish its task.

The very genetic factor that enabled the survival of our ancestors hundreds of thousands of years ago may soon be the source of technological miracles.

REFERENCES

1. Kocourek J. *The Lectins: Properties, Functions and Applications in Biology and Medicine.* San Diego, CA: Academic Press; 1986.

2. Hirschfeld L, Hirschfeld H. *Lancet II.* 1919;:675–679.

3. Snyder L. *Blood Grouping In Relationship to Clinical and Legal Medicine.* 1929.

4. Asimov I, Boyd WC. *Races and People.* New York: Abelard-Schuman; 1955.

5. Ibid.

6. Livingstone FB. On the non-existence of human race. *Current Anthropology.* 1962;3:279–281.

7. Livingstone FB. An analysis of the ABO blood group clines in Europe. *Am J Phys Anthropol.* 1969;31:1–9.

8. Mourant AE. *Blood Groups and Disease.* Oxford, NY: Oxford University Press; 1979.

9. Mourant AE. *Blood Relations: Blood groups and Anthropology.* Oxford, NY: Oxford University Press; 1983.

10. Sato T, Watanabe Y. The Furukawa theory of blood-type and temperament: the origins of a temperament theory during the 1920s [in Japanese]. *The Japanese Journal of Personality.* 1995;3:51–65.

11. Cattell RB. The relation of blood types to primary and secondary personality traits. *The Mankind Quarterly.* 1980;(21):35–51.

12. Cattell RB, Young HB, Houndelby JD. Blood groups and personality traits. *American Journal of Human Genetics.* 1964;16:397–402.

13. Eysenk HJ. National differences in personality as related to ABO blood group polymorphism. *Psychological Reports.* 1977;41:1257–1258.

14. Swan D, et al. The relationship between ABO blood type

and factor of personality among south Mississippi 'Anglo-Saxon' school children. *The Mankind Quarterly.* 1980;20:205–258.

15. Takuma T, Matsui Y. Ketsueki gata surerоetaipu ni tsuite [About blood type stereotype]. *Jinbungakuho.* (Tokyo Metropolitan University) 1985;144:15–30.

16. Rihmer Z, Arato M. ABO blood groups in manic-depressive patients. *J Affect Disord.* 1981;3:1–7.

17. Mendlewicz J, et al. Minireview: molecular genetics in affective illness [review] *Life Sci.* 1993;52:231–242.

18. Mendlewicz J. [Contribution of biology to nosology of depressive states. Neurochemical, endocrine and genetic factors]. *Acta Psychiatr Belg.* 1978;78:724–735.

19. Oruc L, Ceric I, Furac I. [Genetics of manic depressive disorder]. *Med Arh.* 1996;50:45–47.

20. Rinieris PM, Stefanis CN, Rabavilas AD, Vaidakis NM. Obsessive-compulsive neurosis, anancastic symptomatology and ABO blood types. *Acta Psychiatr Scand.* 1978;57:377–381.

21. Rinieris P, Stefanis C, Rabavilas A. Obsessional personality traits and ABO blood types. *Neuropsychobiology.* 1980;6:128–31.

22. Neumann JK, Chi DS, Arbogast BW, Kostrzewa RM, Harvill LM. Relationship between blood groups and behavior patterns in men who have had myocardial infarction. *South Med J.* 1991;84:214–218.

23. Locong AH, Roberge AG. Cortisol and catecholamines response to venisection by humans with different blood groups. *Clin Biochem.* 1985;18:67–69.

24. Neumann JK, Arbogast BW, Chi DS, Arbogast LY. Effects of stress and blood type on cortisol and VLDL toxicity preventing activity. *Psychosom Med.* 1992;54:612–619.

25. Dintenfass L, Zador I. Effect of stress and anxiety on thrombus formation and blood viscosity factors. *Bibl Haematol.* 1975;(41):133–139.

26. Meade TW, Cooper JA, Stirling Y, Howarth DJ, Ruddock V, Miller GJ. Factor VIII, ABO blood group and the incidence of ischaemic heart disease. *Br J Haematol.* 1994;88:601–607.

27. Alexander W. *Br J Exp Path.* 1921;2:66.

28. Mithra PN. *Ind J Med Res.* 1933;20:995–1004.

29. Pautienis PN. *Medicina Kaunas.* 1937;8:1–12.

30. Buchanan Higley. *Br J Exp Path.* 1921;2:227.

31. Ugelli I. *Polyclinico (sez prat).* 1936;(43):1591.

32. Bentall A, Roberts F. *Br J Med.* 1953:799–801.

33. Shahid A, Zuberi SJ, Siddiqui AA, Waqar MA. Genetic markers and duodenal ulcer: *JPMA J Pak Med Assoc.* 1997;47:135–137.

34. Purohit GL, Shukla KC. Correlation of blood groups with gastric acidity in normals. *Indian J. Med Sci.* 1960;(14):522–524.

35. Sievers M. Hereditary aspects of gastric secretory function I. *Amer. J. Med.* 1959;27:246–255.

36. Sievers M. Hereditary aspects of gastric secretory function II. *Amer. J. Med.* 1959;27:256–265.

37. Pals G, Defize J, Pronk JC, et al. Relations between serum pepsinogen levels, pepsinogen phenotypes, ABO blood groups, age and sex in blood donors. *Ann Hum Biol.* 1985;12:403–411.

38. Domar U, Hirano K, Stigbrand T. Serum levels of human alkaline phosphatase isozymes in relation to blood groups. *Clin Chim Acta.* 1991;203:305–313.

39. Meade TW, Cooper JA, Stirling Y, Howarth DJ, Ruddock V, Miller GJ. Factor VIII, ABO blood group and the incidence of ischaemic heart disease. *Br J Haematol.* 1994;88:601–607.

40. Greenwell P. Blood group antigens: molecules seeking a function? *Glycoconj J.* 1997;14:159–173.

41. Dabelsteen E. Cell surface carbohydrates as prognostic markers in human carcinomas. *J Pathol.* 1996;179:358–369.

42. Freitas R. *Basic capabilities.* In: *Nanomedicine.* Vol. 1. 1st ed. Georgetown, TX: Landes Bioscience; 1999.

THREE

Biological Significance of the ABO Blood Groups

The ABO blood groups are an important key to the body's immune system. It controls the influence of viruses, bacteria, infections, chemicals, stress, and the entire assortment of invaders and conditions capable of causing disease and weakening immunity. Through its unique antigens it accomplishes this by serving as a type of biological gatekeeper.

Antigens are chemical markers, typically proteins, found on the cells of our bodies and on most other living things. Any substance can be an antigen; the only requirement is that it be unique enough to allow the immune system an opportunity to determine whether it is "self" or "nonself." When the immune system evaluates an unknown antigen, and recognizes it as a part of the body, the suspect in question is then considered safe and friendly. If not, it is an intruder, and appropriately dealt with. At least a million different substances may provoke immune responses.

All life forms, from the simplest virus to human beings, possess unique antigens. Some of the most numerous antigens in the human body are the ones that determine the ABO blood groups. The different blood group antigens are so sensitive that when they are operating effectively, they are the immune system's greatest security system.

Each blood group possesses a different antigen with its own special chemical structure, and the blood groups are named for their antigen structures. Blood group A has an A antigen on its red blood cells. Blood group B has a B antigen. Blood group AB has both the A and the B antigens. Blood group O has no "true" blood group antigen; the early discoverers of blood groups used the letter O to denote zero, or no real antigen. Because of this it is often referred to as "blood group zero" in Europe. What blood group O does have is an H antigen, but this is not a true blood group antigen as it is hidden in blood groups A, B, and AB as well, which have their own respective antigens on top of it. All human blood, with exceedingly rare exceptions, carry the red cell H antigen. It is present in the greatest amount on group O red cells and in the least amount on group AB cells.

We can visualize the chemical structure of blood groups as antennae of sorts, projecting outward from the surface of our cells into deep space. These antennae are made from long chains of repeating sugars that terminate with a sugar called fucose, which by itself forms the simplest of the blood group antigens, O or H. The group O fucose sugar also serves as a platform for the antigens of the other blood groups, A and B, which are determined by our genetics.

For example, if you are blood group A, you are genetically capable of producing an enzyme that can convert the H antigen into the A antigen. If you are blood group B, you are genetically programmed to change the H antigen into the B antigen. ABs can produce both enzymes, and as you might suspect, group O cannot convert its H into anything. Blood group A is composed of the O sugar, fucose, plus a sugar named *N*-acetyl-galactosamine added to its end. Blood group B is composed of the O sugar, fucose, plus a different sugar, named D-galactosamine, at the end.

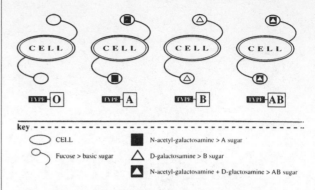

THE FOUR BLOOD TYPES AND THEIR ANTIGENS

Group O is the stalk, fucose; Group A is fucose plus the sugar. N-acetyl-galactosamine; Group B is fucose plus the sugar D-galactosamine; Group AB is fucose plus the A-sugar and the B-sugar.

Antibodies Are Made Against Antigens

When your immune system detects that a foreign antigen has entered the system, it tries to create antibodies to that antigen. These antibodies, specialized chemicals manufactured by the cells of the immune system, are designed to attach to and tag the foreign antigen for destruction.

Antibodies are the cellular equivalent of the military's smart bomb. The cells of our immune system manufacture countless varieties of antibodies, and each is specifically designed to identify and attach to the unique shape of one particular antigen. Antibodies can be thought of as microscopic monkey wrenches that have a constant portion (the handle) that the cells of the immune system can attach to, and a variable portion (the mouth) that can be adjusted to the particular

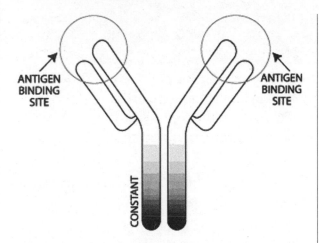

ANTIGEN BINDING SITE

ANTIGEN BINDING SITE

CONSTANT

Antibodies are basic Y-shaped structures, divided into constant and variable regions. The constant region is the base of the antibody. The variable region adjusts according to the shape of the antigen it is meant to bind with.

shape and size of the bolt (antigen) to which it is trying to attach itself.

A continual battle wages between the immune system and intruders that try to change or mutate their antigens into some new form that the body will not recognize. The immune system responds to this challenge with an ever-increasing inventory of antibodies.

Antibodies are denoted by placing the prefix *anti-* in front of the name of the foreign antigen against which the antibody is targeted. For example, antibodies against Human immunodeficiency virus (HIV) are called *anti-HIV antibodies.*

Certain blood groups produce antibodies to other blood group antigens. This is why we often can receive transfusions from some blood groups, but not from others. These anti—other blood group antibodies are among the most potent antibodies in our immune system—because unlike the average measles or flu antibody, which can be

thought of as a single monkey wrench, these antibodies are actually a star-shaped configuration of five monkey wrenches linked together at the center by their handles. Because of this, they can attach to multiple antigens from more than one cell. This produces the curious phenomenon called agglutination (literally, "gluing"), which gives this class of antibody its unique name and class: the hemagglutinins.

The ability of the hemagglutinin antibodies to clump viruses, bacteria, or red blood cells of an opposing blood group is so powerful that it can usually be immediately observed on a glass slide with the unaided eye. This, incidentally, is the most common way that a person's ABO blood group is determined in the laboratory. Most other antibodies in the body require some sort of stimulation for their production, such as a vaccination or infection. The blood group antibodies are different. They are produced automatically, often appearing at birth and reaching almost adult levels by four months of age, often as a result of the inoculation of the young child by foods or microbes that possess the antigen of a different ABO blood group.

When a hemagglutinin antibody encounters the antigen of a microbial interloper, agglutination occurs, because the multiple binding sites of the hemagglutinin can bind with antigens on more than one cell or microbe, producing an interlocking effect. When cells, viruses, parasites, and bacteria are agglutinated, they stick together and clump up, which makes disposing of them all the easier. It is rather like handcuffing criminals together; they become far less dangerous than when they are allowed to move around freely.

Sweeping the system of odd cells, viruses, parasites, and bacteria, the antibodies herd the undesirables together. Unfortunately, when this occurs in large amounts, such as when a person receives an incorrect transfusion, the huge numbers of clumped cells can block the small arteries or clog the filtration devices in the kidneys; this is why transfusion reactions are so deadly.

The relationship of ABO blood group antibodies is in many ways the opposite of the ABO antigens. Group O, which has no true antigen, produces antibodies against all the other blood groups. Since group O produces anti-A and anti-B antibodies, it cannot receive blood from any donor with an A or B antigen. Group O can only receive blood from another O. Group A produces anti-B antibodies and cannot receive blood from a B or AB. Group B produces anti-A antibodies and cannot receive blood from an A or AB. Group AB produces no antibodies, which makes it the "universal receiver," while group O, who produce no antigens for other blood groups to react is the "universal donor."

Our immune system views other blood group antigens as non-self to such an extent that we are genetically programmed to produce an extremely powerful antibody to opposing blood groups—or, rather, to the microorganisms and foods that have these other antigens as well. It is the most powerful immune mechanism in the human body.

Minor Blood Group Systems

Human beings possess as many as 300 independent blood grouping systems, although the ABO system is by far the most important, both from a disease perspective and because it is one of the few blood grouping systems with extensive expression outside the bloodstream. ABO antigens are found in the mucus lining the digestive tract, in digestive secretions, on the white blood cells, and on many of the cells of the reproductive system. Most of the other blood grouping systems, such as the well-known Rhesus (Rh) system, are found exclusively on red blood cells and nowhere else. In addition, unlike the ABO antibodies, these other blood grouping systems do not possess very powerful hemagglutinin antibodies, but rather the more weaker types. For our purposes, only three of them have any real impact, and the second most important system, called the secretor type, is important mainly because it adds another level of sophistication to our understanding of the dynamics of ABO. Two others can be useful in special situations: the Rh factor and the MN blood group systems.

The Lewis Blood Group System and ABH Secretor Status

Although everyone carries an ABO blood group antigen on their blood cells, about 80% of the population also have blood group antigens that float around freely in their body secretions. These people are called secretors, because they "secrete" their blood group antigens into their body fluids, such as saliva, mucus, and sperm. It's possible to ABO-type a secretor from these other body fluids, in addition to their blood.

The other 20% of people who do not secrete

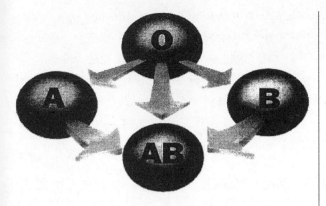

their blood group antigens in other fluids besides blood are called non-secretors. Being a secretor or a non-secretor is independent of your ABO blood group. It is controlled by a different gene. So, one person could be a blood group A secretor, another a blood group A non-secretor. Since the secretor system deals with the secretion of blood group antigens, it is considered proper to call it the ABH secretor system, since even blood group O secretors will secrete H antigen.

Because secretors have more places to put their blood group antigens, they have more blood group expression in their bodies than do non-secretors. Finding out whether you are a secretor or not is as easy as determining your ABO blood group. The most common way to determine secretor status involves testing saliva for the presence of an ABH antigen. If it is found, the person is classed as a secretor (since his or her blood type antigen was secreted in the saliva); if it is absent, the person is classed as a non-secretor.

Another quick and dirty way of determining ABH secretor status is to use the Lewis blood group system. Although it is a proper blood group system in its own right, because of a genetic link-

age between the enzymes that manufacture the Lewis antigens and the genetics of the ABO system, the results of the Lewis typing can often also tell us of a person's ABH secretor status.

In the Lewis system, two possible antigens can be produced, called Lewis^a and Lewis^b (not to be confused with the "A" and "B" of the ABO system). People can type out as one of three varieties: Lewis^{a+b-}, Lewis^{a-b+} and Lewis^{a-b-}.

If you think back to our discussion of ABO antigens, you might remember that everyone starts out with H, but those who are A, B or AB genetically possess the ability to produce enzymes that, in an extra step, allow them to convert their H into A or B. However, group O individuals lack the gene for these enzymes, so they are just left with H.

The Lewis system is rather similar. In this system we all start off making Lewis^a. Many of us, however, possess the genetic ability to produce an enzyme allowing the conversion of all of our Lewis^a into Lewis^b. The ability to convert Lewis^a into Lewis^b is linked genetically with the ability to secrete ABH antigens. Thus all Lewis^{b+} individuals are secretors, and all Lewis^{a+} individuals are non-secretors.

It is common to denote the Lewis system with both the a and b status. Thus a person who is a non-secretor would be designated as Lewis^{a+b-} and a person who is a secretor would be designated Lewis^{a-b+}. The reason for this lies in the fact that a small number of individuals (6% of the white population and 16% of the black population) are genetically incapable of manufacturing Lewis^a in the first place. These individuals are referred to

BLOOD GROUP	GENOTYPE	ENZYMES PRESENT	ANTIGENS	ANTIBODIES
A	AA or Ao	H, A	H, A	anti-B
B	BB or Bo	H, B	H, B	anti-A
AB	AB	H, A, B	H, A, B	none
O	Oo	H	H	anti-B, anti-A

TABLE III. The ABO Blood Group System

as Lewis[a−b−] or "double Lewis negative." For this small percentage of people, the Lewis blood-typing system cannot be used to infer secretor status. However, I have made it a practice to class my double Lewis negative patients as non-secretors, since this small group shares many health problems with non-secretors, and in some can have even more serious consequences.

Since the blood group antigen is an important key to our immune defenses, what are the implications of being unable to secrete blood group antigens in bodily fluids? Quite dramatic, according to a considerable body of scientific research.

In general, non-secretors are far more likely to suffer from an immune disease than secretors, especially when it is provoked by an infectious organism. Non-secretors are dominant in virtually every immune system disorder:

■ Non-secretors are more prone to generalized inflammation than secretors[1,2], although in general their immune responses are not as efficient[3,4].

■ Non-secretors are more prone to both type I and type II diabetes over secretors[5–7].

■ Non-secretors with type I diabetes have much more consistent problems with the yeast *Candida*

albicans, especially in their mouths and upper gastrointestinal tracts[8–10].

■ Non-secretors tend to have more problems with *Helicobacter pylori*, the bacterium thought to cause most stomach ulcers[11].

■ Non-secretors have an increased prevalence of a variety of autoimmune diseases, including ankylosing spondylitis, reactive arthritis, psoriatic arthropathy, Sjögren's syndrome, multiple sclerosis, and Graves' disease[12–14].

■ Non-secretors have an extra risk for recurrent urinary tract infections and more inflammation when they do contract them[15–17].

■ Non-secretors have a higher incidence of heart disease over secretors[18,19].

■ Double Lewis negative individuals (especially men) have a higher incidence of metabolic problems associated with obesity resulting from insulin resistance.[20]

■ Non-secretors have a higher rate of alcoholism over secretors[21,22] and paradoxically are also the group upon which moderate alcohol intake is most likely to have a protective effect[23].

■ Secretor status can influence the accuracy of several common tumor marker tests used to gauge the effectiveness of cancer chemotherapy[24–26].

Often ABO blood group and secretor status will overlap and amplify the effects of each other. For example, it is known that blood group B women develop bladder infections more frequently than the other ABO groups, and that between 55% and 60% of non-secretors have been found to develop renal scars even with the regular use of antibiotic

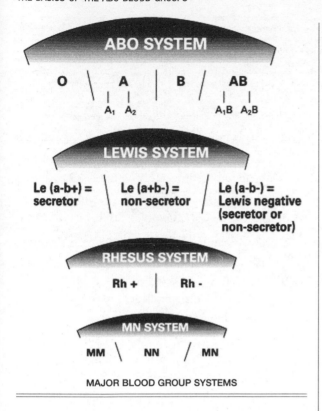

MAJOR BLOOD GROUP SYSTEMS

treatment for urinary tract infections. Thus women who are blood group B non-secretors have the very highest rate of bladder infections, tend to have more scarring of their urinary tracts, and can have a much more difficult time treating their infections with medication. Because of these variations, blood group–related recommendations sometimes differ for secretors and non-secretors independent of ABO blood group.

The Rhesus Blood Group System

From a clinical point of view, the Rhesus (Rh) system is by far the most important system other than ABO. It too is independent of ABO blood

group. The Rh factor is the "positive" or "negative" that appears after the A, B, AB or O in your blood group.

The Rh system is named for the Rhesus monkey, a commonly used laboratory animal, in whose blood it was first discovered. For many years it remained a mystery to doctors why some women who had normal first pregnancies developed complications in their second and subsequent pregnancies, which often resulted in miscarriage and even the death of the mother. In 1939, Dr. Karl Landsteiner discovered that these women were carrying a different blood group than their babies, who took their blood group from the father. The babies were Rh-positive, which meant that they carried the Rh antigen on their blood cells. Their mothers were Rh-negative, which meant that this antigen was missing from their blood. Unlike the ABO system, where the antibodies to other blood types develop from birth, Rh-negative people do not make an antibody to the Rh antigen unless they are first "sensitized." This sensitization usually occurs when blood is exchanged between the mother and infant during birth, so the mother's immune system does not have enough time to react to the first baby. However, should a subsequent conception result in another Rh-positive baby, the mother, now sensitized, will produce antibodies to the baby's blood group. Reactions to the Rh factor can only occur in Rh-negative women who conceive the children of Rh-positive fathers.

Rh incompatibility is the main cause of hemolytic disease of the newborn—the destruction of fetal red corpuscles. It is also a major cause of transfusion reactions. Unlike the antibodies of the

ABO system, each of which is universally present in people lacking the corresponding antigen, antibodies to the Rh antigens are virtually never found except as a result of immunization by pregnancy or transfusion, and reactions appear only at a second exposure to the antigen. Rh-positive women, who represent 85% of the population, have nothing to worry about.

Increasingly, studies are demonstrating that the Rh factor might play a role outside the blood cells. It has been found that the Rh factor might influence one of our primary immune defenses, natural killer (NK) cell activity[27]. While some studies have not found an association, other researchers have observed a higher NK attack against target cells in individuals with Rh-negative blood. It has also recently been demonstrated that certain Rh proteins may correct ammonium transport deficiencies in the kidney[28]. Although much more limited than the wealth of data on the ABO groups, these findings herald a new era in Rh protein research, beyond their role as blood group antigens.

The MN System

Unlike the ABO and Rh blood groups, the MN system is not a major factor in transfusions or organ transplants. For this reason it has been of little interest in the day-to-day practice of medicine. This is deceiving, however, because the MN blood types are of importance to geneticists and anthropologists, because a variety of diseases are associated with them.

The MN system, discovered by Landsteiner and

LEWIS PHENOTYPE	ABO SECRETOR STATUS
Le (a+b−): has Lewis a antigen but not Lewis b	Always ABO non-secretor
Le (a−b+): has Lewis b antigen but not Lewis a	Always ABO non-secretor
Le (a−b−): has neither Lewis a nor Lewis b	Lewis outcome not a determinant of ABO secretor status

TABLE IV. Lewis Types and ABO Secretor Status

his colleagues in 1927, involves three variations—MM, NN, or MN—depending upon whether cells have only the "M" antigen (which would make them MM), the "N" antigen (NN), or both (MN). Around 28% of the population type out as MM, 22% as NN, and 50% as MN.

Because anti-M and anti-N occur only extremely rarely in human serum, there is almost no danger of their causing trouble in blood transfusion. Thus they have been recognized as of little importance in medicine, and testing has largely been left to geneticists. Thus data on the distribution of the M and N groups have built up only very gradually over the years.

The MN system has been shown to have a role in cancer, infection, and heart disease susceptibility. The M antigen is the precursor of one of the most common tumor-associated antigens, the Thomsen-Friedenreich (T) antigen, which is expressed in a variety of cancers, including stomach[29], breast[30], and colon[31], while NN individuals have been found to have a lower incidence of bipolar depression[32] and are supposedly more responsive to dietary regulation of blood lipids (decreased LDL) by the use of a low-fat diet[33]. MM individuals who were also blood group A appear to have a higher incidence of cardiovascular disease[34], while MN individuals appear to have a higher incidence of essential hypertension[35,36] and asthma[37]. M and N blood group antigens appear to inhibit inhibition viral hemagglutination by some influenza virus strains, which may influence susceptibility to certain strains of influenza[38]. It was reported that a disproportionate number of NN individuals (mainly females) were found in an elderly population aged 71 to 80 years[39].

Subgroups

All of the ABO blood groups have subgroups—micro-variations of the primary antigen. For the most part these subgroups are not especially notable, and they're barely detectable in groups O and B. There are over 20 recognized variants of group A—although about 95% of all As are A_1. Most of the variants are found in Africa and probably represent adaptations to local parasites. These include A_2, A_x and A-Bantu.

Of the minor forms of group A, only A_2 is of any practical importance. From population studies it appears to have been an early mutation, or perhaps even the original A. We know that A_2 is found in an inordinately high percentage among the so-called "brown-eyed Laplanders." These are a fairly ancient people, who appear to have headed north to Scandinavia from the area around present-day Armenia, the point at which the A mutation originally developed in large numbers.

Group A_2 has most of the attributes of A_1, but according to some may have represented an offshoot retaining some of the tolerance for fat

largely lost by the more common A_1. Perhaps this represented an adaptation to fish or game, since the area is not suitable for agriculture, though there is no reported difference between A_1 and A_2 in either intestinal enzymes or stomach acid secretion. There is, however, a distinct increase in the occurrence of certain forms of leukemia in A_2. There also appears to be some difference between the A_1 and A_2 subgroups in susceptibility to certain fungal lectins[40].

A_2 differs from A_1 primarily by the number of A antigens found on the cell surface, having between ⅓ and ¼ the number of antigens on the surface[41,42]. Since many parasitic diseases, such as malaria, are known to infect blood group A preferentially, this stepping down of the number of antigens (and hence the number of binding sites for pathogens) may have been a simple matter of selection; the less antigens, the greater the chance for survival and the greater the chance for the gene to propagate.

Blood group antigens are commonly found in the bloodstream, bound to platelets. There appear to be distinct differences between A_1 and A_2 in how this is accomplished.

A_2 is distinguished clinically by the use of a lectin from the plant *Dolichos biflora*, which agglutinates group A_1 but not group A_2 cells. Since A_1 is transfusable into A_2 and vice versa, in conventional medicine they are essentially equivalent.

REFERENCES

1. Klaamas K, Kurtenkov O, Ellamaa M, Wadstrom T. The Helicobacter pylori seroprevalence in blood donors related

to Lewis (a,b) histo-blood group phenotype. *Eur J Gastroenterol Hepatol.* 1997;9:367–370.

2. Sheinfeld J, Schaeffer AJ, Cordon-Cardo C, Rogatko A, Fair WR. Association of the Lewis blood-group phenotype with recurrent urinary tract infections in women. *N Engl J Med.* 1989;320:773–777.

3. Grundbacher FJ. Immunoglobulins, secretor status, and the incidence of rheumatic fever and rheumatic heart disease. *Hum Hered.* 1972;22:399–404.

4. Grundbacher FJ. Genetic aspects of selective immunoglobulin A deficiency. *J Med Genet.* 1972;9:344–347.

5. Peters WH, Gohler W. ABH-secretion and Lewis red cell groups in diabetic and normal subjects from Ethiopia. *Exp Clin Endocrinol.* 1986;88:64–70.

6. Melis C, Mercier P, Vague P, Vialettes B. Lewis antigen and diabetes. *Rev Fr Transfus Immunohematol.* 1978;21:965–971.

7. Petit JM, Morvan Y, Mansuy-Collignon S, et al. Hypertriglyceridaemia and Lewis (A-B-) phenotype in non-insulin-dependent diabetic patients. *Diabetes Metab.* 1997;23:202–204.

8. Thom SM, Blackwell CC, MacCallum CJ, et al. Non-secretion of blood group antigens and susceptibility to infection by Candida species. *FEMS Microbiol Immunol.* 1989;1:401–405.

9. Ben-Aryeh H, Blumfield E, Szargel R, Laufer D, Berdicevsky I. Oral Candida carriage and blood group antigen secretor status. *Mycoses.* 1995;38:355–358.

10. Blackwell CC, Aly FZ, James VS, et al. Blood group, secretor status and oral carriage of yeasts among patients with diabetes mellitus. *Diabetes Res.* 1989;12:101–104.

11. Dickey W, Collins JS, Watson RG, Sloan JM, Porter KG. Secretor status and Helicobacter pylori infection are independent risk factors for gastroduodenal disease. *Gut.* 1993;34:351–353.

12. Shinebaum R. ABO blood group and secretor status in the spondyloarthropathies. *FEMS Microbiol Immunol.* 1989;1:389–395.

13. Shinebaum R, Blackwell CC, Forster PJ, et al. Non-secretion of ABO blood group antigens as a host susceptibility factor in the spondyloarthropathies. *Br Med J (Clin Res Ed).* 1987;294:208–210.

14. Manthorpe R, Staub Nielsen L, Hagen Petersen S, Prause JU. Lewis blood type frequency in patients with primary Sjogren's syndrome. A prospective study including analyses for A1A2BO, Secretor, MNSs, P, Duffy, Kell, Lutheran and rhesus blood groups. *Scand J Rheumatol.* 1985;14:159–162.

15. Sheinfeld J, Schaeffer AJ, Cordon-Cardo C, Rogatko A, Fair WR. Association of the Lewis blood-group phenotype with recurrent urinary tract infections in women. *N Engl J Med.* 1989;320:773–777.

16. May SJ, Blackwell CC, Brettle RP, MacCallum CJ, Weir DM. Non-secretion of ABO blood group antigens: a host factor predisposing to recurrent urinary tract infections and renal scarring. *FEMS Microbiol Immunol.* 1989;1:383–387.

17. Jantausch BA, Criss VR, O'Donnell R, et al. Association of Lewis blood group phenotypes with urinary tract infection in children. *J Pediatr.* 1994;124:863–868.

18. Zhiburt BB, Chepel' AI, Serebrianaia NB. The Lewis antigen system as a marker of IHD risk. *Ter Arkh.* 1997;69:29–31.

19. Slavchev S, Tsoneva M, Zakhariev Z. The secretory type of persons who have survived a myocardial infarct. *Vutr Boles.* 1989;28:31–34.

20. Petit JM, Morvan Y, Viviani V, et al. Insulin resistance syndrome and Lewis phenotype in healthy men and women. *Horm Metab Res.* 1997;29:193–195.

21. Cruz-Coke R. Genetics and alcoholism. *Neurobehav Toxicol Teratol.* 1983;5:179–180.

22. Kojic T, Dojcinova A, Dojcinov D, et al. Possible genetic predisposition for alcohol addiction. *Adv Exp Med Biol.* 1977;85A:7–24.

23. Hein HO, Sorensen H, Suadicani P, Gyntelberg F. Alcohol consumption, Lewis phenotypes, and risk of ischaemic heart disease. *Lancet.* 1993;341:392–396.

24. Vestergaard EM, Hein HO, Meyer H, et al. Reference values and biological variation for tumor marker CA 19-9 in serum for different Lewis and secretor genotypes and evaluation of secretor and Lewis genotyping in a Caucasian population. *Clin Chem.* 1999;45:54–61.

25. Narimatsu H, Iwasaki H, Nakayama F, et al. Lewis and secretor gene dosages affect CA19-9 and DU-PAN-2 serum levels in normal individuals and colorectal cancer patients. *Cancer Res.* 1998;58:512–518.

26. Narimatsu H. Molecular biology of Lewis antigens—histo-blood type antigens and sialyl Lewis antigens as tumor associated antigens. *Nippon Geka Gakkai Zasshi.* 1996;97: 115–122.

27. Lasek W, Jakobisiak M, Plodziszewska M, Gorecki D. The influence of ABO blood groups, Rh antigens and cigarette smoking on the level of NK activity in normal population. *Arch Immunol Ther Exp (Warsz).* 1989;37:287–294.

28. Huang CH, Liu PZ. New insights into the Rh superfamily of genes and proteins in erythroid cells and nonerythroid tissues. *Blood Cells Mol Dis.* 2001;27:90–101.

29. Yoshida A, Sotozono M, Nakatou T, Okada Y, Tsuji T. Different expression of Tn and sialyl-Tn antigens between normal and diseased human gastric epithelial cells. *Acta Med Okayama.* 1998;52:197–204.

30. Tsuchiya A, Kanno M, Kawaguchi T, et al. Prognostic relevance of Tn expression in breast cancer. *Breast Cancer.* 1999;6:175–180.

31. Grosso M, Vitarelli E, Giuffre G, Tuccari G, Barresi G. Expression of Tn, sialosyl-Tn and T antigens in human foetal large intestine. *Eur J Histochem.* 2000;44:359–363.

32. Alda M, Grof P, Grof E. MN blood groups and bipolar disorder: evidence of genotypic association and Hardy-Weinberg disequilibrium. *Biol Psychiatry.* 1998;44:361–363.

33. Birley AJ, MacLennan R, Wahlqvist M, Gerns L, Pangan T, Martin NG. MN blood group affects response of serum LDL cholesterol level to a low fat diet. *Clin Genet.* 1997; 51:291–295.

34. Delanghe J, Duprez D, de Buyzere M, et al. MN blood group, a genetic marker for essential arterial hypertension in young adults. *Eur Heart J.* 1995;16:1269–1276.

35. Turowska B, Gurda M, Wozniak K. ABO, MN, Kell, Hp and Gm1 markers in elderly humans. *Mater Med Pol.* 1991;23:7–12.

36. Gleiberman L, Gershowitz H, Harburg E, Schork MA. Blood pressure and blood group markers: association with the MN locus. *J Hypertens.* 1984;2:337–341.

37. Ksenofontow JP. [Immune responses and blood group genetics in patients with asthma bronchiale (author's transl)]. *Allerg Immunol. (Leipz).* 1977;23:221–225.

38. Vojvodic S. Inhibitory activity of blood group antigens M and N in inhibition of virus hemagglutination reactions of influenza viruses. *Med Pregl.* 2000;53:7–14.

39. Hou M, Stockelberg D, Rydberg L, Kutti J, Wadenvik H. Blood group A antigen expression in platelets is prominently associated with glycoprotein Ib and IIb. Evidence for an A1/A2 difference. *Transfus Med.* 1996;6:51–59.

40. Ying R, Furukawa K. Fungal anti-A agglutinins with different affinities for subgroups A1 and A2 red cells. *Exp Clin Immunogenet.* 1995;12:232–237.

41. Heier HE, Namork E, Calkovska Z, Sandin R, Kornstad L. Expression of A antigens on erythrocytes of weak blood group A subgroups. *Vox Sang.* 1994;66:231–236.

42. Hauser R, Fechner G, Brinkmann B. A1 and A2 blood group substances: are there structural differences? *Z Rechtsmed.* 1990;103:587–591.

FOUR

9q34: The ABO Gene

In 1990, an international consortium of governments launched the Human Genome Project to determine the 3-billion-nucleotide sequence of human DNA. The first completed draft of the genome was reported in February 2001. The implications of these genetic investigations are astounding. It is estimated that mutations in human genes predispose or cause at least 1,500 diseases, from diabetes to asthma to cancer. Scientists believe that the anatomy of the genome is a significant step in the process of identifying and fixing those mutations. In the process, the ABO blood groups have emerged as important genetic markers that play a prominent role in cellular function and dysfunction.

The DNA Code

Each of us shares the same qualities that categorize us as the species *Homo sapiens*. We have the same organ size and structure, the same number of appendages, and many of the same responses to physical stimulation. In fact, genetically we are about 99.9% identical. It's the one-tenth of a percent that makes all the difference.

Our genetic heritage is our biologic hard drive. Embedded within it are the recordings of past "writings" that were saved for use later—along with, in some cases, a few "disk errors."

Traits are inherited because discrete units called genes are passed from parent to offspring when a new organism is conceived. These genes are a unique blueprint for an individual organism, providing all the information needed for the development and life of that species, as well as for the characteristics that make each individual unique.

In general, each gene determines one function, such as the production of an enzyme, which may then go on to produce a protein, hormone, and so on. Complicated processes within the cell are contributed to by the functions of numerous genes. Just as in a machine, where the removal of one part can disrupt the ability of the entire engine to run, so the removal of the influence of one gene can have a severe effect on the life of an organism.

How do we know genes exist? In the late 1800s, an Austrian monk named Gregor Mendel inbred varieties of pea plants and kept careful track of the traits displayed by their offspring. He discovered that the traits of the parent plants were passed on to the progeny plants in strictly reproducible patterns. Mendel postulated that discrete "units of inheritance" determined the traits he examined. He observed that two units of inheritance existed for each trait—one from each parent plant. We now call these units genes.

Genetics is elegant and powerful, but essentially indirect. Inference plays a critical role. Mendel's experiments led him to infer the existence of genes. He never actually saw them. Similarly, the analysis of defects, called mutations, in genes help scientists to infer normal gene function. By seeing what happens to the organism when the function of a gene is missing, scientists can make educated guesses regarding what the normal job of the gene is in the cell.

The Human Genome

The human body contains between 50 and 75 billion cells. The nucleus of each cell contains 23 pairs of chromosomes; 22 are inherited from the mother, 22 are inherited from the father, and two are sex chromosomes—XX for a female, and XY for a male. Within each chromosome there are about 30,000 paired genes composed of DNA (deoxyribonucleic acid), which is the genetic hard drive where information is stored. (Before coding the genome, scientists had long believed there were at least 100,000 genes and were astonished to find less than one-third that number.)

The simplest way to visualize DNA is to picture a spiral staircase. The handrails and balustrade of the staircase are composed of repeated sequences of phosphate and deoxyribose sugar. The steps of the staircase are made of pairs molecules called bases, which repeat themselves again and again. Each of the four pairs are identified by their initial letter—A for adenine, G for guanine, C for cytosine, and T for thymine.

Each of the pairs are connected by hydrogen bonds. Because of the chemical nature of these bonds, A (adenine) and T (thymine) can bind only with each other; and G (guanine) and C (cytosine) can bind only with each other. So four combinations are possible:

A-T

T-A

C-G

G-C

These four combinations are referred to as base pairs. The arrangement and order of these base pairs determines the actual information that DNA carries—much like the arrangement of the 1s and 0s on a computer program assume meaning by virtue of the order they are arranged in. The sequence of bases is read by machinery inside the cell. Various sections of DNA comprise specific genes, which can be read again and again, depending on whether the cell needs to produce what the gene codes for.

A single DNA molecule is composed of approximately 3 billion base pairs, tightly wound into the spiral helix form. Too infinitesimal to be viewed by even the most powerful microscope, the genetic information contained in a single molecule would stretch out uncoiled to about six feet long, and if written down, would fill over 125 massive books the size of the Manhattan telephone directory. The directory would be about 1 million pages long and 210 feet thick, using variations of the four-letter DNA code. DNA is not, however, just a "phone book" of human genes. Most of the genome consists of so-called "junk DNA"—rambling sequences of As, Ts, Gs, and Cs that seem to have been written in gibberish.

The genome has also revealed that the genes composing human DNA are not evenly distributed among the chromosomes. Some chromosomes are densely packed, while others are sparsely populated.

Alleles

What determines a person's unique DNA? Mendel also learned that a particular trait could be characterized by more than one type of information. For example, a gene for flower color could be of the red or white variety. These alternatives for a gene's information are called alleles. Alleles differ in their DNA sequence.

Every person's DNA contains alleles—alternate forms of genes. The alleles determine whether you have blue eyes or brown, are tall or short, have black hair or red, and other distinctions. Alleles are formed by differences in the sequence of base pairs, which can be as long as 10,000 base pairs. Genes with alternate forms are called pol-

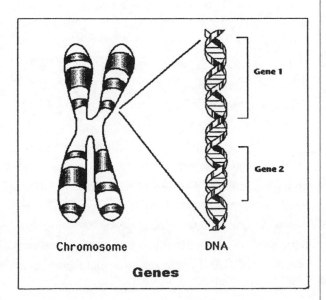

Chromosome   DNA

Genes

ymorphisms, meaning "many forms." Polymorphisms are the presence in a population of two or more genotypes for a given trait.

There are three blood group alleles—A, B, and O. In different combinations they are capable of producing four variations, or alternatives, for your blood group. Since these variations occur within an otherwise highly similar unit (such as a species) they are called polymorphisms.

Think of a gene as a multiple-choice question on an exam, and the gene's alleles as the possible answers to the question. Some alleles have dominant characteristics over others. For example, if a child has one blue eye color allele and one brown eye color allele, the child's eyes will be brown—just as if the child had two brown eye color alleles. Brown is the dominant eye color in humans; blue is the recessive eye color. Needless to say, people with blue eyes have two blue eye color alleles. However, the influence of your blood group allele is far greater than that of the gene that gives you eye color.

Genotype versus Phenotype

The basic genetics of the ABO blood groups is really quite simple, very similar to the way eye or hair color is determined. We are the physical result of our genes; this is called our phenotype. Phenotype is defined as all the physiological, behavioral, biochemical, and other characteristics of an organism that develop through the interaction of their genes and the environment. We get these genes from our parents, and the combination of our parents' genes that we carry is called our genotype. Genotype is defined as the genetic or hereditary information borne by an individual, as distinct from an individual's visible features. In a nutshell, you are your phenotype, and it was your genotype that got you there.

In multiple-allele genes, such as those for the ABO blood groups, one of the two alleles will usually be dominant, which is the key to your physical differences. In the ABO system the A and B alleles are dominant to the O allele (which is actually a blank, or "null" allele), just as in eye color, where the gene for brown eyes is dominant to the gene for blue eyes.

Genes are typically written in italics. Thus if we were referring the A allele, we would express it as *A*. Dominant genes are usually capitalized and recessive genes are usually written in lowercase. Thus a person of blood group A may have either of two possible genotypes: *Ao* or *AA*. All blood group O individuals have the genotype *oo*, while all blood group AB individuals have the genotype *AB*.

For example, if you've received an A allele from your mother and an O allele from your father, your genotype will be *Ao*, but your phenotype will be blood group A. However, you carry a latent O, which in turn can be passed on to your offspring. The distinction between phenotype and genotype is what confuses so many people about blood group genetics. It explains why a blood group A mother and a blood group O father can have a blood group O child, even though you can only become O if you receive an *o* allele from each parent.

The A and B alleles have an interesting relationship with each other: they do not dominate each other, as each does with the null *o* allele; rather they are co-dominant, meaning that if you receive an *A* allele from one parent and a *B* allele from the other, you become blood group AB.

		Dad	
		A	**o**
M o m	**o**	Ao = Type A	oo = Type O
	o	Ao = Type A	oo = Type O

Here's a simple illustration. Called a Punnett square, this tool is used by geneticists to determine possible combinations of phenotype from genotype. Mom (along the left side) is phenotype O (blood type O) and genotype *oo*. Dad (at the top) is phenotype A (blood type A) and genotype *Ao*. As we can see, each offspring has a 50% chance of being either A *(Ao)* or O *(oo)*. Since neither parent carries a B allele, it is impossible for the offspring of these two parents to be either B or AB. This is why blood type can be useful in determining paternity. It cannot confirm that a person is the father of a child; however, in certain circumstances it can confirm that a person is not the father. If the offspring of disputed paternity in the preceding case was either blood group B or AB, we would have to look elsewhere for the father of the child; the combination shown cannot give the child a B antigen.

		Dad	
		A	**B**
M o m	**o**	Ao = Type A	Bo = Type B
	o	Ao = Type A	Bo = Type B

Here's an interesting combination: Mom is blood group O and Dad is blood group AB. In this circumstance, the offspring will be either A or B, as both *A* and *B* alleles are dominant over O. No offspring will possess the blood type of their mother. However, all will possess a recessive *o* that can be passed on to their own offspring, potentially producing O children. This answers another question—why blood group O doesn't disappear over time, since group A and group B have the dominant alleles: There is a constant regenerating supply of the *o* allele in the human gene pool.

		Dad	
		B	**o**
M o m	**A**	AB = Type AB	Ao = Type A
	o	Bo = Type B	oo = Type O

In a third scenario, we can see how a group B father and a group A mother can produce offspring of every group. Thus, although it is a long shot, it is possible for each member of a family to have a different blood type.

TABLE V. Blood Type Inheritance

PARENTS' BLOOD TYPES	POSSIBLE ALLELE COMBINATIONS (GENOTYPE)	POSSIBLE BLOOD TYPES IN CHILDREN (PHENOTYPE)
Both A	AA, Ao	A or O
Both B	BB, Bo	B or O
Both AB	AB	A, B, or AB
Both O	oo	O
One A and one B	AA, Ao, BB, Bo	A, B, AB, or O
One A and one O	AA, Ao, oo	A or O
One A and one AB	AA, Ao, AB	A, B, or AB
One B and one O	BB, BO, oo	B or O
One B and one AB	BB, Bo, AB	A, B, or AB
One AB and one O	AB, oo	A or B

9q34: The ABO Gene

Each chromosome pair is joined at the center at a spot called the centromere. The characteristic banding of chromosomes (shown in the following illustration) is obtained by staining with various dyes. The band width and the order of bands is characteristic of a particular chromosome; a trained geneticist can identify each chromosome (1,2,3 . . . 22, X and Y) by observing its banding pattern under the microscope.

Chromosomes are divided into 2 legs; a "p" leg above the constriction point, and a "q" leg below it. By combining the chromosome number, the p or q leg, and a particular band number, it is possible to construct an address for a particular gene.

Each gene has a particular locus where it can be found. Think of the locus as the location or address of a gene. The gene locus for ABO blood group is located on the q leg of chromosome number 9, around band 34. It is here that the three basic alleles of the ABO blood system are found, which in combination determine whether you are group O, A, B, or AB. But the effect of the ABO blood group gene doesn't just stop there.

If we were to examine the band around 9q34, we would find that the area that determines ABO blood group is densely stained, indicating that there is a lot of thickly packed DNA, which is somewhat odd since the mechanics of ABO selection are fairly simple; the gene codes for the activity of only two enzymes. This brings us to one of the deepest, though least appreciated, aspects of the ABO gene: It can often influence the effect of other, seemingly unrelated genes.

We have already seen an example of this when we looked at the secretor subtype, as the basic mechanics of ABO and secretor status involve genes located on two different chromosomes. Our secretor status, which influences the ability of our bodies to secrete our ABH antigens in free form, is controlled by the secretor gene locus found on chromosome 19 (19q13.3). Interestingly, the gene locus that codes for the manufacture of the H antigen (which determines the O antigen and serves as the building block for A and B antigens) is located on chromosome 19 as well. If you are A, B, or AB, you have active alleles on 9q34; however, if you are blood group O, your DNA has a "null allele" there, so you are left with just the output of chromosome 19 (H) but nothing from 9q34 (A or B).

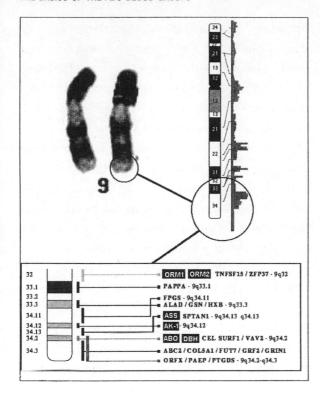

32	ORM1 ORM2 TNFSF15 / ZFP37 - 9q32
33.1	PAPPA - 9q33.1
33.2	FPGS - 9q34.11
33.3	ALAD / GSN / HXB - 9q33.3
34.11	ASS SPTAN1 - 9q34.13 q34.13
34.12	AK-1 9q34.12
34.13	
34.2	ABO DBH CEL SURF1 / VAV2 - 9q34.2
34.3	ABC2 / COL5A1 / FUT7 / GRF2 / GRIN1
	ORFX / PAEP / PTGDS - 9q34.2-q34.3

Gene Linkage

It is often said that great science occurs because good questions are asked. In 1933 T. H. Morgan won the Nobel Prize for work that began in 1910 at Columbia University. In that year he discovered a white-eyed fruit fly mutation. Up to this point it was pretty obvious that genes are on chromosomes. But on which chromosome is a given gene and where on the chromosome is it?

Morgan mated a red-eyed female fly with a white-eyed male and found the offspring to be red-eyed. He concluded that the gene for red eyes must be dominant. Morgan then mated these off-

spring. Now, according to Mendel's laws, there should be three red-eyed flies for each white-eyed fly, and when the flies were analyzed over several months, Morgan counted 3,470 red-eyed flies and 782 white-eyed flies—which was close to the expected one-to-three ratio.

However, Morgan noted a curious feature. None of the females had white eyes. Among the males, 1,011 had red eyes and 782 had white eyes. Further work was able to show that

• White eye color was recessive to red eye color.

• The gene for eye color was carried on the X (female) chromosome.

• There is no gene for eye color on the Y chromosome.

Morgan's work was a vital key to understanding gene linkage, one of the most important concepts in genetics. The concept itself is quite simple: Genes located on the same chromosome tend to be transmitted together. These are referred to as linked genes. The linkage of eye color to sex in the fly is a special case of the general phenomenon of gene linkage, in which two or more genes tend to be inherited together because they are on the same chromosome. In the case of blood groups, several genes are linked to the ABO locus, and tend to transfer in a manner that is dependent on the outcome of one's ABO group (actually, the combination of the ABO alleles).

Adjacent alleles for genes on the same chromosome tend to be coupled more often than expected. This is most likely a consequence of the "founder effect," in which a mutation for a disease arose at an early point in history in a particular population on a particular chromosome, and the allele was consequently linked to a particular adjacent gene marker. This is called *linkage disequilibrium*, since over time we would expect that enough genetic recombination would occur to randomize the relation of the mutant allele with respect to other marker alleles on other chromosomes—that is, to establish linkage equilibrium. Therefore, when linkage disequilibrium is seen, it is likely that inadequate time has passed for equilibrium to be established.

The discovery of a relationship between particular genes and diseases is accomplished through gene linkage studies. Linkage studies examine inherited genetic markers, such as ABO blood group. One of the first examples of gene linkage ever discovered in humans was the coinheritance of ABO blood group with a rare disease called nail-patella syndrome, in which people have abnormal nails and kneecaps. Knowing that the gene causing nail-patella syndrome was linked to blood group told scientists that the gene for nail-patella syndrome is located on chromosome 9—in other words, there is a gene proximity between the gene for blood group and the gene that causes nail-patella syndrome.

By looking at the genetic expression of the ABO blood groups, we can now understand many apparently unrelated physical and mental correlations. Attributes that seem unrelated—such as physiological adaptations to environment, disease, or diet, may have had a survival rationale, and

can be seen as linked traits in genetic memory. If these adaptations were successful and persisted, they would be hard-coded into one of the blood group alleles as a variant strategy for use by later generations.

Blood groups are also valuable markers in gene linkage analysis, and their study has contributed enormously to the mapping of the human genome.

Here are some of the initial findings linking the ABO blood group locus at 9q34 with other genes in close proximity:

BREAST CANCER

In 1984, researchers reporting in the journal *Genetic Epidemiology* presented evidence of a family pedigree in which a major gene for breast cancer susceptibility appeared to link to the ABO gene locus[1]. This supports other studies showing a similarity between the A antigen and a common tumor marker for breast cancer[2].

DOPAMINE METABOLISM

Dopamine beta-hydroxylase (DBH) is associated with the conversion of dopamine into the catecholamines adrenaline and noradrenaline. The gene for DBH virtually sits atop the gene for the ABO blood groups. Several studies have noted the relationship and its corresponding impact, with particular significance for blood group O.

In 1982, researchers measured DBH and catechol-O-methyltransferase (COMT) levels in 162 patients with major affective disorders (depression) and 1,125 of their relatives. A linkage of a locus for DBH to the ABO locus was indicated[3].

In 1988, a report indicated that the previously described activity variation in levels of serum DBH may reflect alterations in either the structure or regulation of the DBH coding. The researchers pointed out that the structural gene for the enzyme is close to the ABO blood group locus, and thus may be influenced by it[4].

A 1988 article published in the *American Journal of Human Genetics* stated that "Previous studies have presented evidence suggesting that levels of dopamine-beta-hydroxylase (DBH) activity are controlled by a gene linked to the ABO blood group locus." The researchers were able to verify this, showing a direct linkage between the gene regulating DBH activity and the gene for ABO blood group locus[5].

Researchers writing in the journal *Biological Psychiatry*, by combining data from a number of other studies, provided evidence for a "susceptibility allele" for affective disorder (depression) near the ABO region on chromosome 9q34, perhaps related to the gene locus for dopamine beta hydroxylase[6].

BLOOD CLOTTING

Lower levels of the blood clotting chemicals factor VIII and von Willebrand factor (vWF) have been reported in individuals with blood group O compared to individuals of other ABO blood groups, which is one reason their rate of heart disease is lower than the other ABO groups. Recent studies have shown that this is probably the result of gene linkage[7].

BLADDER CANCER

The area of the ABO genes (9q34) is an area where genes are commonly lost as cells of the bladder turn cancerous. The loss of ABO antigens is a common occurrence as bladder cells move toward metastasis. Evidence suggests that gene deletions in bladder cancer cells are linked to similar deletions on the ABO locus[8].

MUSCULOSKELETAL INJURY

There may be a genetic linkage between the ABO blood groups and the molecular structure of the tissue of Achilles tendons, as studies have associated a correlation between group O individuals and ruptures of the Achilles tendon[9].

SECRETOR STATUS AND EYE COLOR

A Danish study linked green eye color with being an ABO secretor[10].

NITRIC OXIDE METABOLISM

The amino acid arginine in the form of argininosuccinate is a basic building block in the synthesis of nitric oxide, a molecule critically involved in a plethora of body functions, including brain function, cardiovascular health, and proper immune function. The amino acid citrulline is recycled into argininosuccinate by the action of arginosuccinate synthetase (ASS), whose gene location is known to be very close to the ABO locus[11,12]. Variations in the function of this enzyme may be linked at the genetic level, since variations to inhaled nitric oxide therapy have been shown to occur in individuals who possess a B antigen (blood groups AB and B)[15,14].

ABO Blood Groups: The First Few Hours of Life

Normal cells are differentiated by virtue of having only the genes needed for their particular job activated, and all other genes deactivated, or repressed.

If we turn our thinking for a moment back to the growing embryo, we can get an idea of how this can occur. Embryonic cells (such as one might find in a 2- to 3-week-old fetus) do not yet have the full functionality found in the cells of a mature adult. Initially, unlike the thousands of different highly specific cells found in the normal adult, embryonic cells only come in three varieties:

- Ectoderm cells, which differentiate into the cells of the skin and nerves
- Mesoderm cells, which differentiate into the cells of the muscular system, skeleton, and connective tissues
- Endoderm cells, which become the lining of the digestive system

Since these cells, often called germ cells or germ layers, eventually differentiate into a wide variety of different tissues, they obviously need to repress and de-repress a large number of genes in order to wind up with a highly specialized end product.

The ABO antigens are intimately involved with the process of differentiation. We know that their production is greatly increased in the blood vessel cells of fetal organs, and they are thought to be responsible for specifying the location of future blood vessels in the burgeoning organs, where they serve as differentiation markers. We can almost think of the ABO antigens in the growing fetus as a team of railroad engineers, moving ahead of the construction crew, planning the future location of a railroad track.

One study documented the appearance of ABO blood group antigens in different developing animal embryos. It showed that ABO begins to appear first in endoderm cells, followed by ectoderm cells, and finally by mesoderm cells. Since red blood cells were the last cells to acquire ABO antigens, the authors suggested that ABO antigens should be called tissue antigens rather than blood group antigens[15,16].

This critical embryonic function of ABO blood group is not typically known or understood by the medical community. However, this is probably the single most important reason that blood type antigens appear and disappear in tissues that are about to go aggressively malignant and metastasize[17], a role that is increasingly being linked to ABO blood group antigens[18].

The genetic importance of ABO blood groups is only now emerging as the key to many of the most elusive biological mysteries. We can use this knowledge to maintain health, guard against disease, and even heal already damaged cells. In this respect, the genetic revolution is truly the blood type revolution.

REFERENCES

1. Skolnick MH, Thompson EA, Bishop DT, Cannon LA. Possible linkage of a breast cancer-susceptibility locus to the ABO locus: sensitivity of LOD scores to a single new recombinant observation. *Genet Epidemiol*. 1984;1:363–373.

2. Garratty G. Blood group antigens as tumor markers, parasitic/bacterial/viral receptors, and their association with immunologically important proteins. *Immunol Invest*. 1995;24:213–232.

3. Goldin LR, Gershon ES, Lake CR, et al. Segregation and linkage studies of plasma dopamine-beta-hydroxylase (DBH), erythrocyte catechol-O-methyltransferase (COMT), and platelet monoamine oxidase (MAO): possible linkage between the ABO locus and a gene controlling DBH activity. *Am J Hum Genet*. 1982;34:250–262.

4. Craig SP, Buckle VJ, Lamouroux A, et al. Localization of the human dopamine beta hydroxylase (DBH) gene to chromosome 9q34. *Cytogenet Cell Genet*. 1988;48:48–50.

5. Wilson AF, Elston RC, Siervogel RM, Tran LD. Linkage of a gene regulating dopamine-beta-hydroxylase activity and the ABO blood group locus. *Am J Hum Genet*. 1988;42:160–166.

6. Sherrington R, Curtis D, Brynjolfsson J, et al. A linkage study of affective disorder with DNA markers for the ABO-AK1-ORM linkage group near the dopamine beta hydroxylase gene. *Biol Psychiatry*. 1994;36:434–442.

7. Souto JC, Almasy L, Muniz-Diaz E, et al. Functional effects of the ABO locus polymorphism on plasma levels of von Willebrand factor, factor VIII, and activated partial thromboplastin time. *Arterioscler Thromb Vasc Biol*. 2000;20:2024–2028.

8. Orlow I, Lacombe L, Pellicer I, et al. Genotypic and phenotypic characterization of the histoblood group ABO(H) in primary bladder tumors. *Int J Cancer*. 1998;75:819–824.

9. Leppilahti J, Puranen J, Orava S. ABO blood group and Achilles tendon rupture. *Ann Chir Gynaecol*. 1996;85:369–371.

10. Eiberg H, Mohr J. Major genes of eye color and hair color linked to LU and SE. *Clin Genet*. 1987;31:186–191.

11. Ozelius LJ, Kwiatkowski DJ, Schuback DE, et al. A genetic linkage map of human chromosome 9q. *Genomics*. 1992;14:715–720.

12. Northrup H, Lathrop M, Lu SY, et al. Multilocus linkage analysis with the human argininosuccinate synthetase gene. *Genomics*. 1989;5:442–444.

13. McFadzean J, Tasker RC, Petros AJ. Nitric oxide ABO blood group difference in children. *Lancet*. 1999;353:1414–1415.

14. Weimann J, Bauer H, Bigatello L, Bloch KD, Martin E, Zapol WM. ABO blood group and inhaled nitric oxide in acute respiratory distress syndrome. *Lancet*. 1998;351:1786–1787.

15. Oriol R, Mollicone R, Coullin P, Dalix AM, Candelier JJ. Genetic regulation of the expression of ABH and Lewis antigens in tissues. *APMIS Suppl*. 1992;27:28–38.

16. Szulman AE. Evolution of ABH blood group antigens during embryogenesis. *Ann Inst Pasteur Immunol*. 1987;138:845–847.

17. Sarafian V, Dimova P, Georgiev I, Taskov H. ABH blood group antigen significance as markers of endothelial differentiation of mesenchymal cells. *Folia Med (Plovdiv)*. 1997;39:5–9.

18. Le Pendu J, Marionneau S, Cailleau-Thomas A, Rocher J, Le Moullac-Vaidye B, Clement M. ABH and Lewis histoblood group antigens in cancer. *APMIS*. 2001;109:9–31.

PART TWO

A–Z Blood Group Guide to Health and Medical Conditions

A

ABDOMINAL AORTIC ANEURYSM–*See*

Aneurysm, abdominal aortic

AGING DISEASES–*Conditions that escalate the process of cellular breakdown and shorten lifespan.*

Aging diseases	LONGEVITY AVERAGE		
	SHORT	AVERAGE	LONG
GROUP A			
GROUP B			
GROUP AB			
GROUP O			
NN SUBTYPE (WOMEN)			

Symptoms

- Simple muscle aches
- Arthritis
- Cardiovascular disease
- Hypertension
- Diabetes
- Cancer

About Aging Diseases

All living creatures age. But why do we age? And what can be done to slow down the process?

These questions have fascinated humankind for as long as we can collectively recall. With our sophisticated medical technology and our increased knowledge of the factors that contribute to aging, we are moving ever closer to the answers.

Why do individual aging patterns differ so greatly? Why does the 50-year-old runner, lean and seemingly fit, drop dead of a massive heart attack, while the 89-year-old who has never exercised remains hale and hardy? Why do some people develop Alzheimer's disease or senile dementia, while others do not? At what age does physical deterioration become inevitable? We now understand some pieces of the puzzle. Genetics plays a role—unique variations in chromosomes contribute to susceptibilities that cause deterioration more rapidly in one person than in another. But these studies are incomplete. Although they provide a tantalizing glimpse of the answer, we are still left pondering the scope of the questions.

Lectins and Aging

The action of dietary lectins is directly correlated with the two biggest physiological associations with aging—KIDNEY FAILURE and brain deterioration. As we age, all of us experience a gradual drop in kidney function; by the time the average person reaches age 72, his or her kidneys are operating at only 25% of their original capacity.

Kidney function is a reflection of the volume of blood that is cleansed and re-circulated into the bloodstream. This filtering system is very delicate—large enough for the various fluid elements of blood to move through, but small enough to prevent whole cells from being passed. Lectins have been shown to increase the production of antibodies that are capable of destroying this delicate filter[1]. Lectins that find their way into the bloodstream end up stimulating the production of antibodies, and the antibody/lectin complex can then lodge in the kidneys[2]. The process is similar to having a clogged drain. As more and more agglutination occurs, less and less blood can be cleansed. Over time, the filtration system ceases to function. It is a slow process, but ultimately deadly. Kidney failure is one of the leading causes of physical deterioration in the elderly.

The second major physiological change of aging occurs in the brain, where lectins play an equally destructive role. Scientists have observed that the difference between an old brain and a young brain is that, in an old brain, many elements of neurons get tangled up. This tangling, which leads to dementia and overall deterioration—and which might even be a factor in AL-ZHEIMER'S DISEASE—occurs very gradually over the decades of adult life.

The nerve cells of Alzheimer's patients exhibit a phenomenon called "reactive plasticity," a sort of aberrant sprouting of non-functional side-connections between the nerve cells. The new pathways created have been proposed to be contributors to several neurological disorders. Much of this sprouting is characterized by the profuse production of glycosylated sugars[3], which are precisely the molecules that lectins bind to. In fact, many dietary lectins have been used to map reactive plasticity pathways in brain samples from Alzheimer's patients[4].

A third way that lectins contribute to aging is their effect on hormonal functions. As people age, they have more trouble absorbing and metabolizing nutrients. One common occurrence is the development of a resistance to the effects of the hormone insulin, causing many of the elderly to develop type II (or non-insulin-dependent) diabetes. Many lectins, but probably most significantly the lectin found in wheat, can act as a false insulin, binding to the insulin receptor and blocking the effects of true insulin[5]. In fact, the lectin in wheat has been shown to induce tissue-destroying antibodies that attack the pancreas, destroying the specialized insulin-producing cells[6].

Blood Group Links

The ABO blood group antigens provide a clear road map for the process of aging. As we age, the amount of protective antibodies produced by our antigens declines. These anti–blood group antibodies protect our immune systems from the presence of foreign antigens. Obviously, the decline in their production opens our systems to a series of opportunistic pathogens, and thus to any number of eventually fatal diseases.

Consider the life of the immune system as being divided into three stages. The first stage con-

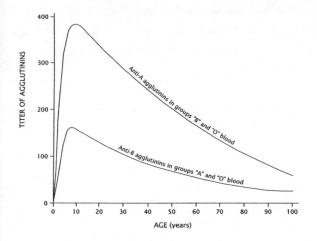

AGGLUTINATION AND THE PROCESS OF AGING

As we age the amount of anti-blood type agglutinins in our blood diminishes, making us more susceptible to disease. A key factor in healthy aging is to maintain high levels of anti-blood type agglutinins.

sists of *education*. As the immune system is exposed to antigens, it begins to learn which is a friend and which is a foe. A functioning immune system will begin to produce antibodies against the foes. The second stage is *maintenance*. If the immune system has learned well, it will remain strong and healthy—effectively warding off foreign antigens. The third stage is *decay*. As we age, our immune defenses weaken. Blood group antigens are less profuse, and provide less protection against foreign antigens. The goal is to delay that final process. If the education process was successful, the maintenance stage will be extended, and the third stage, defensive decline, will be delayed.

Researchers have attempted to learn whether there is a direct link between blood group and longevity. A study of Italian physicians showed a higher percentage of those over the age of 75 were group O[7], while another study showed that group B was associated with a long lifespan[8]. Since blood group B individuals tend to fall almost invariably between A and O with regard to disease susceptibilities, this tempering effect can be expected to translate into a higher percentage of group B individuals attaining a more advanced age.

The NN subtype of the MN blood grouping system may be associated with a slight increase in longevity, especially for women[9].

We do know that each blood group has specific vulnerabilities to age-related conditions.

BLOOD GROUP O:

Group O is at special risk for inflammatory diseases, which affect the elderly.

BLOOD GROUP A:

High cortisol levels are linked to heart attacks and lowered immunity.

Excessive stress hormone levels have been linked to loss of muscle tissue.

As low stomach acid levels decline further, they cause digestive problems.

BLOOD GROUP B:

High cortisol levels are linked to Alzheimer's disease and senile dementia.

Susceptibility to slow-moving viruses creates a risk of immune and neuromuscular problems.

BLOOD GROUP AB:

As low stomach acid levels decline further, they cause digestive problems. Also, there is an increased risk of strokes from embolism, due to increased blood clotting factors.

Declining natural killer (NK) cell activity with age leaves group AB more susceptible to immune system breakdowns.

Therapies, Aging Diseases

BLOOD GROUP A:

1. Immune-Enhancing Protocol
2. Cardiovascular Protocol
3. Cancer Prevention Protocol
4. Antistress Protocol

BLOOD GROUP B:

1. Immune-Enhancing Protocol
2. Liver Support Protocol
3. Antistress Protocol
4. Nerve Health Protocol

BLOOD GROUP AB:

1. Immune-Enhancing Protocol
2. Liver Support Protocol
3. Cardiovascular Protocol

BLOOD GROUP O:

1. Metabolic Enhancement Protocol
2. Liver Support Protocol
3. Anti-Inflammation Protocol

Related Topics

Digestion

Food poisoning

Fungal disease, candidiasis (digestive)

Fungal disease, candidiasis (oral)

Fungal disease, candidiasis (vaginal)

Influenza

Parasitic disease, amoeba

Parasitic disease, *Giardia*

Parasitic disease, hookworm

Toxicity, bowel

Ulcer, *H. pylori*

REFERENCES

1. Coppo R, Amore A, Roccatello D. Dietary antigens and primary immunoglobulin A nephropathy. *J Am Soc Nephrol.* 1992;2(suppl):S173–S180.

2. Coppo R, Amore A, Roccatello D, et al. [Role of food antigens and alcohol in idiopathic nephritis with IgA deposits]. *Minerva Urol Nefrol.* 1991;43:171–174.

3. Espinosa B, Zenteno R, Mena R, Robitaille Y, Zenteno E, Guevara J. O-Glycosylation in sprouting neurons in Alzheimer disease, indicating reactive plasticity. *J Neuropathol Exp Neurol.* 2001;60:441–448.

4. Guevara J, Espinosa B, Zenteno E, Vazquez L, Luna J, Perry G, Mena R. Altered glycosylation pattern of proteins in Alzheimer disease. *J Neuropathol Exp Neurol.* 1998;57:905–914.

5. Livingston JN, Purvis BJ. Effects of wheat germ agglutinin on insulin binding and insulin sensitivity of fat cells. *Am J Physiol.* 1980;238:E267–E275.

6. Kitano N, Taminato T, Ida T, et al. Detection of antibodies against wheat germ agglutinin bound glycoproteins on the islet-cell membrane. *Diabet Med.* 1988;5:139–144.

7. Jorgensen G. ABO blood groups in physicians of 75 years of age. Further evidence in favor of little more fitness on the part of subjects with blood group O. *Minerva Med.* 1974; 65:2881–2886.

8. Dworsky R, Paganini-Hill A, Arthur M, Parker J. Immune responses of healthy humans 83–104 years of age. *J Natl Cancer Inst.* 1983;71:265–268.

9. Turowska B, Gurda M, Wozniak K. ABO, MN, Kell, Hp and

Gm1 markers in elderly humans. *Mater Med Pol.* 1991;23: 7–12.

AGORAPHOBIA–See Anxiety disorders

AIDS–See Viral disease, acquired immune deficiency syndrome (AIDS)

ALCOHOLISM–A dependence on ethanol (ethyl alcohol), leading to physical and mental deterioration and eventual death.

Alcoholism	RISK		
	LOW	AVERAGE	HIGH
GROUP A	███		
GROUP B	███	███	
GROUP AB	███		
GROUP O	███	███	
NON-SECRETOR	███	███	███
MN SUBTYPE	███	███	

Symptoms

Alcohol dependence is associated with three or more of the following symptoms:

- Social withdrawal

- Increased tolerance for alcohol

- Persistent desire to cut down

- Drinking more alcohol than desired

- Time spent getting, drinking, and recovering from alcohol

- Giving up social, occupational, or recreational tasks in order to drink alcohol

- Continued use in spite of physical and psychological problems

About Alcoholism

More than 18 million Americans are alcoholics. Alcoholism is an insidious disease that has a destructive impact on every part of a person's physical, mental, and social life. In addition, everyone who comes in contact with an alcoholic will be affected in some way.

Studies show that alcoholism has a strong genetic component; the biological children of alcoholics are four to five times more likely to be alcoholics as well.

The systemic health consequences of alcoholism include brain degeneration, HEART DISEASE, HYPERTENSION, nutritional deficiencies, and LIVER DISEASE. Only about 3% of the alcohol a person consumes passes through the body and is excreted; the rest is metabolized by the liver and processed in the stomach and small intestines. After heavy and regular alcohol consumption patterns, the alcoholic's liver will begin to deteriorate. The end result can be CIRRHOSIS of the liver, severe malnutrition from malabsorption of foods, and ultimately death.

General Risk Factors and Causes

Although alcoholism is a common disease in Western civilization, it is known in all parts of the world. Evidence now suggests that grain was cultivated for the fermentation of alcohol long before it was used for the production of bread. The desire for alcohol may have been a primary motivation for the first cultivation of grains and the subsequent rise of cities.

Some sources suggest that most alcoholics have a decreased production of adrenocorticotropic hormone (ACTH), the hormone that signals the adrenal glands to produce stress hormones. Almost all alcoholics have some form of hypoglycemia, which they compensate for with stimulants. Typically such individuals will go too long without eating. As a result, alcoholics lack stamina, and use alcohol to dampen adrenaline spikes and provide sugar.

Blood Group Links

In an unfortunate and possibly random cellular twist, the gene that determines secretor status is located on the same part of the DNA as a suspected gene for alcoholism. Nonsecretors seem to be prone to alcoholism[1], and, oddly enough, nonsecretors also seem to derive the most benefit to their hearts from a moderate intake of alcohol. The Copenhagen Male Study, which showed nonsecretors to be at a higher risk for ISCHEMIC HEART DISEASE (a lack of blood flow into the arteries), theorized that moderate consumption of alcohol altered the rate of insulin flow, slowing the accumulation of fat in the blood vessels[2].

It is also clear that alcoholism has a major stress component. A Japanese research team discovered that a greater number of blood group A individuals received treatment for alcoholism than group O or group B. It is thought that group A may have a predilection for alleviating stress by the ingestion of inhibition-releasing chemicals[3].

Although no studies have linked blood group O with alcoholism, there is substantial evidence that group O, because of a link between the ABO gene and the dopamine beta hydroxylase (DBH) gene, tend to have a harder time regulating dopamine, a chemical intimately connected to the activity of the "satiety" or "pleasure" centers of the brain[4,5]. Low levels of DBH can promote pleasure-seeking activity such as alcohol use.

There may be a link between the MN blood group and susceptibility to alcoholism[6]. A study conducted by the Alcohol and Genetics Research Program at the Western Psychiatric Institute and Clinic of Pittsburgh, Pennsylvania, investigated the link between six blood group markers and a putative alcoholism susceptibility gene. Evidence suggested a link between susceptibility to alcoholism and people who have both the N gene and the M gene (MN blood group).

Therapies, Alcoholism

ALL BLOOD GROUPS:

1. If you consume alcohol, avoid the medications cimetidine (Tagamet) and ranitidine (Zantac). They inhibit gastric alcohol dehydrogenase, interfering with alcohol breakdown and substantially increasing blood alcohol levels.

2. Minimize the effects of alcohol by eating cultured foods (PROBIOTICS). For example, a Japanese study showed that natto, a traditional Japanese cultured food product, assisted with the metabolism of alcohol. This suggests that such foods might be useful anti-hangover agents[7].

BLOOD GROUP A:

1. Antistress Protocol

2. Liver Support Protocol

3. Metabolic Enhancement Protocol

Specifics:

L-glutamine: 500 mg twice daily

BLOOD GROUP B:

1. Antistress Protocol

2. Metabolic Enhancement Protocol

3. Liver Support Protocol

Specifics:

Phosphatidylcholine: 500 mg daily

L-carnitine: 300 mg twice daily

BLOOD GROUP AB:

1. Antistress Protocol

2. Metabolic Enhancement Protocol

3. Detoxification Protocol

Specifics:

Phosphatidylcholine: 500 mg daily

L-carnitine: 300 mg twice daily

BLOOD GROUP O:

1. Antistress Protocol

2. Metabolic Enhancement Protocol

3. Detoxification Protocol

Specifics:

Pantethine: 650 mg daily

L-glutamine: 500–750 mg daily

Related Topics

Digestion

Ischemic heart disease

Stress

REFERENCES

1. Stigendal L, Olsson R, Rydberg L, Samuelsson BE. Blood group lewis phenotype on erythrocytes and in saliva in alcoholic pancreatitis and chronic liver disease. *J Clin Pathol.* 1984;37:778–782.

2. Camps FE, Dodd BE, Lincoln PJ. Frequencies of secretors and non-secretors of ABH group substances among 1,000 alcoholic patients. *Br Med J.* 1969;681:457–459.

3. Hill SY, Suggestive evidence of genetic linkage between alcoholism and the MNS blood group. *Alcohol Clin Exp Res.* 1988;12(6):811–814.

4. Wilson AF, Elston RC, Siervogel RM, Tran LD. Linkage of a gene regulating dopamine-beta-hydroxylase activity and the ABO blood group locus. *Am J Hum Genet.* 1988;42:160–166.

5. Sherrington R, Curtis D, Brynjolfsson J, Moloney E, Rifkin L, Petursson H, Gurling H. A linkage study of affective disorder with DNA markers for the ABO-AK1-ORM linkage group near the dopamine beta hydroxylase gene. *Biol Psychiatry.* 1994;36:434–442.

6. DiPadova C, Roine R, Frezza M, Gentry RT, Baraona E, Lieber CS. Effects of ranitidine on blood alcohol levels after ethanol ingestion: comparison with other H2-receptor antagonists. *JAMA.* 1992;267:83–86.

7. Sumi H, Yatagai C, Wada H, Yoshida E, Maruyama M. Effect of Bacillus natto_fermented product (BIOZYME) on blood alcohol, aldehyde concentrations after whisky drinking in human volunteers, and acute toxicity of acetaldehyde in mice. *Arukoru Kenkyuto Yakubutsu Ison.* 1995;30:69–79.

ALLERGIES (general)–*Immune reactions to environmental allergens or foods.*

Allergies (general)	SEVERITY		
	LOW	AVERAGE	HIGH
GROUP A	▓▓		
GROUP B	▓▓	▓▓	▓▓
GROUP AB	▓		
GROUP O	▓▓	▓▓	
SECRETOR	▓▓	▓▓	

Symptoms

- Sneezing
- Runny nose
- Itchy eyes
- Hives
- Headache
- Digestive distress

About Allergies

The word *allergy* means "altered working." It was coined at the beginning of the 20th century, after dogs inoculated with proteins from other animals had altered reactions when they came into contact with that protein again. These reactions were harmful, and sometimes fatal.

Allergies are responses mounted by the immune system to a particular food, inhalant, or chemical. Thus, a true allergy is a reaction that affects the immune system. A sensitivity can include other types of reactions that are not technically allergies, for which the cause has yet to be determined. From a conventional medical point of view, many sensitivities would not be considered allergies. However, because in popular terminology the terms "sensitivity" and "allergy" are often used to mean the same thing, they will be used interchangeably in this section.

According to the National Institute of Allergy and Infectious Diseases (NIAID), people with allergies spend more than $5 billion annually on doctors' visits, allergy shots, and prescription medications.

Many health conditions are related to allergies, such as acne, RHEUMATOID ARTHRITIS, ASTHMA, ATTENTION DEFICIT DISORDERS, and BLADDER INFECTIONS.

The Dynamics of an Allergy Attack

An allergic reaction is the immune system losing control. In addition to attacking its true enemies, such as viruses and bacteria, the immune system of an allergic person also springs into action when an allergen is present. When an allergic person is exposed to an allergen, a special class of antibodies known as immunoglobulin E (IgE) is produced. IgE molecules are specific for the original allergen, and can readily bind to the allergen that caused their production.

Specific IgE molecules travel through the blood and attach to receptors on the surface of mast cells. Mast cells are specialized cells that release histamine, a chemical that produces the classic

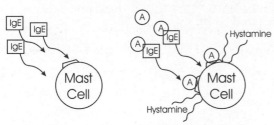

Ige molecules travel through blood and attach to receptors on most cells-specialized cells that release hystamine.

When an allergic person is exposed to an allergen (A), the allergen attaches to the IgE receptors causing mast cells to release histamine. Histamine is responsible for the watery eyes, sneezing, hives and other allergic symptoms

THE DYNAMICS OF AN ALLERGY ATTACK

symptoms of watery eyes, sneezing, welts, and HIVES. Different IgE antibodies are produced for each type of allergen, whether it's latex, pet dander, oak pollen, or ragweed pollen. Once allergen-specific IgE has attached to the mast cell surface, it can remain for weeks or even months, always ready to bind to the original allergen.

The next time the allergen enters the body, the allergic cascade begins, and eventually results in the release of histamines from the mast cell. Different chemicals are produced and released, depending on the allergen. These chemicals target certain areas of the body, producing a wide range of symptoms. These symptoms may occur in just minutes, or up to an hour after contact.

General Risk Factors and Causes

People seem to inherit allergies, most often from their mothers. At least three genes are be-

lieved to be responsible for allergies, but only one has been identified. This gene produces interleukin 4 (IL-4), a growth factor that is required for production of IgE. Overproduction of IL-4 leads to more IgE, which in turn leads to an allergy. Most dietary lectins are known to stimulate production of IL-4[1], which provides the "smoking gun" to a link between highly allergic individuals and an increased sensitivity to dietary lectins.

One theory postulates that the allergic response is a defensive reaction of the immune system against certain innocuous substances that the body mistakes for harmful parasites. This is probably true. IgE is found to increase greatly in response to a PARASITIC INFECTION. Eosinophils (cells that kill parasites such as worms) work in conjunction with IgE. Thus, one of the classic signs of a child with parasites is an itchy nose and watery eyes— the result of the immune system trying to kill the parasite, and meanwhile liberating enough IgE to mimic the symptoms of allergy.

Non-Caucasians tend to have higher levels of IgE than others, and males tend to have higher levels than females. Like the anti-blood-type antibodies, the levels of IgE tend to drop as we age, which perhaps explains why some people grow out of childhood allergies.

As a rule, patients with atopic (inherited) skin diseases, including atopic dermatitis (ECZEMA), have a genetic predisposition for developing IgE antibody-mediated hypersensitivity to inhaled and ingested substances. These allergens are harmless to people who are not atopic. Although an IgE-mediated food allergy may contribute to the symptoms of atopic dermatitis in infants and young children, it is largely independent of the allergic factors among older children and adults.

A marked increase in allergic reactions has been noted with exposure to water-soluble proteins in latex products (e.g., rubber gloves, dental dams, condoms, tubing for respiratory equipment, catheters, and enema tips with inflatable latex cuffs), particularly among medical personnel, patients exposed to latex, and children with SPINA BIFIDA and urogenital birth defects.

Therapies, Allergies

BLOOD GROUP A:

1. Allergy Control Protocol
2. Intestinal Health Protocol
3. Skin Health Protocol

BLOOD GROUP B:

1. Allergy Control Protocol
2. Immune-Enhancing Protocol
3. Skin Health Protocol

BLOOD GROUP AB:

1. Allergy Control Protocol
2. Immune-Enhancing Protocol
3. Skin Health Protocol

BLOOD GROUP O:

1. Allergy Control Protocol
2. Yeast/Fungus Protocol
3. Skin Health Protocol

Related Topics

Asthma

Autoimmune disease (general)

Immunity

REFERENCES

1. Haas H, Falcone FH, Schramm G, et al. Dietary lectins can induce in vitro release of IL-4 and IL-13 from human basophils. *Eur J Immunol.* 1999;29:918–927.

ALLERGIES, ENVIRONMENTAL/HAY FEVER—*Immune reactions to environmental agents; triggered by inhalants or environmental substances, frequently pollens.*

Allergies, environ-mental/hay fever	SEVERITY		
	LOW	AVERAGE	HIGH
GROUP A	▓		
GROUP B	▓	▓	▓
GROUP AB	▓		
GROUP O	▓	▓	
SECRETOR	▓	▓	

Symptoms

- Sneezing
- Congestion
- Runny nose
- Itchy eyes

About Environmental Allergies and Hay Fever

Allergies are the result of the immune system overreacting to normally harmless substances in the environment, termed *allergens*. Common allergens include dust mites and pollen.

Hay fever is the most common environmental allergy syndrome. These seasonal allergies are caused by airborne pollens and mold spores that commonly trigger symptoms. During the spring and fall, seasonal allergic rhinitis sufferers experience increased symptoms of sneezing, CONGESTION, runny nose, and itchiness in the nose, roof of the mouth, throat, eyes, and ears, depending on where they live in the country and the exact allergen.

Pollens are the tiny, egg-shaped male cells of flowering plants. These microscopic, powdery granules are necessary for plant fertilization. The average pollen particle is less than the width of an average human hair. Pollens from plants with bright flowers, such as roses, usually do not trigger allergies. On the other hand, many trees, grasses, and low-growing weeds have small, light, dry pollens that are well-suited for dissemination by wind currents. These are the pollens that trigger allergy symptoms.

Seasonal allergic rhinitis in the early spring is often triggered by the pollens of such trees as oak, western red cedar, elm, birch, ash, hickory, poplar, sycamore, maple, cypress, and walnut. In the late spring and early summer, pollinating grasses—including timothy, bermuda, orchard, sweet vernal, red top, and some blue grasses—often trigger symptoms.

In addition to ragweed—the pollen most responsible for late summer and fall hay fever in North America—other weeds can trigger allergic rhinitis symptoms. These weeds include sagebrush, pigweed, tumbleweed, Russian thistle and cockleweed. Each plant has a period of pollination that does not vary greatly from year to year. However, weather conditions can affect the amount of pollen in the air at any given time. The pollinating season starts later in the spring the farther north one goes.

Blood Group Links

A study of respiratory diseases in Georgians concluded that secretors tend to have higher levels of IgE than non-secretors and thus are more vulnerable to allergies. Blood group B tends to get pollen allergies more often than the other blood types, and blood group O a bit less often.

Group O was found to be at greatest risk for respiratory allergies. The highest resistance to respiratory allergies was found in group AB. In cases of house dust allergy, group O individuals had higher levels of IgE synthesizing B-lymphocytes than the other blood groups. Blood group A had significantly lower levels[1].

Group B has also been associated with a higher incidence of hay fever. In 239 German patients with atopic conditions (atopic dermatitis [eczema], hay fever, allergic rhinitis, bronchial ASTHMA, and acute urticaria) the phenotype and gene distribution of 15 genetic blood polymorphisms, including ABO, MN, and rhesus, were analyzed and compared with those in 151 selected controls (individuals clinically free of allergic conditions and without allergy in their family history). The incidence of blood group B was higher in patients than in controls. These observations were in accordance with the results of previous studies in other populations[2].

In another study, the distribution of ABO blood groups was examined in retrospect in a selected group of 241 patients with grass pollen hay fever. A relative deficiency in blood group O was found, with a shift toward an over-represented B-phenotype as compared to the general population. This shift appeared to be largely due to the contribution from the female patients with pollinosis[3].

Therapies, Environmental Allergies and Hay Fever

BLOOD GROUP A:

1. Allergy Control Protocol

2. Immune-Enhancing Protocol

BLOOD GROUP B:

1. Allergy Control Protocol

2. Pulmonary Support Protocol

BLOOD GROUP AB:

1. Allergy Control Protocol

2. Immune-Enhancing Protocol

BLOOD GROUP O:

1. Allergy Control Protocol

2. Anti-Inflammation Protocol

Related Topics

Asthma

Autoimmune disease (general)

Bronchitis

Immunity

REFERENCES

1. Khetsuriani NG, Gamkrelidze AG. Erythrocyte antigens as immunogenetic markers of respiratory atopic diseases in Georgians. *J Investig Allergol Clin Immunol.* 1995;5:35–39.

2. Brachtel R, Walter H, Beck W, Hilling M. Associations between atopic diseases and the polymorphic systems ABO, Kidd, Inv and red cell acid phosphatase. *Hum Genet.* 1979; 49:337–348.

3. Koers WJ, Houben GF, Berrens L. Blood groups ABO and grass-pollen hay fever. *Allerg Immunol (Leipz).* 1989;35: 167–172.

ALLERGIES, FOOD–*Symptoms occurring repeatedly after eating a specific food, and for which an immunologic basis (immunoglobulin E antibody response to the suspect food) is proved.*

Allergies, food	SEVERITY		
	LOW	AVERAGE	HIGH
GROUP A	■		
GROUP B	■	■	
GROUP AB	■		
GROUP O	■	■	
NON-SECRETOR			■

Symptoms

- Hives

- Eczema

- Gastrointestinal symptoms (irritable bowel, colitis)

- Respiratory symptoms (asthma, allergic rhinitis)

About Food Allergies

Reports of food allergies began to appear in Europe in the early 1900s; since the 1940s, food allergies have been recognized by physicians worldwide. Up to 8% of children (about 2 million) and 2% of adults in the United States are affected by food allergy.

With a true food allergy, an individual's immune system will overreact to an ordinarily harmless food. This is caused by an allergic antibody called immunoglobulin E (IgE), which is found in people with allergies. A food allergy often appears in someone who has family members with allergies, and symptoms may occur after that allergic individual consumes even a tiny amount of the triggering food.

Food allergens—those parts of foods that cause allergic reactions—are usually proteins. Most of these allergens can still cause reactions even after they are cooked or have undergone digestion in the intestines. Numerous food proteins have been studied to establish allergen content. The most common food allergens—responsible for up to 90% of all allergic reactions—are the proteins in cow's milk, eggs, peanuts, wheat, soy, fish, shellfish, and tree nuts.

The most common allergic skin reaction to a food is hives. Hives are red, very itchy, swollen areas of the skin that may arise suddenly and leave quickly. They often appear in clusters, with new clusters appearing as other areas clear. Hives may occur alone, or be accompanied by other symptoms. Food intolerance has been found to be responsible for the symptoms of some patients with irritable bowel syndrome.

Preliminary information suggests that the same phenomenon may take place occasionally in patients with chronic ULCERATIVE COLITIS. The first manifestation may be eczema (atopic dermatitis), alone or in association with gastrointestinal symptoms. By the end of the first year, dermatitis usually has lessened and allergic respiratory symptoms may develop. ASTHMA and allergic RHINITIS can be aggravated by allergy to foods, which can be identified by skin testing.

As children grow, food allergens become less important, and they react increasingly to inhaled allergens. By the time a child with asthma and HAY FEVER is 10 years old, it is rare for a food to provoke respiratory symptoms, even though positive skin tests may persist.

The Allergy–Lectin Connection

Dietary lectins have been shown to induce the production of interleukin-4, which in turn activates IgE[1]. This may explain why one of the more common benefits reported by those who follow the blood type food plans is a lessening of allergic manifestations, SINUSITIS, and asthma. Many bacteria use lectins to attach to host tissue, and these lectins are some of the more highly allergenic parts of the organism. Many food lectins trigger IgE, including the lectins found in bananas, chestnuts, and avocados. They are all implicated in what has been termed "latex fruit allergies." Kiwi fruit lectins also trigger IgE.

Lectins from peas, broad beans, lentils, jack beans, soybeans, peanuts, and wheat germ have been shown to bind directly with IgE and initiate the release of histamine, which can produce a feeling of "spaciness," a condition characterized by an inability to focus and concentrate[2].

Therapies, Food Allergies

BLOOD GROUP A:

1. Allergy Control Protocol

BLOOD GROUP B:

1. Allergy Control Protocol

BLOOD GROUP AB:

1. Allergy Control Protocol

BLOOD GROUP O:

1. Allergy Control Protocol

Related Topics

Autoimmune disease (general)

Celiac disease

Digestion

Lectins

REFERENCES

1. Khetsuriani NG, Gamkrelidze AG. *J Investig Allergol Clin Immunol.* 1995;5:35–39.
2. Kauffmann F, Frette C, Pham QT, Nafissi S, Bertrand JP, Oriol R. *Am J Respir Crit Care Med.* 1996;153:76–82.

ALZHEIMER'S DISEASE–*A progressive neurological degenerative disease, usually afflicting people over age 60.*

Alzheimer's disease	INCIDENCE/RISK/SEVERITY		
	LOW	AVERAGE	HIGH
GROUP A	▨	▨	
GROUP B	▨	▨	
GROUP AB	▨		
GROUP O	▨		
NON-SECRETOR	▨	▨	

Symptoms

Early Stage

- Bouts of forgetfulness
- Loss of concentration
- Short-term memory loss
- Misplacing objects

Later Stage

- Loss of cognitive function
- Inability to recognize friends and family members
- Deterioration of personality

- Inability to recognize familiar surroundings
- Loss of physical function

About Alzheimer's Disease

When Alzheimer's disease was first identified almost a century ago, it was quite rare. But as life expectancy has continued to increase dramatically, Alzheimer's disease has become more common. It is estimated that nearly 20% of people aged 75 to 84 suffer from this devastating condition.

Although there is still no clear understanding of what causes the brain degeneration symptomatic of Alzheimer's disease, autopsy studies have given us a clearer understanding of the type of changes that occur. As the disease progresses, nerve fibers surrounding the memory center of the brain (the hippocampus) become tangled and are no longer able to carry messages to and from the brain. This process is called neurofibrillary tangles.

A second factor is believed to be the buildup of amyloid plaques—that is, plaques that accumulate in the nerve cells, destroying them.

In the early stages, the symptoms of Alzheimer's disease—bouts of forgetfulness and loss of concentration—can be easily missed, as they closely resemble the natural effects of aging. Over time, however, Alzheimer's disease grows progressively more severe, destroying cognitive function, personality, and the ability to function competently.

Most people with Alzheimer's share certain signs of the disease. At its onset, Alzheimer's disease is marked by periods of forgetfulness, especially of recent events or simple directions. But what begins as mild forgetfulness persists and increases. People with Alzheimer's may repeat things and forget conversations or appointments. They routinely misplace things, often putting them in illogical locations. They frequently forget names, and, eventually, they may forget the names of family members and everyday objects such as a comb or a watch.

A person with Alzheimer's may initially have trouble balancing a checkbook, a problem that progresses to the point of trouble understanding and recognizing numbers. It may also be a challenge for those with Alzheimer's to find the right words to express thoughts or even follow conversations. Eventually, reading and writing are also affected. People with Alzheimer's may lose a sense of time and dates. They may find themselves lost in familiar surroundings. Eventually, they may even wander from home.

Solving everyday problems, such as knowing what to do if food on the stove is burning, becomes increasingly impossible. Alzheimer's is characterized by greater difficulty in doing things that require planning, decision making, and judgment. Once-routine tasks that require sequential steps, such as cooking, become a struggle as the disease progresses. Eventually people with Alzheimer's may forget how to do the most basic things, like brushing their teeth.

People with Alzheimer's may also exhibit mood swings. They may express distrust in others, show increased stubbornness, and withdraw socially. Early on, this may be a response to the frustration they feel as they notice uncontrollable changes in their memory. Depression often coexists with Alzheimer's disease. Restlessness is also a common sign. As the disease progresses, people with Alzheimer's may become anxious or aggressive, and may behave inappropriately.

Blood Group Links

Limited studies have been conducted to determine whether there is a relationship between Alzheimer's disease and blood group. To date no direct correlation has been found. However, there is evidence of high plasma cortisol levels in people with senile dementia and Alzheimer's. This may indicate an additional risk factor for blood group A and, to a lesser extent, blood group B.

Therapies, Alzheimer's Disease

ALL BLOOD GROUPS:

1. Phosphatidylserine, which is related to lecithin, is a naturally occurring compound present in the brain. At doses of 100 mg, three times daily, it has been shown to improve mental function in individuals with Alzheimer's disease[1-3].

2. Several clinical trials suggest that acetyl-L-carnitine delays the progression of Alzheimer's disease, improves memory, and enhances overall performance in some individuals with the disease[4-6].

BLOOD GROUP A:

1. Antistress Protocol
2. Immune-Enhancing Protocol

BLOOD GROUP B:

1. Antistress Protocol
2. Cognitive Improvement Protocol
3. Immune-Enhancing Protocol
4. Liver Support Protocol

BLOOD GROUP AB:

1. Antistress Protocol
2. Cognitive Improvement Protocol
3. Immune-Enhancing Protocol
4. Liver Support Protocol

BLOOD GROUP O:

1. Antistress Protocol
2. Immune-Enhancing Protocol
3. Liver Support Protocol
4. Cognitive Improvement Protocol

Specifics:

DMAE (2-dimethylaminoethanol), like choline, may increase levels of the brain neurotransmitter acetylcholine[7,8].

Related Topics

Aging

Diseases

Immunity

Stress

3. Liver Support Protocol
4. Cognitive Improvement Protocol

REFERENCES

1. Priest ND. Satellite symposium on Alzheimer's disease and dietary aluminium. *Proc Nutr. Soc.* 1993;52:231–240.

2. Crook T, Petrie W, Wells C, Massari DC. Effects of phosphatidylserine in Alzheimer's disease. *Psychopharmacol Bull.* 1992;28:61–66.

3. Gindin J, et al. The effect of plant phosphatidylserine on age-associated memory impairment and mood in the functioning elderly. Rehovot, Israel: Geriatric Institute for Education and Research, and Department of Geriatrics, Kaplan Hospital, 1995.

4. Fisman M, Mersky H, Helmes E. Double-blind trial of 2-dimethylaminoethanol in Alzheimer's disease. *Am J Psych.* 1981;138:970–972.

5. Pettegrew JW, Klunk WE, Panchalingam K, et al. Clinical and neurochemical effects of acetyl-L-carnitine in Alzheimer's disease. *Neurobio Aging.* 1995;16:1–4.

6. Salvioli G, Neri M. L-acetylcarnitine treatment of mental decline in the elderly. *Drugs Exp Clin Res.* 1994;20:169–176.

7. Meyer JS, Welch KMA, Deshmuckh VD, et al. Neurotransmitter precursor amino acids in the treatment of multi-infarct dementia and Alzheimer's disease. *J Am Ger Soc.* 1977;7:289–298.

8. Ferris SH, Sathananthan G, Gershon S, et al. Senile dementia. Treatment with Deanol. *J Am Ger Soc.* 1977;25:241–244.

AMENORRHEA–See Menstrual cycle disorders, amenorrhea

AMOEBA–See Parasitic disease, amoeba

AMYOTROPHIC LATERAL SCLEROSIS (ALS)–*Also known as Lou Gehrig's disease; disorders of unknown cause characterized by progressive neuromuscular degeneration.*

Amyotrophic lateral sclerosis (ALS)	INCIDENCE/RISK/SEVERITY		
	LOW	AVERAGE	HIGH
GROUP A	▓		
GROUP B	▓	▓	
GROUP AB	▓		
GROUP O	▓		
NON-SECRETOR	▓		

Symptoms

- Weakness in legs and arms
- Loss of manual dexterity
- Muscle cramps
- Difficulty swallowing
- Problems with speech
- Muscle spasms and twitching

About ALS

Amyotrophic lateral sclerosis (ALS)—a devastating neuromuscular disease that strikes adults in the prime of life—has puzzled physicians since it was first described in medical literature more than 100 years ago. The cause of this deadly disease, which is commonly referred to as Lou Gehrig's disease, is still a bit of a mystery. ALS is a progressive disease that attacks specialized nerve cells called motor neurons, which control the movement of voluntary muscles. ALS causes upper motor neurons, originating from the top of the brain, and lower motor neurons, originating from the lower part of the brain and the spinal cord, to gradually disintegrate, preventing them from delivering chemical signals and the essential nourishment that muscles depend on for normal function.

ALS weakens the body's voluntary muscles, also known as skeletal muscles. The eventual result is total paralysis. Upper motor neuron damage results in weakness, muscle stiffness (spasticity), and exaggerated reflexes. Lower motor neuron damage causes muscle wasting and twitching (fasciculations), in addition to weakness and diminished reflexes. When lower motor neurons in the bottom of the brain, the bulbar region, are affected, the muscles responsible for speech, chewing, and swallowing weaken. When the lower motor neurons in the spinal cord are involved, function is lost in the muscles of the limbs, neck, and trunk.

Some people first experience ALS as a weakness in their legs or arms that makes it difficult for them to walk or do tasks that require manual dexterity. This is referred to as *limb-onset* ALS. In others, the first symptoms may involve problems with speaking or swallowing, which is known as *bulbar-onset* ALS. Many also have muscle twitches, spasms, and cramps, as well as a loss of muscle tissue. Because ALS is progressive, most people with the disease will eventually experience all of these symptoms. Pain isn't associated with ALS during any stage of the illness.

Blood Group Links

ALS is seen in somewhat higher frequency in blood group B and is further proof of the group B tendency to contract unusual, slow-growing viral and neurological disorders. The group B association may explain why many Ashkenazi Jews, with higher rates of blood group B, are afflicted by this disease more than are other ethnic groups. Some researchers believe that ALS is caused by a virus, contracted in youth, that has a B-like appearance. The virus cannot be engaged and defeated by the group B antibodies because it can't produce anti-B antibodies. The virus grows slowly and without symptoms until 20 or more years after it has entered the system. Blood group AB is also at risk for these B-like diseases. Blood groups O and A appear to be relatively immune by virtue of their anti-B antibodies.

Therapies, Amyotrophic Lateral Sclerosis (ALS)

ALL BLOOD GROUPS

There is some evidence that branch chain amino acid therapy (using the amino acids leucine, isoleucine, and valine) may help slow the rate of neuromuscular degeneration. In practice I have seen it work in some patients, though not all. It is inexpensive (these amino acid formulas are often used by body builders) and safe, so it is probably worth a trial.

1. Branch chain amino acid supplement: 1,000 mg each of leucine, isoleucine, and valine, three times daily
2. Methylcobalamin: 400 mcg daily

BLOOD GROUP A:

1. Immune-Enhancing Protocol

2. Nerve Health Protocol

BLOOD GROUP B:

1. Nerve Health Protocol

2. Antiviral Protocol

3. Immune-Enhancing Protocol

BLOOD GROUP AB:

1. Immune-Enhancing Protocol

2. Nerve Health Protocol

BLOOD GROUP O:

1. Immune-Enhancing Protocol

2. Nerve Health Protocol

Related Topics

Arthritis, rheumatoid

Autoimmune disease, general

ANEMIA, IRON DEFICIENCY–*Failure to properly absorb iron.*

Anemia, iron deficiency	INCIDENCE/RISK/SEVERITY		
	LOW	AVERAGE	HIGH
GROUP A			
GROUP B			
GROUP AB			
GROUP O			

Symptoms

Severe anemia can produce the following symptoms:

- Weakness
- Vertigo
- Headache
- Tinnitus
- Spots before the eyes
- Drowsiness
- Irritability

Less frequent symptoms include amenorrhea, loss of libido, gastrointestinal complaints, jaundice, shock, heart failure, and heart attack.

About Iron Deficiency Anemia

Iron deficiency is the most common cause of anemia. It can be caused by a hemorrhage or by an inability to absorb iron properly. In women, pregnancy and heavy menstrual bleeding (MENORRHAGIA) are often the primary cause. In men, slow gastrointestinal absorption of iron is the primary cause.

Blood Group Links

People in blood group A, especially those who are on vegetarian diets, are at increased risk for iron deficiency. The condition is exacerbated by absorption problems due to naturally low levels of hydrochloric acid, which is needed for digestion. Group AB also has low levels of hydrochloric acid.

Therapies, Anemia

ALL BLOOD GROUPS:

Iron citrate: 60 mg/day, best taken around 11:00 A.M.

BLOOD GROUP A:

1. Blood-Building Protocol
2. Liver Support Protocol
3. Intestinal Health Protocol

BLOOD GROUP B:

1. Blood-Building Protocol
2. Liver Support Protocol
3. Intestinal Health Protocol

Specifics:

Aqueous liver extract or desiccated liver tablets: 500 mg with meals, twice daily

BLOOD GROUP AB:

1. Blood-Building Protocol
2. Liver Support Protocol
3. Intestinal Health Protocol

BLOOD GROUP O:

1. Blood-Building Protocol
2. Stomach Health Protocol
3. Intestinal Health Protocol

Specifics:

Fat-soluble liquid chlorophyll supplement: 500 mg twice daily

Related Topics

Anemia, pernicious

Blood cells

Blood clotting disorders

Digestion

ANEMIA, PERNICIOUS–*Vitamin B_{12} deficiency.*

Anemia, pernicious	INCIDENCE/RISK/SEVERITY		
	LOW	AVERAGE	HIGH
GROUP A			▓
GROUP B	▓		
GROUP AB	▓	▓	
GROUP O	▓		

Symptoms

Severe anemia can produce the following symptoms:

- Weakness
- Vertigo
- Headache
- Tinnitus
- Spots before the eyes
- Drowsiness
- Irritability

Less frequent symptoms include amenorrhea, loss of libido, gastrointestinal complaints, jaundice, shock, heart failure, and heart attack.

About Pernicious Anemia

The vitamin B_{12} deficiency that causes pernicious anemia is not related to inadequate dietary consumption. To assimilate vitamin B_{12}, the body requires high levels of stomach acid and the presence of intrinsic factor, a chemical produced by the lining of the stomach that is responsible for the assimilation of the vitamin. Absorption of vitamin B_{12} occurs in the terminal ileum and requires the presence of gastric hydrochloric acid and intrinsic factor. B_{12} is stored in the liver in sufficient quantities to sustain an individual for 3 to 5 years on a B_{12}-deficient diet; typically, pernicious anemia develops insidiously as the liver stores are diminished.

Blood Group Links

A very old association exists between blood group A and pernicious anemia[1-3] although the condition has nothing to do with the vegetarian Type A diet. Pernicious anemia is the result of vitamin B_{12} deficiency secondary to the lack of production of intrinsic factor, so group A has the most difficulty absorbing B_{12} from foods. Group AB also has a tendency toward pernicious anemia, although perhaps not as great as A.

Blood groups O and B tend not to suffer from pernicious anemia; they have high acid production in their stomachs, and sufficient levels of intrinsic factor.

Therapies, Pernicious Anemia

ALL BLOOD GROUPS:

1. Methylcobalamin (active vitamin B_{12}): 400 mcg, A.M. and P.M.

2. Folic acid: 400 mcg, twice daily

BLOOD GROUP A:

1. Blood-Building Protocol

2. Stomach Health Protocol

3. Liver Support Protocol

Specifics:

Vitamin B_{12} administration by injection is most effective.

BLOOD GROUP B:

1. Blood-Building Protocol

2. Stomach Health Protocol

3. Liver Support Protocol

BLOOD GROUP AB:

1. Blood-Building Protocol

2. Stomach Health Protocol

3. Liver Support Protocol

BLOOD GROUP O:

1. Blood-Building Protocol

2. Stomach Health Protocol

3. Liver Health Protocol

Related Topics

Anemia, iron deficiency

Blood cells

Blood clotting disorders

Digestion

REFERENCES

1. Koster KH, Sindrup E, Secle V. *Lancet* 1952.

2. Buckwalter JA, Wohlwend EB, Coler DC. *JAMA* 1956; 1210.

3. "An association between blood group A and pernicious anemia. Collective Series from a number of centers." *Brit Med J.* 1956;723.

ANENCEPHALY–*See Birth defects*

ANEURYSM, ABDOMINAL AORTIC–*A distension of an artery caused by a weakness in the arterial wall.*

Aneurysm, abdominal aortic	INCIDENCE/RISK/SEVERITY		
	LOW	AVERAGE	HIGH
GROUP A			
GROUP B			
GROUP AB			
GROUP O			
MN SUBTYPE			

Symptoms

- Asymptomatic unless severe

- Abdominal pain, radiating to the back or groin

About Abdominal Aortic Aneurysms

An abdominal aortic aneurysm is a permanent localized dilation of the abdominal aorta involving at least a 50% increase in diameter compared to the expected diameter of the artery. The majority of patients with abdominal aortic aneurysms are asymptomatic until the condition is severe. Many times there is a mass located in the abdomen, causing abdominal pain that may radiate to the back or groin. An aneurysm may present in some patients with a rupture, in others with EMBOLISM (obstruction) or THROMBOSIS (clotting). Aortic aneurysms can develop anywhere along the length of the aorta, but 75% are located in the abdominal aorta. Thoracic aortic aneurysms, including those that extend from the descending thoracic aorta into the upper abdomen, account for 25% of aortic aneurysms.

General Risk Factors and Causes

HYPERTENSION and cigarette smoking contribute to the degeneration of the aortic vessels. Trauma, arteritis, and mycotic aneurysms are less frequent causes.

Blood Group Links

Blood groups A and AB have a higher risk for vascular diseases and hypertension, as well as BLOOD CLOTS from excessive clotting factors.

Therapies, Abdominal Aortic Aneurysms

BLOOD GROUP A:

1. Cardiovascular Protocol

2. Antistress Protocol

3. Immune-Enhancing Protocol

Specifics:

Gingko biloba or low-dose aspirin: 1 daily (do not take both)

BLOOD GROUP B:

1. Cardiovascular Protocol

2. Blood-Building Protocol

3. Antistress Protocol

BLOOD GROUP AB:

1. Cardiovascular Protocol

2. Antistress Protocol

Specifics:

Gingko biloba or low-dose aspirin: 1 daily (do not take both)

BLOOD GROUP O:

1. Cardiovascular Protocol

2. Blood-Building Protocol

3. Antistress Protocol

Related Topics

Aneurysm, cerebral

Blood clotting disorders

Cardiovascular disease

Stress

Stroke

ANEURYSM, CEREBRAL–*A cerebrovascular disorder caused by a weakening in the wall of the cerebral artery.*

Aneurysm, cerebral	INCIDENCE/RISK/SEVERITY		
	LOW	AVERAGE	HIGH
GROUP A	▒		
GROUP B	▒	▒	
GROUP AB	▒		
GROUP O	▒	▒	
MN SUBTYPE	▒	▒	

Symptoms

- Sudden and unusually severe headache
- Nausea
- Vision impairment
- Vomiting
- Loss of consciousness

About Cerebral Aneurysm

Cerebral aneurysm is a common cerebrovascular disorder caused by a weakness in the wall of a cerebral artery or vein. The disorder may result from congenital defects or from preexisting conditions such as hypertensive vascular disease and athero-

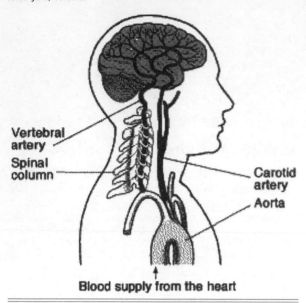

Vertebral artery

Spinal column

Carotid artery

Aorta

Blood supply from the heart

sclerosis (build-up of fatty deposits in the arteries), or from head trauma. Cerebral aneurysms occur more commonly in adults than in children, and are slightly more common in women than in men; however, they may occur at any age.

Before an aneurysm ruptures, the individual may experience such symptoms as a sudden and unusually severe headache, nausea, vision impairment, vomiting, and loss of consciousness; or the individual may be asymptomatic, experiencing no symptoms at all. Rupture of a cerebral aneurysm is dangerous and usually results in bleeding in the brain or in the area surrounding the brain, leading to an intracranial hematoma (a mass of blood—usually clotted—within the skull). Re-bleeding, hydrocephalus (the excessive accumulation of cerebrospinal fluid), vasospasm (spasm of the blood vessels), or multiple aneurysms may also occur.

Blood Group Links

Blood group O and to a lesser extent blood group B have a greater risk of cerebral aneurysm. This risk appears to be related to a lack of sufficient BLOOD CLOTTING factors. In a study of 150 patients with arteriovenous aneurysm, there was a significant absence of aneurysm sufferers who were blood group A, versus an excess in groups O and B. This association was highly significant for men, but was even more significant for women[1].

In another study, among 482 strokes that were the result of cranial bleeding, a significantly higher number of patients were blood groups O and B, as opposed to those who were blood groups A and AB[2].

An older study from 1967 showed a higher rate of groups B and O among 150 Swedish patients who had suffered cerebral aneurysms (bleeding into the cranial cavity). This again points to the lower clotting abilities of groups O and B blood over A and AB[3].

Therapies, Cerebral Aneurysm

ALL BLOOD GROUPS:

If you feel that you are at risk for cerebrovascular accidents, you may want to increase your intake of blue/red/purple pigmented fruits such as elderberries, cherries, and blueberries, which contain antioxidants that can help stabilize the integrity of the vascular system.

BLOOD GROUP A:

1. Cardiovascular Protocol

2. Antistress Protocol

3. Immune-Enhancing Protocol

Specifics:

Gingko biloba or low-dose aspirin: 1 daily (do not take both)

BLOOD GROUP B:

1. Cardiovascular Protocol

2. Antistress Protocol

BLOOD GROUP AB:

1. Cardiovascular Protocol

2. Antistress Protocol

3. Immune-Enhancing Protocol

Specifics:

Gingko biloba or low-dose aspirin: 1 daily (do not take both)

BLOOD GROUP O:

1. Cardiovascular Protocol

2. Antistress Protocol

3. Immune-Enhancing Protocol

Related Topics

Aneurysm, abdominal aortic

Blood clotting disorders

Cardiovascular disease

Stress

Stroke

REFERENCES

1. Ionescu DA, Ghitescu M, Marcu I, Xenakis A. Erythrocyte rheology in acute cerebral thrombosis. Effects of ABO blood groups. *Blut.* 1979;39:351–357.

2. Ionescu DA, Marcu I, Bicescu E. Cerebral thrombosis, cerebral haemorrhage, and ABO blood-groups. *Lancet.* 1976; 1:278–280.

3. Strong RR. Age, sex and ABO blood group distribution of 150 patients with cerebral arteriovenous aneurysms. *J Med Genet.* 1967;29–30.

ANGINA PECTORIS–*Chest pain.*

Angina pectoris	INCIDENCE/RISK/SEVERITY		
	LOW	AVERAGE	HIGH
GROUP A			
GROUP B			
GROUP AB			
GROUP O			
NON-SECRETOR			

Symptoms

- Squeezing pressure, heaviness, or mild ache in the chest (usually behind the breast bone)

- Aching in a tooth, with or without squeezing pressure or heaviness in the chest

- Aching in the neck muscles or jaw

- Aching along one or both arms

- Aching into the back

- A feeling of gas in the upper abdomen and lower chest

- A feeling of choking or shortness of breath
- Paleness and sweating

About Angina Pectoris

Angina pectoris is a recurring pain or discomfort in the chest that occurs when some part of the heart does not receive enough blood. It is a common symptom of coronary heart disease, which occurs when vessels that carry blood to the heart become narrowed and blocked due to ATHEROSCLEROSIS.

An episode of angina is not a HEART ATTACK. Angina pain means that some of the heart muscle is not getting enough blood temporarily—for example, during exercise, when the heart has to work harder. The pain does not mean that the heart muscle is suffering irreversible, permanent damage. Episodes of angina seldom cause permanent damage to heart muscle, but serve as a warning that there are serious problems with the coronary artery circulation.

Less common variations of angina include the following: nocturnal angina (occurs at night during sleep); angina decubitus (occurs at rest and without any clear stimulation; similar to nocturnal angina); unstable angina (also known as preinfarction angina; an intermediate syndrome, indicating acute coronary insufficiency; attacks require less stimulation and are longer and harsher); and variant angina (Prinzmetal's angina; pain while resting, electrocardiogram tracing shows an ST elevation pattern [normal angina typically shows ST depression]).

Blood Group Links

There is a clear-cut association with blood groups A and AB being at increased risk for heart disease. This has been reported continuously in the scientific literature over the last 50 years. It is known that blood group A individuals have higher rates of heart attack across all age groups, genders, and ethnic and national groups.

Therapies, Angina Pectoris

NOTE: Angina is a warning of a potential medical emergency. See your physician.

BLOOD GROUP A:

1. Cardiovascular Protocol
2. Metabolic Enhancement Protocol
3. Antistress Protocol

BLOOD GROUP B:

1. Cardiovascular Protocol
2. Metabolic Enhancement Protocol
3. AntiStress Protocol

BLOOD GROUP AB:

1. Cardiovascular Protocol
2. Antistress Protocol

BLOOD GROUP O:

1. Cardiovascular Protocol
2. Metabolic Enhancement Protocol
3. Antistress Protocol

Related Topics

Atherosclerosis

Cardiovascular disease

Diabetes mellitus, type II

Hypertension

Obesity

Syndrome X

ANKYLOSING SPONDYLITIS–*A systemic rheumatic disorder characterized by inflammation of the axial skeleton and large peripheral joints.*

Ankylosing Spondylitis	INCIDENCE/RISK/SEVERITY		
	LOW	AVERAGE	HIGH
GROUP A	█		
GROUP B	█		
GROUP AB	█		
GROUP O	█		
MN SUBTYPE	█	█	
NON-SECRETOR	█		

Symptoms

The onset of ankylosing spondylitis (AS) is gradual and insidious. Initial symptoms include the following:

- Low back pain, especially in sacroiliac and lumbar areas; may appear to be sciatic pain
- Stiffness on awakening

- Nocturnal pain and stiffness causing insomnia

As the disease advances, symptoms worsen and include the following:

- Spread of pain up the spine, often into the mid-back, neck, and sometimes the hips and shoulders
  - Fatigue
  - Weight loss and anorexia
  - Slight anemia
- Pain on breathing or decreased ability in drawing in deep breath
- Limited mobility of the spine, bent-over stance, increased back curvature, waddling gait

About Ankylosing Spondylitis

AS is a chronic and generally progressive inflammatory arthritic disease that affects the spinal joints and adjacent connective tissue. It's also known as Marie-Strümpell disease.

AS is three times more frequent in men than in women, and begins most often between the ages of 20 and 40. The condition appears to have a genetic component; AS is 10 to 20 times more common in first-degree relatives of AS patients than in the general population. AS sufferers show an increased prevalence of a genetic factor known as HLA-B27.

There are many different rheumatic symptoms of gastrointestinal (GI) disorders, and a whole range of GI symptoms that occur in rheumatologic disorders. Spondyloarthropathies (SpA) are closely related to the GI tract. Bacterial DNA has been detected in some joints that show rheumatic symptoms.

Blood Group Links

ABO non-secretors have a higher incidence of AS. The association between non-secretion and AS strengthens the hypothesis that the root cause may be an infection[1].

Certain bacteria are known to precipitate reactive ARTHRITIS, and may be connected in the pathogenesis of AS as well. Susceptibility to many infectious agents is associated with the ABO blood group or secretor state, or both. In one study, the distribution of the ABO blood group or secretor status, or both, was determined in 87 patients with AS, and 32 with other forms of spondyloarthropathy. The prevalence of non-secretors was significant in the total patient group (47%) and in the subgroup with AS (49%) compared with the unaffected control participants in the study (27%)[2].

Therapies, Ankylosing Spondylitis

ALL BLOOD GROUPS:

1. Treatment plans must address the prevention, delay, or correction of the deformity, as well as the patient's psychosocial and rehabilitation needs. For proper posture and joint motion, daily exercise and other supportive measures (e.g., postural training and thera-peutic exercise) are vital to strengthen the muscle groups that oppose the direction of potential deformities (i.e., strengthen the extensor rather than flexor muscle groups). Reading while lying prone, and thus extending the neck, may help keep the back flexible.

2. Stretching exercises and careful adherence to correct posture are absolutely necessary to maintain as much mobility as possible over time.

3. Surgery is sometimes used to replace a badly affected joint, or to straighten the spine.

BLOOD GROUP A:

1. Arthritis Protocol

2. Antibacterial Protocol

3. Intestinal Health Protocol

4. [If antibiotic therapy is required] Antibiotic Support Protocol

5. [If surgery is required] Surgery Recovery Protocol

BLOOD GROUP B:

1. Arthritis Protocol

2. Anti-Inflammation Protocol

3. Antibacterial Protocol

4. [If antibiotic therapy is required] Antibiotic Support Protocol

5. [If surgery is required] Surgery Recovery Protocol

BLOOD GROUP AB:

1. Arthritis Protocol

2. Antibacterial Protocol

3. Immune-Enhancing Protocol

4. [If antibiotic therapy is required] Antibiotic Support Protocol

5. [If surgery is required] Surgery Recovery Protocol

BLOOD GROUP O:

1. Arthritis Protocol

2. Antibacterial Protocol

3. Anti-Inflammation Protocol

4. [If antibiotic therapy is required] Antibiotic Support Protocol

5. [If surgery is required] Surgery Recovery Protocol

Related Topics

Arthritis, rheumatoid

Autoimmune disease (general)

REFERENCES

1. Shinebaum R. ABO blood group and secretor status in the spondyloarthropathies. *FEMS Microbiol Immunol.* 1989;1: 389–395.

2. Shinebaum R, Blackwell CC, Forster PJ, Hurst NP, Weir DM, Nuki G. Non-secretion of ABO blood group antigens as a host susceptibility factor in the spondyloarthropathies. *Br Med J (Clin Res Ed).* 1987;294:208–210.

ANXIETY DISORDERS–*Conditions involving chronic, debilitating fear; nervousness; and hypervigilance.*

Anxiety disorders	INCIDENCE/RISK/SEVERITY		
	LOW	AVERAGE	HIGH
GROUP A			
GROUP B			
GROUP AB			
GROUP O			

Symptoms

Variable

About Anxiety Disorders

"Anxiety disorder" is a general term referring to a number of conditions:

Panic disorder: Episodic attacks of extreme fear, accompanied by shortness of breath, heart palpitations, hyperventilation, dizziness, and heavy sweating.

Phobia: An irrational fear that prevents normal activities and impedes quality of life. Examples of common phobias are agoraphobia (fear of open spaces—going out of the home) and social phobia (fear of social interaction).

Obsessive-compulsive disorder (OCD): Recurrent or persistent mental images, thoughts, and ideas that provoke repetitive, rigid, self-prescribed behaviors.

Post traumatic stress disorder (PTSD): An extreme and usually chronic emotional reaction to a traumatic event that severely impairs one's life; it is classified as an anxiety disorder because of the similarity of symptoms.

Generalized anxiety disorder (GAD): A clearly identified psychiatric illness, often beginning in childhood, involving excessive, uncontrolled worry.

There is a strong association between anxiety disorders and depression. In one report, over half of patients with depression met the criteria for anxiety disorders. The combination of DEPRESSION and anxiety is a major risk factor for both substance abuse and suicide.

Between 20% and 75% of people with panic attacks also experience major depression. More than two-thirds of OCD patients also suffer from depression.

Generalized anxiety disorder and social phobia are more likely to precede depression, whereas panic disorder and agoraphobia are more likely to follow depression. People with PTSD are four to seven times more likely to be depressed than are people without PTSD.

According to one interesting year 2000 study of teenagers, anxiety disorders were associated with later BIPOLAR DISORDERS (MANIC DEPRESSION) in adulthood; conversely, manic behavior in adoles-

cence appeared to increase the risk for adult anxiety disorders.

Anxiety can be mediated by abnormalities of the neurotransmitter system. Risk factors include social and financial problems, medical illness, family history, and lack of social support.

Blood Group Links

A number of studies have documented that blood group A is more prone to anxiety disorders than the other blood groups. This is most likely related to higher levels of cortisol, and lower levels of melatonin[1].

In one study, determination of ABO blood types was carried out in 72 (35 female and 37 male) patients with obsessive-compulsive neurosis, 73 (35 female and 38 male) patients with phobic neurosis, 75 (54 female and 21 male) patients with hysteria, and a random sample of 600 individuals (268 female and 332 male) drawn from the general population. The results provided evidence of a positive association between obsessive-compulsive neurosis and blood group A, and a corresponding negative association with blood group O. There was also a positive association between hysteria and blood group A and a corresponding negative association with blood group O. Moreover, gender did not appear to modify the ABO blood group distribution. The researchers reported that these findings were supportive of the view that hereditary factors in the neurotic individual may influence the clinical form of neurosis[2].

Therapies, Anxiety Disorders

BLOOD GROUP A:

1. Antistress Protocol

2. Cognitive Improvement Protocol

BLOOD GROUP B:

1. Antistress Protocol

2. Cognitive Improvement Protocol

BLOOD GROUP AB:

1. Antistress Protocol

2. Cognitive Improvement Protocol

BLOOD GROUP O:

1. Antistress Protocol

2. Cognitive Improvement Protocol

Related Topics

Depression, bipolar

Depression, unipolar

Obsessive-compulsive disorder

Stress

REFERENCES

1. Catapano F, Monteleone P, Fuschino A, Maj M, Kemali D. Melatonin and cortisol secretion in patients with primary obsessive-compulsive disorder. *Psychiatry Res.* 1992;44:217–225.

2. Rinieris P, Rabavilas A, Lykouras E, Stefanis C. Neuroses and ABO blood types. *Neuropsychobiology.* 1983;9:16–18.

ARTERIOSCLEROSIS–*See Atherosclerosis; Coronary artery disease*

ARTHRITIS, OSTEO–*A condition involving inflammation or deterioration of the joints.*

Osteoarthritis	INCIDENCE/RISK/SEVERITY		
	LOW	AVERAGE	HIGH
GROUP A	▓	▓	
GROUP B	▓		
GROUP AB	▓	▓	
GROUP O	▓		

Symptoms

- Painful movement
- Joint inflammation
- Joint stiffness

About Osteoarthritis

Osteoarthritis, a degenerative type of arthritis, develops when the linings of the joints wear down. Although it's associated with aging and injury (it used to be called "wear-and-tear arthritis"), its true cause remains unknown.

Osteoarthritis first appears asymptomatically at age 20. By age 40, almost all people have some pathologic changes in their weight-bearing joints.

Unlike some types of arthritis such as rheumatoid arthritis, osteoarthritis is not systemic; it does not spread through the entire body. Instead,

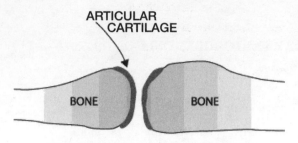

ARTICULAR CARTILAGE

BONE   BONE

Osteoarthritis occurs when articular cartilage,
the firm rubbery protein material covering the end
of the bone, breaks down. Articular cartilage is like a cushion
between bones. Without it, bones will grind together.

it concentrates in one or several joints where deterioration occurs. Osteoarthritis affects joints differently, depending on their location in the body. It is commonly found in joints of the fingers, feet, knees, hips, and spine.

General Risk Factors and Causes

Osteoarthritis occurs in almost all vertebrates, including animals supported in the water. In bats and sloths, two mammals that customarily hang upside down, osteoarthritic changes are not seen. Generally, the cause is unknown, but prolonged overuse is thought to aid in the development of osteoarthritis. It is interesting that operators of pneumatic hammer drills and long-distance running champions have no corresponding increase in osteoarthritis compared with age- and gender-matched control individuals.

X-ray studies in the United States and Great Britain reveal that almost 50% of the adult population has osteoarthritis. Men and women are equally affected, but males generally get it earlier.

Blood Group Links

Compared to a control group of blood donors from the same geographical area, there was a significant lack of blood group O among the arthritic patients. It is suggested that there may be a heritable component in the susceptibility to develop osteoarthritis in an otherwise normal hip joint[1].

In another study, a comparative analysis of the distribution of the blood groups of the ABO system was conducted with 1,731 patients with syndromes of spinal osteochondrosis. It was demonstrated that there were significantly fewer patients with spinal osteochondrosis (bone and cartilage inflammation) who were blood group O, and a greater number of blood group A. The revealed regularities may be considered as evidence of the influence of the genotype on the development of spinal osteochondrosis, as well as one of the mechanisms determining the immune response in this disease[2].

CLINICAL NOTE: BLOOD GROUPS A AND AB

Blood groups A and AB, who have a higher risk of BLOOD CLOTS, should note that VENOUS THROMBOEMBOLISM (clots in the leg veins) is a common complication of hip replacement surgery. In 79 patients having hip or knee surgery, the 41 patients who were not Type O had significantly elevated levels of clotting proteins than did the type O patients. The authors of the study suggested that ABO blood group be considered a prime risk factor for vein clots in patients receiving hip or knee replacement surgery[3].

Therapies, Osteoarthritis

ALL BLOOD GROUPS:

Ginger shows moderate abilities for inhibiting the COX2 enzyme, which is the target of many newer arthritis medications.

1. Ginger extract: 500 mg twice daily, away from food; or 1 tsp fresh ginger juice taken two to three times daily

2. Glucosamine/chondroitin sulfate combination: 650 mg twice daily

3. Avoid solanine (found in nightshade plants)

BLOOD GROUP A:

1. Arthritis Protocol

2. Anti-Inflammation Protocol

3. Intestinal Health Protocol

4. [If surgery is required] Surgery Recovery Protocol

BLOOD GROUP B:

1. Arthritis Protocol

2. Anti-Inflammation Protocol

3. Intestinal Health Protocol

4. [If surgery is required] Surgery Recovery Protocol

BLOOD GROUP AB:

1. Arthritis Protocol

2. Anti-Inflammation Protocol

3. Intestinal Health Protocol

4. [If surgery is required] Surgery Recovery Protocol

BLOOD GROUP O:

1. Arthritis Protocol

2. Anti-Inflammation Protocol

3. Intestinal Health Protocol

4. [If surgery is required] Surgery Recovery Protocol

Related Topics

Arthritis, rheumatoid

Autoimmune disease (general)

Inflammation

REFERENCES

1. Lourie JA. Is there an association between ABO blood groups and primary osteoarthrosis of the hip? *Ann Hum Biol.* 1983;10:381–383.

2. Ritsner MS, Shmidt IR, Shekhner IA, Gurkov IV, Stankov IA. Analysis of the distribution of ABO system blood groups among patients with spinal osteochondrosis syndromes. *Zh Nevropatol Psikhiatr.* 1979;79:409–413.

3. Iturbe T, Cornudella R, De Miguel R, Varo MJ, Gutierrez M. ABO blood group and improvement of preoperative fragment prothrombin 1,2 in orthopaedic surgery. *Lancet.* 1999; 353:2158.

ARTHRITIS, RHEUMATOID–*A painful, debilitating inflammatory condition involving the breakdown and destruction of multiple joints.*

Rheumatoid arthritis	INCIDENCE/RISK/SEVERITY		
	LOW	AVERAGE	HIGH
GROUP A	▨		
GROUP B	▨		
GROUP AB	▨		
GROUP O		▨	
NON-SECRETOR	▨		

Symptoms

- Swelling and stiffness in the joints
- Extreme debilitation
- Pain
- Fever
- Swelling
- A purple hue in involved joints

About Rheumatoid Arthritis

Rheumatoid arthritis is a chronic autoimmune condition that can afflict adults of any age. The joints typically involved are in the hands, feet, wrists, ankles, and knees—although its devastating effects can tax the entire body. These include swelling and stiffness in the joints, which may advance to extreme debilitation.

Rheumatoid arthritis is unlikely to be due to a single cause, but rather a combination of genetic and environmental factors that trigger an abnormal immune response—where the body attacks its own tissues.

General Risk Factors and Causes

Generally, rheumatoid arthritis is considered an autoimmune condition. Possible contributing factors are the following:

1. Food sensitivities
2. Heavy metal toxicity
3. High fat diet
4. Hypothyroidism
5. Free radical damage

Blood Group Links

The link between blood group O and rheumatoid arthritis has been considered in a variety of mechanisms. Studies examining the antibodies made against the joint tissue, typically found in rheumatoid arthritis, have shown that they have key differences from normal antibodies. Normal antibodies have the sugar galactose as the carbohydrate-side chain. Antibodies in rheumatoid arthritis appear to be somewhat defective. Instead of galactose, the carbohydrate found on the side-chain is *N*-acetyl glucosamine, the sugar for which the wheat germ lectin is highly specific. The adoption of a wheat-free diet appears to have some use in mollifying the effect of the antibody[1].

Thus, glucosamine and chondroitin, the two sugars most commonly used in alternative medicine to treat arthritis (the so called "arthritis cure"), may have lectin-blocking actions as the basis for their effectiveness. It is worth noting again that glucosamine binds wheat germ lectin very effectively, while chondroitin replicates the blood type A antigen in very long linkages (polymerized). In either case, it is very likely that both function as sacrificial molecules, reacting with lectins and preventing these same lectins from reacting with the inflamed tissue. In fact, the basis of the "arthritis cure" may well be that it chemically mimics the effect of a low-lectin diet. The aberrant antibody in rheumatoid arthritis, fintergalactose-free immunoglobulin, has also been shown to have a high degree of reactivity with the lectin found in the common lentil bean (*Lens culinaris*). It has been found that a very good experimental model of human rheumatoid arthritis can be produced in laboratory rabbits by injecting their joints with this lentil lectin[2].

The link between rheumatoid arthritis and blood group O may also be related to inflammation of the gut. It is a widespread clinical observation that inflammation of the gut is frequently associated with inflammation of the joints and vice versa. In one study, evidence was provided that the interaction of dietary lectins with enterocytes and lymphocytes (immune mediators) may facilitate the translocation of both dietary and gut-derived pathogenic antigens to peripheral tissues, which in turn causes persistent peripheral antigenic stimulation. In genetically susceptible individuals, it was spec-

ulated that this antigenic stimulation might ultimately result in the expression of overt rheumatoid arthritis via molecular mimicry, a process whereby foreign peptides, similar in structure to endogenous peptides, may cause antibodies or T-lymphocytes to cross-react with both foreign and endogenous peptides, thereby breaking immunological tolerance. It was proposed that by eliminating dietary elements—particularly lectins, which adversely influence both enterocyte and lymphocyte structure and function—the peripheral antigenic stimulus (both pathogenic and dietary) would be reduced, and thereby result in a diminution of disease symptoms in certain patients with rheumatoid arthritis[3,4].

Clinical and genetic results were analyzed for 47 patients with rheumatoid arthritis who had had upper gastrointestinal (GI) endoscopy examinations. Fifty-three percent of patients with rheumatoid arthritis had PEPTIC ULCERS and/or peptic erosions. Sixty percent of patients with ulcers and/or erosions had a history of peptic ulcer disease.

Although a greater number of patients with ulcers and/or erosions were taking regular aspirin or indomethacin, a comparable number of patients with abnormal and normal endoscopies were using nonsteroidal anti-inflammatory drugs, such as ibuprofen. Nineteen of the 25 patients (76%) with ulcers and/or erosions were blood group O. Patients with abnormal and normal endoscopy results had similar frequencies of GI complaints and fecal blood loss. GI symptoms and occult fecal blood loss, therefore, are not prominent features of upper GI disease in rheumatoid arthritis. It was determined that ABO blood group screening might be helpful in determining which patients with rheumatoid arthritis are at risk for developing peptic ulcers and/or erosions[5].

Researchers determined that the relationship among active H. PYLORI infection, blood group O, and peptic ulcer might also be helpful in identifying a subpopulation of patients taking NSAIDs who are at risk of developing peptic ulcers[6].

Therapies, Rheumatoid Arthritis

BLOOD GROUP A:

1. Arthritis Protocol

2. Chronic Illness Recovery Protocol

3. Intestinal Health Protocol

4. [If surgery is required] Surgery Recovery Protocol

BLOOD GROUP B:

1. Arthritis Protocol

2. Chronic Illness Recovery Protocol

3. Intestinal Health Protocol

4. [If surgery is required] Surgery Recovery Protocol

BLOOD GROUP AB:

1. Arthritis Protocol

2. Immune-Enhancing Protocol

3. Intestinal Health Protocol

4. [If surgery is required] Surgery Recovery Protocol

BLOOD GROUP O:

1. Arthritis Protocol

2. Chronic Illness Recovery Protocol

3. Anti-Inflammation Protocol

Specifics:

Ginger shows moderate abilities for inhibiting the COX2 enzyme, which is the target of many newer arthritis medications.

Ginger extract: 500 mg twice daily, away from food; or 1 tsp fresh ginger juice taken two to three times daily

Related Topics

Arthritis, osteo

Autoimmune disease (general)

Inflammation

REFERENCES

1. Tertti R, Jarvinen H, Lahesmaa R, Yli-Kerttula U, Toivanen A. ABO and Lewis blood groups in reactive arthritis. *Rheumatol Int.* 1992;12:103–105.

2. Hoss VK, Raabe G, Muller P [Lectin arthritis: a new arthritis model]. *Allerg Immunol (Leipz).* 1976;22:311–316.

3. Braun J, Sieper J. Rheumatologic manifestations of gastrointestinal disorders. *Curr Opin Rheumatol.* 1999;11:68–74.

4. Cordain L, Toohey L, Smith MJ, Hickey MS. Modulation of immune function by dietary lectins in rheumatoid arthritis. *Br J Nutr.* 2000;83:207–217.

5. Semble EL, Turner RA, Wu WC. Clinical and genetic characteristics of upper gastrointestinal disease in rheumatoid arthritis. *J Rheumatol.* 14:692–699.

6. Henriksson K, Uribe A, Sandstedt B, Nord C. Helicobacter pylori infection, ABO blood group, and effect of misoprostol on gastroduodenal mucosa in NSAID-treated patients with rheumatoid arthritis. *Dig Dis Sci.* 1993;38:1688–1696.

ASTHMA–*Closing of the airway in response to an intrinsic or extrinsic stimulus.*

Asthma	INCIDENCE/RISK/SEVERITY		
	LOW	AVERAGE	HIGH
GROUP A	█		
GROUP B	█		█
GROUP AB	█		
GROUP O	█	█	
MN SUBTYPE	█	█	
NON-SECRETOR	█	█	

Symptoms

- Coughing

- Wheezing

- Extreme difficulty in breathing

- A tightening sensation over the anterior neck or upper chest

About Asthma

Asthma is most common in children under 10 years old, and is twice as common in males. It affects about 3% of the general population. Factors involved with asthmatic reactions include a variety of stimuli: exercise; emotional upset; food sensitivities; inhalation of cold air or irritating substances (smoke, gas, chemical and paint fumes); suppression of previously more minor diseases such as ECZEMA or OTITIS MEDIA with drug therapy; and reactions to specific allergens, such as pollens (see ALLERGIES).

There are two kinds of asthma:

Extrinsic asthma: Also called atopic asthma, this is considered to be IgE-mediated. That is, it is caused by an antigen-antibody reaction. Attacks are mostly initiated by exposure to allergens: dust, molds, pollens, animal dander, and foods.

Intrinsic asthma: This form does not seem related to an antigen-antibody complex. Rather, the bronchial reaction is due to other factors, such as cold air, exercise, infection, emotional upset, and irritating inhalants.

Most patients have a mixture of the two kinds, although it is thought that extrinsic asthma is more common in infants and children. An unrecognized food allergy is a contributing factor for at least 75% of childhood asthmatics, and about 40% of adult asthmatics[1].

The signs and symptoms of asthma vary widely. Some asthmatics have symptoms all the time, whereas others have asymptomatic periods followed by severe episodes. Mild symptoms may include slight coughing followed by minor wheezing. Sometimes symptoms start with some coughing and progress into severe coughing, often accompanied by extreme difficulty in breathing. In children, a tightening sensation over the anterior neck or upper chest is an early sign of an impending attack. Often a certain stressor—such as exercise, breathing cold air, or some noxious agent—may initiate the onset of an attack. Over a long period of time, asthma can wear out the body's adrenal and immune functions, and cause severe FATIGUE and susceptibility to infection.

Blood Group Links

Blood group B is associated with greater severity of chronic inflammatory diseases of the lungs. Asthma from chronic lung inflammation is also more common in group B. In a study population of Soviet Georgians, 293 patients who had respiratory allergies, 83 patients who had bronchial asthma, and 215 healthy individuals were examined to determine the relationship between respiratory diseases and ABO blood group, Rh status, MN status, and secretor status. Researchers found that markers for bronchial asthma and pollinosis showed that the risk for the development of severe bronchial asthma was higher in blood group B patients, and mild-to-moderate in blood group O patients. The MN blood group was also associated with an increased incidence of bronchial asthma[1].

In a study of 228 coal miners, researchers looked for a connection between ABO blood group and secretor status and lung function, wheezing, and asthma, considering the potential modifying effect of environmental factors on these associations. Asthma was significantly related to non-secretor phenotype. Significantly lower lung function and higher prevalences of wheezing and asthma were observed in non-secretor patients of blood group O[2].

There is also a stress-related factor in asthma, which lowers lung function in blood group A and to a lesser extent in blood group B. High levels of stress can cause a perceived narrowing of the breathing tubes. In one study, adult asthma sufferers were asked to perform difficult math tests, or watch highly emotional videos. Between 15% and 30% of the patients reported an increased tightening of their airways[3].

Therapies, Asthma

BLOOD GROUP A:

1. Allergy Control Protocol

2. Pulmonary Support Protocol

3. Stomach Health Protocol

BLOOD GROUP B:

1. Allergy Control Protocol

2. Pulmonary Support Protocol

3. Antistress Protocol

Specifics:

Avoid aspirin and nonsteroidal anti-inflammatory drugs (NSAIDs)

Magnesium: 400 mg/day, associated with improved pulmonary function of asthmatic patients. Intravenous magnesium works very well for acute asthmatic conditions.

Flax oil: 1–2 tbsp/day

BLOOD GROUP AB:

1. Allergy Control Protocol

2. Pulmonary Support Protocol

3. Antistress Protocol

4. Intestinal Health Protocol

BLOOD GROUP O:

1. Allergy Control Protocol

2. Pulmonary Support Protocol

3. Anti-Inflammation Protocol

4. Intestinal Health Protocol

Specifics:

Avoid aspirin and nonsteroidal anti-inflammatory drugs (NSAIDs)

Flax oil: 1–2 tbsp/day

Related Topics

Allergies (general)

REFERENCES

1. Kauffmann F, Frette C, Pham QT, Nafissi S, Bertrand JP, Oriol R. *AM J Respir Crit Care Med.* 1996;153:76–82.

2. Cohen BH, Bias WB, Chase GA, et al. Is ABH nonsecretor status a riskfactor for obstructive lung disease. *Am J Epidemiol.* 1980;3:285–291.

3. Brachtel R, Walter H, Beck W, Hilling M. Associations between atopic diseases and the polymorphic systems ABO, Kidd, Inv and red cell acid phosphatase. *Hum Genet.* 1979; 49:337–348.

ASTROCYTOMA–*See Cancer, glioma and other brain tumors*

ATHEROSCLEROSIS–*Hardening of the arteries, also known as coronary artery disease.*

Atherosclerosis	INCIDENCE/RISK/SEVERITY		
	LOW	AVERAGE	HIGH
GROUP A			
GROUP B			
GROUP AB			
GROUP O			
NON-SECRETOR			

Symptoms

- Chest pain
- Shortness of breath
- Tightness in the chest, with tingling in the left arm and shoulder

About Atherosclerosis

Atherosclerosis (*athero* from the Greek for "gruel or fat" and *sclerosis* from the Greek for "hard"—thus the term hardening of the arteries) is a slow, progressive disease that can affect large and medium-sized arteries. Often, it doesn't affect people until they are in their fifties or sixties; however, the condition may start in childhood and progress rapidly. It is a sobering thought that early signs of atherosclerosis, such as fatty streaks or lipid deposits, are sometimes found in the aortas of children as young as 3 years.

Atherosclerosis can restrict the flow of blood to the heart, which often triggers heart attacks—the leading cause of death in Americans and Europeans. Atherosclerosis of the arteries supplying the legs causes a condition called INTERMITTENT CLAUDICATION.

If a clot develops in a coronary artery, cutting off blood to the heart muscle, it is called a coronary thrombosis. This causes a HEART ATTACK because the heart muscle cannot get life-sustaining oxygen through the restricted bloodstream, and it begins to die. That's why the medical name for a heart attack is MYOCARDIAL INFARCTION: *myocardial* refers to the heart, and *infarction* means dead muscle.

It is unknown exactly how atherosclerosis begins or what causes it, although some scientists believe that it begins when the innermost layer of the artery, called the *endothelium*, becomes damaged. Regardless of the original provocation, fats, cholesterol, fibrin, platelets, cellular debris, and calcium are deposited in the artery wall over time. These substances can stimulate the cells of the artery wall to produce still other substances that result in further accumulation of cells causing atherosclerotic lesions, called *plaque*.

The specific kind of artery and the location of the plaque varies with each person. Plaque may partially or totally block the blood's flow through an artery, causing bleeding into the plaque or formation of a blood clot (thrombus) on the plaque's surface. If either of these occurs and blocks the entire artery, a heart attack or stroke (brain attack) may result.

The genesis of CARDIOVASCULAR DISEASE may well lie with an immunologic event, such as an infection, and its further development may depend on other risk factors, such as elevated CHOLESTEROL. Even more striking, the other risk factors may themselves depend on an initiating event, such as damage to the artery lining from a chronic infection.

An increasingly recognized cause of cardiovascular disease is chronic, low-grade infection. Subclinical infections with chlamydia pneumoniae, H. PYLORI, chronic BRONCHITIS, and chronic dental infections and GUM DISEASE have been linked to elevated serum levels of an inflammatory modulator called C reactive protein, and have been implicated as risk factors for cardiovascular disease. Elevated serum levels of C reactive protein can also be detected in the presence of chronic low-grade systemic inflammation. This is probably of major significance as a risk factor for non-secretors.

Genetics and lifestyle issues play a role. Other means of initiating damage to the artery wall include the effects of super-oxide free radicals, which react with the delicate lining. Smoking, for example, dramatically increases the activity of free radicals.

Overall, atherosclerosis is an enormous problem, responsible for $50–$100 billion annually in health care costs and lost wages.

General Risk Factors and Causes

People with elevated cholesterol levels are much more likely to have atherosclerosis than people with low cholesterol levels. Thus, many important nutritional approaches to protecting against atherosclerosis are aimed at lowering serum cholesterol levels. People with DIABETES are also at very high risk for atherosclerosis, as are people with elevated levels of TRIGLYCERIDES.

Blood Group Links

Blood groups A and AB are at greater overall risk of atherosclerosis. A 1994 Polish study of cardiac bypass surgery patients with highly advanced arteriosclerosis of the coronary arteries found a significantly higher number of cases with blood group AB, and far fewer with blood group O[1].

Blood groups A and AB have "thicker" blood, more likely to deposit plaque in the arteries—one reason why blood groups A and AB are more prone to CORONARY ARTERY DISEASE.

In another study, serum lipoprotein and lipid levels in patients with intermittent claudication were examined according to ABO blood group. A predominance of blood group A (61%) was again found[2].

An excess of blood group A was found in a group of 125 patients suffering from venous thrombosis in a Brazilian population[3]. ABO nonsecretors may have a higher incidence of atherosclerosis[4].

Therapies, Atherosclerosis

BLOOD GROUP A:

1. Cardiovascular Protocol

2. Metabolic Enhancement Protocol

3. Antistress Protocol

BLOOD GROUP B:

1. Cardiovascular Protocol

2. Metabolic Enhancement Protocol

3. Antistress Protocol

BLOOD GROUP AB:

1. Cardiovascular Protocol

2. Metabolic Enhancement Protocol

3. Antistress Protocol

BLOOD GROUP O:

1. Cardiovascular Protocol

2. Metabolic Enhancement Protocol

3. Antistress Protocol

Related Topics

Cardiovascular disease

Cholesterol

Coronary artery disease

Diabetes mellitus, type II

Triglycerides

REFERENCES

1. Slipko Z, Latuchowska B, Wojtkowska E. [Body structure and ABO and Rh blood groups in patients with advanced coronary heart disease after aorto-coronary by-pass surgery]. *Pol Arch Med Wewn.* 1994;91:55–60.

2. Landé KE, Sperry WM. Human atherosclerosis in relation to the cholesterol content of the blood serum. *Archives of Pathology.* 1936;22:301–312.

3. Paterson JC, Armstrong R, Armstrong EC. Serum lipid levels and the severity of coronary and cerebral atherosclerosis

in adequately nourished men, 60 to 69 years of age. *Circulation*. 1963;27:229–236.

4. Mathur KS, and others. Serum cholesterol and atherosclerosis in man. *Circulation*. 1961;23:847–852.

ATTENTION DEFICIT DISORDERS (ADD/ADHD)–*Syndromes characterized by hyperactivity, inattention, distractibility, and impulsivity.*

Attention deficit disorders (ADD/ADHD)	INCIDENCE/RISK/SEVERITY		
	LOW	AVERAGE	HIGH
GROUP A			
GROUP B			
GROUP AB			
GROUP O			

Symptoms

- Hyperactivity

- Emotional instability

- Motor impairment

- Inattention

- Poor concentration and inability to finish things

- Learning disabilities

About Attention Deficit Disorders

Attention deficit disorder (ADD) and attention deficit hyperactivity disorder (ADHD) currently rank as among the most over-diagnosed and over-medicated conditions in our society. The characterization of the symptoms tends to be vague, and often is applied to behaviors that all children exhibit at one time or another. Because of the attendant publicity surrounding these disorders, parents and teachers often pressure doctors to prescribe medications such as Ritalin or Depakote when a child is difficult to control or has trouble learning. In one study of fifth graders in two different cities, 18% to 20% of the boys were on Ritalin, suggesting a rush to medicate children who exhibited any difficulties whatsoever. In any case, drugs only treat the symptoms, not the problem—the well-known underlying causes, including elevated stress hormones, autoimmune syndromes, and an uncontrolled, sugar-heavy diet, are ignored.

Legitimate cases of ADD and ADHD must be taken seriously, however. A child with one of these conditions can experience severe difficulties that are carried into adulthood. Adult cases of ADD/ADHD often go undiagnosed.

General Risk Factors and Causes

The underlying causes include elevated stress hormones and autoimmune syndromes. Smoking during pregnancy should be strictly avoided, as it increases the risk of giving birth to a child who develops ADD[1]. Exposure to lead and other heavy-metals has been linked to ADD. If other therapies do not seem to be helping a child with ADD, the possibility of heavy-metal exposure can be explored with a nutritionally oriented health practitioner.

Blood Group Links

High catecholamine levels and DOPAMINE IM-BALANCES have been associated with hyperactivity. Many of the symptoms associated with these conditions are common to blood group O. Research shows that many ADHD children also suffer from hypersensitivity and allergies, which are autoimmune problems also common to blood group O[2].

ADD and ADHD have also been associated with chronic EAR INFECTIONS, a condition most common in group A children. New research suggests that decreased levels of C4B, or complement, the immune protein responsible for aiding in the destruction of bacteria, may be a marker for ADHD. Blood group A children often exhibit low levels of complement. There is also some evidence that hyperactivity is related to high cortisol levels in group A children[3].

Therapies, Attention Deficit Disorders (ADD/ADHD)

ALL BLOOD GROUPS:

Traditionally, hyperactivity is treated with drugs such as Ritalin. Once again, drugs only treat the symptoms, not the problem; they completely ignore the well-known underlying causes, including elevated stress hormones, autoimmune syndromes, and an uncontrolled sugar-heavy, fat-laden diet.

Calcium: 500–750 mg daily

BLOOD GROUP A:

1. Cognitive Improvement Protocol

2. Antistress Protocol

Specifics:

Bacopa monnieri (Brahmi): 100–150 mg daily; this Ayurvedic herb is a premiere cerebral antioxidant

BLOOD GROUP B:

1. Cognitive Improvement Protocol

2. Antistress Protocol

3. Allergy Control Protocol

Specifics:

Magnesium: 500 mg daily

BLOOD GROUP AB:

1. Cognitive Improvement Protocol

2. Antistress Protocol

Specifics:

Magnesium: 500 mg daily

BLOOD GROUP O:

1. Cognitive Improvement Protocol

2. Antistress Protocol

3. Allergy Control Protocol

Specifics:

Pycnogenol: 60–100 mg daily loading dose for 2 weeks, then cut in half. Vitamin B_6: 20–30 mg/kg

Related Topics

Allergies (general)

Immunity

Stress

REFERENCES

1. Locong AH, Roberge AG. Cortisol and catecholamines response to venisection by humans with different blood groups. *Clin Biochem.* 1985;18:67–69.
2. Scerbo AS, Kolko DJ. Salivary testosterone and cortisol in disruptive children: relationship to aggressive, hyperactive, and internalizing behaviors. *J Am Acad Child Adolesc Psychiatry.* 1994;33:1174–1184.

ATRIAL ARRHYTHMIA—*See Cardiovascular disease*

AUTISM—*Also called Asperger's disorder. A neurological malfunction or brain disorder that prevents the formation of normal relationships with the exterior world.*

Autism	INCIDENCE/RISK/SEVERITY		
	LOW	AVERAGE	HIGH
GROUP A			
GROUP B			
GROUP AB			
GROUP O			

Symptoms

- Absence or impairment of imaginative and social play
- Impaired ability to make friends with peers
- Impaired ability to initiate or sustain a conversation
- Stereotyped, repetitive, or unusual use of language
- Restricted patterns of interests that are abnormal in intensity or focus
- Inflexibility with regard to changes in routine or rituals
- Preoccupation with parts of objects

About Autism

Autism is a mysterious mental disorder that afflicts 400,000 children in the United States alone. It develops in toddlers after deceptively normal infancies that are free of the developmental abnormalities that are early and obvious hallmarks of severe mental retardation or cerebral palsy. Around the age of 18 months or 2 years, the child does not attain developmental milestones. Normal communication between parent and child lapses. Autistic children often fail to make eye contact, and their speech is rudimentary. They may be prone to explosive tantrums, or engage in repetitive mechanical behavior such as rocking or shutting off all the lights in a room again and again. Although autism varies in severity, its key features are improper sensory integration, lack of subtlety of emotional expression (flatness can quickly give way to agitation), and limited communication ability.

Autistic children seldom are able to lead independent lives without heavy remedial education, dedicated parental care, and sometimes institutionalization and drug therapy. It appears that the most helpful test in delineating the syndrome is the standard IQ test. Most autistic children are shown to be retarded, and generally will maintain the same traits into adulthood. However, some of these children, who have normal IQs and exhibit communicative language by 5 years of age, may develop some remarkable talents, such as near-genius musical or mathematical skills, while still remaining socially withdrawn.

General Risk Factors and Causes

The causes of autism are unknown, although maternal RUBELLA infection is thought to play a role in some cases. No relationship between autism and reactions to vaccines and other external factors has been clearly proven.

Blood Group Links

Although there is not yet a published study, an informal accounting shows a marked prevalence of blood group A among autistic children. Some positive results have been seen using the Blood Type Diet in some group A children with autism. Since the type A diet limits several dietary lectins that are thought to interfere with secretin, it is not too far-fetched to consider that improvement in these children may have actually resulted from enhancement of their own secretin metabolism.

Secretin stimulates the liver to produce bile, and triggers the pancreas to begin secreting pancreatic juice. As with the stomach juices, pancreatic juice and bile are heavily impregnated with ABO blood group antigens. It has been shown that wheat germ agglutinin (but not soybean) inhibited secretin production by about 57%. The effects of wheat germ agglutinin were completely suppressed by administration of the lectin-blocking sugar N-acetyl-D-glucosamine[1].

One study on secretin and autism reported that three children with autism and gastrointestinal problems had improved gastrointestinal function after secretin infusion, and that the children became more sociable and communicative[2].

Therapies, Autism

ALL BLOOD GROUPS

1. Fragile X syndrome, a collection of inborn metabolic errors that include autistic tendencies, has been reported to be somewhat responsive to folic acid.

2. The Ayurvedic herb Bacopa (sometimes called Brahmi) has been used in several cases of autism with promising effect. Bacopa is an Ayurvedic medicine used in India for memory enhancement, epilepsy, insomnia, and as a mild sedative. This herb commonly grows in marshy areas throughout India. Some studies have shown that Bacopa has antioxidant effects specific to the cerebral tissue.

3. Low-lectin diet

4. Deflect (specific A, B, O, or AB formula): 1–2 capsules with each meal

BLOOD GROUP A:

1. Liver Support Protocol

2. Cognitive Improvement Protocol

BLOOD GROUP B:

1. Liver Support Protocol

2. Cognitive Improvement Protocol

BLOOD GROUP AB:

1. Liver Support Protocol

2. Cognitive Improvement Protocol

BLOOD GROUP O:

1. Liver Support Protocol

2. Cognitive Improvement Protocol

Related Topics

Digestion

Liver disease

Rubella (German measles)

REFERENCES

1. Mikkat U, Damm I, Schroder G, Schmidt K, Wirth C, Weber H, Jonas L. Effect of the lectins wheat germ agglutinin (WGA) and Ulex europaeus agglutinin (UEA-I) on the alpha-amylase secretion of rat pancreas in vitro and in vivo. *Pancreas.* 1998;16:529–538.

2. Horvath K, Stefanatos G, Sokolski KN, Wachtel R, Nabob L, Tildon JT. Improved social and language skills after secretin administration in patients with autistic spectrum disorders. *Journal of the Association for Academic Minority Physicians.* 1998;9:9–15.

AUTOIMMUNE DISEASE (general)–*Conditions of hyperimmunity, where the immune system attacks itself.*

Autoimmune disease (general)	INCIDENCE/RISK/SEVERITY		
	LOW	AVERAGE	HIGH
GROUP A			
GROUP B			
GROUP AB			
GROUP O			
RH NEGATIVE			
NON-SECRETOR			

Symptoms

Variable

About Autoimmune Disease

Auto is the Greek word for "self." If a person is suffering from an autoimmune disease, the immune system mistakenly attacks itself, targeting its own cells, tissues, and organs. There are many different autoimmune diseases, and they can each affect the body in different ways. For example, the autoimmune reaction is directed against the brain (or the control of the central nervous system) in MULTIPLE SCLEROSIS, and against the gut in CROHN'S DISEASE. Ultimately, damage to certain tissues by the immune system may be permanent, as with the destruction of the insulin-producing cells of the pancreas in type I DIABETES MELLITUS.

Much of the damage done by autoimmune disease is the result of immune complexes, an insoluble lattice network of antibodies bound to antigens in the bloodstream. Immune complexes are harmful when they accumulate and initiate inflammation. Immune complexes, immune cells, and inflammatory molecules can block blood flow and ultimately destroy organs such as the insulin-secreting islet of Langerhans in the pancreas or the kidney in people with SYSTEMIC LUPUS ERYTHEMATOSUS. One of the major jobs of the complement system is to remove immune complexes. The different types of molecules of the complement system make immune complexes more soluble. Complement molecules prevent the formation and reduce the size of immune complexes, so they do not accumulate in the wrong places, such as the organs and tissues of the body.

Many of the autoimmune diseases are rare. As a group, however, autoimmune diseases afflict millions of Americans. Autoimmune diseases tend to strike women more often than men; in particular, they affect women during their childbearing years. Some autoimmune diseases occur more frequently in certain minority populations. For example, lupus is more common in women of African and Hispanic ancestry than among Caucasian women of European ancestry. RHEUMATOID ARTHRITIS and scleroderma affect a higher percentage of residents in some Native American communities than the overall U.S. population.

Some autoimmune diseases are known to begin or worsen with certain triggers, such as viral infections. Sunlight not only acts as a trigger for lupus but can worsen the course of the disease. It is important to be aware of the factors that can be avoided to help prevent or minimize the amount of damage from the autoimmune disease. Other less understood influences affecting the immune system and the course of autoimmune diseases include aging, chronic stress, hormones, and pregnancy.

Blood Group Links

Blood group O has a moderately high risk for inflammation-related diseases such as FIBROMYALGIA and RHEUMATOID ARTHRITIS.

ABO non-secretors appear to have an increase in the prevalence of a variety of autoimmune diseases, including ANKYLOSING SPONDYLITIS, reactive ARTHRITIS, SJÖGREN'S SYNDROME, MULTIPLE SCLEROSIS, and GRAVES' DISEASE. This susceptibility to autoimmune problems appears to be most pronounced among Lewis (a−b−) phenotypes[1-3].

Therapies, Autoimmune Disease

ALL BLOOD GROUPS:

1. Low-lectin diet
2. Deflect (specific A, B, O, or AB formula): 1–2 capsules with each meal

BLOOD GROUP A:

1. Anti-Inflammation Protocol
2. Detoxification Protocol

BLOOD GROUP B:

1. Immune-Enhancing Protocol
2. Nerve Health Protocol
3. Antiviral Protocol

BLOOD GROUP AB:

1. Immune-Enhancing Protocol

2. Nerve Health Protocol

3. Fatigue-Fighting Protocol

BLOOD GROUP O:

1. Detoxification

2. Anti-Inflammation Protocol

3. Intestinal Health Protocol

Related Topics

Ankylosing spondylitis

Arthritis, rheumatoid

Autoimmune disease, fibromyalgia

Autoimmune disease, multiple sclerosis

Autoimmune disease, myasthenia gravis

Autoimmune disease, sarcoidosis

Autoimmune disease, Sjögren's syndrome

Autoimmune disease, systemic lupus erythematosus

Chronic fatigue syndrome

Diabetes mellitus, type I

Inflammation

Thyroid disease, Graves'

REFERENCES

1. Shinebaum R. ABO blood group and secretor status in the spondyloarthropathies. *FEMS Microbiol Immunol.* 1989;1: 389–395.

2. Shinebaum R, Blackwell CC, Forster PJ, et. al. Non-secretion of ABO blood group antigens as a host suscepti-

bility factor in the spondyloarthropathies. *Br Med J (Clin Res Ed).* 1987;294:208–210.

3. Manthorpe R, Staub Nielsen L, Hagen Petersen S, Prause JU. Lewis blood type frequency in patients with primary Sjögren's syndrome. A prospective study including analyses for A1A2BO, Secretor, MNSs, P, Duffy, Kell, Lutheran and rhesus blood groups. *Scand J Rheumatol.* 1985;14:159–162.

AUTOIMMUNE DISEASE, FIBROMYAL-GIA—*A group of common nonarticular disorders characterized by aching pain, tenderness, and stiffness of muscles, areas of tendon insertions, and adjacent soft tissue structures.*

Fibromyalgia	INCIDENCE/RISK/SEVERITY		
	LOW	AVERAGE	HIGH
GROUP A	■		
GROUP B	■		
GROUP AB	■		
GROUP O	■	■	
NON-SECRETOR	■	■	■

Symptoms

- Chronic, widespread musculoskeletal pain

About Fibromyalgia

The name fibromyalgia comes from *fibro* meaning fibrous tissues such as tendons and ligaments, *my* meaning muscles, and *algia* meaning pain. Fibromyalgia syndrome has had a long, if rather obscure, history as an illness. Fibromyalgia syndrome (also called "FMS" or "FM") is a complex, chronic condition that causes widespread pain and fatigue, as well as a variety of other symptoms. Unlike arthritis, fibromyalgia does not cause pain or swelling in the joints themselves; rather, it produces pain in the soft tissues located around joints, skin, and organs throughout the body. Because fibromyalgia produces few symptoms that are outwardly noticeable, it has been nicknamed "the invisible disability" or the "irritable everything" syndrome.

The pain of fibromyalgia usually consists of diffuse aching or burning described as "head to toe," and it is often accompanied by muscle spasm. Its severity varies from day to day and can change location, becoming more severe in the parts of the body that are used the most (that is, the neck, shoulders, and feet). In some people, the pain can be intense enough to interfere with work and ordinary daily tasks; in others, it causes only mild discomfort. Likewise, the fatigue of fibromyalgia also varies from person to person, ranging from a mild, tired feeling, to the exhaustion of a flu-like illness. The good news is that fibromyalgia is neither crippling nor fatal.

Fibromyalgia is not an easy disease to identify. The most common diagnostic criteria uses the following parameters:

History of widespread pain above and below the waist and on both sides of the body

Chronic, widespread, musculoskeletal pain for longer than 3 months in all four quadrants of the body

Axial skeletal pain—in the cervical spine, anterior chest, thoracic spine, or low back

Pain in 11 of 18 tender point sites on palpation with the fingers

With fibromyalgia, doctors investigate 18 tender points; a patient must be positive in 11 of the 18 for this diagnosis. Approximately four kilograms of pressure (about 9 lbs.) is applied to a tender point, and if the patient indicates that the points are tender, then the point is considered positive.

General Risk Factors and Causes

Although the cause of fibromyalgia syndrome is not currently known, research has already uncovered significant information. It is becoming increasingly clear that there is a breakdown in the pain perception system in fibromyalgia patients; it is not yet known whether the problem is related to an increase in pain perception (which occurs even though the stimuli sent from the various parts of the body are basically normal), or a "hyper" response to real pain stimuli. A great deal of interest has been directed at the neuroendocrine system and to the abnormal status of such NEUROTRANSMITTERS/neurochemicals as calcitonin-gene-related peptide, noradrenaline, endorphins, dopamine, histamine, and GABA. The hormones of the hypothalamus, pituitary, and adrenal glands are suspected as being dysfunctional as well.

Blood Group Links

Blood group O is highly susceptible to fibromyalgia, especially with consumption of wheat. Wheat germ lectins exacerbate the tendency for

HYPERIMMUNITY, which is a characteristic of AU-TOIMMUNE DISEASES. Of the foods known to induce joint INFLAMMATION, grains certainly top the list. In some cases, avoidance of grains is the only dietary maneuver required, especially in the early stages. Our most common grains contain lectins, and many of these lectins are specifically attracted to the sugars that are found abundantly in connective tissue, particularly N-acetyl glucosamine (NAG). Wheat germ lectin, in particular, has an affinity for NAG.

Therapies, Fibromyalgia

ALL BLOOD GROUPS:

1. Low-lectin diet
2. Deflect (specific A, B, O, or AB formula): 1–2 capsules with each meal
3. Vitamin B_6: 50 mg three times a day

BLOOD GROUP A:

1. Immune-Enhancing Protocol
2. Nerve Health Protocol
3. Fatigue-Fighting Protocol

BLOOD GROUP B:

1. Immune-Enhancing Protocol
2. Nerve Health Protocol
3. Antiviral Protocol

BLOOD GROUP AB:

1. Immune-Enhancing Protocol
2. Nerve Health Protocol
3. Fatigue-Fighting Protocol

BLOOD GROUP O:

1. Fatigue-Fighting Protocol
2. Anti-Inflammation Protocol
3. Nerve Health Protocol

Specifics:

Vitamin B_1: thiamin deficiency symptoms closely resemble many of the symptoms experienced by fibromyalgia patients; possibly this is related to the reduced activity of some thiamin-dependent enzymes.

Related Topics

Autoimmune disease (general)

Infectious disease

Inflammation

Lectins

AUTOIMMUNE DISEASE, MULTIPLE SCLEROSIS–*A slowly progressive disease, resulting in multiple and varied neurologic symptoms and signs, usually with remissions and exacerbations.*

Multiple sclerosis	INCIDENCE/RISK/SEVERITY		
	LOW	AVERAGE	HIGH
GROUP A	▓		
GROUP B	▓	▓	
GROUP AB	▓	▓	
GROUP O	▓		
NON-SECRETOR	▓	▓	
RH POSITIVE	▓		
DUFFY A−B+	▓		

Symptoms

- Vision problems
- Muscle weakness
- Difficulty with coordination and balance
- Fatigue

About Multiple Sclerosis

Although MS was first diagnosed in 1849, the earliest known description of a person with possible MS dates from 14th century Holland. An unpredictable disease of the central nervous system, MS can range from relatively benign to somewhat disabling. It can become devastating when communication between the brain and other parts of the body is disrupted. The vast majority of patients are mildly affected, but in the worst cases MS can render a person unable to write, speak, or walk.

The initial symptom of multiple sclerosis (MS) is often blurred or double vision, red–green color distortion, or even blindness in one eye. Inexplicably, visual problems tend to clear up in the later stages of MS. Inflammatory problems of the optic nerve may be diagnosed as retrobulbar optic neuritis. At one time or another, 55% of MS patients will have an attack of optic neuritis; it will be the first symptom of MS in approximately 15%. This has led to general recognition of optic neuritis as an early sign of MS, especially if tests also reveal abnormalities in the patient's spinal fluid.

Most MS patients experience muscle weakness in their extremities, and difficulty with coordination and balance during the course of the dis-

ease. These symptoms may be severe enough to impair walking or even standing. In the worst cases, MS can produce partial or complete paralysis. Spasticity—an involuntary increase in muscle tone leading to stiffness and spasms—is common, as is FATIGUE. Fatigue may be triggered by physical exertion and improve with rest, or it may take the form of a constant, persistent tiredness.

During an MS attack, inflammation occurs in areas of the white matter of the central nervous system in random patches called plaques. This process is followed by destruction of myelin, the fatty covering that insulates nerve cell fibers in the brain and spinal cord. Myelin facilitates the smooth, high-speed transmission of electrochemical messages between the brain, the spinal cord, and the rest of the body; when it is damaged, neurological transmission of messages may be slowed or blocked completely, leading to diminished or lost function. The name "multiple sclerosis" signifies both the number (multiple) and condition (*sclerosis*, from the Greek term for scarring or hardening) of the demyelinated areas in the central nervous system.

No one knows exactly how many people have MS. At any point in time, it is believed that approximately 250,000 to 350,000 people in the United States have MS. This estimate suggests that approximately 200 new patients are diagnosed each week.

General Risk Factors and Causes

Most people experience their first symptoms of MS between the ages of 20 and 40, but a diagnosis is often delayed. This is due to both the transitory nature of the disease and the lack of a diagnostic test. Specific symptoms and changes in the brain must develop before the diagnosis can be confirmed. Although scientists have documented cases of MS in young children and elderly adults, the symptoms rarely begin before age 15 or after age 60. Caucasians are more than twice as likely as others to develop MS. In general, women are affected at almost twice the rate of men; however, among patients who develop the symptoms of MS at a later age, the gender ratio is more balanced.

Periodically, scientists receive reports of MS "clusters." The most famous of these MS epidemics took place in the Faeroe Islands north of Scotland in the years following the arrival of British troops during World War II. Despite intense study of this and other clusters, no direct environmental factor has been identified. Nor has any definitive evidence been found to link daily stress to MS attacks, although there is evidence that attacks worsen after acute viral illnesses.

Blood Group Links

MS is an example of the blood group B tendency to contract unusual, slow-growing viral and neurological disorders. The blood group B association may explain why many Ashkenazi Jews, with high rates of group B blood, suffer from these diseases. Some researchers believe that MS is caused by a virus contracted in youth that has a B-like appearance. The virus cannot be engaged and defeated by the B immune system because it cannot produce anti-B antibodies[1].

Blood group AB is at greater risk of rapidly progressing MS. Researchers have studied genetic markers in MS patients who were born in Mexico, had no family history of MS, were middle-class, and had a high-level education. When their blood systems were analyzed and compared with results of 295 control individuals, the study found an excess of AB group carriers among the MS patients[2].

One study showed a marked predominance of non-secretors among MS sufferers. The researchers noted that "inspired by the widely discussed problem of a possible genetic background of multiple sclerosis, we have undertaken a trial of determining the relationship between the hereditary trait conveyed by a single gene, i.e., the salivary secretion or nonsecretion of blood type substances, and the occurrence of this disease. The investigations have shown that in the population of western Poland the non-secretors of blood type substances into their saliva have a statistically significant higher chance of developing multiple sclerosis than secretors of these substances"[3].

Rh-positive individuals show an increased incidence of MS. In one study, the Rh-positive factor was present in 95.55% of the MS patients, whereas the Rh-negative factor was found in only 4.45%[4].

The Duffy blood group antigen is also considered predictive of MS. An increased rate of the Duffy phenotype (a−b+) has been reported among MS patients versus the population control. Individuals with this phenotype have a three times greater risk of developing disseminated sclerosis than those with the Duffy phenotype (a+b−). The Duffy antigen (b+) may be a potential genetic marker for MS in the Armenian population[5].

Of Special Note

Blood from MS patients show a deficit of intestinal alkaline phosphatase (serum type Pp2) by comparison with normal sera. This is not due to variation in ABO frequency, since the specimens from MS patients and normal individuals match for ABO frequency; nor is it due to differences in secretor frequency. Rather, it represents a real deficit for Pp2 in MS patients, which is particularly noticeable in the blood group O individuals[6].

Therapies, Multiple Sclerosis

BLOOD GROUP A:

1. Immune-Enhancing Protocol
2. Nerve Health Protocol
3. Chronic Illness Recovery Protocol

BLOOD GROUP B:

1. Antiviral Protocol
2. Nerve Health Protocol
3. Chronic Illness Recovery Protocol

BLOOD GROUP AB:

1. Antiviral Protocol
2. Nerve Health Protocol

BLOOD GROUP O:

1. Anti-Inflammation Protocol
2. Nerve Health Protocol
3. Chronic Illness Recovery Protocol

Related Topics

Autoimmune disease (general)

Immunity

Lectins

REFERENCES

1. Warner HB, Merz GS, Carp RI. Blood group frequencies in multiple sclerosis populations in the United States. *Neurology*. 1980;30:671–673.
2. Gorodezky C, Najera R, Rangel BE, Castro LE, Flores J, Velazquez G, Granados J, Sotelo J. Immunogenetic profile of multiple sclerosis in Mexicans. *Hum Immunol*. 1986;16: 364–374.
3. Markovic S, Bozicevic D, Simic D, Brzovic Z. Genetic markers in the blood of multiple sclerosis patients. *Neurol Croat*. 1991;41:3–12.
4. Darbinian VZ, Nersisian VM, Martirosian IG. [Genetic markers of erythrocyte blood groups in multiple sclerosis among the Armenian population]. *Zh Nevropatol Psikhiatr Im S S Korsakova*. 1983;83:42–46.
5. Wender M, Przybylski Z, Stawarz M, Chmielewska U. Salivary secretion of blood group substances in multiple sclerosis patients. *Eur Neurol*. 1981;20:52–55.
6. Papiha SS, Roberts DF. Serum alkaline phosphatase in patients with multiple sclerosis. *Clin Genet*. 1975;7:77–82.

AUTOIMMUNE DISEASE, MYASTHENIA GRAVIS—*An acquired autoimmune disorder recognized by easy muscle fatigability and weakness.*

Myasthenia gravis	INCIDENCE/RISK/SEVERITY		
	LOW	AVERAGE	HIGH
GROUP A	▓		
GROUP B	▓	▓	
GROUP AB	▓		
GROUP O	▓		
NON-SECRETOR	▓	▓	▓
RH NEGATIVE	▓		
DUFFY A−B+	▓	▓	

Symptoms

- Easy muscle fatigability and weakness

About Myasthenia Gravis

The incidence of myasthenia gravis is 2 to 5 people per million each year. Although the disease may strike anyone at any age, the two most affected patient groups are adolescents and younger adults, especially females; and adults over 40, who also have a higher risk of associated conditions. The cause of MG seems to be a deficiency of the acetylcholine receptors at the motor endplate of the muscles. Absence of these receptors decreases the muscle response. The disease affects specific external ocular muscles, or affects the cranial nerves more generally. As the disease progresses, weakness often spreads over the entire body. During the first 3 years the progression of the disease is rapid; most deaths occur during this time. Although remissions are seen in about 25% of patients, they do not usually last long.

Blood Group Links

Individuals with group B and Rh-negative blood have an increased incidence of MG. The distribution of ABO blood groups and rhesus factor was studied in patients with MG as compared with an unaffected population. There was a statistically significant association of MG with the Rh-negative phenotype; generalized myasthenia was found to be concurrent with thymoma with the B blood group[1].

Therapies, Myasthenia Gravis

BLOOD GROUP A:

1. Chronic Illness Recovery Protocol
2. Nerve Health Protocol
3. Fatigue-Fighting Protocol

BLOOD GROUP B:

1. Antiviral Protocol
2. Nerve Health Protocol
3. Chronic Illness Recovery Protocol

BLOOD GROUP AB:

1. Immune-Enhancing Protocol
2. Nerve Health Protocol

BLOOD GROUP O:

1. Immune-Enhancing Protocol
2. Nerve Health Protocol

Related Topics

Autoimmune disease (general)

Immunity

Stress

REFERENCES

1. Stringa SG, Bianchi C, Andrada JA, Comini E, Gaviglio AM, Casala A. Immunologic response to A and B erythrocytic antigen. *Arch Dermatol.* 1976;112:489–492.

AUTOIMMUNE DISEASE, SARCOIDOSIS–

A multisystem disorder of unknown cause, involving various organs or tissues, with symptoms depending on the site and degree of involvement.

Sarcoidosis	INCIDENCE/RISK/SEVERITY		
	LOW	AVERAGE	HIGH
GROUP A	███	███	
GROUP B	███		
GROUP AB	██		
GROUP O	███		
NON-SECRETOR	███	███	

Symptoms

Patients may be asymptomatic, or may have the following symptoms:

- Cough
- Shortness of breath
- New skin lesions
- Pain or irritation of the eyes
- General fatigue
- Malaise
- Fever
- Night sweats
- Bell's palsy, a partial facial paralysis

About Sarcoidosis

Sarcoidosis is a multisystem disease of unknown cause that commonly affects younger and middle-aged adults. The disease frequently presents with shortness of breath, general malaise, eye irritation, and skin lesions. Other organs may be involved, including the liver, spleen, lymph nodes, heart, and central nervous system. Sarcoidosis is found worldwide, but there is an increased prevalence among women of Scandinavian, Japanese, Irish, and African descent.

Sarcoidosis can be relatively mild, requiring no treatment. This form often goes into spontaneous remission. The more severe form is chronic, recurring throughout life, and may affect major organs.

Blood Group Links

Blood group O is associated with the most benign clinical course of sarcoidosis. Blood group A is associated with a more severe form of the disease[1].

Therapies, Sarcoidosis

BLOOD GROUP A:

1. Immune-Enhancing Protocol

BLOOD GROUP B:

1. Immune-Enhancing Protocol

BLOOD GROUP AB:

1. Immune-Enhancing Protocol

BLOOD GROUP O:

1. Immune-Enhancing Protocol

Related Topics

Autoimmune disease (general)

Immunity

REFERENCES

1. Blackwell CC. The role of ABO blood groups and secretor status in host defences. *FEMS Microbiol Immunol.* 1989;1: 341–349.

AUTOIMMUNE DISEASE, SJÖGREN'S SYNDROME—*A chronic, systemic inflammatory disorder of unknown cause, characterized by dryness of the mouth, eyes, and other mucous membranes, and often associated with rheumatic disorders sharing certain autoimmune features (for example, rheumatoid arthritis, scleroderma, and systemic lupus erythematosus).*

Sjögren's syndrome	INCIDENCE/RISK/SEVERITY		
	LOW	AVERAGE	HIGH
GROUP A	▓		
GROUP B	▓		
GROUP AB	▓		
GROUP O	▓		
NON-SECRETOR	▓	▓	

Symptoms

Variable

About Sjögren's Syndrome

In 1933, Swedish physician Henrik Sjögren observed a large number of his female patients were experiencing dry eyes and mouths along with their arthritic symptoms. The condition became known as Sjögren's syndrome. Sjögren's syndrome is an ARTHRITIS-related disease that can affect several organs. Its most common effect is on the moisture-producing glands, including those of the eyes and mouth jaw; it can cause extremely dry eyes (sometimes described as the feeling of sand in the eyes or a burning sensation), an extremely dry mouth and throat, dental cavities from lack of saliva, enlarged glands, vaginal dryness, fatigue, and joint pain, stiffness, and swelling. Less common symptoms include rash, numbness, and inflammation of the lungs, kidneys, or liver.

General Risk Factors and Causes

A major risk factor for developing Sjögren's is being a postmenopausal woman. It occurs less commonly in younger women, children, or men of any age. Other risk factors include having an AUTOIMMUNE DISEASE such as LUPUS, vasculitis, THYROID DISEASE, scleroderma, and/or a family member with Sjögren's. An association has been found between HLA-DR3 antigens and primary Sjögren's syndrome in Caucasians.

Blood Group Links

A greater frequency of Lewis negative phenotype (Le (a−b−)) is seen among individuals with primary Sjögren's syndrome than among the general population[1].

Therapies, Sjögren's Syndrome

BLOOD GROUP A:

1. Detoxification Protocol
2. Menopause Support Protocol

BLOOD GROUP B:

1. Chronic Illness Recovery Protocol
2. Anti-Inflammation Protocol
3. Menopause Support Protocol

BLOOD GROUP AB:

1. Immune-Enhancing Protocol
2. Menopause Support Protocol

BLOOD GROUP O:

1. Immune-Enhancing Protocol
2. Anti-Inflammation Protocol
3. Menopause Support Protocol

Related Topics

Autoimmune disease (general)

Immunity

Inflammation

REFERENCES

1. Manthorpe R, Staub, Nielsen L, et al. Lewis blood type frequency in patients with primary Sjögren's syndrome. A prospective study including analyses for A1A2BO, Secretor, MNSs, P, Duffy, Kell, Lutheran, and Rhesus blood groups. *Scand, J. Rheumatol.* 1985;14:159–162.

AUTOIMMUNE DISEASE, SYSTEMIC LUPUS ERYTHEMATOSUS (LUPUS)–*A chronic inflammatory connective tissue disorder of unknown cause that can involve joints, kidneys, serous surfaces, and vessel walls.*

Lupus	INCIDENCE/RISK/SEVERITY		
	LOW	AVERAGE	HIGH
GROUP A	▓		
GROUP B	▓	▓	
GROUP AB	▓		
GROUP O	▓		
NON-SECRETOR	▓	▓	

Symptoms

- Fever
- Skin rash
- Anemia
- Photosensitivity
- Arthritis
- Psychiatric disorders

About Lupus

Lupus means "wolf," and *erythematosus* means "redness." In 1851, doctors coined this name for the disease because they thought the facial rash that frequently accompanies lupus looked like the bite of a wolf. There are two major types of lupus: discoid and systemic.

Discoid lupus erythematosus (DLE) is characterized by a SKIN RASH only. It occurs in about 20% of patients who have systemic lupus erythematosus. The lesions are patchy, crusty, sharply defined skin plaques that may scar. These lesions are usually seen on the face or other sun-exposed areas. DLE may cause patchy, bald areas on the scalp, and hypopigmentation or hyperpigmentation in older lesions. A biopsy of a lesion will usually confirm the diagnosis. Topical and intralesional corticosteroids are usually effective for localized lesions; antimalarial drugs may be needed for more generalized lesions. DLE only rarely progresses to systemic lupus erythematosus.

Systemic lupus erythematosus (SLE) is an inflammatory immune disease characterized by excessive production of autoantibodies that are directed against the body's own tissues. It is nine times more common in women, and more common still in those of African, Hispanic, and Asian ancestry. Most typically the disease strikes after puberty or before menopause. Lupus is also related to abnormalities in the metabolism of estrogen, progesterone, and androgens.

In addition to the symptoms previously listed, people with lupus often display psychiatric manifestations, such as depression and difficulty concentrating. In fact, patients are often diagnosed with psychiatric disorders before the lupus is discovered.

General Risk Factors and Causes

Individuals of African, Hispanic, Asian, or Native American ancestry have a higher prevalence of lupus. There are some recognizable genetic markers. There is a hereditary deficiency of immune modulators such as complement. There is also a polymorphism in the Fc gamma-Rlla gene, which may be an important risk factor in SLE.

Blood Group Links

Lupus is most common in blood group B, and is characterized by an inappropriate isohemagglutinin response to stimulation with the B antigen. Literally, normal antigens of blood group B are agglutinated[1,2].

Therapies, Lupus

BLOOD GROUP A:

1. Immune-Enhancing Protocol
2. Anti-Inflammation Protocol
3. Chronic Illness Recovery Protocol

BLOOD GROUP B:

1. Immune-Enhancing Protocol
2. Detoxification Protocol
3. Chronic Illness Recovery Protocol

BLOOD GROUP AB:

1. Immune-Enhancing Protocol
2. Detoxification Protocol
3. Chronic Illness Recovery Protocol

BLOOD GROUP O:

1. Immune-Enhancing Protocol
2. Anti-Inflammation Protocol
3. Chronic Illness Recovery Protocol

Related Topics

Autoimmune disease (general)

Immunity

REFERENCES

1. Stringa SG, Bianchi C, Andrada JA, Comini E, Gaviglio AM, Casala A. Immunologic response to A and B erythrocytic antigen. *Arch Dermatol.* 1976;112:489–492.
2. Ottensooser F, Leon N, de Almeida TV. ABO blood groups and isoagglutinins in systemic lupus erythematosus. *Rev Bras Pesqui Med Biol.* 1975;6:421–425.

B

BACTERIAL DISEASE (general)– *The result of harmful bacteria that gain entry into the system and produce cell-damaging toxins.*

Symptoms

Variable, depending on bacterial agent. Common symptoms include:

- Fever
- Chills
- Diarrhea
- Gastroenteritis
- Nausea and vomiting

About Bacteria

There are two categories of infectious agents: bacterial and viral. Bacterial infections are caused by invading organisms in the environment, food, and by contact with people who are infected.

Over the last hundred years or so, people have grown accustomed to associating bacteria with human or animal disease. This is a misunderstanding, as the vast majority of bacteria do not cause disease. Many species are beneficial, producing antibiotics and nutrients. There are over 400 different bacteria that normally live quietly and beneficially in the large intestine. The soil teems with free-living bacteria that perform many essential functions for the biosphere, such as fixing nitrogen for use by plants.

Even among bacteria that are capable of causing disease, few are continual threats. Many free-living bacteria, or members of the normal flora, are potentially pathogenic in certain types of individuals. This holds true especially for those whose immune systems are compromised, such as cancer patients receiving chemotherapy. But most of the time bacteria is harmless, and even beneficial.

Administration of broad-spectrum antibiotics has a profound effect on the normal flora, and can result in the growth of antibiotic-resistant bacteria. Disruption of the normal flora from long-term antibiotic use can lead to fungal infections, such as candidiasis, or to antibiotic-associated colitis caused by the bacteria *Clostridium difficile.*

Many bacteria are categorized by the terms *gram-positive* and *gram-negative*. The terms refer to a staining procedure used to visualize bacteria

Common Harmful Bacteria and Their Blood Group Preferences

	TYPE O	TYPE A	TYPE B	TYPE AB	SUBTYPES
E. coli	Susceptible to strains that cause diarrhea.	Susceptible to the most severe intestinal reactions.	Susceptible to strains causing gastroenteritis.	Susceptible to strains causing gastroenteritis.	
Shigella			Most susceptible	Most susceptible	
Giardia		Most susceptible			
Candida	Most susceptible				Non-secretors most susceptible
Amoeba			Most susceptible		

under a microscope. Bacteria that appear blue are called gram-positive bacteria; those that stain pink are called gram-negative.

Blood Group Links

Blood groups have an important influence on the growth of particular strains of intestinal bacteria. Many bacteria consume blood group antigens, which are found extensively in the large intestine. The upper colon contains large amounts of blood group antigens; these gradually diminish, until, by the very end of the colon, there is little or no blood group antigen to be found. This is probably because they are used as a food source by the colon bacteria.

The composition of the normal flora varies somewhat from individual to individual. Some bacterial species may be carried only transiently. Most are fairly permanent. Animal experiments have shown that it can be extremely difficult to alter the composition of the normal flora in the gut of a healthy person. Many of the common bacteria choose to live in the colon of one blood group or another. Sometimes this is because the bacteria can mimic the blood group of their host, and so are viewed as normal by the host's immune system. In other circumstances, bacteria have a taste for one particular blood group's antigen over others, and prefer to nibble mucus containing that antigen. Some bacteria more easily adhere to the mucus of one blood group over others because they themselves make lectins, which they use to attach to the walls of the colon; these lectins are usually specific for one blood group.

The ability of blood group to determine aspects of the gut bacterial ecosystem is not unique to secretors. Non-secretors also have a preponderance of blood group–friendly bacteria and produce similar enzymes that degrade blood type antigens.

Therapies, Bacterial Disease (General)

BLOOD GROUP A:

1. Antibacterial Protocol

2. Antibiotic Support Protocol

BLOOD GROUP B:

1. Antibacterial Protocol

2. Antibiotic Support Protocol

BLOOD GROUP AB:

1. Antibacterial Protocol

2. Antibiotic Support Protocol

BLOOD GROUP O:

1. Antibacterial Protocol

2. Antibiotic Support Protocol

Related Topics

Digestion

Food poisoning

Fungal disease, candidiasis (digestive)

Fungal disease (oral)

Fungal disease (vaginal)

Infectious disease

Parasitic disease (amoeba)

Parasitic disease (*Giardia*)

Parasitic disease (hookworm)

Toxicity, bowel

Ulcer, *H. pylori*

BACTERIAL DISEASE, CHOLERA—*An acute infection by* Vibrio cholerae *involving the entire small bowel.*

Cholera	SEVERITY/SUSCEPTIBILITY		
	LOW	AVERAGE	HIGH
GROUP A	▓	▓	
GROUP B	▓	▓	
GROUP AB	▓		
GROUP O	▓	▓	▓

Symptoms

- Diarrhea
- Vomiting
- Intense thirst
- Muscle cramps
- Weakness
- Sunken eyes
- Wrinkling of skin on the fingers

About Cholera

Cholera still accounts for an enormous number of deaths worldwide. In the early 1900s, it was still common in the slums of many modern cities such as London and New York. In ancient times, cholera epidemics routinely decimated large cities. Several of the highly lethal plagues that were the scourge of the Roman Empire are now thought to have been cholera.

Poverty and lack of basic sanitation measures are among the main contributing factors to the current and past cholera epidemics. Cholera is most commonly spread by contact with infected feces, generally by drinking water or eating food contaminated with raw sewage that contains the cholera bacterium. The disease spreads most rapidly in areas with inadequate treatment of sewage and drinking water. The cholera bacterium can also live in brackish rivers and coastal waters, so raw shellfish have been a source of cholera. In the United States, cases of cholera have developed after eating raw or undercooked shellfish from the Gulf of Mexico.

Cholera can be subclinical; a mild, uncomplicated episode of DIARRHEA; or a full-blown, potentially lethal disease. Abrupt, painless, watery diarrhea and vomiting are usually the initial symptoms. The resultant severe water and electrolyte depletion leads to intense thirst, muscle cramps, weakness, and marked loss of tissue turgor—the normal state of turgidity and tension in living cells—resulting in sunken eyes and wrinkling of the skin on the fingers. The manifestations of cholera can be dire, and result from the loss of fluids in watery stools rich in sodium, chloride, bicarbonate, and potassium, depleting the system of its most vital balancing elements. If untreated, cholera results in blood poisoning, KIDNEY FAILURE, and heart failure. The incubation period for cholera is 1 to 3 days.

Blood Group Links

Cholera offers a huge selective disadvantage for blood group O, as it is the blood group that is almost guaranteed to suffer the most severe form of cholera infection. It has been speculated that the low number of Os in comparison to As in Mediterranean cities with ancient roots may be a result of selection, as group O people die more frequently from cholera. This constant selective pressure of cholera targeting group O may account in part for the extremely low prevalence of O genes, and the high prevalence of B genes among people living in the Ganges Delta of India. Group AB has the highest degree of protection from cholera infections. When they contract cholera, their symptoms are the least severe, and their recovery is almost always assured[1].

In 1991, at the onset of a cholera epidemic in Trujillo, Peru, a household survey determined that group O was strongly associated with the most severe cases of cholera[2]; infected persons had more diarrhea-like stools per day than persons of other blood groups, were more likely to report vomiting and muscle cramps, and were almost eight times more likely to require hospital treatment. In an independent study, similar findings were reported: Individuals with the most severe diarrhea were more often group O (68%), compared with those who had asymptomatic infections[3].

Therapies, Cholera

ALL BLOOD GROUPS:

Adhere to safe-travel guidelines. If you are traveling to an underdeveloped country, adhere to the following guidelines:

- Avoid raw or undercooked meat and seafood.

- Avoid raw vegetables and fruit, unless peeled.

- Avoid tap water and ice made from tap water.

- Avoid buying food from street vendors.

- Take along water-purifying tablets (available in pharmacies and sporting goods stores) if you're going to be hiking or backpacking through undeveloped areas.

- Check travel guides for restaurants that have high food safety standards.

- Use bottled water for drinking and brushing your teeth, even in hotels. Carbonated water may be the safest, since carbonation appears to kill some of the microorganisms. Be sure that the bottles have been properly sealed.

BLOOD GROUP A:

1. Antibacterial Protocol
2. Antibiotic Support Protocol
3. Immune-Enhancing Protocol

BLOOD GROUP B:

1. Antibacterial Protocol
2. Antibiotic Support Protocol
3. Chronic Illness Recovery Protocol

BLOOD GROUP AB:

1. Antibacterial Protocol
2. Antibiotic Support Protocol
3. Immune-Enhancing Protocol

BLOOD GROUP O:

1. Antibacterial Protocol
2. Antibiotic Support Protocol

3. Intestinal Health Protocol

Related Topics

Bacterial disease (general)

Digestion

Food poisoning

Fungal disease, candidiasis (digestive)

Fungal disease, candidiasis (oral)

Fungal disease, candidiasis (vaginal)

Infectious disease

REFERENCES

1. Mourant AE. *Blood Types and Disease*. Oxford, NY: Oxford University Press, 1979.
2. Swerdlow DL, Mintz ED, Rodriguez M, et al. Severe life-threatening cholera associated with blood group O in Peru: implications for the Latin American epidemic. *J Infect Dis.* 1994;170:468–472.
3. Glass RI, Holmgren J, Haley CE, et al. Predisposition for cholera of individuals with O blood group. Possible evolutionary significance. *Am J Epidemiol.* 1985;121:791–796.

BACTERIAL DISEASE, DIPHTHERIA–*An acute, contagious disease caused by* Corynebacterium diphtheriae.

Diphtheria	SEVERITY/SUSCEPTIBILITY		
	LOW	AVERAGE	HIGH
GROUP A			
GROUP B			
GROUP AB			
GROUP O			

Symptoms

Variable

About Diphtheria

Diphtheria is an acute, contagious disease caused by *Corynebacterium diphtheriae*, characterized by the formation of a fibrinous pseudomembrane, usually on the respiratory mucosa, and by myocardial and neural tissue damage. The incubation period ranges between 1 and 4 days. Initially, the patient with tonsillar diphtheria has only a mild sore throat, difficulty swallowing, a low-grade fever, increased heart rate, and a high white blood cell count. Nausea, vomiting, chills, headache, and fever are more common in children.

Diphtheria is spread chiefly by contact with the secretions of infected persons. Humans are the only known reservoir for *C. diphtheriae*. Sporadic cases generally result from exposure to carriers who may never have had apparent disease. Infection can occur in immunized persons and is most common and severe in those partially immunized. Communicability in untreated persons usually lasts for about 2 weeks. In patients who have been treated with appropriate antimicrobial drugs, communicability usually lasts 4 days. Occasionally, people will be chronic carriers even after antimicrobial treatment.

Cutaneous diphtheria (infection of the skin) can occur when a wound is colonized by *C. diphtheriae*. Lacerations, abrasions, ULCERS, burns, and other wounds are potential reservoirs of the organism. Skin carriage of *C. diphtheriae* is also a silent reservoir of infection. Poor personal and community hygiene contribute to the spread of cutaneous diphtheria. The infection seems to favor warm climates, but the disease is not restricted to tropical zones—large outbreaks have occurred in less temperate climates. In the United States, indigent adults and impoverished groups such as Native Americans living in endemic areas are particularly at risk. There are special risks for those who are not immunized and for the people who have compromised immune systems.

Blood Group Links

In Russia, antidiphtheritic antibodies were studied in the blood serum of a Kiev region population capable of blood donation (984 persons). Over a year's time, antidiphtheritic antibodies were found to be present in the blood serum of men and women of different blood groups (by ABO system). Antidiphtheritic antibodies with high titers were most often found in autumn, winter, and spring in people of the A (II), B (III), and AB (IV) blood groups[1].

Therapies, Diphtheria

ALL BLOOD GROUPS:

Diphtheria has been reported in the former Soviet Union, Albania, Haiti, Dominican Republic, Ecuador, Brazil, Philippines, Indonesia, and many countries in Africa and Asia. Travelers to these areas should be sure their immunizations are up to date. Active immunization with diphtheria-tetanus-pertussis (DTP) vaccine should be routinely given to all children. Be advised, however, that diphtheria antitoxin is derived from horses; hence, a skin (or conjunctival) test to rule out sensitivity should always precede administration.

Adhere to safe-travel guidelines. If you are traveling to an underdeveloped country, adhere to the following guidelines:

- Avoid raw or undercooked meat and seafood.
- Avoid raw vegetables and fruit, unless peeled.
- Avoid tap water and ice made from tap water.
- Avoid buying food from street vendors.
- Take along water-purifying tablets (available in pharmacies and sporting goods stores) if you're hiking or backpacking through undeveloped areas.
- Check travel guides for restaurants that have high food safety standards.
- Use bottled water for drinking and brushing your teeth, even in hotels. Carbonated water may be the safest, since carbonation appears to kill some of the microorganisms. Be sure that the bottles have been properly sealed.

In addition to rigorous attention to hygiene and avoidance of contaminated foods, your best defense is a healthy immune system. Nutrition is a major contributor to the functioning of the immune system, which in turn influences whether the body can maintain peak resistance to infection. Specifically, it makes sense to restrict sugar, because sugar interferes with the ability of white blood cells to destroy bacteria. Alcohol interferes with a wide variety of immune defenses. Exces-

sive dietary fat also reduces natural killer cell activity.

Promoting the growth of friendly bacteria is key. By eating foods teeming with favorable bacteria, you gain significant health advantages, including improved digestive and immune function and better resistance to infections from unfavorable bacteria. Favorable bacteria can be found in cultured foods or taken in supplement form.

BLOOD GROUP A:

1. Basic Antibacterial Protocol
2. Basic Antibiotic Therapy Enhancement Protocol

BLOOD GROUP B:

1. Antibacterial Protocol
2. Antibiotic Support Protocol

BLOOD GROUP AB:

1. Antibacterial Protocol
2. Antibiotic Support Protocol

BLOOD GROUP O:

1. Antibacterial Protocol
2. Antibiotic Support Protocol

Related Topics

Bacterial disease (general)

Food poisoning

Parasitic disease, amoeba

Parasitic disease, *Giardia*

Parasitic disease, hookworm

Toxicity, bowel

Ulcer, *H. pylori*

REFERENCES

1. Fedorovs'ka OO, Nazarchuk LV, Myronenko VI, Mel'nyk OA. The antidiphtheria immunity of the eligible donor population. *Fiziol Zh.* 1997;43:109–112.

BACTERIAL DISEASE, *E. COLI*–*Inflammation of the lining of the stomach and intestines, predominantly manifested by upper gastrointestinal tract symptoms (anorexia, nausea, vomiting), diarrhea, and abdominal discomfort.*

E. coli	SEVERITY/SUSCEPTIBILITY		
	LOW	AVERAGE	HIGH
GROUP A (intestinal)			
GROUP B (gastroenteritis)			
GROUP AB (gastroenteritis)			
GROUP O (diarrhea)			

Symptoms

- Urinary tract infections
- Prostatitis
- Gastroenteritis

About *E. coli*

The symptoms of *Escherichia coli* infection can range from urinary tract infections and prostatitis, to recurring gastroenteritis. *E. coli* organisms can cause bowel inflammation and watery or bloody diarrhea. The extraintestinal site most often infected by *E. coli* is the urinary tract, which is generally colonized from the outside. *E. coli* is an important cause of bacteremia, which often occurs without an overt portal of entry.

There are many variant strains of *Escherichia coli* living in the lower intestinal tract, and the vast majority are well-tolerated by the immune system. There are so many different strains because they are very good at exchanging genetic information, and can mutate at an astounding rate. This ability to mutate resulted in the potentially lethal new O157:H7 variant of *E. coli* that was first recognized in 1982, which can generate diarrheal disease.

E. coli O157:H7 is an emerging cause of foodborne illness, and it results in an estimated 10,000 to 20,000 cases of infection in the United States each year. Unlike the many harmless strains of *E. coli* that coexist in our digestive tracts, *E. coli* O157:H7 produces a powerful toxin that can cause severe illness. Infection will often result in bloody diarrhea, and occasionally progress to KIDNEY FAILURE.

The overwhelming cause of *E. coli* infection is exposure to undercooked, contaminated ground beef. Among the large outbreaks of *E. coli* O157:H7 that have been reported in the United States, a 1993 outbreak that resulted in more than 600 reported cases and four deaths was linked to undercooked hamburgers.

Though vegan enthusiasts tend to emphasize meat as a cause of *E. coli* infection, animal products are not alone in initiating the spread of this infection. Since 1995, raw sprouts have been associated with 13 outbreaks of food-borne disease due to *E. coli* or Salmonella. Contamination of the sprouts themselves, rather than improper handling, is believed to have been the source of the problem. In 1996, more than 6,000 schoolchildren in Japan developed *E. coli* O157:H7 infection after eating contaminated radish sprouts.

E. coli can also be spread by person-to-person contact, so it can and does occur within families and childcare centers. Infection can also occur after drinking raw milk, and after swimming in or ingesting sewage-contaminated water.

In most cases, the infection is limited to diarrhea and cramps, although in advanced cases, the diarrhea can be bloody and debilitating. In fewer than 2% to 7% of those infected, particularly in the very young and the very old, a disorder called hemolytic uremic syndrome (HUS) will develop. A bacterial toxin damages small blood vessels in the kidney, reduces platelet counts, and destroys red blood cells. Kidney function can be greatly impaired, to the degree that dialysis may be necessary. There are no currently available treatments that can prevent HUS once a person is infected with the organism.

This organism is an opportunistic pathogen, causing disease in patients who have defects in host resistance as a result of other disease (e.g., CANCER, DIABETES, CIRRHOSIS) or who have received treatment with corticosteroids, radiation, antineoplastic drugs, or antibiotics.

E. coli bacteremia and meningitis are common in newborns, particularly preterm infants.

Blood Group Links

It appears that many of the variants of *E. coli* have developed individualized tastes for different ABO blood groups. Even their "strategies" differ.

BLOOD GROUP A—ATTACHMENT

Many of the bad forms of *E. coli* express rope-like bundles of filaments, termed bundle-forming pili (BFP), which allow them to attach to the lining of the intestines. These particular *E. coli* have suction cup-like lectins on their pili that attach to the various sugars (glycoproteins or glycolipids), comprising the polysaccharides of the intestinal mucus lining. Many of these sugars are, in fact, particular ABO antigens. For example, certain strains of *E. coli* that colonize the human digestive tract express lectins specific for different glycolipids, called a "globoseries." One such glycolipid, globo-A, is restricted to individuals of blood type A with a positive secretor state[1,2].

BLOOD GROUPS B AND AB—MIMICRY

It appears that many forms of *E. coli* capable of causing diarrhea are immunologically B-like. That is, they possess an antigen on their surface that resembles the antigen that conveys group B blood. Several studies show a higher number of group B and AB people, who cannot manufacture anti-B antibodies, being afflicted with gastroenteritis. In one study, 148 Egyptian patients were studied for parasitic and bacterial infections in relation to ABO blood groups. There were a significantly greater number of blood group B who had cases of *E. coli* (46.15%). The expected frequency of group B should have been around 11%[3].

It has been hypothesized for years that the reason certain individuals manufacture antibodies to other blood types is a result of "inapparent immunization" by bacterial antigens in the gut. The hypothesis that naturally occurring anti-B (in those individuals who are blood group O or A) protects against B-like *E. coli* infection was verified in a second study[4], which examined the blood types of 115 patients with *E. coli* infection, and compared them with three "control" populations: 138 patients with infection due to other organisms; 23,135 hospitalized patients; and 40,038 normal blood donors. The incidence of group B and AB, who cannot make anti-B antibodies, in the *E. coli* infection group was significantly higher than groups A and O, who can manufacture anti-B antibodies.

BLOOD GROUP O — INTERACTION

There is an association between blood group O and the severity of the diarrhea that results from *E. coli* infection. During studies of diarrhea due to *E. coli* in 316 adult volunteers, ABO and Rh blood type determinations were done to look for differences in the severity of illness in association with certain blood groups. Volunteers with group O blood had a significantly higher attack rate for diarrhea than did persons with other blood types[5]. The researchers speculated that there was an interaction between blood group O and the toxin produced by the bacteria.

OF SPECIAL NOTE

There is certainly no substitute for avoidance. However, infection with *E. coli* might at least result in one positive outcome: People recovering from *E. coli*–induced enteritis apparently have higher levels of anti–Thomsen-Friedenreich (T) antibodies. Since the TF antigen is often expressed in cancer cells, it is possible that an *E. coli* infection might protect against certain cancers.

Therapies, *E. coli*

ALL BLOOD GROUPS:

To prevent *E. coli* contamination:

- Avoid eating an undercooked hamburger or other ground beef product in a restaurant.
- Drink only pasteurized milk, juice, or cider.
- Wash fruits, sprouts, and vegetables thoroughly, especially those that will not be cooked.
- Keep raw meat separate from ready-to-eat foods.
- Wash hands, counters, and utensils with hot soapy water after contact with raw meat.
- Never place cooked hamburgers or ground beef on the same plate that held the raw patties.

BLOOD GROUP A:

1. Antibacterial Protocol
2. Immune-Enhancing Protocol
3. Antibiotic Support Protocol

BLOOD GROUP B:

1. Antibacterial Protocol
2. Immune-Enhancing Protocol
3. Antibiotic Support Protocol

BLOOD GROUP AB:

1. Antibacterial Protocol

2. Immune-Enhancing Protocol

3. Antibiotic Support Protocol

BLOOD GROUP O:

1. Antibacterial Protocol

2. Immune-Enhancing Protocol

3. Antibiotic Support Protocol

Related Topics

Bacterial disease (general)

Food poisoning

Immunity

Infectious disease

REFERENCES

1. Yang N, Boettcher B. Development of human ABO blood group A antigen on *Escherichia coli* Y1089 and Y1090. *Immunol Cell Biol.* 1992;70(6):411–416.

2. Lindstedt R, Larson G, Falk P, Jodal U, Leffler H, Svanborg C. The receptor repertoire defines the host range for attaching *Escherichia coli* strains that recognize globo-A. *Infect Immun.* 1991;59:1086–1092.

3. Gabr NS, Mandour AM. Relation of parasitic infection to blood group in El Minia Governorate, Egypt. *J Egypt Soc Parasitol.* 1991;21:679–683.

4. Wittels EG, Lichtman HC. Blood group incidence and *Escherichia coli* bacterial sepsis. *Transfusion.* 1986;26:533–535.

5. Black RE, Levine MM, Clements ML, Hughes T, O'Donnell S. Association between O blood group and occurrence and severity of diarrhea due to *Escherichia coli. Trans R Soc Trop Med Hyg.* 1987;81:120–123.

BACTERIAL DISEASE, GONORRHEA–*Infection of the epithelium of the urethra, cervix, rectum, pharynx, or eyes by* Neisseria gonorrhoeae.

Gonorrhea	SEVERITY/SUSCEPTIBILITY		
	LOW	AVERAGE	HIGH
GROUP A			
GROUP B (Gastroenteritis)			
GROUP AB (Gastroenteritis)			
GROUP O (diarrhea)			
NON-SECRETORS			

Symptoms

Women:

- Vaginal discharge
- Pelvic inflammation and pain
- Abnormal menstrual bleeding
- Rectal itching
- Painful or difficult urination

Men:

- Discharge from the penis
- Painful or difficult urination

About Gonorrhea

Approximately 400,000 cases of gonorrhea are reported to the U.S. Centers for Disease Control and Prevention (CDC) each year in this country. Gonorrhea is caused by the *Neisseria gonorrhoeae* microorganism. This is a sexually transmitted bacterium, and the risk of contracting the infection heightens with multiple sexual partners. Newborns can be infected when passing through the infected birth canal of the mother.

Symptoms usually appear between 2 and 21 days after infection. Untreated in women, the infection can lead to ectopic pregnancy and infertility.

Blood Group Links

The genetically determined inability to secrete the water-soluble glycoprotein form of the ABO blood group antigens into saliva and other body fluids is a recognized risk factor for infection by the *N. gonorrhoeae* bacterium. ABO non-secretors are consistently over-represented among individuals contracting this infection. This over-representation is even greater among individuals who are carriers of the infection[1]. Secretory immune capabilities and other factors appear to contribute to the relative protection against colonization by *N. gonorrhoeae* enjoyed by ABO secretors. ABO non-secretors typically have low levels of salivary gamma M immunoglobulin (IgM), and, both the gamma A immunoglobulin (IgA) and IgM antibodies produced by ABO secretors are more effective at providing protection against this microorganism[2].

Therapies, Gonorrhea

ALL BLOOD GROUPS:

When exposed to the bacterium, any person can contract gonorrhea. The only protection is to avoid unsafe sexual contact. If gonorrhea is contracted, antibiotic therapy is necessary. Historically, penicillin has been used to treat gonorrhea, but four types of antibiotic resistance have emerged. Newer classes of antibiotics or combinations of drugs must be used to treat the resistant strains.

BLOOD GROUP A:

1. Antibacterial Protocol
2. Antibiotic Support Protocol

BLOOD GROUP B:

1. Antibacterial Protocol
2. Antibiotic Support Protocol

BLOOD GROUP AB:

1. Antibacterial Protocol
2. Antibiotic Support Protocol

BLOOD GROUP O:

1. Antibacterial Protocol
2. Antibiotic Support Protocol

Related Topics

Bacterial disease (general)

Fungal disease (all)

Viral disease, hepatitis

REFERENCES

1. Blackwell CC, Weir DM, James VS, et al. Secretor status, smoking, and carriage of Neisseria meningitidis. *Epidemiol Infect.* 1990;104:203–209.

2. Zorgani AA, Stewart J, Blackwell CC, Elton RA, Weir DM. Inhibitory effect of saliva from secretors and non-secretors on binding of meningococci to epithelial cells. *FEMS Immunol Med Microbiol.* 1994;9:135–142.

BACTERIAL DISEASE, *KLEBSIELLA PNEUMONIAE*–*A severe pulmonary infection, caused by infection with* Klebsiella *bacteria.*

Klebsiella *pneumoniae*	SEVERITY/SUSCEPTIBILITY		
	LOW	AVERAGE	HIGH
GROUP A			
GROUP B (INCIDENCE)			
GROUP AB (VIRULENCE)			
GROUP O			

Symptoms

- Severe pneumonia
- Lung abscesses
- Emphysema

About *Klebsiella*

Klebsiella bacterial infections are most common in diabetics and alcoholics. As a rule, *Klebsiella* causes infection in the same sites as does *Escherichia coli*, and they are also an important cause of bacteremia. These infections are usually acquired in the hospital, mainly by patients with diminished host resistance. For this reason, infants in special-care nurseries—who often are sick, preterm, have a low birth weight, and require many supportive invasive procedures—frequently receive antimicrobial therapy. Colonizing bacterial flora tend to be gram-negative organisms.

Klebsiella pneumoniae can cause a rare pulmonary infection characterized by severe PNEUMONIA (sometimes with expectoration of dark brown or red currant-jelly-like sputum), lung abscess formation, and emphysema.

Blood Group Links

Blood group B is associated with a higher overall risk of bacterial infections, especially *Klebsiella*, whereas blood group AB has been shown to encounter greater virulence when infected with *Klebsiella*. Since infection with this strain is associated with diabetes and alcoholism, blood group A and non-secretors should be cautious as well[1].

Therapies, *Klebsiella*

ALL BLOOD GROUPS:

Klebsiella infection is normally contracted in hospitals, when individuals are at their most vulnerable, so it is important to prepare for any hospital visit by making sure your immune system is as strong as possible.

BLOOD GROUP A:

1. Antibacterial Protocol
2. Antibiotic Support Protocol

BLOOD GROUP B:

1. Antibacterial Protocol
2. Antibiotic Support Protocol

BLOOD GROUP AB:

1. Antibacterial Protocol

2. Antibiotic Support Protocol

BLOOD GROUP O:

1. Antibacterial Protocol

2. Antibiotic Support Protocol

Related Topics

Bacterial disease (general)

Bronchitis

Infectious disease

Toxicity, bowel

REFERENCES

1. Kostiuk OP, Chernyshova LI, Slukvin II. Protective effect of Lactobacillus acidophilus on development of infection, caused by *Klebsiella pneumoniae* [in Russian]. *Fiziol Zh.* 1993;39:62–68.

BACTERIAL DISEASE, MENINGITIS–*Severe, life-threatening infection caused by one of several bacterial strains.*

Bacterial meningitis	SUSCEPTIBILITY		
	LOW	AVERAGE	HIGH
GROUP A			
GROUP B			
GROUP AB			
GROUP O			
NON-SECRETORS			

Symptoms

Meningitis can be either viral or bacterial. Viral meningitis is the most common form, and its symptoms are less severe. Bacterial meningitis is more severe, and even life-threatening. Symptoms of bacterial meningitis include:

- Fever, stiff neck/back, and vomiting

- High fever and chills

- Changes in consciousness, including irritability, confusion, lethargy, stupor, delirium, coma (may occur in more serious disease)

- Skin rash (with meningococcal infections)

- Infants: fever, vomiting, shrill/metallic/high-pitched cry; bulging fontanelle; seizures

About Bacterial Meningitis

Bacterial meningitis can be caused by several strains, including *Haemophilus influenzae, Streptococcus pneumoniae,* Group A streptococci, *Escherichia coli, Pseudomonas,* or *Staphylococcus. H. influenzae* is usually the associated microorganism in children 2 months to 3 years old. Pneumococcal meningitis occurs mostly in the over-40 population.

Meningococcal disease is an infection in the fluid and membranes covering the brain and spinal cord. It can be extremely serious. It is spread through coughs and sneezes, and is particularly dangerous for children. Vaccines are recommended for travelers in the so-called "meningitis belt," which are the countries in sub-Saharan Africa extending from Nigeria to Somalia. Countries that experienced outbreaks in the year 2000 included Central African Republic, Niger, Ethiopia, and Sudan. The CDC no longer recommends repeat vaccinations for travelers to Saudi Arabia, Nepal, India, Mongolia, Kenya, Burundi, and Tanzania, where outbreaks were previously reported.

Bacterial meningitis is more severe, and even life-threatening. Bacterial meningitis moves very swiftly through the system, and can become deadly within a 24-hour period if not treated. Bacterial meningitis can be fatal if diagnosed late, or in neonates, the elderly, or the debilitated. In children who survive this infection, 10% will experience neurologic deficits, especially hearing loss.

Blood Group Links

Non-secretors of ABO blood group antigens are over-represented among patients with meningococcal diseases. In one study, total serum and salivary gamma G immunoglobulin (IgG), IgA, and IgM, and levels of these antibodies specific for *Neisseria lactamica* and *meningitidis* were analyzed in 357 of the pupils and staff of a secondary school in which an outbreak of meningitis had occurred. Non-secretors had significantly lower levels of salivary IgM specific for *N. lactamica* and five meningococcal isolates. Researchers determined that secretory IgM played an important role in protecting mucosal surfaces in infants[1], and that non-secretors are more vulnerable to infection.

Further confirmation of non-secretor status as a risk factor for meningococcal disease occurred during a communitywide investigation of a prolonged outbreak of bacterial meningitis in Stonehouse, Gloucestershire. The ABO blood group and secretor status of almost 5,000 residents was determined. The proportion of non-secretors in the Stonehouse population was significantly higher than the proportion of non-secretors among blood donors in the southwest region and in England generally. Seven of 13 Stonehouse residents with meningococcal disease who were tested were found to be non-secretors, a high proportion[2].

Therapies, Bacterial Meningitis

ALL BLOOD GROUPS:

If meningitis is contracted, antibiotic therapy is necessary.

BLOOD GROUP A:

1. Antibacterial Protocol
2. Antibiotic Support Protocol

BLOOD GROUP B:

1. Antibacterial Protocol
2. Antibiotic Support Protocol

BLOOD GROUP AB:

1. Antibacterial Protocol
2. Antibiotic Support Protocol

BLOOD GROUP O:

1. Antibacterial Protocol
2. Antibiotic Support Protocol

Related Topics

Bacterial disease (general)

Infectious disease

REFERENCES

1. Zorgani AA, Stewart J, Blackwell CC, Elton RA, Weir DM. Secretor status and humoral immune responses to Neisseria lactamica and Neisseria meningitidis. *Epidemiol Infect.* 1992;109:445–452.

2. Blackwell CC, Weir DM, James VS, Cartwright KA, Stuart JM, Jones DM. The Stonehouse study: secretor status and carriage of Neisseria species. *Epidemiol Infect.* 1989;102:1–10.

BACTERIAL DISEASE, PNEUMONIA–*An acute infection of lung parenchyma including alveolar spaces and interstitial tissue.*

Bacterial pneumonia	SUSCEPTIBILITY		
	LOW	AVERAGE	HIGH
GROUP A			
GROUP B			
GROUP AB			
GROUP O			

Symptoms

Variable

About Pneumonia

Pneumonia is an inflammation of the lung caused by infection with bacteria, viruses, and other organisms. It is sometimes defined by its distribution as lobar (when it occurs in one lobe of the lungs) or bronchopneumonia (when it is more patchy), but these categories are not gener-ally useful to the physician in determining the cause and treatment of pneumonia. Organisms that cause pneumonia are the important factors. Usually they enter the lungs after being inhaled into the airways. Sometimes the normally harmless bacteria present in the mouth may be aspirated into the lungs, usually if the gag reflex is suppressed. Pneumonia may also be caused from infections that spread to the lungs through the bloodstream from other organs.

Bacteria or other infectious agents that evade the airway defense system are attacked in the air sacs of the lungs (the alveolar sacs) by defenders from the body's immune system, particularly macrophages, large white blood cells that literally eat foreign particles. These strong defense systems normally keep the lung sterile. If these defenses are weakened or damaged, then bacteria or other organisms, such as viruses, fungi, and parasites, can gain the upper hand, producing pneumonia.

The most common cause of pneumonia is the bacterium *Streptococcus pneumoniae.* It accounts for up to half of all cases of community-acquired bacterial pneumonia. Because it is such a common cause of the disease, the bacteria is often called pneumococcus and the pneumonia it causes is called pneumococcal pneumonia. *Staphylococcus aureus,* the other major gram-positive bacterium responsible for pneumonia, accounts for about 10% of bacterial cases. It is uncommon in healthy adults but can develop about 5 days after viral influenza, usually in susceptible individuals such as people with weakened immune systems, very young children, hospitalized patients, and injection drug users.

The symptoms of bacterial pneumonia develop abruptly and may include chest pain, fever, shaking, chills, shortness of breath, and rapid breathing and heartbeat. Symptoms of pneumonia indicating a medical emergency include high fever, a rapid heart rate, low blood pressure, bluish skin (cyanosis), and mental confusion. Coughing up sputum containing pus or blood is an indication of serious infection. Severe abdominal pain may accompany pneumonia occurring in the lower lobes of the lung. Breathing may become labored and heavy.

Older people may have fewer or different symptoms than younger people. An elderly person who experiences even a minor COUGH and weakness for more than a day should seek medical help. Some may exhibit confusion, lethargy, and general deterioration.

Risk factors for developing pneumonia include upper respiratory tract infections, malnutrition, hospitalization, debility or immobilization, ALCOHOLISM, exposure, coma, inhalation of bacterial agents, foreign object aspiration into the lungs, decreased cough reflex (e.g., from smoking), EMPHYSEMA or BRONCHITIS, major bony abnormalities or deformities (e.g., severe kyphoscoliosis), bronchial tumors, and treatment with immunosuppressive drugs.

The infection spreads into the blood in 20% to 30% of cases; when this occurs, up to 30% of those patients die.

Blood Group Links

Blood group B is highly susceptible to the most common cause of pneumonia, the bacterium *S. pneumoniae.* Streptococcal disease occurs more often in type Bs than other blood types, resulting in STREP THROAT, or more serious illnesses such as TOXIC SHOCK SYNDROME, bacteremia, and pneumonia. A severe form of streptococcal disease occurs primarily among neonates. The consequences of this infection can be SEPSIS, pneumonia, and MENINGITIS. Neurologic complications can also occur, resulting in loss of sight or hearing, and mental retardation. Death occurs in 6% of infants and 16% of adults. There is also a connection between blood type B and neonatal group B streptococcal infection. This association is strong enough to be demonstrated even based on the mother's blood type; that is, a type-B infant with a type-B mother has double the risk[1].

Therapies, Pneumonia

ALL BLOOD GROUPS:

A vaccine (Pneumovax) is available and is recommended for people who have DIABETES or steroid-dependent ASTHMA, and for alcoholics, smokers, and those who have had their spleen removed.

BLOOD GROUP A:

1. Antibacterial Protocol
2. Antibiotic Support Protocol

BLOOD GROUP B:

1. Antibacterial Protocol
2. Antibiotic Support Protocol

BLOOD GROUP AB:

1. Antibacterial Protocol
2. Antibiotic Support Protocol

BLOOD GROUP O:

1. Antibacterial Protocol

2. Antibiotic Support Protocol

Related Topics

Bacterial disease (general)

Bronchitis

Immunity

Infectious disease

Influenza

REFERENCES

1. Haverkorn MK, Goslings WR. Streptococci, ABO blood groups, and secretor status. *Am J Hum Genet.* 1969;21:360–375.

BACTERIAL DISEASE, *SHIGELLA*–*Infection caused by contaminated food.*

Shigella	VIRULENCE		
	LOW	AVERAGE	HIGH
GROUP A			
GROUP B			
GROUP AB			
GROUP O			

Symptoms

- Sudden onset of fever
- Irritability
- Drowsiness
- Anorexia
- Nausea
- Vomiting
- Diarrhea
- Abdominal pain and distention
- Blood, pus, and mucus in fecal stool

About *Shigella*

The source of *Shigella* infection is the excreta of infected individuals, so the bacteria may be indirectly spread by contaminated food. The incubation period is 1 to 4 days.

Blood Group Links

Blood group B is most susceptible to *Shigella* infection. A study on the distribution of ABO blood groups was carried out on 85 patients with clinically and bacteriologically proven shigellosis. A significant association of blood group B was observed with shigellosis cases in comparison to controls from whom no *Shigella* species or other enteropathogen could be isolated.

In 1991, a study done in India linked the gastrointestinal pathogen *Shigella* to blood groups that cannot manufacture anti-B antibodies (groups B and AB). The study was conducted on 85 patients with clinically and bacteriologically proven *Shigella* infection. A significant association with blood group B was observed in comparison to individuals who had no *Shigella* infection[1].

Therapies, *Shigella*

ALL BLOOD GROUPS:

Adhere to food safety guidelines:

- Drink only pasteurized milk, juice, or cider.
- Wash fruits, sprouts, and vegetables thoroughly, especially those that will not be cooked.
- Keep raw meat separate from ready-to-eat foods.
- Wash hands, counters, and utensils with hot soapy water after contact with raw meat.
- Never place cooked hamburgers or ground beef on the same plate that held the raw patties.
- Rinse meat and poultry with cold water before cooking to remove some of the bacteria.
- Cook poultry until there is no pink meat. If you use a meat thermometer, check to see that the meat reaches an internal temperature of 180° to 185°F (82.2° to 85°C). Make sure to insert the thermometer into the thickest part of the chicken—the thigh, away from the bone—to get the most accurate reading.

Adhere to safe-travel guidelines. If you are traveling to an underdeveloped country, adhere to the following guidelines:

- Avoid raw or undercooked meat and seafood.
- Avoid raw vegetables and fruit, unless peeled.
- Avoid tap water and ice made from tap water.
- Avoid buying food from street vendors.
- Take along water-purifying tablets (available in pharmacies and sporting goods stores) if you are hiking or backpacking through undeveloped areas.
- Check travel guides for restaurants that have high food safety standards.
- Use bottled water for drinking and brushing your teeth, even in hotels. Carbonated water may be the safest, since carbonation appears to kill some of the microorganisms. Be sure that the bottles have been properly sealed.

BLOOD GROUP A:

1. Antibacterial Protocol
2. Antibiotic Support Protocol

BLOOD GROUP B:

1. Antibacterial Protocol
2. Antibiotic Support Protocol

BLOOD GROUP AB:

1. Antibacterial Protocol
2. Antibiotic Support Protocol

BLOOD GROUP O:

1. Antibacterial Protocol
2. Antibiotic Support Protocol

Related Topics

Bacterial disease (general)

Food poisoning

Infectious disease

Toxicity, bowel

REFERENCES

1. Sinha AK, Bhattacharya SK, Sen D, Dutta P, Dutta D, Bhattacharya MK, Pal SC Blood group and shigellosis. *J Assoc Physicians India*. 1991;39:452–453.

BACTERIAL DISEASE, STAPHYLOCOCCAL INFECTION–*Infection with* Staphylococcus aureus.

Staphylococcal Infection	SUSCEPTIBILITY		
	LOW	AVERAGE	HIGH
GROUP A (INCIDENCE)			
GROUP B			
GROUP AB (VIRULENCE)			
GROUP O			
RH NEGATIVE			

Symptoms

Staphylococcal (staph) infections can be caused by bacterial or viral microorganisms. Symptoms may include:

- Redness
- Fever
- Signs of malaise such as lethargy or anorexia

About Staph Infections

Staphylococcus aureus (S. aureus) is a gram-positive bacterium, responsible for about 10% of all cases of bacterial PNEUMONIA. It is uncommon in healthy adults but can develop about 5 days after viral influenza, usually in susceptible individuals such as people with weakened immune systems, very young children, hospitalized patients, and injection drug users.

Blood Group Links

Blood group A is prone to more malignant staphylococcal (staph) infections. In one study, 326 employees of four medical institutions (one regional hospital, two city hospitals, and a maternity clinic) were examined for the presence of *S. aureus* every 3 months over a period of 3 years. The results of these examinations were compared with the distribution of the blood groups in the ABO system among the carriers of staph organisms. Constant and malignant carrier states were detected mainly in persons with blood group A[1].

Considerable evidence has been accumulated showing that carbohydrate-containing blood group substances represent prime candidates for the specific interaction with microbial surface lectins in infectious diseases. Accordingly, clinical studies have proved that urinary tract infections by *Staphylococcus saprophyticus* can be positively correlated with a patient's blood type. Apparently, the blood type antigens (terminal carbohydrates) represent receptors recognized by *S. saprophyticus* and *Pseudomonas aeruginosa* surface lectins. The group A carbohydrate pattern is important for colonization. Blood group AB is associated with the most virulent infection when the urinary tract is involved[2].

When the blood of 100 adults living in Budapest was examined for certain bacterial antibodies, they were found to be lower in the Rh-negative than the Rh-positive persons[3]. Additionally, there is further evidence of an increased susceptibility for Rh-negative individuals.

Therapies, Staph Infections

BLOOD GROUP A:

1. Antibacterial Protocol

2. Antibiotic Support Protocol

BLOOD GROUP B:

1. Antibacterial Protocol

2. Antibiotic Support Protocol

BLOOD GROUP AB:

1. Antibacterial Protocol

2. Antibiotic Support Protocol

BLOOD GROUP O:

1. Antibacterial Protocol

2. Antibiotic Support Protocol

Related Topics

Bacterial disease (general)

Immunity

Infectious disease

Toxicity, bowel

REFERENCES

1. Geisel J, Steuer MK, Ko HL, Beuth J. The role of ABO blood groups in infections induced by Staphylococcus sap-rophyticus and Pseudomonas aeruginosa. *Zentralbl Bakteriol.* 1995;282:427–430.

2. Beuth J, Ko HL, Tunggal L, Pulverer G. Urinary tract infections caused by Staphylococcus saprophyticus. Increased incidence depending on the blood group. *Dtsch Med Wochenschr.* 1992;117:687–691.

3. Veres, J. Natural antibodies in healthy adults. *Acta Microbiol Acad Sci Hung.* 1975;22:65–73.

BACTERIAL DISEASE, TUBERCULOSIS–

A chronic, recurrent infection, most commonly detected in the lungs.

Tuberculosis	SUSCEPTIBILITY/VIRULENCE		
	LOW	AVERAGE	HIGH
GROUP A	░		
GROUP B (ASIANS GREATEST INCIDENCE)	░	░	░
GROUP AB	░	░	
GROUP O (VIRULENCE)	░	░	
RH NEGATIVE (EUROPEANS WORST OUTCOME)	░	░	░

Symptoms

▪ A bad cough that lasts longer than 2 weeks

▪ Pain in the chest

▪ Coughing up blood or sputum (phlegm from deep inside the lungs)

▪ Weakness or fatigue

▪ Weight loss

▪ Lack of appetite

- Chills
- Fever
- Night sweats

About Tuberculosis

At the turn of the twentieth century, TB was the leading cause of death in the United States. This infection is caused by bacteria called *Mycobacterium tuberculosis*, which can attack any part of the body, but usually attacks the lungs. In the 1940s, scientists discovered the first of several drugs now used to treat TB, which resulted in a slow and steady decline in TB infection in the United States. However, a more powerful, drug-resistant TB has been making a comeback. Since 1984, the number of TB cases reported in the United States has increased, with more than 25,000 cases reported in 1993.

TB is spread through the air from one person to another, generally by an infected person either coughing or sneezing. In most people who breathe in TB bacteria and become infected, the body keeps the bacteria, at least initially, in check. The bacteria become inactive, but they remain alive in the body and can become active later. Many people who have TB infection never develop TB disease. In these people, the TB bacteria remain inactive for a lifetime without causing disease. But in others, especially people who have weak immune systems, the bacteria becomes active and causes TB disease. Those at greatest risk include urban dwellers, the homeless, migrant workers, people living in institutions (such as prisons or nursing homes). Health care workers and others who have close contact with infected individuals are at risk.

Children traveling to developing countries may be at increased risk for tuberculosis infection and should be screened when they return. High rates of TB are found in Mexico, China, Hong Kong, Taiwan, Central America, the Philippines, Vietnam, India, Haiti, and South Korea. There have also been a few reports of tuberculosis among airline passengers exposed to TB during long flights. The bacille Calmette-Guérin (BCG) vaccine is used in most developing countries to reduce the severe consequences of tuberculosis in children. Its effectiveness has varied from 0 to 76% in major studies, however; it is not routinely used in the United States.

There is no visible onset of the disease; signs become apparent when a lesion is large enough to be seen on an x-ray. Fever, malaise, and weight loss are very gradual and often go unnoticed. A TB skin test is the only way to find out if you have a TB infection. A skin test can be procured at the health department or at your doctor's office.

Blood Group Links

Tuberculosis runs a much more aggressive and detrimental course in blood group O, while blood group A is afforded the highest degree of protection. A further complicating factor appears to be ethnic background. Group Os of European lineage have a greater susceptibility and a poorer outcome than group Os from other backgrounds. Among Asians, group B has higher rates of infection and severer forms of tuberculosis. Rh-positive or Rh-negative blood type might have some impact on tuberculosis survival as well. Research demonstrates that more Rh-negative persons have died from tuberculosis, while a higher percentage of Rh-positive persons have survived.

Therapies, Tuberculosis

ALL BLOOD GROUPS:

The best defense against TB is to avoid contact with someone who has active TB. If you're at high risk, get a skin test every 6 months. It takes 72 hours after a skin test has been given to indicate whether you've been infected with the TB bacteria. However, a skin test may not be positive until you've had the TB bacteria in your system for several weeks.

BLOOD GROUP A:

1. Antibacterial Protocol
2. Antibiotic Support Protocol

BLOOD GROUP B:

1. Antibacterial Protocol
2. Antibiotic Support Protocol

BLOOD GROUP AB:

1. Antibacterial Protocol
2. Antibiotic Protocol

BLOOD GROUP O:

1. Antibacterial Protocol
2. Antibiotic Support Protocol

Related Topics

Bacterial disease (general)

Infectious disease

BACTERIAL DISEASE, TYPHOID—*A systemic disease caused by* Salmonella typhi *and characterized by fever, prostration, abdominal pain, and a rose-colored rash.*

Typhoid	SUSCEPTIBILITY		
	LOW	AVERAGE	HIGH
GROUP A	▓	▓	▓
GROUP B (MEN)	▓	▓	▓
GROUP AB	▓	▓	▓
GROUP O	▓		
RH NEGATIVE	▓	▓	▓

Symptoms

- Fever
- Headache
- Malaise
- Abdominal discomfort/bloating/constipation
- Diarrhea
- Dry cough
- Confusion
- Lethargy
- Cervical adenopathy
- Bradycardia
- Conjunctivitis

About Typhoid

Typhoid is an acute systemic illness unique to humans, caused by *Salmonella typhi*. It is a classic example of a FEVER caused by the *Salmonella* family of bacteria. It is endemic in some developing nations where sanitation is poor. The majority of cases in North America are acquired after travel to such regions. The most common means of transmission are fecal to oral through ingestion of contaminated food, most often poultry, water, and milk. The incubation period varies from 7 to 21 days. Typhoid must be considered in any patient who has a fever after having traveled to tropical parts of the world, or who has been exposed to a chronic carrier.

Blood Group Links

Blood group A appears to be more susceptible to typhoid bacilli infection. Blood groups of the ABO system were studied in 186 chronic carriers of typhoid bacilli, and in 392 patients with typhoid fever from various districts of Uzbekistan. In comparison with healthy persons, group A had a higher number of infections than did group O. These data demonstrated the predisposition of persons with blood group A to the chronic typhoid carrier state. It was a characteristic of the Asian part of the country. In comparison, there were significantly fewer persons with blood group O who were infected, and more with blood group AB. The researchers suggested a correlation between the specific blood type and the typhoid infection[1].

The B antigen appears to be protective for women, but may also be responsible for an increase in susceptibility in men. Rh-negative people have an increased risk of becoming ill with typhoid.

Therapies, Typhoid

ALL BLOOD GROUPS:

Adhere to safe-travel guidelines. If you are traveling to an underdeveloped country, adhere to the following guidelines:

- Avoid raw or undercooked meat and seafood.
- Avoid raw vegetables and fruit, unless peeled.
- Avoid tap water and ice made from tap water.
- Avoid buying food from street vendors.
- Take along water-purifying tablets (available in pharmacies and sporting goods stores) if you are hiking or backpacking through undeveloped areas.
- Check travel guides for restaurants that have high food safety standards.
- Use bottled water for drinking and brushing your teeth, even in hotels. Carbonated water may be the safest, since carbonation appears to kill some of the microorganisms. Be sure that the bottles have been properly sealed.

To prevent *Salmonella* poisoning:

- Rinse meat and poultry with cold water before cooking to remove some of the bacteria.
- Cook poultry until there is no pink meat. If you use a meat thermometer, check to see that

the meat reaches an internal temperature of 180° to 185°F (82.2° to 85°C). Make sure to insert the thermometer into the thickest part of the chicken—the thigh, away from the bone—to get the most accurate reading.

- Keep utensils and cutting boards used to prepare meat and poultry separate from those used to prepare fruit and vegetables. For example, if you prepare a mixed chicken and vegetable dish, use a separate knife and cutting board for the chicken, and another for the vegetables.

- Wash thoroughly all the utensils you use to prepare raw meat and poultry with hot, soapy water. Dishwasher water is hot enough.

- Keep wood cutting boards clean by washing them every few days with a diluted bleach-and-water solution. The bleach should kill any bacteria.

- Don't partially cook meat ahead of time.

In addition to rigorous attention to hygiene and avoidance of contaminated foods, your best defense is a healthy immune system. Nutrition is a major contributor to the functioning of the immune system, which in turn influences whether the body can maintain peak resistance to infection. Specifically, it makes sense to restrict sugar, because sugar interferes with the ability of white blood cells to destroy bacteria. Alcohol interferes with a wide variety of immune defenses. Excessive dietary fat also reduces natural killer cell activity.

Promoting the growth of friendly bacteria is key. By eating foods teeming with favorable bacteria, you gain significant health advantages, including improved digestive and immune function

and better resistance to infections from unfavorable bacteria. Consume friendly bacteria in cultured foods or take in supplement form.

BLOOD GROUP A:

1. Antibacterial Protocol
2. Antibiotic Support Protocol
3. Immune-Enhancing Protocol

BLOOD GROUP B:

1. Antibacterial Protocol
2. Antibiotic Support Protocol
3. Immune-Enhancing Protocol

BLOOD GROUP AB:

1. Antibacterial Protocol
2. Antibiotic Support Protocol

BLOOD GROUP O:

1. Antibacterial Protocol
2. Antibiotic Support Protocol

Related Topics

Bacterial disease (general)

Food poisoning

Immunity

Infectious disease

References

1. Nevskii MV, Lerenman MI, Iusupov KI, Aminzada ZM, Vedenskaia VA. [Blood groups of the ABO system of chronic carriers of typhoid bacteria and typhoid patients in Uzbekistan]. *Zh Mikrobiol Epidemiol Immunobiol.* 1976;8:66–69.

BACTERIAL DISEASE, *YERSINIA* (PLAGUE)–*An acute, severe infection appearing most commonly in a bubonic or pneumonic form, caused by the bacillus* Yersinia pestis.

Yersinia (plague)	SUSCEPTIBILITY		
	LOW	AVERAGE	HIGH
GROUP A	▓		
GROUP B	▓		
GROUP AB	▓		
GROUP O	▓		▓

Symptoms

- Acute gastroenteritis
- Arthritis
- Septicemia
- Acute diarrhea

About Plague

Plague occurs primarily in wild rodents (such as rats, mice, squirrels, and prairie dogs). Massive human epidemics have occurred, such as the Black Death of the Middle Ages. Plague continues to flare among humans sporadically. It has been reported worldwide, including outbreaks in Vietnam and Zambia in the 1990s. In the United States, 90% of cases of human plague have been in the southwestern states, especially New Mexico, Arizona, California, and Colorado.

Yersinia is transmitted through food, water, and person-to-person contact. The usual course is severe and often fatal.

Bubonic plague is the most common form. Plague bacteria are carried by rodents and transmitted by fleas. Plague is transmitted from rodents to humans by the bite of an infected flea. Human-to-human transmission occurs by inhaling droplet nuclei from the coughs of patients with bubonic or septicemic plague who have pulmonary lesions (primary pneumonic plague).

Most plagues are transmitted by handling infected animals. An exception is the Indian pneumonic plague, which can be passed in the air, although the risk of picking it up is very low. The source is often ingestion of contaminated food.

Blood Group Links

Yersinia produces an antigen that mimics the H antigen of blood group O, and O does not produce antibodies against it[1]. Without doubt many of those who did succumb to the plague in medieval times were blood group O[2], and the effect was probably to redress the population balance toward more blood group A.

Therapies, *Yersinia* (Plague)

ALL BLOOD GROUPS:

Adhere to safe-travel guidelines. If you are traveling to an underdeveloped country, adhere to the following guidelines:

- Avoid raw or undercooked meat and seafood.
- Avoid raw vegetables and fruit, unless peeled.

- Avoid tap water and ice made from tap water.

- Avoid buying food from street vendors.

- Take along water-purifying tablets (available in pharmacies and sporting goods stores) if you are hiking or backpacking through undeveloped areas.

- Check travel guides for restaurants that have high food safety standards.

- Use bottled water for drinking and brushing your teeth, even in hotels. Carbonated water may be the safest, since carbonation appears to kill some of the microorganisms. Be sure that the bottles have been properly sealed.

Travelers should wear insect repellents and avoid handling any animals. People traveling to countries with plague outbreaks may consider taking preventive antibiotics, tetracycline or doxycycline. (Children would take sulfonamides.) A vaccine is also available and should be considered for travelers to high-risk regions.

BLOOD GROUP A:

1. Antibacterial Protocol

2. Antibiotic Support Protocol

BLOOD GROUP B:

1. Antibacterial Protocol

2. Antibiotic Support Protocol

BLOOD GROUP AB:

1. Antibacterial Protocol

2. Antibiotic Support Protocol

BLOOD GROUP O:

1. Antibacterial Protocol

2. Antibiotic Support Protocol

3. Immune-Enhancing Protocol

Related Topics

Bacterial disease (general)

Infectious disease

REFERENCES

1. Kaneko K, et al. Prevalence of O agglutinins against the epizootic strains of Yersinia pseudo tuberculosis serovars IB and IVA in barn rats. *Nippon Juigaku Zasshi.* 1982;44:375–377.

2. Zhukov-Berezhnilov NN, Adamov AK, Anisimov PI, Bochko GM, Podopletov II. Heterogenetic antigens of plague and cholera microbes, similar to antigens of human and animal tissues [in Russian]. *Biull Eksp Biol Med.* 1972;73:63–65.

BAD BREATH–*See Halitosis*

BARRETT'S ESOPHAGUS–*A pre-cancerous condition in the cells lining the esophagus.*

Barrett's esophagus	INCIDENCE		
	LOW	AVERAGE	HIGH
GROUP A (WITH GERD)			
GROUP B			
GROUP AB			
GROUP O			

Symptoms

- Heartburn

- Regurgitation

- Trouble swallowing
- Chest pain
- Bronchospasm
- Laryngitis
- Chronic cough
- Loss of dental enamel

About Barrett's Esophagus

Barrett's esophagus involves pre-cancerous changes in the cells lining the esophagus. This pre-cancerous condition afflicts between 10% and 20% of people who suffer from chronic GASTROE-SOPHAGEAL REFLUX DISEASE (GERD). Barrett's esophagus can be a precursor to both ESOPHAGEAL CANCER and STOMACH CANCER.

GERD can be caused by a number of conditions. Hiatal hernia due to acid trapping may be a cause of reflux. Infection with H. PYLORI has also been linked to GERD. Cigarette smoking, and excessive alcohol and coffee all lower pressure on the lower esophageal sphincter. In children, Down syndrome, mental retardation, cerebral palsy, or a repaired tracheal esophageal fistula may predispose a child to esophageal irritation. However, the more common reason so many people are afflicted with chronic HEARTBURN is poor dietary habits.

In the United States, over the 1980s and 1990s, the incidence of esophageal cancer increased more rapidly than any other type of cancer. Unfortunately, patients who develop esophageal cancer subsequent to Barrett's esophagus typically have a poor prognosis, because the cancer is often discovered at an advanced stage for which a cure is difficult.

Blood Group Links

Barrett's esophagus has been linked to blood group A, as have stomach and esophageal cancers. Barrett's esophagus and esophageal cancer also have a positive association with Lewis (a+b−) non-secretor phenotypes[1].

Barrett's esophagus has also been linked to the ulcer-causing bacteria *H. pylori*, which is implicated in the development of gastric ulcers. *H. pylori* predominantly afflicts group O not group A. However, pre-malignant cells secrete copious amounts of blood group antigens, and many people who are phenotypically group A are genotypically AO, and thus can secrete the O antigen as well as the A antigen. In addition, low stomach acid, common in group A, increases the growth of bacteria[2].

Therapies, Barrett's Esophagus

ALL BLOOD GROUPS:

1. Avoid lying down directly after meals.
2. Walk upright, not in a stooped position that causes esophageal pressure.
3. Don't wear tight-fitting garments.
4. Avoid drugs that increase pressure on the lower esophageal sphincter.
5. If you are overweight, lose weight to help in decreasing the pressure.

BLOOD GROUP A:

1. Stomach Health Protocol
2. Immune-Enhancing Protocol
3. Cancer Prevention Protocol

BLOOD GROUP B:

1. Stomach Health Protocol

2. Immune-Enhancing Protocol

BLOOD GROUP AB:

1. Stomach Health Protocol

2. Immune-Enhancing Protocol

3. Cancer Prevention Protocol

BLOOD GROUP O:

1. Stomach Health Protocol

2. Immune-Enhancing Protocol

3. Antibacterial Protocol

Related Topics

Cancer (general)

Cancer, esophageal

Cancer, stomach

Digestion

Gastroesophageal reflux disease (GERD)

REFERENCES

1. Mufti SI, Zirvi KA, Garewal HS. Precancerous lesions and biologic markers in esophageal cancer. *Cancer Detect Prev.* 1991;15:291–301.

2. Torrado J, Ruiz B, Garay J, et al. Blood-group phenotypes, sulfomucins, and Helicobacter pylori in Barrett's esophagus. *Am J Surg Pathol.* 1997;21:1023–1029.

BENIGN PROSTATIC HYPERPLASIA–*See Prostatic hyperplasia, benign*

BIPOLAR DEPRESSION–*See Depression, bipolar*

BIRTH DEFECTS–*Conditions, often severe or fatal, arising from abnormal fetal development.*

About Birth Defects

Prenatal diagnosis of birth defects may be possible by the use of ultrasonography, amniocentesis, or chorionic villus sampling. Obstetric factors that may suggest an anomaly include breech presentation; polyhydramnios, which may result from difficulty in swallowing (e.g., due to severe central nervous system disorders such as anencephaly) or blockage of the gastrointestinal tract (e.g., due to esophageal atresia); and oligohydramnios (rupture of amniotic membranes), which may be caused by low urine output due to genitourinary anomalies.

Among the most common birth defects are:

Anencephaly: A neural tube defect, resulting in the inability of the fetus to develop a brain.

Cystic fibrosis: Failure of the pancreas to produce digestive enzymes.

Down syndrome: The development of an extra chromosome in each cell.

Spina bifida: A neural tube defect, causing deformity of the spinal column.

General Risk Factors and Causes

Risk factors include genetics, nutrient deficiencies (e.g., folic acid), environmental influences on fetuses, and maternal exposure to teratogenic substances, and drug and alcohol use during pregnancy.

Blood Group Links

Blood group incompatibility, which may occur between a blood group O mother and a blood group A father, has been implicated in several common birth defects, including hydatiform mole, choriocarcinoma, spina bifida, and anencephaly. Several studies suggest that these disorders are caused by maternal blood group incompatibility with the fetal nervous system tissue and blood tissue.

The Rh Factor and Hemolytic Disease of the Newborn

Hemolytic (blood destroying) disease of the newborn is the primary condition related to the rhesus factor. It is a condition that only afflicts the offspring of Rh-negative women.

Some 50 years ago, researchers discovered that Rh-negative women, who were missing the Rh antigen, faced a special problem when their babies were Rh-positive and carried the Rh antigen on their blood cells. Unlike the major blood group system, where the antibodies to other blood types develop from birth, Rh-negative people do not make an antibody to the Rh antigen unless they are first sensitized. This sensitization usually occurs when blood is exchanged between the mother and infant during birth; the mother's immune system does not have enough time to react to the first baby, and so that baby suffers no consequences. However, should a subsequent concep-

tion result in another Rh-positive baby, the mother, now sensitized, will produce antibodies to the baby's blood type, potentially causing birth defects and even infant death. Fortunately, there is a vaccine that has been developed for this condition, which is given to Rh-negative women after the birth of their first child, and then after every subsequent birth.

Therapies, Birth Defects

BLOOD GROUP A:

1. Female Balancing Protocol
2. Male Health Protocol

BLOOD GROUP B:

1. Female Balancing Protocol
2. Male Health Protocol

BLOOD GROUP AB:

1. Female Balancing Protocol
2. Male Health Protocol

BLOOD GROUP O:

1. Female Balancing Protocol
2. Male Health Protocol

Related Topics

Infertility

BLADDER CANCER–*See Cancer, bladder*

BLADDER INFECTION–*See Cystitis*

Blood Cells

Blood is composed of 60% plasma and 40% cells and platelets.

Plasma a straw-colored liquid that is mostly water, transports most of the molecules needed by cells, as well as their waste products.

Red blood cells account for blood's characteristic color. These cells are designed to carry oxygen. A mature red blood cell lacks a nucleus and mitochondria; instead, the cell is almost entirely filled with molecules of hemoglobin, a protein structure that collects oxygen in the lungs and releases it in the tissues. Each hemoglobin molecule contains four long protein chains, each wrapped around a much smaller molecule called heme. Each heme molecule contains a single atom of iron, which enables it to combine with oxygen molecules. One hemoglobin molecule can hold up to four oxygen molecules. Because mature red blood cells lack nuclei, they cannot repair themselves, and will die off within a few months. Thus, the body must continually manufacture new red blood cells to replace those that die. All blood cells are produced by bone marrow, the spongy material in the middle of bones. Bone marrow contains a small number of cells called hematopoietic stem cells, the building blocks for all other blood cells.

White blood cells are larger, nearly colorless, and less plentiful than red blood cells. White blood cells perform the vital function of defending the body against foreign invaders such as viruses and bacteria. Different types of white blood cells perform different functions. Granulocytes attack invading microbes by engulfing and digesting them. Monocytes settle in the lymph nodes and organs, where they trap microbes that manage to slip through the initial defenses. Lymphocytes occur in two forms: B lymphocytes and T lymphocytes, also known as B cells and T cells. These cells produce antibodies in response to the detection of foreign antigens.

Platelets are tiny disks, smaller than red blood cells. They are fragments of much larger cells found in bone marrow. Platelets contain chemicals that initiate the blood clotting process. When tissue is torn, the plasma launches a complex chain of chemical reactions. Ultimately, the fibrinogen protein in plasma is converted to fibrin molecules, which clump together to form a mesh at the injury site. This mesh traps red blood cells and platelets, forming a clot.

BLOOD CLOTTING DISORDERS– *The inability of blood to properly clot following damage to blood vessels.*

Blood clotting disorders	SEVERITY		
	LOW	AVERAGE	HIGH
GROUP A			
GROUP B			
GROUP AB			
GROUP O			
NON-SECRETORS			

Symptoms

- Easy bruising
- Long bleeding time
- Clots

Minor trauma can result in extensive tissue hemorrhages and hemarthroses, which, if improperly managed, can result in crippling musculoskeletal deformities. Bleeding into the base of the tongue, causing airway compression, may be life threatening; it requires prompt, vigorous replacement therapy. Even a trivial blow to the head requires replacement therapy to prevent intracranial bleeding.

About Blood Clotting

When blood vessels are cut or damaged, the loss of blood from the system must be stopped before shock and possible death occur. This is accomplished by solidification of the blood at the wound site, a process called coagulation or clotting. The bloodstream contains special non-living components called platelets, which are responsible for blood's clotting abilities. In its most simple sense, a blood clot consists of a plug of platelets enmeshed in a network of insoluble protein molecules called fibrin.

Platelet aggregation and fibrin formation both require the enzyme thrombin. Clotting also requires calcium, which is why blood banks use a chelating agent to bind the calcium in donated blood so that the blood will not clot in the bag.

There are at least a dozen other protein clotting factors, and most of these circulate in the blood as inactive enzyme precursors. Many of the well-known bleeding disorders (such as hemophilia) result from the absence of one or more of these clotting factors.

The various clotting factors act as a cascade, originating with injury to the blood vessel, and ending with the conversion of inactive prothrombin into thrombin, which activates the platelets to aggregate, forming the clot. This begins when damaged cells make a surface protein called tissue factor, which activates dormant clotting factors present in blood. Each activated clotting factor converts still other inactive factors into active ones, much like a phone tree might cascade out to alert people of an emergency. Thus, what begins as a tiny, localized event rapidly expands into a cascade of activity.

Blood Group Links

Unlike the other factors, factor VIII is not an enzyme. Factor VIII normally circulates in the plasma bound to VON WILLEBRAND FACTOR (vWF). When thrombin is activated by injury to the vessel wall, it chops factor VIII free from von Willebrand factor and activates it. Von Willebrand factor goes on to bind to the ruptured blood vessel surface, where it stimulates platelets to stick together. Active factor VIII (now called factor VIIIa) reacts with another factor (factor IXa) and calcium to help localize the site of clot formation to the injured vessel.

High levels of factor VIII have been linked to CORONARY ARTERY DISEASE, and this may in part explain why coronary artery disease shows a higher rate of occurrence in blood groups A and AB. For example, there is evidence that hemophiliacs experience less coronary artery disease than expected, so high factor VIII levels may contribute to the incidence of coronary artery disease by increasing one's potential for developing blood clots.

ABO non-secretors are reported to have shorter bleeding times and a tendency toward higher factor VIII and vWF. This relationship appears to be another example of blood type synergy between ABO and secretor/non-secretor phenotypes. In fact, secretor genetics appear to interact with ABO genetics to influence as much as 60% of the variance of the plasma concentration of vWF, with secretors (Lewis (a−b+)) having the lowest vWF concentrations[1,2].

Blood group O is most likely to have problems with clotting, having the lowest concentration of von Willebrand antigen (vWF:Ag) and factor VIII antigen (VIII:Ag)—especially O secretors. Blood group O non-secretors will have a higher concentration of both vWF:Ag and VIII:Ag, providing them with a better ability to clot[3].

Based upon these findings, researchers have suggested that the Lewis (a−b−) phenotype (and blood groups A, B, and AB especially), by virtue of their association with raised levels of factor VIII and von Willebrand factor, might be at a higher risk for future thrombotic disease and HEART DISEASE[4].

A study at St. Bartholomew's Hospital, London linked the relationship between blood group, factor VIII activity, von Willebrand factor antigen and ISCHEMIC HEART DISEASE in 1,393 men aged 40 to 64 years. The incidence of heart disease was significantly higher in those of blood group AB than in those of groups O, A, or B, particularly for fatal events. In addition, they theorized that blood type AB may be a genetic marker of characteristics influencing other risks for heart disease such as short stature, as the type AB men studied were on average about 2 cm shorter than the men in the other groups[5].

Measurements of von Willebrand factor antigen and factor VIII in a group of 40 blood donors (20 of group O, 20 of group A) showed reduced levels of both clotting factors in group O, compared with the other blood groups. The data suggest an influence of blood group antigens on the interaction between von Willebrand factor and platelets[6].

A study of pairs of twins showed that the concentration of factor VIII was lowest in group O individuals, higher in A2 individuals, and highest in A1 and B individuals. The authors concluded that "thirty percent of the genetic variance of VIII was due to the effect of ABO blood type. The ABO locus is therefore a major locus for the determination of factor VIII concentration"[7].

Blood group ABO antigens are known to be carried by glycoproteins found on platelets. Besides these proteins, blood group A antigen was expressed on other platelet proteins as well[8,9]. Thus, it appears that the genetic expression of blood type in blood group A individuals has some intimate effect on the function of their platelets.

To investigate possible associations between ABO blood system and coagulability levels, fibrinolysis, total lipids, cholesterol, and triglycerides, the plasma and serum of 300 Rh-positive male blood donors were tested. Analysis of the laboratory data showed a lower coagulability in O blood group individuals. This result was obtained in coagulation tests specific for factor VIII level. In addition, a higher sensitivity to the in vitro heparin anticoagulant effect in O group individuals was confirmed. Although these conclusions are specific for individuals of African ancestry, the same effects were not observed in Caucasians. None of the other laboratory tests revealed any differences related to either blood group or race[10].

In Caucasian men with blood groups A, B, or AB, and the Lewis (a−b−) phenotype, significantly higher levels of factor VIII and von Willebrand factor were observed, as compared to those with other Lewis phenotypes (Le[a+b−] or Le[a−b+]). Two-way analysis of variance indicated a significant interaction between blood group and Lewis phenotype in terms of relationship to factor VIII. A similar trend was observed in men of African ancestry with blood groups A, B, or AB, and phenotype Lewis (a−b−) for factor VIII and von Willebrand factor and in women with blood groups A, B, or AB, and phenotype Lewis (a−b−) for factor VIII. The researchers concluded that the Lewis (a−b−) phenotype and blood groups A, B, and AB, by virtue of their association with raised levels of factor VIII and von Willebrand factor, may be risk markers for future atherothrombotic disease[11].

Blood Group and Rheology

Rheology is the science of deformation and flow. One common factor between solids, liquids, and all materials whose behavior is intermediate between solid and liquid is that if we apply a stress or load on any of them they will deform or strain. For our purposes we will use the term to describe the dynamics between blood clotting (moving toward a solid state) or blood thinning (moving toward a liquid state). It might be tempting to substitute the word viscosity for rheology when talking about blood types and clotting, but it does not cover the "dynamics" of how, when, and why blood can change texture; it only distinguishes one texture state from another. As we will see, your blood type has a very potent effect on the rheology of your blood.

There are profound differences between the blood types with regard to the rheology of their clotting chemistries. These differences are significant reasons why the blood types tend to polarize with regard to their tendencies: Blood groups A and AB have blood that clots more easily, and groups O and B have blood that does not clot as readily.

Differences between the blood types in blood thickness have been also reported in studies of DEPRESSION[12], HIGH BLOOD PRESSURE[13], STRESS[14], DIABETES[15], HEART ATTACK and THYROID DISEASE[16], KIDNEY FAILURE[17], and MELANOMA[18].

Therapies, Blood Clotting Disorders

BLOOD GROUP A:

1. Cardiovascular Protocol

2. Liver-Support Protocol

3. Antistress Protocol

BLOOD GROUP B:

1. Blood-Building Protocol

2. Cardiovascular Protocol

3. Immune-Enhancing Protocol

Specifics:

Avoid aspirin. If necessary, use other non-steroidal anti-inflammatory drugs (NSAIDs) that have a lesser, more transient effect than aspirin on platelet function.

Regular dental care is essential to avoid tooth extractions and other dental surgery.

Build your vitamin K stores. Vitamin K is essential to blood clotting. Eat lots of greens, especially kale, spinach, and collard greens, and supplement your diet with liquid chlorophyll.

At least a week prior to surgery, begin a daily protocol of 2,000 mg vitamin C, and 30,000 IU vitamin A. These vitamins promote wound healing.

BLOOD GROUP AB:

1. Blood-Building Protocol

2. Cardiovascular Protocol

3. Antistress Protocol

BLOOD GROUP O:

1. Blood-Building Protocol

2. Cardiovascular Protocol

3. Metabolic Enhancement

Specifics:

Avoid aspirin. If necessary, use other nonsteroidal anti-inflammatory drugs (NSAIDs) that have a lesser, more transient effect than aspirin on platelet function.

Regular dental care is essential to avoid tooth extractions and other dental surgery.

Build your vitamin K stores. Vitamin K is essential to blood clotting. Eat lots of greens, especially kale, spinach, and collard greens, and supplement your diet with liquid chlorophyll.

At least a week prior to surgery, begin a daily protocol of 2,000 mg vitamin C, and 30,000 IU vitamin A. These vitamins promote wound healing.

Related Topics

Cardiovascular disease

Stroke

REFERENCES

1. Wahlberg TB, Blomback M, Magnusson D. Influence of sex, blood group, secretor character, smoking habits, acetylsalicylic acid, oral contraceptives, fasting and general health state on blood coagulation variables in randomly selected young adults. *Haemostasis.* 1984;14:312–319.

2. Orstavik KH. Genetics of plasma concentration of von Willebrand factor. *Folia Haematol Int Mag Klin Morphol Blutforsch.* 1990;117:527–531.

3. Orstavik KH, Kornstad L, Reisner H, Berg K. Possible effect of secretor locus on plasma concentration of factor VIII and von Willebrand factor. *Blood.* 1989;73:990–993.

4. Green D, Jarrett O, Ruth KJ, Folsom AR, Liu K. Relationship among Lewis phenotype, clotting factors, and other cardiovascular risk factors in young adults. *J Lab Clin Med.* 1995;125:334–339.

5. Meade TW, Cooper JA, Stirling Y, Howarth DJ, Ruddock V, Miller GJ. Factor VIII, ABO blood group and the incidence of ischaemic heart disease. *Br J Haematol.* 1994; 88:601–607.

6. Sweeney JD, Labuzetta JW, Hoernig LA, Fitzpatrick JE. Platelet function and ABO blood group. *Am J Clin Pathol.* 1989;91:79–81.

7. Orstavik KH, Magnus P, Reisner H, Berg K, Graham JB, Nance W. Factor VIII and factor IX in a twin population. Evidence for a major effect of ABO locus on factor VIII level. *Am J Hum Genet.* 1985;37:89–101.

8. Stockelberg D, Hou M, Rydberg L, Kutti J, Wadenvik H. Evidence for an expression of blood group A antigen on platelet glycoproteins IV and V. *Transfus Med.* 1996;6: 243–248.

9. Hou M, Stockelberg D, Rydberg L, Kutti J, Wadenvik H. Blood group A antigen expression in platelets is prominently associated with glycoprotein Ib and IIb. Evidence for an A1/A2 difference. *Transfus Med.* 1996;6:51–59.

10. Colonia VJ, Roisenberg I. Investigation of associations between ABO blood groups and coagulation, fibrinolysis, total lipids, cholesterol, and triglycerides. *Hum Genet.* 1979; 48:221–230.

11. Green D, Jarrett O, Ruth KJ, Folsom AR, Liu K. Relationship among Lewis phenotype, clotting factors, and other cardiovascular risk factors in young adults. *J Lab Clin Med.* 1995;125:334–339.

12. Dintenfass L, Zador I. Blood rheology in patients with depressive and schizoid anxiety. *Biorheology.* 1976;13:33–36.

13. Dintenfass L, Bauer GE. Dynamic blood coagulation and viscosity and degradation of artificial thrombi in patients with hypertension. *Cardiovasc Res.* 1970;4:50–60.

14. Dintenfass L, Zador I. Effect of stress and anxiety on thrombus formation and blood viscosity factors. *Bibl Haematol.* 1975;41:133–139.

15. Dintenfass L, Davis E. Genetic and ethnic influences on blood viscosity and capillaries in diabetes mellitus. *Microvasc Res.* 1977;14:161–172.

16. Dintenfass L, Forbes CD. Effect of fibrinogen on aggregation of red cells and on apparent viscosity of artificial thrombi in haemophilia, myocardial infarction, thyroid disease, cancer and control systems: effect of ABO blood groups. *Microvasc Res.* 1975;9:107–118.

17. Dintenfass L, Stewart JH. Formation, consistency, and degradation of artificial thrombi in severe renal failure. Effect of ABO blood groups. *Thromb Diath Haemorrh.* 1968;20: 267–284.

18. Dintenfass L. Some aspects of haemorrheology of metastasis in malignant melanoma. *Haematologia (Budap).* 1977;11:301–307.

Blood Transfusion

The American blood supply is reasonably safe, and patients who need blood can accept it with confidence, according to Food and Drug Administration (FDA) experts. But this doesn't mean that blood is entirely risk-free. Blood is human tissue, a biological product, so it carries a degree of risk. Estimates of the risk of infection with HIV, the virus responsible for AIDS, range from 1 in 61,000 to 1 in 225,000 transfused units—or potentially 90 to 300 infections among some 18 million blood products used each year. The risk from transfusion, however, is far less than the risk involved in not using blood when it's needed. There are no known cases of anyone contracting AIDS from donating their blood.

Using Your Own Blood for Transfusion

Patients who are likely to require a transfusion during an upcoming surgery may decide to donate their own blood for possible reinfusion. The FDA recommends this practice, called autologous transfusion, whenever possible for elective surgery. Use of your own blood reduces the chance of infection or other adverse reactions. The practice also decreases the demand on the public blood supply. In addition, autologous transfusion allows blood lost during surgery to be replaced more quickly, because the process of donating blood in itself stimulates the bone marrow to produce new blood cells.

Conditions that might prevent someone from donating blood for others don't necessarily prevent autologous blood donation. For example, people who have had hepatitis may give blood to themselves. Autologous donation may be inadvisable for some patients, such as those with severe heart and blood vessel disease whose condition may be worsened by donating a unit or two of blood. Although the fluid lost from donation replenishes within 24 hours, replacement of red blood cells, with their life-giving oxygen, can take up to 2 months. For patients giving multiple autologous donations over several weeks, iron supplements may be prescribed to help increase the red blood cell count.

Recycling Blood during Surgery

When an operation is expected to involve a large loss of blood, the surgical team may recover the patient's blood and reinfuse it during the surgery. This practice, called intraoperative blood collection, or salvage, has been widely used in open-chest surgery. Another salvage method filters the blood. After filtration, the unwashed blood is transferred into a bag for reinfusion. Factors that make blood recycling inadvisable include cancer or infection.

Hemodilution

Blood dilution (hemodilution) is a practice to prevent loss of red blood cells. The patient has blood drawn before surgery, and is immediately given intravenous fluids to make up for the drawn blood, which is saved to be reinfused after the operation. The idea is that during the operation any blood the patient loses will have been diluted, and therefore fewer red blood cells are lost.

Directed Donations

In directed donations, friends or family donate blood for a specific patient, usually a relative. Such donors must go through all the standard donor screening and testing procedures. Several states have passed laws establishing directed donation as a procedure that must be followed when requested, except in an emergency. Some people may feel it's always safer to receive blood from a relative or friend than from the general blood supply, but experts say this is not necessarily the case. Although matching a patient's blood type may be easier when the donor is a relative rather than someone else, such patients have a high risk of developing graft-versus-host disease, a complication caused by the donor and recipient sharing certain tissue-type substances. In this disease, lymphocyte white blood cells from the transfused blood multiply and react against the recipient's tissues.

Artificial Blood

No one knows for sure whether researchers will ever develop an ideal artificial oxygen carrier as an alternative to blood transfusion. But promising possibilities are being worked on, and new ideas are being researched. However, blood is extremely complex, so a true substitute may never be realized.

Drugs

A number of approved drugs and biological agents can lessen the need for or serve as alternatives to blood transfusion. These drugs prevent or control bleeding, or stimulate the bone marrow to produce more red blood cells in patients with anemia, or on medications that suppress the function of the bone marrow, such as the anti-AIDS drug AZT.

Body Composition

What Is Body Composition, and Why Is It Important?

Your body is made up of water, fat, protein, carbohydrate, and various vitamins and minerals. If you have too much fat—especially if a lot of it is located in your waist area—you're at higher risk for health problems, including HIGH BLOOD PRESSURE, HIGH CHOLESTEROL, DIABETES, HEART DISEASE, and STROKE.

Body composition is one measure of a person's overall physical fitness. Obesity is now recognized as a major independent risk factor for heart disease. Other measures are cardiovascular endurance (fitness of the heart and lungs), and muscular strength and flexibility.

The waist circumference and the body mass index (BMI) are indirect measures for assessing a person's body composition. The waist-to-hip ratio (WHR) is another index of body fat distribution. However, WHR is less accurate than waist circumference and is no longer a recommended measure.

What Is the Waist Circumference?

The waist circumference is a simple measure around a person's natural waist (just above the navel). A high-risk waistline is defined as more than 35 inches (88 cm) for women, and more than 40 inches (102 cm) for men.

What Is the Body Mass Index (BMI)?

The body mass index is a formula to assess a person's body weight relative to height. It's a useful, indirect measure of body composition, because it correlates highly with body fat in most people. Weight in kilograms is divided by height in meters squared (kg/m^2). In studies by the National Center for Health Statistics, BMI values less than 18.5 are considered underweight. BMI values from 18.5 to 24.9 are healthy. "Overweight" is defined as a body mass index of 25.0 to less than

30.0. A BMI of approximately 25 kg/m² corresponds to about 10% over ideal body weight. People with BMIs in this range have a moderate risk of heart and blood vessel disease. Obesity is defined as a BMI of 30.0 or greater (based on criteria of the World Health Organization), or about 30 pounds overweight. People with BMIs of 30 or more are at high risk of cardiovascular disease. Extreme obesity is defined as a BMI of 40 or greater.

Some well-trained people with dense muscle mass may have a high BMI score but very little body fat. For them the waist circumference, the skinfold or fatfold measurements, or more direct methods of measuring body fat may be more useful measures.

How Do You Find Your Body Mass Index?

1. Use a weight scale on a hard, flat, uncarpeted surface. Wear very little clothing and no shoes.

2. Obtain your weight to the nearest pound and write it down.

3. With your eyes facing forward and your heels together, stand very straight against a wall. Your buttocks, shoulders, and the back of your head should be touching the wall.

4. Use a ruler held at a right angle to the wall to mark your height at the highest point of your head. Then use a yardstick held flat against the wall to measure from the floor to the point you marked with the ruler. Write down your height in inches to the nearest quarter inch.

5. Find your height in feet and inches in the first column of the Body Mass Index Risk Levels table below. The range of weights that corresponds to minimal risk, moderate risk (overweight), and high risk (obese) is shown in the three columns for each height.

Height	MINIMAL RISK (BMI under 25) Healthy	MODERATE RISK (BMI 25.0–29.9) Overweight	HIGH RISK (BMI 30 and above) Obese
4'10"	118 lbs. or less	119–142 lbs.	143 lbs. or more
4'11"	123 or less	124–147	148 or more
5'0"	127 or less	128–152	153 or more
5'1"	131 or less	132–157	158 or more
5'2"	135 or less	136–163	164 or more
5'3"	140 or less	141–168	169 or more
5'4"	144 or less	145–173	174 or more
5'5"	149 or less	150–179	180 or more
5'6"	154 or less	155–185	186 or more
5'7"	158 or less	159–190	191 or more
5'8"	163 or less	164–196	197 or more
5'9"	168 or less	169–202	203 or more
5'10"	173 or less	174–208	209 or more
5'11"	178 or less	179–214	215 or more
6'0"	183 or less	184–220	221 or more
6'1"	188 or less	189–226	227 or more
6'2"	193 or less	194–232	233 or more
6'3"	199 or less	200–239	240 or more
6'4"	204 or less	205–245	246 or more

To calculate your exact BMI number, multiply your weight in pounds by 705, divide by your height in inches, then divide again by your height in inches.

(Chart adapted from Obesity Education Initiative: Clinical Guidelines on the Identification, Evaluation, and Treatment of Overweight and Obesity in Adults, National Institutes of Health, National Heart, Lung, and Blood Institute, Preprint June 1998)

BOWEL TOXICITY–_See Toxicity, bowel (indicanuria); Toxicity, bowel (polyamines)_

BRAIN TUMOR–_See Cancer, glioma and other brain tumors_

BREAST CANCER–_See Cancer, breast_

BRONCHITIS–_An inflammation of the bronchi (the airways in the lungs)._

Bronchitis	SEVERITY/SUSCEPTIBILITY		
	LOW	AVERAGE	HIGH
GROUP A (severity)	░	░	
GROUP B	░		
GROUP AB	░		
GROUP O	░		
NON-SECRETORS (susceptibility)	░	░	░

Symptoms

- Persistent, productive cough
- Tightness in the chest
- Wheezing
- Difficulty breathing
- Fever

About Bronchitis

Bronchitis is an acute or chronic inflammation of the bronchial tubes that results in mucus production, COUGHING, FEVER, CHEST PAIN, sore throat, and difficulty breathing. Acute bronchitis is usually caused by an infection, and often follows a cold or the flu.

Acute bronchitis is an infection in the passages that carry air from the throat to the lung, causing a cough that produces phlegm. In such cases, the airway tubes have become inflamed and collected mucus. In 95% of cases, acute bronchitis is caused by a virus and is spread from person to person through coughing. In some cases other tiny microbes called _Mycoplasma_ or _Chlamydia_ may be responsible. The cough usually lasts for about 1 week to 10 days, but in about half of patients coughing can last for up to 3 weeks; 25% of patients continue to cough for over 1 month.

Chronic bronchitis is an inflammation and degeneration of the air passages of the lung. The underlying culprit is most often tobacco smoke. In fact, cigarette smoking is the most common cause of chronic bronchitis. Other causes include pollution and repeated infections of air passages of the lung.

Many people, most of them smokers, develop EMPHYSEMA (destruction of the air sacs) along with chronic bronchitis. Chronic bronchitis results in abnormal air exchange in the lung and causes permanent damage to the respiratory tract. It's much more serious than acute bronchitis. Chronic bronchitis is not contagious.

Blood Group Links

In general, blood groups A and AB have more bronchial infections than blood groups O and B. This may result from improper diets, which produce excessive mucus in their respiratory passages. This mucus facilitates the growth of blood-type mimicking bacteria, such as the A-like *Pneumococcus* bacteria in groups A and AB, and the B-like *Haemophilus* bacteria in groups B and AB.

A 1951 study of 400 postmortems at the Royal Hospital for Sick Children, Glasgow, observed that there was an excess of children who were blood group A dying under 2 years of age from bronchopneumonia—a severe lung infection that develops from bronchitis[1].

Non-secretors are at greater risk for chronic bronchitis. In a study of cigarette smokers in the Northwick Park Heart Study in Northwest London, England, secretors of ABO antigen had a higher mean peak expiratory flow rate than did non-secretors. The relationship was independent of other factors known to affect peak expiratory flow rate[2].

Researchers are just beginning to discover some other blood group connections that are more complex. For example, it appears that blood group A children born to group A fathers and group O mothers die more frequently of bronchopneumonia early in life. It is thought that some form of sensitization occurs at birth between the group A infant and the mother's anti-A antibodies, which inhibit the infant's ability to fight the *Pneumococcus* bacteria. There are no solid data yet to confirm the reason that this occurs, but information of this kind can spark research interest in a potential vaccine.

Therapies, Bronchitis

BLOOD GROUP A:

1. Pulmonary Support Protocol
2. Antibacterial Protocol
3. Immune-Enhancing Protocol

BLOOD GROUP B:

1. Pulmonary Support Protocol
2. Antibacterial Protocol
3. Immune-Enhancing Protocol

BLOOD GROUP AB:

1. Pulmonary Support Protocol
2. Antibacterial Protocol
3. Immune-Enhancing Protocol

BLOOD GROUP O:

1. Pulmonary Support Protocol
2. Antibacterial Protocol
3. Immune-Enhancing Protocol

Related Topics

Common cold

Infectious disease

Influenza

Pneumonia

REFERENCES

1. Struthers D. *Brit J Prev Soc Med.* 1951.
2. Haines AP, Imeson JD, Meade TW. ABH secretor status and pulmonary function. *Am J Epidemiol.* 1982;115:367–370.

BRONCHOPNEUMONIA–*See Bacterial disease, pneumonia*

C

CANCER (general)–*A general term for a group of more than 100 diseases characterized by the uncontrolled growth and spread of abnormal cells.*

Cancer (general)	RISK		
	LOW	AVERAGE	HIGH
GROUP A			
GROUP B			
GROUP AB			
GROUP O			
NON-SECRETOR			

About Cancer

As we age, so do the cells of our bodies. All organs of the body are made up of cells capable of normal division; they produce more cells when the body calls upon itself to manufacture them. If cells divide when new ones aren't needed, these cells form a mass of excess tissue called a tumor. As a tumor grows, nutrients are provided by direct diffusion from the circulation. Local tissue invasion can result in pressure on normal tissues, which can lead to inflammation, or the tumor may produce substances (e.g., collagenase) that lead to enzymatic destruction of tissues. Tumors can be benign (non-cancerous) or malignant (cancerous).

As with many other diseases, both genetic and environmental factors are implicated in the cause and development of human cancers. Cancer-causing biological, chemical, and physical agents are referred to as carcinogens, and the process of a carcinogen-instigating cancer is called carcinogenesis. Recent advances in the molecular biology of cancer, stemming from the study of cancer-causing viruses (oncoviruses) and transforming DNA, are providing new ways of investigating cancer-forming genes (oncogenes) and cellular pathways that are involved in the mechanisms of viral, chemical, and physical carcinogenesis.

Carcinogens are grouped into two categories. Direct-acting carcinogens are carcinogenic on their own. Procarcinogens must be converted metabolically inside the body into carcinogens. Paradoxically, most forms of chemotherapy for cancer are direct-acting carcinogens as well. Procarcinogens include aflatoxin (the toxin from mold), many chemical dyes, nitrosamines from smoked foods in the diet, and some metals such as nickel. Carcinogenesis can take years or decades to finally result in a tumor. This latent period between an exposure to a carcinogen and cancer formation is explained by studies showing that carcinogenesis is divisible into two stages, tumor initiation and tumor promotion.

A living creature is the result of a complex symphony of various specialized cells, each of which has a particular job to do. Like a modern city, which could not function without its specialized members such as police, firefighters, sanitation workers, and shopkeepers, the body can only function properly if there are adequate numbers of very specialized cells, each with its particular part to play.

What makes a cell become one particular type or another is what particular part of its DNA is turned on or off. A grossly oversimplified way of considering this would be to think about a cell currently residing on your fingernail. That type of cell is programmed to be very hard and somewhat waterproof, two specialized functions that would not be very helpful if found in your brain. There, you need specialized cells that can conduct electrical charges and stretch out for very long distances. The fingernail cell's DNA has only the information needed to be a fingernail cell activated; all other parts of the cell's DNA are turned off. In essence it is a fingernail cell that has only those genes left active. A nerve cell is a nerve cell for the same reason; the genes that would have made it a fingernail cell, or a hair cell, or a muscle cell have all been turned off—or, as it is termed in biology, the genes have been repressed.

Cell function and specialization results in large part from controlling on the genetic level what a cell can or cannot do. Normal cells are called differentiated because they have the same characteristics as all other cells of that cell type. Hair cells look very much like other hair cells, and when they reproduce, they make other hair cells. In this nicely ordered way of things, life goes on. The body goes to great trouble to keep cells differentiated, since the loss of this control is the first step in a process of cellular anarchy that can eventually lead to malignancy.

Differentiation is also called tumor grade. The evaluation of differentiation of cells shows the degree of malignancy. Cells with a high level of differentiation are normal cells with specific functions. Cells with low levels of differentiation are more dangerous in respect to malignancy.

Characteristics of a Cancer Cell

- Cancer cells have a typically round appearance, instead of the normal flat appearance.

- The cancer cells do not adhere to one another as normal cells do. This is due to the reduction in surface adhesion molecules on the cancer cell's surface. The major adhesion molecules lost are the ABO antigens.

- There is limited contact inhibition of movement. Normal cells terminate movement when in contact with one another; cancer cells don't.

- The cells have less anchorage dependence. So they are free to invade other tissues and enter the blood and lymph systems (metastasis).

- Cancer cells are not inhibited by the density of surrounding tissue. Cells are able to pile up on top of one another.

- Extracellular growth factors are not required for proliferation, because cells are able to produce their own growth factors. Certain blood type an-

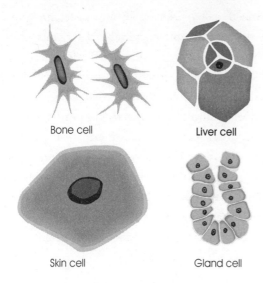

Bone cell

Liver cell

Skin cell

Gland cell

CELL DIFFERENTATION

The DNA code of every cell contains all of the information needed for that cell to be any other kind of cell. What gives a cell its unique ability to perform the function for which it is intended is that only the information for that cell is turned on. So a gland cell performs only the function of glands, the bone cell performs only the function of bones, and so on. These different cells all have distinct appearances.

tigens can interact with cancer cell growth factors. The lifespan is indefinite, because apoptosis (programmed cell death) is inhibited.

In medicine, it is typical to grade tumors according to the degree of differentiation, which is usually determined by a pathologist looking at slides of the tissue. The more differentiated a tumor cell is, the more effectively the body's immune response to it can be. Thus, a well-differentiated tumor will have cancer cells that more or less still resemble each other; an antibody, or killer cell, can be programmed to look for a tumor antigen (or tumor "marker") that should be consistently found on every cell in the tumor. As the tumor cells become more undifferentiated,

they no longer resemble each other enough to allow for a potent immune response. In essence, the immune system would have to make a new and different antibody for each different tumor cell—an impossible job. For that reason well-differentiated tumor cells (such as MELANOMA cells) tend to respond to immunotherapy better than poorly differentiated ones.

Here are the common stages of differentiation normally used by pathologists.

STAGE	DEGREES OF CELL DIFFERENTIATION
Normal	Cells are highly differentiated.
G1	The lowest tumor grade; cells are well differentiated. A good response to treatment is usually expected.
G2	Cells are moderately differentiated. Troubling, but still responsive to appropriate treatment.
G3	Cells are poorly differentiated. This is a poor result, and will require aggressive treatment.
G4	Cells are undifferentiated. This is the worst case in respect to malignancy of the cells. These cells are the most dangerous. They are in essence "junk cells" with no positive function. Aggressive treatment options must be employed.

Normal cells are differentiated by virtue of having only the genes needed for their particular job activated, and all other genes deactivated, or repressed. How do tumors lose differentiation? As tumors mutate, the mutations begin to activate latent, repressed genes that are normally turned off. This is called de-repression, and as it occurs, cells very often regress to forms much like those found in embryonic tissue. Embryonic cells (such as one might find in a 2- or 3-week-old fetus) do not yet have the full functionality found in the cells of a mature adult. Initially, unlike the thousands of different, highly specific cells found in the normal adult, there are only three types of embryonic cells:

- *Ectoderm cells:* which differentiate into the cells of the skin and nerves

- *Mesoderm cells:* which differentiate into the cells of the muscular system, skeleton, and connective tissues

- *Endoderm cells:* which differentiate into the cells lining the digestive system

Since these cells (often called germ cells or germ layer) eventually differentiate into a wide variety of different tissues, they need to repress and de-repress a large number of genes to wind up with a highly specialized end product. As a cancer cell mutates and loses control of its normally controlled genetic material, it deteriorates regressively and begins to resemble these early embryonic cell forms. Many cancer cells begin to manufacture glycoprotein antigens that are typically found only in embryonic tissue; many of these are used diagnostically, such as the CEA (carcinogenic embryonic antigen), which can be used to gauge the progression of several types of cancer.

Blood Group Links

ABO blood group antigens are intimately involved with the process of differentiation. We know that their production is regulated in the blood vessel cells of the fetal organs, and they are theorized to be responsible for specifying the location of future blood vessels in the burgeoning organs, where they serve as differentiation markers. This is a very important function of the ABO blood group, and is for the most part not known or understood by the majority of the medical community. However, this critical embryonic function is probably the single most important reason that blood group antigens appear and disappear in tissues that are about to become aggressively malignant and metastasize[1].

Studies have shown that blood group A has higher levels of the p53 tumor suppressor gene in certain cancers, especially those of the digestive tract. Although one might think that higher levels of a gene that suppresses tumors might be a good thing, the general consensus holds that it tends to be associated with signs that the tumor is becoming more invasive. Higher levels of the p53 suppressor gene have also been linked to the likelihood that the tumor has begun to develop disturbances in its production of blood group antigens, weakening its resistance[2].

Although there are well over a thousand published findings on the associations between blood types and disease, many are based entirely on statistical analyses. Most of the earlier studies have been controversial, usually because they were small studies that may have had inadequate controls, or been analyzed incorrectly. Nevertheless, it is difficult to argue with the general pattern that emerges from the large body of statistical data on malignancy, coagulation, and infection. Some of the findings on microbe receptors and their association with important immune proteins are most convincing, and suggest that blood type antigens do play an important biological role. Interestingly, it is a role that is often completely unrelated to the red blood cell. Cancers in general tend to be associated with blood group A, and slightly less so with blood group B.

Perhaps the greatest focus of current research on the ABO blood group antigens resides in the field of molecular oncology. Recent findings in membrane chemistry, tumor immunology, and infectious disease have provided a compelling scientific rationale for several blood type associations. Because of this, there is an increase in acceptance of the earlier statistical findings.

The huge interest in blood groups stems from the developing awareness that blood group antigens are important components in the process of cell maturation and control. As an example, the appearance or disappearance of blood group antigens is a hallmark of malignancy in many common cancers.

Several tumor antigens or tumor markers are the known product of certain blood type precursors. Many of these tumor antigens are A-like, which helps in part to explain the striking number of associations with blood group A and AB. On the contrary, autoimmune disorders tend to be associated with blood group O. The contrast with the cancer–group A association is an interesting one in view of the suggestion of earlier immunologists that there is a fundamental antithesis between the two classes of disease. The heightened surveillance and overactive immune activity tend to result in less malignancy, whereas overly tolerant immune activity tends to encourage it. These observations suggest a more general hypothesis that in the tissues of all people, both nor-

mal and cancerous, there are A-like antigens present at a biochemical level that are usually inaccessible to the immune system. However, when stimulated by an autoimmune process, or the immune response to a growing cancer, the antigen becomes accessible. At that point, a blood group A person, who cannot make anti-A antibodies, will be more likely than a blood type O person to tolerate the cancer, but the A person's immune system will be less likely than that of a blood type O person to attack the body's own tissues.

The cancer–group A link is far from an absolute. There are several tumors that show a consistent association with groups O and B. This implies that cancer is a condition associated with derangement of blood type activity in general, and the expression of A-like antigens on the surface tumors is just simply the most common of these derangements.

Blood Group Antigens and Cancer Cell Adhesion

When cancer spreads away from the primary site it is called metastasis. Metastasis is a complex phenomenon consisting of several sequential steps:

1. Invasion of primary sites
2. Entry into the blood or lymphatic vessels
3. Transport
4. Migration from the blood vessel into the tissues, and growth at the target sites

The results show that certain types of carbohydrate antigen expressions in cancer cells are profoundly related not only to the mode of metastatic spread and the organ distribution pattern of metastasis, but also to the prognosis of cancer patients. Lymphatic metastasis is related to the expression of Tn antigens and Tn-like antigens (see IMMUNITY) where no conspicuous similarities have been found in the hematogenous metastasis-related carbohydrates among the cancers. The expressions of blood group antigens such as ABO, Lewis, and MN, including their precursors, appear to be strong prognostic indicators of these cancers, although the relation of these antigens to each cancer varies. Adhesion molecules and/or carbohydrates may be one of the determinants of cancer metastasis and prognosis, at least in part[3].

The reason that deletion or reduction of the A or AB antigens in tumors of A or B individuals correlates with malignancy and metastatic potential may be due to the lack of adhesiveness that a cancer cell achieves when it loses blood group antigens. Findings in human colon cancer patients have indicated that the degree of motility and the proliferation of colon tumor cells are directly associated with the deletion or reduction of the A antigen. As cells lose the A-like antigen, they seem also to lose the ability to express many of the cell adhesion proteins, such as the integrins, which normally express an A-like antigen on their receptors and control cell movement[4].

The loss of blood group antigen results in the tumor cells gaining the ability to move and circulate through the body, because the blood type antigens are needed for the cell's integrin receptors to work properly as the adhesive glue that holds cells together. This link between blood group and cell adherence is probably as elemental to the development of cancer as it is to life itself. A growing fetus needs the ability to spawn new organs and grow an effective blood supply to feed them; in these instances, the loss of blood group antigens would allow for this migration of embryonic cells to the sites of future organs and blood vessels. In fact, many of the embryonic cell tumor markers (such as the CEA) are expressed almost in parallel with the loss of blood group antigens. The greater the loss of blood group antigens, the greater the production of embryonic tumor antigens. In malignancy, which in many ways is the process of a cell losing function and reverting back to its embryonic state, the loss of blood group antigens means uncontrolled migration, and that indicates metastasis.

Loss of blood group antigens doesn't occur in all tumors. In fact, it is usually the reverse of what happens under normal conditions. Tissues and organs that in normal circumstances manufacture blood group antigens (like those of the colon) will tend to lose them when undergoing malignant change[5]. Other organs like the thyroid, which do not make blood group antigens when normal, will tend to gain them when turning cancerous. Sometimes, such as in the case of the thyroid and the colon, changes taking place in the blood group antigen expression in one organ will influence the expression of blood group antigens in another[6].

T and Tn: Pan-Carcinogenic Antigens

Many malignant cells (such as those found in breast and stomach cancer) develop a tumor marker called the Thomsen-Friedenreich (T) antigen. This antigen is suppressed in normal healthy cells, much like a rock is covered over by water at high tide. The T antigen only becomes unsuppressed as a cell moves toward malignancy, much like the covered rock in our example becomes exposed as the tide lowers. It is so rare to find the T antigen in healthy tissue that we actually have antibodies against it. It is even more unusual to find a Tn antigen on a healthy cell. Tn is actually a precursor to T antigen, or a less well-developed T antigen.

It has been estimated that in about 90% of all cancers (and in some LEUKEMIAS) T and Tn antigens are expressed and uncovered. As a general rule, an orderly expression of T antigens on a cancer cell usually indicates a cancer with a relatively favorable outlook. However, a prevalence of Tn antigens on a cancer cell usually denotes a highly aggressive, metastatic cancer, irrespective of the organ involved or the form of cancer.

Cancer cells differ radically from healthy cells in the fine architecture of their cell surfaces. A healthy cell surface looks like a well-tended yard, with groomed bushes, shrubs, and flowers. A cancer cell looks like someone has taken a chain saw to the yard, and leveled the bushes, shrubs, and flowers down to their stumps. So, in a very simplistic way, a cancer cell clearly looks like a different yard than a healthy one (your immune system, in this case).

In this example, the T and Tn antigens are the stumps found in cancer, while the well-groomed yard has bushes, shrubs, and flowers that correspond to the ABO markers and other antigens found on healthy cells. The difference between the yards is largely because a cancer cell is unable to completely assemble a normal, healthy cell membrane structure like a blood group ABO antigen.

As a general rule, well-differentiated cancers usually have a preponderance of T antigens and less of the Tn antigens. However, as a cancer cell becomes poorly differentiated, Tn antigen expression predominates. One of the functions of these T and Tn antigens is to promote cancer cell adhesion—the ability of the cancer cell to stick to other cells, including healthy ones. This process of adhesion is a critically important part of cancer cell invasion and metastasis. When it comes to T and Tn antigens, there is good news. Everyone has preexisting anti-T and anti-Tn antibodies—a built-in immune system response against cells with these markers. These anti-T and anti-Tn antibodies are primarily induced by your intestinal flora. Blood group will often influence the amount and activity of these antibodies against T and Tn antigens.

The T and Tn antigens show some structural similarity to the A antigen (even though it is derived from the M blood type antigen)[7]. Not surprisingly, blood group A individuals have the least aggressive antibody immune response against the T and probably Tn antigens. In fact, the T and Tn antigens, and blood group A antigens are actually immunologically considered to be quite similar because of their shared terminal sugar (N-acetyl-galactosamine), and so might be readily confused by the immune system of blood group A individuals. This finding has led researchers to conclude that the Tn antigen is, in a broad sense, an A-like antigen. The hypothesis: because of the lower level of antibody against T and Tn antigens, and because of this tendency for the immune system of blood group A to be disinclined to attack Tn antigens, blood group A is at an immunological disadvantage in attacking any cell bearing the T and Tn antigenic markers[8].

Blood group A cancer patients had the greatest and most uniform suppression of the level of Thomsen-Friedenreich antigen agglutinins, irrespective of age, cancer stage, or tumor morphology, and lower levels of anti-B isohemagglutinins. This is probably at least a part of the explanation for the poorer outcomes in many cancers among blood group A individuals.

Ideally, the immune system is naturally predisposed to fight against cells with incomplete or abnormal structures—just as it would against an invading virus. Blood groups A and AB start with a bit of an immune disadvantage, due to this structural similarity to the T antigen.

Coagulation and Cancer:
Another Group A Weakness

The A-like cancer hypothesis is a strong one, well supported in the literature. However, several other aspects of the blood group A antigen, in addition to the T and Tn antibody limitation, appear to convey additional susceptibility to malignancy. Perhaps the second most potent pathway by which blood group A is rendered more prone to severe complications for malignancy is by virtue of their thicker blood, or tendency toward aggregation.

Von Willebrand factor and factor VIII: It has been noted that cancer cells can often hitch a ride on circulating platelets as they begin to spread, or metastasize. This is due to an aberrant platelet glycoprotein receptor expressed by human tumor cells that appears to participate in the adhesive interactions required for the metastatic process. Von Willebrand factor (vWF) and factor VIII are serum proteins that are a sort of molecular glue that platelets use to attach to blood clotting proteins along the lining of the blood vessels. It is also required for this aberrant platelet glycoprotein to bind to cancer cells. Plasma specimens from patients with disseminated metastases showed that their plasma levels of von Willebrand factor and factor VIII were elevated (vWF almost double) above those of normal individuals, apparently because they lack adequate amounts of an enzyme required to cleave vWF and factor VIII into their inactive forms. Because of this, cancer patients with widely disseminated metastasis have levels of platelet activity upward of 150% greater than that of normal individuals.

Fibrinogen: As with STRESS, THYROID DISEASE, HEART DISEASE, and DIABETES, studies have shown that cancer patients who are blood group A have higher levels of blood viscosity than cancer patients who are group O. This appears to be the result of higher levels of the clotting protein fibrinogen. Fibrinogen is an acute phase protein important to the inflammatory response and to wound healing. It is known to be elevated in cancer patients, where its presence is believed to shorten survival and contribute to weight loss. As with vWF and factor VIII, fibrinogen serves as part of the adherence cascade by which cancer cells can attach to platelets and the walls of the blood vessels as a prelude to metastatic spread.

This helps explain why older studies have

shown that cancer patients who are on blood thinning medication have a lower incidence of METASTASIS[9]. Blood group A is associated with higher levels of vWF and factor VIII over the other blood types, which probably accounts for their "thicker blood." Similarly, group A has a tendency toward higher levels of fibrinogen, which might also help cancer cells to metastasize. In the case of malignancy, vWF and factor VIII probably help metastasizing cancer cells adhere to platelets, while also having the secondary effect of inducing metastasis as well.

Growth Factors and Group A Risk

One little-known or appreciated effect of blood group A antigen is its ability to attach to the receptor for "growth factors" that are found in much higher concentration on tumor cells than on normal ones. Growth factors are proteins that act on nearby cells in a way not dissimilar to hormones. As a matter of fact, the best known growth factor is insulin itself. Growth factors are very powerful regulatory agents, and their production is normally highly controlled. Growth factors have varied effects, acting not only as regulators of cell proliferation but also as inducers of secretion of chemical attractants and stimulants to cell differentiation. Over the course of our lives, our body changes in a variety of dynamic ways: Our bones elongate, men develop facial hair, women's breasts grow larger. Growth factors are active in every situation where some sort of tissue remodeling must occur, such as embryonic development, response to injury, puberty, inflammation, and, unfortunately, cancer.

All the above processes require cells to proliferate (hyperplasia), enlarge (hypertrophy), and sometimes die (apoptosis), and a major role of the growth factors is to coordinate the activities of the different cell types in remodeling tissues in an organized fashion.

There is a close relation between growth factor action and oncogenes, genes that were discovered because of their association with the transformation of cells to the malignant state. The idea that growth factors may be related to cancer was given strong support by the finding that the actual products that are the physical result of many oncogenes are related either to growth factors or their receptors. Overproduction of these growth factors as a result of oncogene activity contributes to the loss of the body's ability to regulate growth, which results in cancerous cell growth.

Epidermal growth factor (EGF): A growth factor normally synthesized to help tissue to repair itself, EGF also has important effects on the growth of prostate, colon, breast, and several other cancer types. These cancers are characterized by cells that have an excessively high concentration of EGF receptors (EGF-R) on their surfaces[10]. So it appears that EGF-R expression plays an important role in the pathogenesis of human cancer, including but not limited to oral, brain, pancreatic, breast, lung, and colorectal cancers[11–14].

Basically, the larger number of EGF-R on the cancer cell means that the cell can bind an excessive number of these molecules. It may be that this excessive dose of growth factor is critical to tumor growth. In fact, it is now clear that the growth of breast cancer is regulated by growth factor receptors (EGFR and Her-2/neu), and that their upregulation is associated with impaired prognosis.

Because of its deregulation in many cancers (BLADDER, BREAST, CERVICAL, COLON, ESOPHAGEAL, HEAD AND NECK, LUNG, and PROSTATE), EGF-R has been selected as a prime target for chemoprevention.

The EGF-R bears an antigenic determinant that is closely related to the human blood group A carbohydrate structure. An increase in the number of high-affinity EGF binding sites was observed in donors with blood group A1-erythrocytes as compared to red cells taken from donors with blood groups O and B[15].

It is now very well-documented that the blood group A antigen can bind to EGF-R as well. So it is not unlikely that free A antigen in blood group A and AB individuals (especially if they are secretors) can find their way onto these excess EGF-R and act to simulate cell growth. Like von Willebrand and factor VIII, excessive activation of the EGF-R results in cancer cells that become more mobile and able to develop new and additional blood supplies (angiogenesis)[16].

Blood Group and Natural Killer Cells

Natural killer (NK) cells function to destroy cells infected with cancer or a virus. In virtually every type of cancer investigated, NK activity is low. As a matter of fact, if we were to make one blanket statement about cancer patients, irrespective of the form of cancer, or the patient's blood type, race, gender, or age, it would be that by virtue of having cancer, we can predict that this person will have NK cell activity significantly lower than that found in normal, healthy individuals.

The prognostic significance of NK cell function in cancer, with regards to predicting relapses, poor responses to treatment, and survival time, has been receiving increasing emphasis in medical literature. Compromised NK cell function has been linked to the development and metastasis of cancer, as well as patient survival time. A sampling of cancers known to be associated with low NK cell activity include breast cancer, prostate cancer, RENAL CANCER, STOMACH CANCER, lung cancer, colon cancer, BRAIN CANCER, and leukemia. Let's examine NK cell activity in two of the most common forms of cancer: breast and prostate cancer.

In breast cancer, a negative correlation is seen between NK cell activity levels and the maximum tumor diameter. NK cell activity is also predictive of advanced disease and the spread of disease in women with breast cancer. Destruction of cancer cells by NK cells is much lower in women with advanced disease (stages II, III, and IV) than in women with limited disease (stage I).

In prostate cancer, changes in NK activity have been reported to be reliably associated with both the likelihood of metastasis and tumor response to therapy, matching in its reliability the tumor markers reflective of prostate cancer (PSA and TPS). In both treated and untreated patients with prostate cancer, a lower NK cell activity level means a greater likelihood of cancer cells escaping containment and finding their way into the circulation (this is not a good thing, since your survival depends on keeping the cancer contained to its original site). The level of NK cell activity also provides a direct reflection of the body's response to treatment: Normalization of NK cell activity is found in patients in remission following appropriate treatment. As a matter of fact, at least in prostate cancer, the laboratory work done to determine NK activity levels will often provide more useful information with respect to outcomes in advanced disease than the routinely used tumor marker assessments.

The genetics of blood type might influence NK cell activity. And while many factors are involved in the individual variation in NK cell function, again we find a role of blood group antigenic structures. Lowered NK cell activity has been shown to have a familial association in melanoma suggesting a possible genetic contribution. A significant relationship between Lewis antigen expression and resistance to NK cell destruction is found on target cells (meaning that the Lewis antigens being present on a cell make it a less likely target for NK cell destruction. Cell surface A and O antigens also increase resistance to lysis, while the pan-carcinogenic precursor structures (T and Tn antigens, discussed on page 168) increase the sensitivity of tumor cells to be destroyed by NK cells. So blood group antigen expression on target cells certainly influences the ability of NK cells to bind and destroy those cells. Although information is not unequivocal, higher NK activity has been associated with blood group AB when compared either to blood group A alone, or to blood group AB and O taken together as a group. In general, the lowest NK cell activity has been associated with blood group A. Rh blood type might also influence NK cell activity. Although some studies have not found an association, other researchers have observed a higher natural NK cytotoxicity against target cells in individuals with Rh-negative blood type[17-26].

Therapies, Cancer

ALL BLOOD GROUPS:

Important therapeutic note:

Without question, the best way to protect yourself from cancer is to follow the Blood Type Diet and reduce your stress levels. Over the years, I've developed a number of supplementary strategies. However, I want to emphasize that none of the suggestions in this section are meant to replace the recommendations of your surgeons and oncologists. My experience is that the best approach to take with an adversary like cancer is to place as many independent and mutually supportive strategies at your disposal as possible. My patients are routinely using the best that conventional medicine has to offer. I advise you to do the same. The strategies we will discuss are accessory strategies, which attack cancer from an angle currently ignored or not emphasized within conventional medicine. Some of these angles are actually being explored, and I suspect they will eventually be incorporated into the mainstream. Until that time, view these strategies as additional fences placed around a bad neighbor's yard.

If you are suffering from a cancerous condition, I do not encourage you to use these strategies by themselves. My experience is that the most successful outcomes are the result of using the best of conventional medicine, supplemented with the best of natural medicine.

BLOOD GROUP A:

1. Cancer Prevention Protocol

2. Chemotheraphy Adjunct Protocol

3. Surgery Recovery Protocol

4. Chronic Illness Recovery Protocol

BLOOD GROUP B:

1. Cancer Prevention Protocol

2. Chemotheraphy Adjunct Protocol

3. Surgery Recovery Protocol

4. Chronic Illness Recovery Protocol

BLOOD GROUP AB:

1. Cancer Prevention Protocol

2. Chemotheraphy Adjunct Protocol

3. Surgery Recovery Protocol

4. Chronic Illness Recovery Protocol

BLOOD GROUP O:

1. Cancer Prevention Protocol

2. Chemotheraphy Adjunct Protocol

3. Surgery Recovery Protocol

4. Chronic Illness Recovery Protocol

Related Topics

Autoimmune disease

Immunity

Also refer to individual cancers by name

REFERENCES

1. Sarafian V, Dimova P, Georgiev I, Taskov H. ABH blood group antigen significance as markers of endothelial differentiation of mesenchymal cells. *Folia Med (Plovdiv).* 1997;39:5–9.

2. Palli D, Caporaso NE, Shiao YH, et al. Diet, Helicobacter pylori, and p53 mutations in gastric cancer: a molecular epidemiology study in Italy. *Cancer Epidemiol Biomarkers Prev.* 1997;6:1065–1069.

3. Kawaguchi T. [Adhesion molecules and carbohydrates in cancer metastasis]. *Rinsho Byori.* 1996;44:1138–1146.

4. Ichikawa D, Handa K, Hakomori S. Histo-blood group A/B antigen deletion/reduction vs. continuous expression in human tumor cells as correlated with their malignancy. *Int J Cancer.* 1998;76:284–289.

5. Sarafian V, Popov A, Taskov H. Expression of A, B, and H blood group antigens and carcinoembryonic antigen in human tumours. *Zentralbl Pathol.* 1993;139:351–354.

6. Vowden P, Lowe AD, Lennox ES, Bleehen NM. Thyroid blood group isoantigen expression: a parallel with ABH isoantigen expression in the distal colon. *Br J Cancer.* 1986; 53:721–725.

7. Hirohashi S. Tumor-associated carbohydrate antigens related to blood group carbohydrates. *Gan To Kagaku Ryoho.* 1986;13(pt 2):1395–1401.

8. Kurtenkov O, Klaamas K, Miljukhina L. The lower level of natural anti-Thomsen-Friedreich antigen (TFA) agglutinins in sera of patients with gastric cancer related to ABO(H) blood group phenotype. *Int J Cancer.* 1995;60: 781–785.

9. Oleksowicz L, Bhagwati N, DeLeon-Fernandez M. Deficient activity of von Willebrand's factor-cleaving protease in patients with disseminated malignancies. *Cancer Res.* 1999;59:2244–2250.

10. Ciardiello F, Tortora G. Interactions between the epidermal growth factor receptor and type I protein kinase A: biological significance and therapeutic implications. *Clin Cancer Res.* 1998;4:821–828.

11. Shapiro WR, Shapiro JR. Biology and treatment of malig-

nant glioma [review]. *Oncology (Huntingt)*. 1998;12:233–240.

12. Kurpad SN, Zhao XG, Wikstrand CJ, Batra SK, McLendon RE, Bigner DD. Tumor antigens in astrocytic gliomas. *Glia*. 1995;15:244–256.

13. Neal DE, Mellon K. Epidermal growth factor receptor and bladder cancer: a review. *Urol Int*. 1992;48:365–371.

14. Defize LH, Arndt-Jovin DJ, Jovin TM, et al. A431 cell variants lacking the blood group A antigen display increased high affinity epidermal growth factor-receptor number, protein-tyrosine kinase activity, and receptor turnover. *J Cell Biol*. 1988;107:939–949.

15. Engelmann B, Schumacher U, Haen E. Epidermal growth factor binding sites on human erythrocytes in donors with different ABO blood groups. *Am J Hematol*. 1992;39:239–241.

16. Ueda M, Ueki M, Terai Y, et al. Biological implications of growth factors on the mechanism of invasion in gynecological tumor cells. *Gynecol Obstet Invest*. 1999;48:221–228.

17. Brenner BG, Margolese RG. The relationship of chemotherapeutic and endocrine intervention on natural killer cell activity in human breast cancer. *Cancer*. 1991;68:482–488.

18. Garner WL, Minton JP, James AG, Hoffmann C. Human breast cancer and impaired NK cell function. *J Surg Oncol*. 1983;24:64–66.

19. Parra S, Pinochet R, Vargas R, Sepulveda C, Miranda D, Puente J. Natural killer cytolytic activity in renal and prostatic cancer [in Spanish]. *Rev Med Chil*. 1994;122:630–637.

20. Aparicio-Pages NM, Verspaget HW, Pena SA, Lamers CB. Impaired local natural killer cell activity in human colorectal carcinomas. *Cancer Immunol Immunother*. 1989;28:301–304.

21. Fulton A, Heppner G, Roi L, Howard L, Russo J, Brennan M. Relationship of natural killer cytotoxicity to clinical and biochemical parameters of primary human breast cancer. *Breast Cancer Res Treat*. 1984;4:109–116.

22. Lasek W, Jakobisiak M, Plodziszewska M, Gorecki D. The influence of ABO blood groups, Rh antigens and cigarette smoking on the level of NK activity in normal population. *Arch Immunol Ther Exp (Warsz)*. 1989;37:287–294.

23. Hersey P, Edwards A, Trilivas C, Shaw H, Milton GW. Relationship of natural killer-cell activity to rhesus antigens in man. *Br J Cancer*. 1979;39:234–240.

24. Blottiere HM, Burg C, Zennadi R, et al. Involvement of histo-blood-group antigens in the susceptibility of colon carcinoma cells to natural killer-mediated cytotoxicity. *Int J Cancer*. 1992;52:609–618.

25. Lasek W, Jakobisiak M, Plodziszewska M, Gorecki D. The influence of ABO blood groups, Rh antigens and cigarette smoking on the level of NK activity in normal population. *Arch Immunol Ther Exp (Warsz)*. 1989;37:287–294.

26. Pross HF, Baines MG. Studies of human natural killer cells. I. In vivo parameters affecting normal cytotoxic function. *Int J Cancer*. 1982;29:383–390.

CANCER, BLADDER—*Tumors that occur most often in the elderly, thought to be associated with smoking or chemical exposure.*

Bladder cancer	RISK		
	LOW	AVERAGE	HIGH
GROUP A	▓	▓	
GROUP B	▓	▓	▓
GROUP AB			
GROUP O	▓		
NON-SECRETOR	▓	▓	

Symptoms

- Microscopic hematuria

- Blood in the urine

- Frequent urination

- Pain and burning with urination
- Pelvic pain
- A palpable mass

About Bladder Cancer

Bladder cancer is the sixth most common cancer in the United States. About 12,400 people will die every year of this disease. Bladder cancer is more common among men than among women. When found and treated early (as often happens), the chances for survival are very good. The 5-year survival rate for early bladder cancer is 94%. If the cancer has spread to nearby pelvic organs, the rate is 49%, and if distant organs are involved it drops to 6%.

There are three forms of bladder cancer:

- Transitional cell carcinoma (TCC) is by far the most common form of bladder cancer. It accounts for about 90% of these cancers. There are subgroups of TCC. Some of these are more likely to spread than others.

- Squamous cell carcinomas account for about 8% of bladder cancers. Under a microscope, these cancer cells look very much like skin cancer cells. Nearly all cancers of this type are likely to invade deeper layers of the bladder. Squamous cell carcinoma of the bladder has a poor prognosis because it is usually highly infiltrative and is found at a more advanced stage.

- Adenocarcinomas account for only about 1% to 2% of bladder cancers. They are also very likely to involve deeper layers of the bladder.

The causes of bladder cancers are not entirely understood. Risk factors include severe chronic CYSTITIS, ALCOHOLISM, tobacco smoking, and radiation exposure. Chemicals used in a variety of industries—including dye, rubber, leather, paint, and textile manufacturing—may be risk factors for bladder cancer.

With bladder cancer, often there are no symptoms in the early stages. Microscopic hematuria may be the earliest sign. Later, blood in the urine, frequent urination, and pain and burning with urination occur. Pelvic pain occurs with advanced disease. A mass may be palpable with manual examination.

Diagnosis of bladder cancer is made with cytoscopy, the placement of a lens into the bladder that allows a view. If abnormalities are seen, a biopsy is performed. In patients with superficial malignancies, death from bladder cancer is very rare. In patients with deeply invasive lesions of the bladder musculature, survival is poor (about 50% at 5 years), but adjuvant chemotherapy may improve these results.

Early superficial MALIGNANCIES (including superficial invasion of the bladder musculature) can be completely removed by transurethral resection and fulguration. Recurrence at the same or another site in the bladder is relatively common and may be reduced by repeated bladder instillations of chemotherapeutic drugs.

Blood Group Links

Bladder cancer cases for both sexes show a marked frequency of blood groups B and A, as well as an overall preference for non-secretors.

One study of transitional cell cancers of the bladder and urethra showed a high rate of reaction when the cancer cells were treated with antibodies to group A blood[1]. This implies that these types of tumors may be A-like in appearance.

It has also been shown that bladder cancer occurs with a high frequency in people who suffer from recurrent BLADDER and KIDNEY INFECTIONS—conditions that afflict blood group B more often than other blood groups.

Rh-positive individuals have more invasive tumors of the upper urinary tract.

Transitional cell carcinomas of the urinary bladder show variable blood group antigen reactivity even in the noninvasive stage. A correlation exists between the tumor reactivity and subsequent clinical course: when the expected blood group antigen(s) is retained, the clinical course is favorable; absence of the expected antigen(s) denotes an aggressive potential.

Therapies, Bladder Cancer

ALL BLOOD GROUPS:

The most effective preventive measures include the following:

1. Don't smoke. Smoking has been isolated as a major risk factor for bladder cancer.

2. Avoid chemical exposure. If you work in a chemical environment, wear protective clothing.

3. Moderate your levels of alcohol consumption.

4. Since bladder cancer is a disease of the elderly, maintain general health strategies

throughout life, according to your blood type, that will strengthen immunity.

BLOOD GROUP A:

1. Cancer Prevention Protocol
2. Chemotherapy Adjunct Protocol
3. Surgery Recovery Protocol
4. Chronic Illness Recovery Protocol

BLOOD GROUP B:

1. Cancer Prevention Protocol
2. Chemotherapy Adjunct Protocol
3. Antiviral Protocol
4. Surgery Recovery Protocol
5. Chronic Illness Recovery Protocol

BLOOD GROUP AB:

1. Cancer Prevention Protocol
2. Chemotherapy Adjunct Protocol
3. Surgery Recovery Protocol
4. Chronic Illness Recovery Protocol

BLOOD GROUP O:

1. Cancer Prevention Protocol
2. Chemotherapy Adjunct Protocol
3. Surgery Recovery Protocol
4. Chronic Illness Recovery Protocol

Related Topics

Cancer (general)

Cystitis

Immunity

REFERENCES

1. Limas C, Lange P. Altered reactivity for A, B, H antigens in transitional cell carcinomas of the urinary bladder. A study of the mechanisms involved. *Cancer*. 1980;46:1366–1373.

CANCER, BRAIN–*See Cancer, glioma and other brain tumors*

CANCER, BREAST–*Cancerous conditions of the breasts, milk ducts, and lymphatic nodes.*

Breast cancer	RISK		
	LOW	AVERAGE	HIGH
GROUP A			
GROUP B			
GROUP AB			
GROUP O			
SECRETOR			

Symptoms

- A new lump or mass

A lump that is painless, hard, and has irregular edges is more likely to be cancer. But some rare cancers are tender, soft, and rounded. Other signs of breast cancer include the following:

- A swelling of part of the breast
- Skin irritation or dimpling

- Nipple pain or the nipple turning inward
- Redness or scaliness of the nipple or breast skin
- A discharge other than breast milk

About Breast Cancer

Breast cancer is the most common cancer among women. And while the mortality rates are falling slightly for some subpopulations of women, it is still a potentially lethal adversary. Standard treatment can vary, but procedures such as lumpectomy surgery (removal of the tumor and some surrounding tissue), mastectomy (removal of the whole breast), chemotherapy, radiation, and hormone-blocking therapy are the norm, with any combination of the above strategies potentially employed.

Five-year breast cancer survival rates vary significantly based on size of tumor and extent of metastasis:

> 80%—tumor was smaller than 2 cm with no metastases
>
> 65%—tumor was larger than 2 cm with no metastases
>
> 40%—tumor was greater than 5 cm with no metastases
>
> 10%—distant metastases

Blood Group Links

ABO blood group exerts a significant influence on susceptibility and outcomes.

In 1984 scientists discovered a gene for breast

cancer susceptibility linked to ABO susceptibility, located on band q34 of chromosome 9. This discovery of a genetic connection confirms an increasing body of statistical evidence connecting blood group to breast cancer[1].

Some researchers have stated that blood groups were shown to possess a predictive value independent of other known prognostic factors for breast cancer.

Substantial research shows that blood group A women are over-represented among breast cancer patients, and that this trend occurs even among women thought to be at low risk for cancer. One of the most significant risk factors for a rapidly progressing breast cancer is also blood group A. Blood group A women have been observed to have poorer outcomes once they are diagnosed with breast cancer. On the other hand, blood group O status implies a slight degree of resistance against breast cancer; even among breast cancer patients, group O showed a significantly lower risk of death. Blood group AB has a slight increase in susceptibility over A, and is associated with poorer outcomes and earlier deaths. Blood group B has a reduced risk, which is particularly evident among women who do not have a family history of breast cancer. However, if there is a family member with breast cancer, the protection normally associated with being a blood group B is lost. Group B women who currently have or have had breast cancer have a higher statistical likelihood of a recurrence.

The association between blood type A and breast cancer was evaluated in 648 patients with family histories of the disease, 1,897 general patients, 4,577 institutional blood donor controls, and 14,508 extramural blood donor controls. The familial patients were classified into three pedigree groups in which the lifetime breast cancer risks to first-degree relatives ranged from 11% to 32%. In the pedigree group associated with a relatively low risk to relatives, the authors saw a significant excess of blood type A individuals when compared with either control group. The general patient population, which was considered to refer to a general series of patients, also showed an excess of blood type A individuals[2].

Breast cancer shows a weaker association with being a non-secretor[3].

Therapies, Breast Cancer

ALL BLOOD GROUPS:

Adhere to breast cancer screening guidelines. The earlier breast cancer is found, the better the chances for successful treatment. The American Cancer Society recommends the following guidelines for finding breast cancer early:

1. Women 40 and over should have a mammogram every year.

2. Between the ages of 20 and 39, women should have a clinical breast exam every 3 years. After age 40, women should have a breast exam by a health professional every year.

3. All women over 20 should do breast self-examination (BSE) every month. The best time for this is 7 days after the beginning of the menstrual cycle.

BLOOD GROUP A:

1. Cancer Prevention Protocol

2. Surgery Recovery Protocol

3. Chronic Illness Recovery Protocol

BLOOD GROUP B:

1. Cancer Prevention Protocol

2. Surgery Recovery Protocol

3. Chronic Illness Recovery Protocol

BLOOD GROUP AB:

1. Cancer Prevention Protocol

2. Surgery Recovery Protocol

3. Chronic Illness Recovery Protocol

BLOOD GROUP O:

1. Cancer Prevention Protocol

2. Surgery Recovery Protocol

3. Chronic Illness Recovery Protocol

Related Topics

Cancer (general)

Immunity

REFERENCES

1. Skolnick MH, Thompson EA, Bishop DT, Cannon LA. Possible linkage of a breast cancer-susceptibility locus to the ABO locus: sensitivity of LOD scores to a single new recombinant observation. *Genet Epidemiol.* 1984;1:363–373.

2. Anderson DE, Haas C. Blood type A and familial breast cancer. *Cancer.* 1984;54:1845–1849.

3. Nagata C, Kabuto M, Kurisu Y, Shimizu H. Decreased se-rum estradiol concentration associated with high dietary intake of soy products in premenopausal Japanese women. *Nutr Cancer* 1997;29:228–233.

CANCER, CERVICAL–<i>See Cancer, gynecological tumors</i>

CANCER, COLON–<i>Tumors of the colon; together with rectal tumors, they're often referred to as colorectal cancers.</i>

Colon cancer	RISK		
	LOW	AVERAGE	HIGH
GROUP A			
GROUP B			
GROUP AB			
GROUP O			

Symptoms

- Rectal bleeding

- Abdominal pain

- Change in bowel habits and/or the size, shape, or color of stool—especially gradually increasing constipation and black stool

- Acute obstruction: colicky (spasmodic) pain, increasing abdominal distention, failure to pass stools or gas

- Weight loss

- Anorexia

About Colon Cancer

Colon cancer will cause about 48,100 deaths and rectal cancer about 8,600 deaths each year. Nine out of 10 people whose colorectal cancer is found and treated at an early stage before it has spread will live at least 5 years. Once the cancer has spread to nearby organs or lymph nodes, the 5-year survival rate goes down to 65%. For people whose colorectal cancer has spread to distant parts of the body such as the liver or lungs, the 5-year survival rate is 8%.

The onset of symptoms is very gradual and depends on the tumor location, size, type, and complications. Often the first sign of colon cancer comes when the tumor irritates an adjacent organ, such as the urinary bladder or the stomach; or if it leads to bowel perforation and peritonitis. Symptoms differ according to the tumor's location:

Right colon: There may be a palpable mass through the abdominal wall, along with fatigue and weakness from anemia due to a concealed hemorrhage. A change in bowel habits is usually a late sign.

Left colon: A change in bowel habits is more apparent—including alternating constipation with diarrhea, and overtly bloody stools.

Rectum: The primary symptom is defecation with bloody stools.

The prognosis varies with the extent of the disease, the location in bowel, the degree of wall infiltration, and whether there is local or distant METASTASIS. In patients with cancer limited to the mucosa, the 5-year survival rate is 70%; with spread to the lymph nodes, it drops to 30%.

From Polyp to Cancer

Polyps are usually benign growths that develop in the colon. They vary in size and appearance; some look like a wart when small, and a cherry on a stem or fig when they grow. They are important because with time they can become cancerous. Polyps of the colon and rectum are almost always benign and usually produce no symptoms. They may, however, cause painless rectal bleeding or bleeding not apparent to the naked eye. The incidence of polyps increases with age. The cumulative risk of cancer developing in an unremoved polyp is 2.5% at 5 years, 8% at 10 years, and 24% at 20 years after the initial discovery and diagnosis. Polyps larger than 1 cm have a greater cancer risk associated with them than smaller polyps. It has been shown that the removal of polyps by colonoscopy reduces the risk of getting colon cancer significantly.

Risk factors for colon cancer include a high meat diet and corresponding low intake of fresh fruits and vegetables.

Blood Group Links

Being either blood group A or blood group AB should be considered an important risk factor for colorectal cancer[1].

The amount of blood group antigen made in the colon is highest in the upper colon (the cecum), and diminishes gradually so as to virtually disappear by the very end of the colon (the rectosigmoid). In colon cancer, the exact opposite happens. The cells of the upper colon lose the ability to produce ABO antigens, while the cells of the lower colon start to manufacture them. In immunology the term "horror autotoxicus" is used to indicate that the immune system has an innate disinclination to attack the body; thus, an ability to mimic the markers on cells that are normally used by the immune system to determine whether a cell is healthy or malignant is a potent way to derail the immune response. For example, the expression of blood group antigens was found to correlate with the degree of effectiveness of the immune system's natural killer (NK) cells. The higher the amount of blood group antigen on the tumor cells, the lower the aggressiveness of the tumor-killing NK cells of the immune system[2,3,4].

Cancer cells often manufacture antigens that are typically made only in fetal development and repressed throughout adult life. The opposite of this is also true. That is, when a cell starts to lose genetic control over itself, it can also lose the ability to manufacture the antigens that are made when that same cell is healthy.

Since the production of surface antigens is intimately linked with the process of each cell attaching to its neighbor, it is likely that the addition or deletion of blood group antigens from the surface of colon cancer cells is somehow related to their ability to spread, or metastasize[5]. It has even been reported that colorectal cancer cells can manufacture blood type antigens of a different blood group than their host. The production of B antigen in normally type A or O individuals

with colon cancer has been most often reported. In fact, in one case the detection of an unwarranted B antigen led to the diagnosis of a previously undetected tumor[6].

Colon cancer cells of the rectosigmoid, the area that most often develops colon cancer, manufacture large amounts of group A antigen, even in people who are not group A. Also, the amount of group A antigen made seems to correlate with the potential for metastasis, or spread.

Blood Group and Tumor Markers

Physicians often monitor a tumor marker called CEA, or "carcinoembryonic antigen," when gauging the progression of colon cancer. Like most tumor markers, CEA is a glycoprotein, the same class of molecule as blood group antigens. It appears that expression of blood group A antigen is intimately related to synthesis of CEA.

In 1987 researchers looked at the expression of blood group antigens in relation to the production of CEA in human colon carcinoma cells of different ABO blood groups. All tumor cells made A and B antigens, regardless of the patient's original blood group. However, tumor cells from group O patients had lower expression of both A and B antigens and high production of CEA. Cells from patients with group A blood had low to undetectable CEA production and high expression of both A and B antigens[7].

In 1995 an article published in the *Journal of Cell Biochemistry* reported that "altered expression of ABO blood group substances is a common feature of human colorectal carcinoma, yet it remains unclear how these structural changes influence the biological properties of tumor cells."

Certain chemically induced rat colon tumors display many features of human cancer, thereby providing a potentially useful model to study the role of blood group substances in colon cancer progression. Using antibodies developed for chemically induced tumors of the colon, the researchers found that these same antibodies reacted to the epitope (binding site) that is also expressed in blood group A human colon carcinoma cell lines but not in cell lines whose donors were blood group B. The researchers offered that "blood group A-specific lectins may provide a useful tool for early detection of colon cancer"[8].

It is interesting that the A antigens made by cancer cells in the lower colon are embryonic variations not seen typically in adults. In one study, four variants of the A antigen were found in human colon cancer cells, but of these only one was found in adults; the other three were variants of blood group A typically only found in fetal tissue[9]. This is significant, as one of the primary roles blood group antigens play in the developing fetus involves shaping the architecture of developing tissue and organs by serving as cell-to-cell attachment and detachment points. The question is, does the redevelopment of these "fetal" forms of blood group A permit tumor cells to develop the ability to detach from the primary site and spread through the body? Only more research will tell.

There is a strange but documented link between the expression of blood group antigens in tumors of the thyroid and lower colon[10]. Blood group A individuals with a history of thyroid tumors, either benign or malignant, may be at especially high risk of developing cancer of the lower colon.

Blood Group and the Tn Antigen

Malignant cells in colon cancer develop a tumor marker called the Thomsen-Friedenreich (T) antigen. This antigen is suppressed in normal healthy cells, and only becomes unsuppressed as a cell moves toward malignancy. It is so rare to find the T antigen in healthy tissue that we actually have antibodies against it. It is even more unusual to find a Tn antigen, the precursor to T or a less well-developed T antigen, on a healthy cell.

As a general rule, an orderly expression of T antigens on a cancer cell usually indicates a cancer with a relatively favorable outlook. However, a prevalence of Tn antigens on a cancer cell usually denotes a highly aggressive, metastatic cancer, irrespective of the organ involved or the form of cancer. In addition to colon cancer, Tn is also expressed in ULCERATIVE COLITIS[11], which may help explain why chronic ulcerative colitis is a risk factor for the subsequent development of colon cancer.

The Thomsen-Friedenreich (T) antigen and Tn antigen show some structural similarity to the A antigen (even though it is derived from the M blood type antigen). Not surprisingly, blood group A individuals have the least aggressive antibody immune response against the T and probably Tn antigens. In fact, the T and Tn antigens and the A antigens are actually immunologically considered to be quite similar because of their shared terminal sugar (N-acetyl-galactosamine), and so might be readily confused by the immune system of blood group A individuals. This finding has led researchers to conclude that the Tn antigen is, in a broad sense, an A-like antigen. The hypothesis: because of the lower level of antibody against T and Tn antigens, and because of this tendency for the immune system of group A to be disinclined to attack Tn antigens, blood group A is at an immunological disadvantage in attacking any cell bearing the T and Tn antigenic markers.

Therapies, Colon Cancer

ALL BLOOD GROUPS:

Adhere to the colon cancer screening guidelines as part of your overall physical health screening program. The three types of screening are fecal occult blood testing (FOBT), flexible sigmoidoscopy, or the colonoscopy for detection.

The FOBT looks for blood in the stool that might be associated with cancer. In some instances, the presence of blood is caused by hemorrhoids. In other cases, cancer might not be accompanied by blood in the stool.

The flexible sigmoidoscopy, which examines the bottom third of the colon, could miss a cancer farther up. *The New England Journal of Medicine* has featured two large studies that reported that the flexible sigmoidoscopy missed too many precancerous growths in a sample of 5,000 patients.

Colonoscopy is the most thorough screening test, so it is also the best test for colon cancer. Colonoscopy is an examination of the entire colon (5 feet in length) with a slender, flexible, lighted tube, looking for abnormal cells that could develop into cancer.

BLOOD GROUP A:

1. Cancer Prevention Protocol
2. Chemotherapy Adjunct Protocol
3. Intestinal Health Protocol
4. Surgery Recovery Protocol
5. Chronic Illness Recovery Protocol

BLOOD GROUP B:

1. Cancer Prevention Protocol
2. Chemotherapy Adjunct Protocol
3. Intestinal Health Protocol
4. Surgery Recovery Protocol
5. Chronic Illness Recovery Protocol

BLOOD GROUP AB:

1. Cancer Prevention Protocol
2. Chemotherapy Adjunct Protocol
3. Intestinal Health Protocol
4. Surgery Recovery Protocol
5. Chronic Illness Recovery Protocol

BLOOD GROUP O:

1. Cancer Prevention Protocol
2. Chemotherapy Adjunct Protocol
3. Intestinal Health Protocol
4. Surgery Recovery Protocol
5. Chronic Illness Recovery Protocol

Related Topics

Cancer (general)

Colitis, ulcerative

Crohn's disease

Immunity

Lectins

Polyps, colon

REFERENCES

1. Slater G, Itzkowitz S, Azar S, Aufses AH Jr. Clinicopathologic correlations of ABO and Rhesus blood type in colorectal cancer. *Dis Colon Rectum.* 1993;36:5–7.

2. Salem RR, Wolf BC, Sears HF, et al. Expression of colorectal carcinoma-associated antigens in colonic polyps. *J Surg Res.* 1993;55:249–255.

3. Blottiere HM, Burg C, Zennadi R, et al. Involvement of histo-blood-group antigens in the susceptibility of colon carcinoma cells to natural killer-mediated cytotoxicity. *Int J Cancer.* 1992;52:609–618.

4. Schoentag R, Primus FJ, Kuhns W. ABH and Lewis blood group expression in colorectal carcinoma. *Cancer Res.* 1987;47:1695–1700.

5. Kawaguchi T. [Adhesion molecules and carbohydrates in cancer metastasis]. *Rinsho Byori.* 1996;44:1138–1146.

6. Northoff H, Wolpl A, Bewersdorf H, Faulhaber JD. An ABO-blood group abnormality leading to the detection of a colon-carcinoma. *Blut.* 1983;46:161–164.

7. Cooper HS, Marshall C, Ruggerio F, Steplewski Z. Hyperplastic polyps of the colon and rectum. An immunohistochemical study with monoclonal antibodies against blood groups antigens (sialosyl-Lea, Leb, Lex, Ley, A, B, H). *Lab Invest.* 1987;57:421–428.

8. Laferte S, Prokopishyn NL, Moyana T, Bird RP. Monoclonal antibody recognizing a determinant on type 2 chain blood group A and B oligosaccharides detects oncodevelopmental changes in azoxymethane-induced rat colon tumors and human colon cancer cell lines. *Cancer J Cell Biochem.* 1995;57:101–119.

9. Itzkowitz SH. Blood group-related carbohydrate antigen expression in malignant and premalignant colonic neoplasms. *J Cell Biochem Suppl.* 1992;16G:97–101.

10. Vowden P, Lowe AD, Lennox ES, Bleehen NM. Thyroid blood group isoantigen expression: a parallel with ABH isoantigen expression in the distal colon. *Br J Cancer.* 1986;53:721–725.

11. Freed DL, Green FH. Do dietary lectins protect against colonic cancer? *Lancet.* 1975;2:1261–1262.

CANCER, COLORECTAL—*See Cancer, colon*

CANCER, ENDOMETRIAL—*See Cancer, uterine*

CANCER, ESOPHAGEAL—*Cancer of the esophagus.*

Esophageal cancer	RISK		
	LOW	AVERAGE	HIGH
GROUP A	███	███	███
GROUP B	███		
GROUP AB	███	███	███
GROUP O	███		

Symptoms

- Difficulty swallowing
- Chest pain
- Weight loss
- Vocal cord paralysis and hoarseness

About Esophageal Cancer

About 12,500 people will die of the disease each year. This cancer is about three times more common among men than among women and three times more common among individuals of African ancestry than among Caucasians. There are two main types of esophageal cancer. One type grows in the cells that form the top layer of the lining of the esophagus. These are called squamous cells, and cancer that starts there is known as squamous cell carcinoma. Squamous cell cancer can grow anywhere along the length of the esophagus. It accounts for about half of all esophageal cancer. The other type of cancer of the esophagus starts near the opening to the stomach. It begins in the cells of Barrett's esophagus and is called adeno-carcinoma. Adenocarcinoma cannot start unless squamous cells have been changed by acid reflux.

Esophageal cancer usually presents with pro-gressive dysphagia (difficulty swallowing) over several weeks, as the lumen of the esophagus be-comes constricted. The first stage involves diffi-culty swallowing solid food, and the sensation that food is sticking on the way down the esophagus. The second stage involves difficulty swallowing semisolid food. Finally, there is difficulty swallow-ing liquid food and saliva; this progression over time suggests the presence of a growing malignant process rather than a spasm, benign ring, or peptic stricture. Chest pain usually radiates to the back.

Weight loss, even when the patient maintains a good appetite, is almost universal. Compression of the recurrent laryngeal nerve may lead to vocal cord paralysis and hoarseness.

Scientists believe that some risk factors such as smoking and drinking cause damage to the cells that line the esophagus. Likewise, long-term ir-ritation of the lining of the esophagus from re-flux can promote cancer formation. There is also some evidence that certain viruses can increase the risk of esophageal cancer.

Blood Group Links

Groups A and AB seem to have a higher inci-dence of esophageal cancer over the other blood groups.

Up to 20% of those with chronic GERD will go on to develop the precancerous condition called BARRETT'S ESOPHAGUS—and up to 10% of those will have an increased risk of developing esoph-ageal cancer. Furthermore, patients who develop esophageal cancer subsequent to Barrett's esoph-agus typically have a poor prognosis because the cancer is often discovered at an advanced stage.

Therapies, Esophageal Cancer

BLOOD GROUP A:

1. Cancer Prevention Protocol
2. Chemotherapy Adjunct Protocol
3. Stomach Health Protocol
4. Surgery Recovery Protocol
5. Chronic Illness Recovery Protocol

BLOOD GROUP B:

1. Cancer Prevention Protocol
2. Chemotherapy Adjunct Protocol
3. Stomach Health Protocol
4. Surgery Recovery Protocol
5. Chronic Illness Recovery Protocol

BLOOD GROUP AB:

1. Cancer Prevention Protocol

2. Chemotherapy Adjunct Protocol

3. Stomach Health Protocol

4. Surgery Recovery Protocol

5. Chronic Illness Recovery Protocol

BLOOD GROUP O:

1. Cancer Prevention Protocol

2. Chemotherapy Adjunct Protocol

3. Stomach Health Protocol

4. Surgery Recovery Protocol

5. Chronic Illness Recovery Protocol

Related Topics

Barrett's esophagus

Cancer (general)

Gastroesophageal reflux disease (GERD)

Immunity

CANCER, GALLBLADDER–*Tumors of the gallbladder.*

Gallbladder cancer	RISK		
	LOW	AVERAGE	HIGH
GROUP A			
GROUP B			
GROUP AB			
GROUP O			

Symptoms

- Abdominal pain
- Nausea and/or vomiting
- Jaundice
- Gallbladder enlargement

About Gallbladder Cancer

Gallbladder cancer is a disease of the elderly. Between 6,000 and 7,000 new cases of gallbladder cancer are diagnosed each year in the United States, usually among people over 70 years old. They are nearly three times as likely to be women than men. Gallbladder cancer is more common among Caucasian women than among women of African ancestry. It is also more common among individuals of Mexican and Native American ancestry than among the general population as a whole.

Few gallbladder cancers are found early, before they have spread to other tissues and organs. Many early cancers are found incidentally when a person's gallbladder is removed as treatment for gallstones. At later stages, symptoms may include the following:

Abdominal pain: More than half of all gallbladder cancer patients have abdominal pain at the time of diagnosis. Most often this is in the right upper part of the abdomen.

Nausea and/or vomiting: At the time of their diagnosis, more than half of all people with gallbladder cancer report vomiting as a symptom.

Jaundice: Almost half of all gallbladder cancer patients have jaundice when they are diagnosed.

Gallbladder enlargement: Sometimes bile duct blockage causes bile to accumulate in the gallbladder, causing it to become larger than usual. This enlargement can sometimes be felt by the doctor during a physical exam, and can also be detected by imaging studies such as ultrasound.

Blood Group Links

Group B seems to have a higher incidence of gallbladder cancer over the other blood groups. This is probably related to group B's susceptibility to slow-growing viruses and bacterial diseases, which compromise the immune system.

Therapies, Gallbladder Cancer

BLOOD GROUP A:

1. Cancer Prevention Protocol
2. Chemotherapy Adjunct Protocol
3. Liver Support Protocol
4. Surgery Recovery Protocol
5. Chronic Illness Recovery Protocol

BLOOD GROUP B:

1. Cancer Prevention Protocol
2. Chemotherapy Adjunct Protocol
3. Liver Support Protocol
4. Surgery Recovery Protocol
5. Chronic Illness Recovery Protocol

BLOOD GROUP AB:

1. Cancer Prevention Protocol
2. Chemotherapy Adjunct Protocol
3. Liver Support Protocol
4. Surgery Recovery Protocol
5. Chronic Illness Recovery Protocol

BLOOD GROUP O:

1. Cancer Prevention Protocol
2. Chemotherapy Adjunct Protocol
3. Liver Support Protocol
4. Surgery Recovery Protocol
5. Chronic Illness Recovery Protocol

Related Topics

Cancer (general)

Gallstones

Liver disease (general)

Immunity

CANCER, GLIOMA AND OTHER BRAIN TUMORS—*Tumors of the brain, spinal cord, and nervous system.*

Cancer, glioma	RISK		
	LOW	AVERAGE	HIGH
GROUP A			
GROUP B			
GROUP AB			
GROUP O			

Symptoms

- Numbness and/or weakness of both legs
- Abnormal positioning of the body
- Headache
- Nausea
- Vomiting
- Blurred vision

About Brain Gliomas

Glioma is a term referring to three types of brain tumors:

Astrocytoma: Most tumors that arise within the brain itself start in brain cells called astrocytes. These tumors are called astrocytomas. Most astrocytomas cannot be cured because they spread widely throughout the surrounding normal brain tissue. Sometimes astrocytomas spread along the cerebrospinal fluid pathways. However, with only very rare exceptions, astrocytomas do not spread outside of the brain or spinal cord.

Oligodendroglioma: These tumors start in brain cells called oligodendrocytes. They spread or infiltrate in a manner similar to astrocytomas and, in most cases, cannot be completely removed by surgery. However, a small number of oligodendrogliomas are associated with long-term survivals of 30 or 40 years. Oligodendrogliomas may spread along the cerebrospinal fluid pathways but rarely spread outside the brain or spinal cord.

Ependymoma: These tumors arise from the ependymal cells that line the ventricles. Ependymomas may block the exit of cerebrospinal fluid from the ventricles, causing the ventricle to become very large in a condition called hydrocephalus. Unlike astrocytomas and oligodendrogliomas, ependymomas characteristically do not spread or infiltrate into normal brain tissue. As a result, some but not all ependymomas can be completely removed and cured by surgery. Spinal cord ependymomas have the greatest chance of surgical cure. Ependymomas may spread along the cerebrospinal fluid pathways but do not spread outside the brain or spinal cord.

Whether a brain cancer is detected early usually depends on its location within the brain. Cancers located in more important areas of the brain may cause symptoms earlier than those located in less important areas of the brain. Brain and spinal cord tumors often interfere with the specific functions of the region they develop in. For example, spinal cord tumors often cause numbness and/or weakness of both legs, and tumors of the basal ganglia typically cause abnormal movements and abnormal positioning of the body. Tumors within any part of the brain may cause pressure to rise within the skull. Increased pressure within the skull may cause headache, nausea, vomiting, or blurred vision. Headache is a common symptom of brain tumor, occurring in about 50% of patients.

Blood Group Links

A positive, consistent, and often very strong association has been found between blood group A and brain and nervous system tumors. A weaker association for these forms of cancer exists for group B. Conversely, it has been a consistent finding that being group O is a favorable prognostic factor for brain and nervous system cancers.

Additionally, ABO blood group has found to be of prognostic value in gliomas. In one study of oligodendroglioma patients, those with blood group A had a distinctly poorer prognosis than patients with O or B blood. The survival data from this unselected series indicated that cerebral oligodendrogliomas have a less favorable prognosis than has generally been believed[1].

In another study, the distribution of ABO blood groups was analyzed statistically in 271 patients treated for glioblastoma multiforme. The control group included 500 patients treated for craniocerebral trauma. A statistically significant difference was observed in the distribution of ABO blood groups between these patient groups, with higher frequency of group A and lower of group O in the patients with glioblastoma multiforme[2].

The efficacy of postoperative chemotherapy and immunochemotherapy was analyzed according to the survival period from study of patients who underwent operation for malignant (III–IV degree malignancy) gliomas. In analyzing the efficacy of various schedules of combined treatment, the investigators took into consideration the patients' ABO blood group because it is known that many antineoplastic antibiotics contain structures that are marked by cross-reaction with the ABO isoantigens. The results of the study showed that the use of polychemotherapy and levamisole in neuro-oncological patients with A(II) and AB(IV) blood group promising. Levamisole and the antineoplastic antibiotic reumycin proved to be authentically effective in patients with A(II) blood group and ineffective in those with O(I) blood group. The data obtained are recommended for use in individual selection of the schedule of chemotherapy and immunochemotherapy in patients of different ABO blood groups[3].

The exception to the overall preference of group A and B is pituitary adenomas. Pituitary adenoma has been shown to be associated with an increased occurrence of group O blood over the other blood groups. In an analysis of 282 brain tumors of all types compared with 55,089 control individuals from the Boston population, the percentage of adenoma of the pituitary was significantly increased in group O (almost 62% of all adenomas) versus all other brain tumors, which showed an overall excess of group A[4].

Therapies, Glioma, and Other Brain Tumors

BLOOD GROUP A:

1. Cancer Prevention Protocol

2. Chemotherapy Adjunct Protocol

3. Surgery Recovery Protocol

4. Chronic Illness Recovery Protocol

BLOOD GROUP B:

1. Cancer Prevention Protocol

2. Chemotherapy Adjunct Protocol

3. Surgery Recovery Protocol

4. Chronic Illness Recovery Protocol

BLOOD GROUP AB:

1. Cancer Prevention Protocol

2. Chemotherapy Adjunct Protocol

3. Surgery Recovery Protocol

4. Chronic Illness Recovery Protocol

BLOOD GROUP O:

1. Cancer Prevention Protocol

2. Chemotherapy Adjunct Protocol

3. Surgery Recovery Protocol

4. Chronic Illness Recovery Protocol

Related Topics

Cancer (general)

Immunity

REFERENCES

1. Turowski K, Czochra M. [ABO blood groups in glioblastoma multiforme]. *Neurol Neurochir Pol.* 1979;13:173–176.

2. Mork SJ, Lindegaard KF, Halvorsen TB, et al. Oligodendroglioma: incidence and biological behavior in a defined population. *J Neurosurg.* 1985;63:881–889.

3. Romodanov SA, Gnedkova IA, Lisianyi NI, Glavatskii AI. [Efficacy of chemotherapy and immunochemotherapy in neuro-oncologic patients of various blood groups (ABO system)]. *Zh Vopr Neirokhir Im N N Burdenko.* 1989;(1):17–20.

4. Mayr E, Diamond L, Levine RP, Mayr M. Suspected correlation between blood group frequency and pituitary adenoma. *Science.* 1956;(9):932–934.

CANCER, GYNECOLOGICAL TUMORS–

Neoplasm of the female reproductive tract.

Gynecological tumors	RISK		
	LOW	AVERAGE	HIGH
GROUP A	▓	▓	
GROUP B	▓		
GROUP AB	▓	▓	▓
GROUP O	▓	▓	

Various cancers can occur in the female reproductive tract: Endometrial cancer, ovarian cancer, cervical cancer, vulvar cancer, vaginal cancer, fallopian tube cancer, and gestational trophoblastic disease.

Blood Group Links

A retrospective analysis of 968 women affected by gynecological tumors was conducted to assess any difference in survival among patients with different blood groups. Data were presented on 237 cases of endometrial cancer, 92 cases of ovarian cancer, and 639 cases of invasive cervix cancer, detailing the women's ABO blood group antigenic phenotypes, the stage of the cancer, and the treatment they received. With regard to endometrial cancer, a better 5-year and 10-year survival is associated with blood group O when compared with blood group A. This finding is more evident when 5-year survival is considered among patients affected by ovarian cancer. With regard to cervical cancer, analysis showed that a little better than 5-year survival is associated with the O blood phenotype. The study confirmed the evidence of an association between the A blood group and gynecological tumors. Endometrial and ovarian cancer occur more frequently in women with blood group A, than in women with other blood groups. Moreover, for the same tumors, blood group A is associated with a poor prognosis[1,2].

Related Topics

Cancer (general)

Immunity

REFERENCES

1. Marinaccio M, Traversa A, Carioggia E, et al. [Blood groups of the ABO system and survival rate in gynecologic tumors]. *Minerva Ginecol.* 1995;47:69–76.

2. Milunicova A, Jandova A, Skoda V. [The secretion of ABH group substances by women with gynecologic carcinomas]. *Z Immunitatsforsch Allerg Klin Immunol.* 1969;139:90–93.

CANCER, HEAD, NECK, AND SALIVARY GLANDS–*Primarily oral tumors.*

Cancer of the head, neck, and salivary glands	RISK		
	LOW	AVERAGE	HIGH
GROUP A			
GROUP B			
GROUP AB			
GROUP O			
NON-SECRETORS			
SECRETORS (salivary)			
TYPE A2 (larynx)			

Blood Group Links

NOTE: There have been statistical studies related to these cancers and blood groups, but little is known about their full relationships or the implications for treatment. Many of these studies remain contradictory or are subject to further investigation.

Cancer of the lip is significantly associated with blood group A. Cancers of the tongue, gums, and cheeks also have a blood group A association. Cancers of the salivary glands are strongly associated with blood group A, and weakly with blood group B—although studies are few and have yielded contradictory results[1].

Blood group O seems to have substantial protection against this type of cancer. Cancer of the salivary glands also appear to have an association with being a secretor.

As a general rule, a higher intensity of oral disease is found among ABO non-secretors. So it is not surprising that when it comes to precancerous, or cancerous changes to tissue of the mouth and esophagus, non-secretors seem to fare worse than secretors. This oral disease susceptibility is reflected in the occurrence of epithelial dysplasia, for example, which is found almost exclusively in the non-secretor group[2].

Cancers of the larynx and hypopharynx are associated with blood groups A, B, and AB. The A2 blood type (a less common variant of group A) is significantly more frequent in patients with glottis cancer.

Structural changes to squamous cell cancers of the head and neck are quite common. ABO blood groups are expressed in normal tissue of this region. However, once squamous cell cancer develops, the A antigen disappears in about one-third of group A and AB individuals, and the O antigen is expressed in carcinoma cells from all the blood groups. These cancers generally have a poor prognosis. The T and Tn antigens also become commonly expressed in these cancers.

Ductular epithelium and the epithelial components of benign Warthin's tumors have ABO antigens, whereas the loss of antigen in the epithelial portion of the malignant Warthin's tumor is characteristic of epithelial cancerous dedifferentiation. Loss of antigen in adenoid cystic and undifferentiated carcinomas of the parotid supports the concept that antigen is absent in epithelially derived malignant tumors[3].

Therapies, Cancer of the Head, Neck, and Salivary Glands

BLOOD GROUP A:

1. Cancer Prevention Protocol
2. Chemotherapy Adjunct Protocol
3. Surgical Recovery Protocol
4. Chronic Illness Recovery Protocol

BLOOD GROUP B:

1. Cancer Prevention Protocol
2. Chemotherapy Adjunct Protocol
3. Surgery Recovery Protocol
4. Fatigue-Fighting Protocol

BLOOD GROUP AB:

1. Cancer Prevention Protocol
2. Immune-Enhancing Protocol
3. Surgery Recovery Protocol
4. Fatigue-Fighting Protocol

BLOOD GROUP O:

1. Cancer Prevention Protocol
2. Chemotherapy Adjunct Protocol
3. Surgery Recovery Protocol
4. Chronic Illness Recovery Protocol

Related Topics

Cancer (general)

REFERENCES

1. Garrett JV, Nicholson A, Whittaker JS, Ridway JC. Blood-groups and secretor status in patients with salivary-gland tumours. *Lancet.* 1971;2:1177–1179.
2. Vidas I, Delajlija M, Temmer-Vuksan B, Stipetic-Mravak M, Cindric N, Marieie D. Examining the secretor status in the saliva of patients with oral pre-cancerous lesions. *J Oral Rehabil.* 1999;26:177–182.
3. Woltering EA, Tuttle SE, James AG, Sharma HM. ABO (H) cell surface antigens in benign and malignant parotid neoplasms. *J Surg Oncol.* 1983;24:177–179.

CANCER, LEUKEMIA – *Malignant neoplasms of blood-forming tissues.*

Leukemia	RISK		
	LOW	AVERAGE	HIGH
GROUP A	░	░	░
GROUP B	░	░	
GROUP AB	░	░	░
GROUP O (males)	░		
Type A₂	░	░	░

Symptoms

- Weight loss
- Fever
- Loss of appetite
- Anemia, a shortage of red blood cells, causes
- Shortness of breath
- Excessive tiredness
- A "pale" color to the skin

About Leukemia

Leukemia is cancer of the white blood cells. This cancer starts in the bone marrow but can then spread to the blood, lymph nodes, the spleen, liver, central nervous system, and other organs. Leukemia is a complex disease with four different types and subtypes. There are four types of leukemia:

Acute means rapidly growing. Although the cells grow rapidly, they are not able to mature properly.

Chronic refers to a condition where the cells look mature but they are not completely normal. The cells live too long and cause a build-up of certain kinds of white blood cells.

Lymphocytic are leukemias that develop from lymphocytes in the bone marrow.

Myelogenous leukemia develops from either of two types of white blood cells: granulocytes or monocytes.

Most signs and symptoms of acute leukemia result from a shortage of normal blood cells due to crowding out of normal blood cell–producing bone marrow by the leukemia cells. As a result, people do not have enough properly functioning red blood cells, white blood cells, and blood platelets. As a result, individuals will experience the following symptoms:

- Anemia, a shortage of red blood cells, causes shortness of breath, excessive tiredness, and a pale color to the skin.
- Leukemia often causes enlargement of the liver and spleen, two organs located on the right and left side respectively, of the abdomen. Enlargement of these organs would be noticed as a fullness, or even swelling, of the belly.
- Leukemia may spread to the lymph nodes, causing swelling; or to the skin, causing rashes; or to the gums, causing swelling, pain, and bleeding.

Blood Group Links

Loss of A, B, and O antigens from the surface of red blood cells has been a recurrent observation in patients with hematologic malignancy (blood cancers), particularly those malignancies in which the myeloid lineage is involved. In fact, a study found that 55% of patients of blood group A, B, or AB had a proportion of red cells with decreased expression of A or B antigens compared with no changes in 127 healthy A, B, and AB individuals. In most cases, the changes were not detected by routine serologic (blood) typing. The loss of A or B antigens was the primary change in 28% of patients. In 17% of patients, loss of A or B antigens was an indirect consequence of loss of the precursor H (O) antigen. Alterations involving both the H (O) and the A or B antigens were seen in 10% of patients. Loss of H was also detected in 21% of group O patients whereas none of 51 healthy O individuals showed changes. Alterations of ABO antigens can now be considered a common event in myeloid malignancy[1].

Acute leukemia is more common in males at almost every age, and this fact remains unexplained. A study was carried out in northeast peninsular Malaysia to examine whether there was a difference in ABO blood group distribution between males and females with acute leukemia. The ABO blood groups of 109 male and 79 female patients with acute leukemia were compared with those of 1,019 normal individuals (controls). In the control population, 39.7% were group O. Among males with acute leukemia, 39.4% were group O, whereas among females with acute leukemia, the proportion was 24.1%. The same trend to a lower proportion of group O among females was seen if the group was divided into adult/pediatric or lymphoblastic/myeloblastic groups, though these differences were not statistically sig-

nificant. If these findings can be confirmed by other studies, they suggest the presence of a "sex-responsive" gene near to the ABO gene locus on chromosome 9, which relatively protects group O women against acute leukemia. The existence of such a gene might also partly explain why acute leukemia, and possibly other childhood cancers, are more common in males[2].

Among leukemia patients, a significant increase in the frequency of the A2 phenotype was found in chronic lymphocytic leukemia[3].

Therapies, Leukemia

BLOOD GROUP A:

1. Cancer Prevention Protocol
2. Chemotherapy Adjunct Protocol
3. Surgery Recovery Protocol
4. Chronic Illness Recovery Protocol

BLOOD GROUP B:

1. Cancer Prevention Protocol
2. Chemotherapy Adjunct Protocol
3. Surgery Recovery Protocol
4. Chronic Illness Recovery Protocol

BLOOD GROUP AB:

1. Cancer Prevention Protocol
2. Chemotherapy Adjunct Protocol
3. Surgery Recovery Protocol
4. Chronic Illness Recovery Protocol

BLOOD GROUP O:

1. Cancer Prevention Protocol
2. Chemotherapy Adjunct Protocol

3. Surgery Recovery Protocol

4. Chronic Illness Recovery Protocol

Related Topics

Cancer (general)

Immunity

REFERENCES

1. Marsden KA, Pearse AM, Collins GG, Ford DS, Heard S, Kimber RI. Acute leukemia with t(1;3)(p36;q21), evolution to t(1;3)(p36;q21), t(14;17)(q32;q21), and loss of red cell A and Le(b) antigens. *Cancer Genet Cytogenet.* 1992;64:80–85.
2. Jackson N, Menon BS, Zarina W, Zawawi N, Naing NN. Why is acute leukemia more common in males? A possible sex-determined risk linked to the ABO blood group genes. *Ann Hematol.* 1999;78:233–236.
3. Janardhana V, Propert DN, Green RE. ABO blood groups in hematologic malignancies. *Cancer Genet Cytogenet.* 1991; 51:113–120.
4. Bianco T, Farmer BJ, Sage RE, Dobrovic A. Loss of red cell A, B, and H antigens is frequent in myeloid malignancies. *Blood.* 2001;97:3633–3639.

CANCER, LIVER–*Tumors of the liver.*

Liver cancer	RISK		
	LOW	AVERAGE	HIGH
GROUP A			
GROUP B			
GROUP AB			
GROUP O			

Symptoms

Liver cancer is often not found early because there are seldom any signs or symptoms. In later stages, symptoms include:

- Weight loss
- Lack of appetite
- Pain in the stomach area
- Sudden jaundice

About Liver Cancer

Many cases of liver cancer can be prevented. Worldwide, preventing infection with HEPATITIS B AND C can reduce the risk of liver cancer. There is now a vaccine to prevent hepatitis B, and children especially should be vaccinated. Using protection during sex and not sharing needles lowers the chances of getting hepatitis. Not abusing alcohol will help lower the number of cases of CIRRHOSIS of the liver, a risk factor for liver cancer. Changing the way certain grains are stored in other countries could reduce contact with aflatoxins. Also, laws to protect workers from harmful chemicals can lower the risk. These measures have already been taken in many countries.

Also beware of:

- Anabolic steroids: These are male hormones. They are sometimes given for medical reasons, but some athletes also take them to increase their strength.
- Arsenic: In some parts of the world, drinking

water contains traces of arsenic. This can increase the risk of liver cancer.

▪ Tobacco: Some studies suggest a link between tobacco use and liver cancer. Tobacco is carcinogenic, and smoking is clearly linked to many other cancers.

Blood Group Links

Liver cancer may show an increased incidence of group A. Liver hemangiomas are known to be more common in group A over the other blood groups.

Therapies, Liver Cancer

ALL BLOOD GROUPS:

Most liver cancer can be prevented by adhering to the Blood Type Diet, moderating alcohol intake, and reducing your exposure to toxic substances.

BLOOD GROUP A:

1. Cancer Prevention Protocol
2. Chemotherapy Adjunct Protocol
3. Liver Support Protocol
4. Surgery Recovery Protocol
5. Chronic Illness Recovery Protocol

BLOOD GROUP B:

1. Cancer Prevention Protocol
2. Chemotherapy Adjunct Protocol
3. Liver Support Protocol

4. Surgery Recovery Protocol
5. Chronic Illness Recovery Protocol

BLOOD GROUP AB:

1. Cancer Prevention Protocol
2. Chemotherapy Adjunct Protocol
3. Liver Support Protocol
4. Surgery Recovery Protocol
5. Chronic Illness Recovery Protocol

BLOOD GROUP O:

1. Cancer Prevention Protocol
2. Chemotherapy Adjunct Protocol
3. Liver Support Protocol
4. Surgery Recovery Protocol
5. Chronic Illness Recovery Protocol

Related Topics

Cancer (general)

Immunity

Liver disease

CANCER, LUNG–*Tumors of the lung.*

Lung cancer	RISK		
	LOW	AVERAGE	HIGH
GROUP A (under 50)			
GROUP B (bronchial)			
GROUP AB			
GROUP O			

Symptoms

- A cough that does not go away
- Chest pain, often made worse by deep breathing
- Hoarseness
- Weight loss and loss of appetite
- Bloody or rust-colored sputum (spit or phlegm)
- Shortness of breath
- Fever without a known reason
- Recurring infections such as bronchitis and pneumonia
- New onset of wheezing

About Lung Cancer

Lung cancer is the leading cause of cancer death for both men and women though it is slightly more common in men. More people die of lung cancer than of colon, breast, and prostate cancers combined. Lung cancer is fairly rare in people under the age of 40. The average age of people found to have lung cancer is 60.

The lung is a site for both primary tumors and, very often, METASTASES from other organs (breast, colon, kidney, thyroid, testes, bone, and prostate). Most lung cancers are clearly associated with cigarette smoking, which explains the continual rise in lung cancers in women paralleling their increase in smoking. Primary lung malignancy is the most common cause of death from cancer.

Since most people with early lung cancer do not have any symptoms, only about 15% of lung cancers are found in the early stages. Although most lung cancers do not cause symptoms until they have spread, you should report any of the preceding symptoms to your doctor right away. Often these problems are caused by some other condition, but if lung cancer is found, prompt treatment could extend your life and relieve symptoms.

Blood Group Links

Lung cancer is closely associated with cigarette smoking although additional environmental or individual factors might regulate a person's susceptibility to that disease. As a third genetic host factor, the ABO blood group frequencies were evaluated in 263 lung cancer patients. The frequency ratio of group A to group O was significantly higher as compared to 41,423 blood donors. The ratio of A to tended to be especially high in young patients not older than 50 years. In bronchial cancer, the ratio of B to O was significantly higher than expected. The conclusion was that ABO blood groups seem to influence lung cancer susceptibility[1].

Therapies, Lung Cancer

NOTE: Although there appear to be secondary and tertiary links between lung cancer and blood groups, it would be misleading to suggest that blood group is a significant factor in the development of lung cancer. The primary cause of lung cancer is smoking, followed by the regular inhalation of toxic substances.

BLOOD GROUP A:

1. Cancer Prevention Protocol

2. Chemotherapy Adjunct Protocol

3. Surgery Recovery Protocol

4. Chronic Illness Recovery Protocol

BLOOD GROUP B:

1. Cancer Prevention Protocol

2. Chemotherapy Adjunct Protocol

3. Surgery Recovery Protocol

4. Chronic Illness Recovery Protocol

BLOOD GROUP AB:

1. Cancer Prevention Protocol

2. Chemotherapy Adjunct Protocol

3. Surgery Recovery Protocol

4. Chronic Illness Recovery Protocol

BLOOD GROUP O:

1. Cancer Prevention Protocol

2. Chemotherapy Adjunct Protocol

3. Surgery Recovery Protocol

4. Chronic Illness Recovery Protocol

Related Topics

Cancer (general)

REFERENCES

1. Roots I, Drakoulis N, Ploch M, et al. Debrisoquine hydroxylation phenotype, acetylation phenotype, and ABO blood groups as genetic host factors of lung cancer risk. *Klin Wochenschr.* 1988;66(suppl):87–97.

CANCER, LYMPHOMA–*Tumors of the lymphoid tissue.*

Lymphoma	RISK		
	LOW	AVERAGE	HIGH
GROUP A			
GROUP B			
GROUP AB			
GROUP O			

Symptoms

Variable

About Lymphomas

There are two main types of lymphomas. Hodgkin's lymphoma or Hodgkin's disease is named after Dr. Thomas Hodgkin, who first described it as a new disease in 1832. All other types of lymphoma are called non-Hodgkin's lymphomas. These two types of lymphoma can usually be distinguished from each other by examining the cancerous tissue under a microscope. In some cases, additional tests to identify specific chemical components of the lymphoma cells or tests of the cells' DNA may be needed.

Hodgkin's lymphoma: Hodgkin's disease is a type of cancer that starts in lymphatic tissue. Lymphatic tissue includes the lymph nodes and other organs that are part of the body's lymph system, which forms blood and protects against germs. Because lymphatic tissue is found in many parts of the body, Hodgkin's disease can start almost anywhere. This disease causes the lymphatic tissue to become enlarged and press on nearby structures. The cancer can spread through the lymphatic vessels. If it gets into the blood vessels it can then spread to almost any other place in the body.

There are no screening tests to find Hodgkin's disease early, and some people with the disease have no symptoms at all. When they do occur, symptoms can include enlarged, painless lymph nodes. But in most people, especially children, enlarged lymph nodes are caused by an infection or other illness, not cancer. If you (or your child) have lymph nodes over an inch in size and no recent infection, it is best to have them checked by the doctor.

Other symptoms of Hodgkin's disease can be caused by the swelling of lymph nodes inside the chest, creating pressure on the windpipe. These symptoms can include coughing or shortness of breath. Some people have fever, drenching night sweats, or weight loss. The fever can come and go over periods of several days or weeks.

Non-Hodgkin's lymphoma: Non-Hodgkin's lymphoma is cancer that starts in lymphoid tissue (also called lymphatic tissue). The lymphatic system is important for filtering germs and cancer cells as well as fluid from the extremities and internal organs. Other types of cancer—lung or colon cancers, for example—can develop in other organs and then spread to lymphoid tissue. But these cancers that can spread to lymph nodes are not lymphomas. Lymphomas start in the lymphoid tissue and can spread to other organs.

Non-Hodgkin's lymphoma is the fifth most common cancer in this country, excluding non-MELANOMA skin cancers. Since the early 1970s, the incidence rates for non-Hodgkin's lymphoma have nearly doubled; the increase was a result of both better methods of detection and an actual increase in the number of new cases. During the 1990s, the rate of increase appeared to slow and may be beginning to decline.

Although some types of non-Hodgkin's lymphoma are among the most common childhood cancers, over 95% of non-Hodgkin's lymphoma cases occur in adults. The average age at diagnosis is in the early 40s. The risk of developing non-Hodgkin's lymphoma increases throughout life, and the elderly have the highest risk. The increasing average age of the American population is expected to contribute to the increase in non-Hodgkin's lymphoma cases during the next few years. Non-Hodgkin's lymphoma is more common in men than in women. Caucasians are affected more often than people of African or Asian ancestry.

Non-Hodgkin's lymphoma that involves easily seen or palpated lymph nodes close to the surface of the body (lymph nodes on the sides of the neck, in the groin or underarm areas, above the collar bone, etc.) are usually noticed by the patient, a family member, or a health care professional.

When the lymphoid tissue inside the abdomen is involved, the abdomen can be swollen, sometimes so much it may resemble pregnancy in a woman. This may be due to large collections of fluid or tumor. Sometimes the cancer damages the lining layer of the abdominal cavity and causes large amounts of fluid to build up. When lymphoma causes swelling of lymphoid tissue near the intestines, passage of feces through the compressed area may be blocked. The pressure or blockage can also cause discomfort or abdominal pain.

When lymphoma starts in the thymus, irritation or compression of the nearby trachea can cause coughing, shortness of breath, or even suffocation. The superior vena cava (SVC) is the large vein that carries blood from the head and arms back to the heart. It passes near the thymus and lymph nodes inside the chest. Growth of lymphoma may compress this vein. This causes swelling of the head and arms known as SVC syndrome. This can also affect the brain and can be life threatening. Patients with SVC syndrome need to be treated as soon as possible.

In addition to symptoms and signs resulting from local effects of cancer growth, non-Hodgkin's lymphoma can produce generalized symptoms such as unexplained weight loss, fever, profuse sweating (enough to soak clothing), particularly at night, or severe itchiness. Oncologists sometimes call these generalized effects "B symptoms." The presence of B symptoms is associated with a poor prognosis and is related to an increased tumor burden (more cancer cells) in some patients.

Blood Group Links

There are only highly preliminary data linking blood groups to lymphoma. EPSTEIN-BARR VIRUS may play a role in the development of Hodgkin's disease, placing blood group B at a somewhat elevated risk. Group O is associated with the best clinical outcome. More investigation is needed before conclusions can be reached.

Therapies, Lymphoma

BLOOD GROUP A:

1. Cancer Prevention Protocol
2. Chemotherapy Adjunct Protocol
3. Surgery Recovery Protocol
4. Chronic Illness Recovery Protocol

BLOOD GROUP B:

1. Cancer Prevention Protocol
2. Chemotherapy Adjunct Protocol
3. Antiviral Protocol
4. Surgery Recovery Protocol
5. Chronic Illness Recovery Protocol

BLOOD GROUP AB:

1. Cancer Prevention Protocol
2. Chemotherapy Adjunct Protocol
3. Surgery Recovery Protocol
4. Chronic Illness Recovery Protocol

BLOOD GROUP O:

1. Cancer Prevention Protocol
2. Chemotherapy Adjunct Protocol
3. Surgery Recovery Protocol
4. Chronic Illness Recovery Protocol

Related Topics

Cancer (general)

Epstein-Barr virus

Immunity

CANCER, MELANOMA–*Tumors of the skin.*

Melanoma	RISK		
	LOW	AVERAGE	HIGH
GROUP A			
GROUP B			
GROUP AB			
GROUP O			

Symptoms

▪ A change in any pigmented lesion, including hypo or hyperpigmentation, bleeding, scaling, size change, and any texture change.

About Melanoma

The median age for skin cancers is 53 years old, but it has the highest annual incidence rate of any cancer among Caucasians between the ages of 25 to 29. More than 50% of all individuals with melanoma are between the ages of 20 to 40. The only genetic predisposition is in the familial dysplastic nevus syndrome. If an affected person's family history includes one relative with melanoma, the risk of developing melanoma is 100%. Skin pigmentation is the only other risk factor transmitted genetically up. Also there is twice the risk for people who had adolescent blistering sunburns; or a fair complexion, freckling, blue eyes and blond hair; and those who have had any previous pigmented lesions (especially for dysplastic nevi) and intermittent ultraviolet light exposure.

An important symptom is any change in any pigmented lesion, including hypopigmentation or hyperpigmentation, bleeding, scaling, size, and texture. The overwhelming majority of melanoma arises in the skin, but it may also present as a primary lesion in any tissue pigmentation. Metastatic spread may be to any region in the body. Lentigo maligna is a cutaneous lesion that is the slowest growing malignant melanoma and has the least tendency to metastasize. It occurs most often on the face, beginning as a circumscribed macular patch of model pigmentation showing shades of dark brown, tan, or black. There is also an ocular melanoma that effects the eye; it is a progressive lesion of malignant origin.

Blood Group Links

When the records of 168 patients with malignant melanoma were reviewed with regard to the incidence of the major blood groups, blood group A was encountered in 39.9%, group B in 7.7%, group AB in 3%, and group O in 49.4%. Although blood group O had a higher frequency compared to that of the general Caucasian population of various series, the difference was not significant. Patients with blood group A had a median survival of 67.7 months, whereas patients with blood group O had a median survival of 46.6 months. The improved survival for blood group A remained significant only in female patients, when the sexes were considered separately. However, group A had an incidence of 24% in early Clark's lesions while that incidence in group O was 9.8%. Female patients had longer median survival (86 months) than male patients (44 months)[1].

Fifteen polymorphic systems of the blood (ABO, MNSs, Rhesus, P, Kell, Duffy, Kidd, Hp, Gc, Gm, Inv, aP, PGM1, EsD, and 6-PGD) were examined in 191 unrelated male and female patients suffering from malignant melanoma. These polymorphic systems were compared with the corresponding phenotype and gene frequencies of controls from the same geographical area (Rhineland-Palatinate). The only associations discovered were the ABO and Gm polymorphisms: The incidence of O and Gm(-1) phenotypes in patients was obviously higher than in controls. These observations agree with the findings in other population samples from Germany and Bulgaria[2].

Therapies, Melanoma

ALL BLOOD GROUPS:

PREVENTION

Avoid solar radiation from exposure to the sun. The best protection against the sun is proper clothing. Wear clothes made of tightly woven fabrics. Clothing made of loosely woven fabric or wet clothes can expose your skin to 30% more ultraviolet radiation. Wear long sleeves and pants. Wear a hat with a broad brim to protect your neck and ears (a baseball cap only protects your forehead). Apply sunscreen to sun-exposed skin.

Don't go out without sunscreen. Sunscreen lotion is generally divided into two categories: physical sunscreens and chemical sunscreens. Physical sunscreens reflect ultraviolet radiation away from the skin while chemical sunscreens absorb ultraviolet radiation. Examples of physical sunscreens include zinc oxide and titanium dioxide. Although physical sunscreens are generally better at blocking the different kinds of ultraviolet radiation, they tend to be more "messy"—some can melt with heat and/or discolor clothing. Chemical sunscreens tend to become invisible when they are rubbed on the skin; because they are invisible it's easy to miss an area of skin, which limits their effectiveness. Many products also come in a water-resistant formulation. Many chemical sunscreens also can cause eye irritation, and there is a higher chance of allergic reactions to chemical sunscreens, as opposed to physical sunscreens.

Choose a sunscreen with an SPF (sun protection factor) of at least 15. That means it provides 15 times more protection against ultraviolet radiation than no sunscreen at all. For persons with a fair complexion, a sunscreen with an SPF of 30 to 40 may be preferable.

TREATMENT

The standard method of early treatment for melanomas is excisional biopsy—the surgical removal of a mole that is thought to be melanoma. Your doctor will cut out the suspected melanoma, being careful to remove the depth of the mole as well as the portion above the skin. The excised tissue will be sent to a lab where a pathologist will look at it under a microscope to determine the nature of the tissue. If the body tissue removed in the biopsy is determined to be melanoma, your doctor will excise the remaining skin around the original site that was cut out to ensure clear margins. This means that the skin around the melanoma is noncancerous.

BLOOD GROUP A:

1. Cancer Prevention Protocol
2. Chemotherapy Adjunct Protocol
3. Skin Health Protocol
4. Surgery Recovery Protocol
5. Chronic Illness Recovery Protocol

BLOOD GROUP B:

1. Cancer Prevention Protocol
2. Chemotherapy Adjunct Protocol
3. Skin Health Protocol
4. Surgery Recovery Protocol
5. Chronic Illness Recovery Protocol

BLOOD GROUP AB:

1. Cancer Prevention Protocol
2. Chemotherapy Adjunct Protocol
3. Skin Health protocol
4. Surgery Recovery Protocol
5. Chronic Illness Recovery Protocol

BLOOD GROUP O:

1. Cancer Prevention Protocol
2. Chemotherapy Adjunct Protocol
3. Skin Health Protocol
4. Surgery Recovery Protocol
5. Chronic Illness Recovery Protocol

Related Topics

Cancer (general)

Immunity

REFERENCES

1. Karakousis CP, Evlogimenos E, Suh O. Blood groups and malignant melanoma. *J Surg Oncol.* 1986;33:24–26.
2. Walter H, Brachtel R, Hilling M. On the incidence of blood group O and Gm(-1) phenotypes in patients with malignant melanoma. *Hum Genet.* 1979;49:71–81.

CANCER, OVARIAN—*Tumors of the ovary.*

Ovarian cancer	RISK		
	LOW	AVERAGE	HIGH
GROUP A			
GROUP B			
GROUP AB			
GROUP O			
Rh-POSITIVE			

Symptoms

- Swelling of the abdomen
- Unusual vaginal bleeding
- Pelvic pressure
- Back pain
- Leg pain
- Digestive problems such as gas, bloating, indigestion, or long-term stomach pain

About Ovarian Cancer

Ovarian cancer is the sixth most common cancer in women. It ranks fifth as the cause of cancer death in women. Ovarian cancer causes more deaths than any other reproductive organ cancer. Most women who have ovarian cancer are post-menopausal.

The chances of survival from ovarian cancer are better if the cancer is found early. If the cancer is found and treated before it has spread outside the ovary, 95% of women will survive at least 5 years. However, only 25% of ovarian cancers are found at this early stage.

There is a familial risk factor for ovarian cancer. A woman who has a first-degree relative, i.e., a mother or a sister with a history of ovarian cancer, her risk for disease increases from 1.4% to 5.0%. With two or more such relatives, the lifetime risk becomes 7%. In families with hereditary ovarian cancer syndrome, the risk rises to 40% to 50%.

Small ovarian tumors are difficult for even the most skilled examiner to feel. Early cancers of the ovaries tend to cause symptoms that are relatively nonspecific. These symptoms include swelling of the abdomen (due to a mass or accumulation of fluid), unusual vaginal bleeding, pelvic pressure, back pain, leg pain, and digestive problems such as gas, bloating, indigestion, or long-term stomach pain. Most of these symptoms can also be caused by other less serious conditions. By the time ovarian cancer is considered as a possible cause of these symptoms, it may have already spread beyond the ovaries. Also, some types of ovarian cancer can rapidly spread to the surface of nearby organs. Nonetheless, prompt attention to symptoms can improve the odds of early diagnosis and successful treatment. If you have symptoms of ovarian cancer, report them to your health care provider right away.

Blood Group Links

The distribution of ABO blood group and Rh factor was studied in 175 women with ovarian tumors and cysts, compared with healthy controls. An increased probability of the majority of the ovarian tumor types among AB blood group females was noted, compared with other groups (O, A, and B). The probability of ovarian tumors becoming malignant proved to be least in B group females. A considerably increased relative ovarian tumor and cyst morbidity was noted among Rh-positive females compared with Rh-negative ones[1].

In the period from 1955 to 1979, 337 patients with carcinoma of the ovary were reported to the Icelandic Cancer Registry. ABO blood groups for 192 of the patients were available and showed a significant excess of blood group A; significantly fewer patients of blood group B were found than expected[2].

Therapies, Ovarian Cancer

ALL BLOOD GROUPS:

Screening: Women with a high risk of developing epithelial ovarian cancer, such as those with a very strong family history of this disease, may be screened with transvaginal sonography (an ultrasound test performed with a small instrument placed in the vagina) and blood tests. Transvaginal sonography is helpful in finding a mass in the ovary, but it does not accurately predict which masses are cancers and which are benign diseases of the ovary. Blood tests for ovarian cancer may include measuring the amount of CA-125 (also known as OC-125). The amount of this protein is increased in the blood of many women with ovarian cancer. However, some noncancerous diseases of the ovaries can also increase the blood levels of CA-125 and some ovarian cancers may not produce enough CA-125 to cause a positive test. When these tests are positive, it may be necessary to do more x-ray studies or to take samples of fluid from the abdomen or tissue from the ovaries to find out whether a cancer is really present.

BLOOD GROUP A:

1. Cancer Prevention Protocol

2. Chemotherapy Adjunct Protocol

3. Surgery Recovery Protocol

4. Chronic Illness Recovery Protocol

BLOOD GROUP B:

1. Cancer Prevention Protocol

2. Chemotherapy Adjunct Protocol

3. Surgery Recovery Protocol

4. Chronic Illness Recovery Protocol

BLOOD GROUP AB:

1. Cancer Prevention Protocol

2. Chemotherapy Adjunct Protocol

3. Surgery Recovery Protocol

4. Chronic Illness Recovery Protocol

BLOOD GROUP O:

1. Cancer Prevention Protocol

2. Chemotherapy Adjunct Protocol

3. Surgery Recovery Protocol

4. Chronic Illness Recovery Protocol

Related Topics

Cancer (general)

Cancer, gynecological tumors

Immunity

REFERENCES

1. Rybalka AN, Andreeva PV, Tikhonenko LF, Koval'chuk NA. [ABO system blood groups and the rhesus factor in tumors and tumorlike processes of the ovaries]. *Vopr Onkol.* 1979;25:28–30.

2. Bjarnason O, Tulinius H. Tumours in Iceland. 9. Malignant tumours of the ovary. A histological classification, epidemiological considerations and survival. *Acta Pathol Microbiol Immunol Scand [A].* 1987;95:185–192.

CANCER, PANCREATIC–*Tumors of the pancreas.*

Pancreatic cancer	RISK		
	LOW	AVERAGE	HIGH
GROUP A			
GROUP B			
GROUP AB			
GROUP O			

Symptoms

- Jaundice

- Pain in the abdominal (stomach) area or the middle to upper back area

- Weight loss over a number of months, accompanied by loss of appetite and severe tiredness

- Digestive problems, with pale, bulky, and greasy stools

- Swollen gallbladder

- Blood clots

- Diabetes

About Pancreatic Cancer

The incidence of pancreatic cancer has tripled over the last 40 years. There is no known cause, although chronic pancreatitis, smoking, certain chemicals (metal, and gas), coffee, alcohol, and DIABETES MELLITUS (in women) are risk factors. It is a rare cancer, accounting for only 2% to 3% of all cancers; however, it accounts for 10% of all fatal abdominal malignancies, and is now the fourth most common fatal cancer in the United States. It is three to four times more common in men, and is seen between the years of 35 and 70, with the peak at about 60.

Pancreatic cancer is a quickly metastasizing malignancy that is usually surgically untreatable by the time of diagnosis. The prognosis is extremely unfavorable; the 5-year survival rate is only 9%, and it is rare for a patient to live beyond 5 years.

By the time a person has symptoms of pancreatic cancer, the tumor has often reached a large size and the cancer may have spread to other organs.

Blood Group Links

Blood group B and blood group A have the highest incidence of pancreatic cancer. Group O is associated with the lowest risk (29). Since pancreatic juice is liberally laced with blood type antigens, the expression of group A and group B antigens must have some effect in inhibiting the immune response.

Few investigations have discussed an association between ABO blood groups and pancreatic cancer. In one study, the ABO blood groups distribution of 224 patients with histologically-confirmed pancreatic cancer was compared with that of two control groups: 7,086 patients with various diseases and 7,320 voluntary blood donors. An increased number of pancreatic cancers were found among the patients with blood group B and a decreased number in patients with blood group O, when compared with the two control groups.

Therapies, Pancreatic Cancer

ALL BLOOD GROUPS:

Especially if there is a family history of pancreatic cancer:

1. Avoid exposure to metals.

2. Limit or avoid consumption of alcohol and coffee.

3. Don't smoke.

BLOOD GROUP A:

1. Cancer Prevention Protocol
2. Chemotherapy Adjunct Protocol
3. Liver Support Protocol
4. Surgery Recovery Protocol
5. Chronic Illness Recovery Protocol

BLOOD GROUP B:

1. Cancer Prevention Protocol
2. Chemotherapy Adjunct Protocol
3. Liver Support Protocol
4. Surgery Recovery Protocol
5. Chronic Illness Recovery Protocol

BLOOD GROUP AB:

1. Cancer Prevention Protocol
2. Chemotherapy Adjunct Protocol
3. Liver Support Protocol
4. Surgery Recovery Protocol
5. Chronic Illness Recovery Protocol

BLOOD GROUP O:

1. Cancer Prevention Protocol
2. Chemotherapy Adjunct Protocol
3. Liver Support Protocol
4. Surgery Recovery Protocol
5. Chronic Illness Recovery Protocol

Related Topics

Cancer (general)

Immunity

Liver disease

CANCER, PROSTATE–_The development of abnormal cells in the prostate that multiply at an uncontrollable rate._

Prostate cancer	RISK		
	LOW	AVERAGE	HIGH
GROUP A			
GROUP B			
GROUP AB			
GROUP O			
SECRETORS			

Symptoms

The most common signs of a prostate problem, which may be early signs of cancer, include:

- Painful, frequent, urgent, or hesitant urination
- Trouble fully emptying the bladder
- Frequent need to urinate during the night
- Sluggish urine flow
- Sharp pain in the pelvic region or rectum
- Blood in the urine

About Prostate Cancer

Prostate cancer is the most common cancer, excluding skin cancers, in American men. One man in six will be diagnosed with prostate cancer during his lifetime, but only one man in 30 will die of this disease. Men of African ancestry are more likely to have prostate cancer than are Caucasians or men of Asian ancestry.

Prostate cancer usually takes its time, advancing very slowly through four stages.

Stage A: The cancer is microscopic, there are no symptoms, and it cannot be detected by a digital rectal exam. A prostate-specific antigen (PSA) test might show elevated antigen levels, as will a biopsy.

Stage B: There are probably no notable symptoms, although a doctor can normally detect a lump or an unnaturally hard area on the prostate's outer lobes. This information is obtained during a rectal examination. At this point, the cancer hasn't advanced beyond the prostate. Stage B cancers are usually divided into two subgroups. Stage B-1 means that the cancer is confined to one lobe of the prostate. In Stage B-2, the cancer has spread to both lobes.

Stage C: By this stage, there's a good chance that the cancer has advanced beyond the prostate, and has initially invaded surrounding tissues. There might be some urinary problems. Stage C prostate cancer can be detected by a digital rectal or other standard exam. Stage C-1 is the less severe of the two C stages, because the cancer's involvement with other tissues is still minimal. In Stage C-2, the cancer has caused some blockage of the urethra, and has made its presence known by impeding the flow of the urine.

Stage D: The cancer is no longer confined to the prostate, and has spread widely throughout the body, potentially involving the lymph nodes, lungs, and bones. This is the most serious stage of all cancers. It has four subgroupings. In Stage D-0,

other than elevated prostate enzyme levels, there are no other visible manifestations that the cancer has progressed. In Stage D-1, there is clear evidence that the cancer has spread to the lymph nodes in the immediate area surrounding the prostate. In Stage D-2, the cancer has metastasized to other sites in the body, notably the other lymph nodes, the bones, or other organs.

General Risk Factors and Causes

Prostate disease, especially cancer, is sometimes confusing, since even the known risk factors are so poorly understood. For example, it is known that African-Americans have a higher incidence of prostate cancer than Caucasians, but this may be environmental, not genetic, since African nationals have a low incidence. (Men of Hispanic and Japanese ancestry also have a low incidence of prostate cancer.) Cadmium miners have a higher rate of prostate cancer than the general population, but the reason is not known. It's also still a mystery why men who have had vasectomies seem to experience more prostate cancer than the general population.

Blood Group Links

Men of blood groups A and AB have a higher risk of developing prostate cancer. Secretors tend to have a greater incidence of prostate cancer than non-secretors.

Therapies, Prostate Cancer

ALL BLOOD GROUPS:

The prostate-specific antigen (PSA) test is a simple and inexpensive blood test. The protein in the seminal fluid is produced in the prostate, but circulated throughout the body. When PSA levels are elevated in the bloodstream, there's the possibility of a problem. The reading shows how many nanograms (1 nanogram equals 1 billionth of a gram) of PSA are present per milliliter of blood. As a rule, up to four nanograms is considered acceptable, although doctors also watch for rapid changes in the PSA over short periods. For example, if your PSA reading is 2.5 one year, then rises to 3.5 the next, it might raise a red flag even though it is within the normal range.

BLOOD GROUP A:

1. Cancer Prevention Protocol
2. Chemotherapy Adjunct Protocol
3. Surgery Recovery Protocol
4. Chronic Illness Recovery Protocol

BLOOD GROUP B:

1. Cancer Prevention Protocol
2. Chemotherapy Adjunct Protocol
3. Surgery Recovery Protocol
4. Chronic Illness Recovery Protocol

BLOOD GROUP AB:

1. Cancer Prevention Protocol
2. Chemotherapy Adjunct Protocol
3. Surgery Recovery Protocol
4. Chronic Illness Recovery Protocol

BLOOD GROUP O:

1. Cancer Prevention Protocol
2. Chemotherapy Adjunct Protocol
3. Surgery Recovery Protocol
4. Chronic Illness Recovery Protocol

Related Topics

Cancer (general)

Prostatic hyperplasia, benign

CANCER, RECTAL–*See Cancer, colon*

CANCER, STOMACH–*Tumors of the stomach.*

Stomach cancer	RISK		
	LOW	AVERAGE	HIGH
GROUP A			
GROUP B			
GROUP AB			
GROUP O			

Symptoms

- Weight loss
- Iron-deficiency anemia

About Stomach Cancer

Cancer of the stomach is responsible for approximately 13,000 deaths and 24,000 new cases per year in the United States. Worldwide, over half a million deaths result from stomach cancer annually. Although the stomach cancer rate in the United States and the number of deaths from this disease fell dramatically from the 1940s to the 1990s, it is still a potent killer. The disease is found most often in people over age 55. It affects men twice as often as women, and is more common in individuals of African ancestry than in Caucasians. Also, stomach cancer is more common in some parts of the world—such as Japan, Korea, parts of Eastern Europe, and Latin America—than in the United States. The diets in these parts of the world contain many foods that are preserved by drying, smoking, salting, or pickling. Scientists believe that eating foods preserved in these ways may play a role in the development of stomach cancer. Fresh foods, especially fresh fruits and vegetables, may protect against this disease.

Stomach cancer may initially manifest with mild symptoms. All the common signs associated with stomach problems may arise but are usually not as severe as those caused by ulcers. The most common first sign is of a metastasis while the primary malignancy remains silent. Weight loss and iron-deficiency anemia may be present.

Blood Group Links

Stomach cancer was one of the earliest diseases ever shown to be associated with blood groups, an association first discovered in the early 1950s[1-3]. Originally, it was thought that the tendency for blood group A toward low stomach acid may have been the provocative factor, but other causes may be more important. The genetic ability for cells of the stomach to turn cancerous has been shown to be linked to the ABO gene locus itself, on chromosome 9q34. In this case, the A allele itself is contributing to the genetic mutations in the stomach, another instance of the link between a blood group and disease not being the result of a physical expression of blood type, per se, but rather a genetic linkage.

The Thomsen-Friedenreich Antigen

Many malignant cells, such as those found in stomach cancer, develop a tumor marker called the Thomsen-Friedenreich (T) antigen. This antigen is suppressed in normal healthy cells, but becomes unsuppressed as a cell moves toward malignancy. It is so rare to find the Tn antigen in healthy tissue that most people actually have an antibody to it.

The T antigen is exuberantly expressed in cells of the stomach that turn cancerous. About one-third of all Japanese express some T antigen in apparently normal stomach tissue, and this may also help explain why stomach cancer rates in Japan are among the highest in the world[4].

The Thomsen-Friedenreich antigen shows some structural similarity to the A antigen. Perhaps this explains why, of all the blood groups, blood group A stomach cancer patients carry the least amount of the anti-T antibody. Since gastric juice is typically loaded with blood group antigens anyway, it is not unlikely that groups A and AB would be at a disadvantage at recognizing the T antigens as cancer markers, or mounting a defense if they did[5,6].

Therapies, Stomach Cancer

BLOOD GROUP A:

1. Cancer Prevention Protocol
2. Chemotherapy Adjunct Protocol
3. Surgery Recovery Protocol
4. Chronic Illness Recovery Protocol

BLOOD GROUP B:

1. Cancer Prevention Protocol
2. Chemotherapy Adjunct Protocol
3. Surgery Recovery Protocol
4. Chronic Illness Recovery Protocol

BLOOD GROUP AB:

1. Cancer Prevention Protocol
2. Chemotherapy Adjunct Protocol
3. Surgery Recovery Protocol
4. Chronic Illness Recovery Protocol

BLOOD GROUP O:

1. Cancer Prevention Protocol
2. Chemotherapy Adjunct Protocol
3. Surgery Recovery Protocol
4. Chronic Illness Recovery Protocol

Related Topics

Barrett's esophagus

Cancer (general)

Immunity

REFERENCES

1. Aird I, Bental HH, Mehigan JA, Roberts JA Fraser. *Brit Med J.* 1954;(2):315.
2. Walther WW, Raeburn C, Case J. *Lancet.* 1956;(2):970.
3. Wallace J. *Brit Med J.* 1954;(2):254.
4. Hirohashi S. Tumor-associated carbohydrate antigens related to blood group carbohydrates. *Gan To Kagaku Ryoho.* 1986;13(2):1395–1401.
5. Kurtenkov O, Klaamas K, Miljukhina L. The lower level of natural anti-Thomsen-Friedenreich antigen (TFA) agglutinins in sera of patients with gastric cancer related to ABO(H) blood group phenotype. *Int J Cancer.* 1995;60:781–785.
6. Clausen H, Stroud M, Parker J, Springer G, Hakomon S. Monoclonal antibodies directed to the blood group A associated structure, galactosyl-A: specificity and relation to the Thomsen-Friedenreich antigen. *Mol Immunol.* 1988;25:199–204.

CANCER, THYROID–*Tumors of the thyroid.*

Thyroid cancer	RISK		
	LOW	AVERAGE	HIGH
GROUP A			
GROUP B			
GROUP AB			
GROUP O			

Symptoms

▪ A lump or swelling in the front of the neck or in other parts of the neck.

About Thyroid Cancer

Cancer of the thyroid is a disease in which malignancies are found in the tissues of the thyroid gland. It is more common in women than in men. Most patients are between 25 and 65 years old. People who have been exposed to large amounts of radiation, or who have had radiation treatment for medical problems in the head and neck have a higher chance of getting thyroid cancer, although the cancer may not appear until 20 years or longer after radiation treatment.

There are four main types of cancer of the thyroid: papillary, follicular, medullary, and anaplastic.

▪ *Papillary:* The most commonly seen thyroid cancer, it is found two to three times more often in women than in men. Although seen more frequently in the young, it is a more serious malignancy in the elderly. It is often seen in patients who have had radiation exposure or HASHIMOTO'S THYROIDITIS.

▪ *Follicular:* Responsible for approximately 25% of thyroid tumors, it is seen more often in the elderly patient. It also is more common in females and has a history of radiation associated with its onset. As follicular cancer spreads through the blood, it more easily causes distant metastases and is therefore more malignant.

▪ *Medullary:* Most likely to have a strong genetic factor, it is related to a gene abnormality.

▪ *Anaplastic:* It is faster growing and more inclined to spread rapidly to other organs.

Blood Group Links

Blood group A has a propensity for thyroid cancer, while blood group O appears to be protected. Similar to many other cancers, the fine structure of various antigens is altered between healthy and cancerous cells. As a general rule, loss of A and B antigens, and the appearance of greater numbers of Tn antigens are characteristic of thyroid cancers, and are associated with a tendency for malignancy[1-3].

Therapies, Thyroid Cancer

ALL BLOOD GROUPS:

Four types of conventional treatment are used:

▪ Surgery (taking out the cancer and/or thyroid gland)

▪ Radiation therapy (using high-dose x-rays or other high-energy rays to kill cancer cells)

▪ Hormone therapy (using hormones to stop cancer cells from growing)

▪ Chemotherapy (using drugs to kill cancer cells)

In addition, the following dietary guidelines are recommended. Consume foods rich in iodine, silicon, and phosphorus: kelp, dulse, Swiss chard, turnip greens, egg yolks, wheat germ, cod roe, lecithin, sesame seed butter, seeds and nuts, and raw goat's milk.

BLOOD GROUP A:

1. Cancer Prevention Protocol
2. Chemotherapy Adjunct Protocol
3. Surgery Recovery Protocol
4. Chronic Illness Recovery Protocol

BLOOD GROUP B:

1. Cancer Prevention Protocol
2. Chemotherapy Adjunct Protocol
3. Surgery Recovery Protocol
4. Chronic Illness Recovery Protocol

BLOOD GROUP AB:

1. Cancer Prevention Protocol
2. Chemotherapy Adjunct Protocol
3. Surgery Recovery Protocol
4. Chronic Illness Recovery Protocol

BLOOD GROUP O:

1. Cancer Prevention Protocol
2. Chemotherapy Adjunct Protocol
3. Surgery Recovery Protocol
4. Chronic Illness Recovery Protocol

Related Topics

Cancer (general)

Immunity

Thyroid disease, Graves'

Thyroid disease, Hashimoto's thyroiditis

Thyroid disease, hyperthyroidism

Thyroid disease, hypothyroidism

REFERENCES

1. Vowden P, Lowe AD, Lennox ES, Bleehen NM. Thyroid blood group isoantigen expression: a parallel with ABH isoantigen expression in the distal colon. *Br J Cancer.* 1986; 53:721–725.

2. Klechova L, Gosheva-Antonova T. [ABO and Rh blood group factors in thyroid gland diseases]. *Vutr Boles.* 1980; 19:75–79.

3. Toyoda H, Kawaguchi Y, Shirasawa K, Muramatsu A. Familial medullary carcinoma of the thyroid through 3 generations. *Acta Pathol Jpn.* 1977;27:111–121.

CANCER, UTERINE–*Tumors of the uterus.*

Uterine cancer	RISK		
	LOW	AVERAGE	HIGH
GROUP A	■	■	
GROUP B	■		
GROUP AB	■	■	
GROUP O	■		
NON-SECRETOR	■		■

Symptoms

- Postmenopausal bleeding

About Uterine Cancer

Uterine cancer is the most common gynecological cancer in women and the third most common female cancer overall (after breast and colorectal). It is seen primarily in postmenopausal women between 50 to 60 years old. Predisposing factors include OBESITY, DIABETES, HIGH BLOOD PRESSURE, INFERTILITY, a history of IRREGULAR PERIODS, late onset of MENOPAUSE (over 52 years old), and use of estrogen therapy (unopposed estrogens) in a woman who still has her uterus. Overall, the general 5-year survival rate for endometrial (uterine lining) cancer is somewhat favorable.

Almost 63% of women will be alive after 5 years of treatment with no sign of the cancer; 28% will die within 5 years; and 9% will be alive but have the disease. However, in the United States, the 5-year survival rate for stage I tumors reaches 90%.

Postmenopausal bleeding is the most frequent sign of endometrial cancer. See a doctor if any spotting occurs.

Blood Group Links

Normal endometrial tissue does not contain blood group antigens. However, over one-half of endometrial cancers have detectable blood group antigens. An increased rate of expression of Lewis group antigens, particularly Lewis (b) antigen, is also observed in endometrial cancers compared with its expression in normal endometria.

Therapies, Uterine Cancer

BLOOD GROUP A:

1. Cancer Prevention Protocol
2. Chemotherapy Adjunct Protocol
3. Surgery Recovery Protocol
4. Chronic Illness Recovery Protocol

BLOOD GROUP B:

1. Cancer Prevention Protocol
2. Chemotherapy Adjunct Protocol
3. Surgery Recovery Protocol
4. Chronic Illness Recovery Protocol

BLOOD GROUP AB:

1. Cancer Prevention Protocol
2. Chemotherapy Adjunct Protocol
3. Surgery Recovery Protocol
4. Chronic Illness Recovery Protocol

BLOOD GROUP O:

1. Cancer Prevention Protocol
2. Chemotherapy Adjunct Protocol
3. Surgery Recovery Protocol
4. Chronic Illness Recovery Protocol

Related Topics

Cancer (general)

Cancer, gynecological tumors

CANCER, VAGINAL–*See Cancer, gynecological tumors*

CANCER, VULVAR–*See Cancer, gynecological tumors*

CANDIDA ALBICANS–*See Fungal disease, candidiasis*

CANDIDIASIS–*See Fungal disease, candidiasis*

CARBOHYDRATE INTOLERANCE–*See Insulin resistance (Syndrome X)*

CARDIOVASCULAR DISEASE–*Disorders of the heart and blood vessel system, including coronary artery disease (CAD), heart attack, hypertension, and stroke.*

Cardiovascular disease	RISK		
	LOW	AVERAGE	HIGH
GROUP A			
GROUP B			
GROUP AB			
GROUP O			
NON-SECRETOR			

Symptoms

Characteristically there are few symptoms of cardiovascular disease, and the condition remains silent until there is a cardiovascular event, such as stenosis (narrowing), thrombosis (clotting), or aneurysm (widening) of an artery or chamber.

There are many conditions that exist in relationship to CARDIOVASCULAR DISEASE, including essential HYPERTENSION, coronary ARTERIOSCLEROSIS, congestive heart failure, CEREBROVASCULAR ACCIDENT, atrial arrhythmias, ventricular arrhythmias, and ANEURYSMS.

About Cardiovascular Disease

The human heart weighs only 10.5 ounces (about the size of an average fist) and is hollow. This is not really very big considering the job it does. In some animals such as horses the heart size is much greater. The heart is also bigger in champion endurance athletes as a result of genetics and training.

In each 24-hour period, the human heart beats over 100,000 times and pumps about 2,000 gallons of blood—enough to fill an oil tanker. In a 70-year lifetime, an average human heart beats more than 2.5 billion times. It has been speculated that the lifespan of any particular species is relative to the absolute number of heartbeats over the course of its life; smaller sized, short-lived species have very high heart rates, while larger, longer-lived species have much slower heart rates.

In a sense, the heart is really two hearts, the left heart and the right. Both sides pump the same amount of blood, but to different locations of the body, and at different pressures. The right ventricle pumps low-oxygen blood from the body to the lungs where it is oxygenated. This is a short trip and requires little pressure development, so the right ventricle is rather thin walled, like a fireplace bellows.

The left ventricle is the real workhorse, pumping oxygenated blood that has returned from the lungs to the entire body. This job requires being able to move blood through an incredible maze of blood vessels at tremendously greater pressure. The left heart muscle is thicker as a result.

The circulatory system, composed of heart and blood vessels, contains five quarts of blood. The heart pumps these five quarts through 60,000 miles of veins and arteries. The round trip takes about 1 minute, and sometimes the blood reaches a speed of 10 miles per hour.

The heart is an amazingly resilient organ. Alexis Carrel, the famous experimental biologist who received the 1912 Nobel Prize in Physiology for Medicine, concluded that, given an optimum supply of nutrients and oxygen, the human heart is capable of functioning perfectly for over two centuries! The most common forms of heart disease do not result from a wearing-out of the heart, but rather from a breakdown in the supply of nutrients to the heart, usually the result of disease in the arteries on which the heart relies.

General Risk Factors and Causes

As we age, our vessels become less pliant. Therefore, aging itself is a risk factor for cardiovascular disease. Additional risk factors include HYPERTENSION, tobacco use, DIABETES, OBESITY, physical inactivity, a family history of premature arteriosclerosis, and HIGH CHOLESTEROL—especially decreased high-density lipoproteins (HDL) and increased low-density lipoproteins (LDL).

Although the health of the cardiovascular system relies on a complex blend of several important factors, including diet, exercise, stress, and other lifestyle issues, one unrecognized but very important component of the puzzle involves genetics, in particular blood group genetics.

Blood Group Links

Your blood group influences the workings of the cardiovascular system in several ways. It influences the ability to metabolize dietary fats, which has important effects on the heart and circulation.

ABO blood group directly influences the viscosity or thickness of blood, which has powerful implications for circulation. Blood group genetics have a direct effect upon the chemical response to stress—an important risk factor for heart disease.

Although each blood group can develop elements of cardiovascular disease, they appear to do so for different reasons. Some of the causes of heart disease in one blood group may be obvious, such as the link between blood group A and cholesterol. Others, such as the effects of high triglycerides and INSULIN RESISTANCE in blood group O, are less well known. Yet it makes good sense to look for different causes of action in different people, since the conventional wisdom that heart disease is always the result of a high fat, high protein diet can and has been effectively challenged by a number of studies.

The ability to understand your risk factors for cardiovascular disease in light of the specifics of your blood group gives a powerful predictive ability that is absent when you are evaluating the abundant and often contradictory literature on lifestyle and heart disease.

Not every risk factor for heart disease has a blood group component. For example, untreated high blood pressure, diabetes, or smoking will increase your odds of developing cardiovascular disease no matter what your blood type is. Quitting smoking and undergoing frequent blood pressure and diabetes screenings with appropriate treatment, if necessary, will contribute to your success in modifying other, blood group–specific risk factors.

Heart Disease and Blood Group Differences

Blood group O and blood group B are less likely to generate heart disease as a result of high cholesterol. Their pathway is CARBOHYDRATE INTOLERANCE. Blood groups A and AB follow a more conventional path, through high cholesterol. Each of these pathways leads to a very different lifestyle plan and diet to stay heart healthy.

A and AB: The Blood Group–Cholesterol Factor

A number of studies show that blood groups A and AB are more likely to be at risk of heart disease and death by virtue of elevated cholesterol.

The relationship between blood type and total serum cholesterol level was examined in a Japanese population to determine whether elevated cholesterol levels are associated with blood group A, as had been demonstrated in many Western European populations. The results showed that cholesterol levels were very significantly elevated in the group A group compared to the others[1].

A study examining a total of 380 marker/risk factor combinations found positive associations between blood group A and both total serum cholesterol and LDL cholesterol, while a negative association was found between blood group B and total serum cholesterol as a risk factor for heart disease[2].

A Hungarian study measured the cholesterol of 653 patients who underwent coronary angiography between 1980 and 1985 at the Hungarian Institute of Cardiology. The results showed the numbers of blood group A patients were smaller than would be normally expected from the Hungarian population. The study also found that there were differences between the blood types as to the areas of the vessels where the narrowing of the coronary arteries had occurred[3].

Several forms of elevated lipoproteins are inherited. One of the more common forms of hyperlipoproteinemia is called type IIB, and it is characterized by increased LDL and VLDL (very low density lipoproteins). Type IIB hyperlipoproteinemia results in premature hardening of the arteries, obstruction of the carotid artery (the artery that supplies blood to the head and brain), PERIPHERAL ARTERY DISEASE, HEART ATTACK, and STROKE. Since all of these disorders show higher rates of occurrence in blood group A, it is not surprising that studies have found a significant connection between hyperlipoproteinemia IIB and group A in both newborns and in patients who have suffered heart attacks[4].

O and B: The Blood Group–Carbohydrate Intolerance Factor

For blood groups O and B, the leading risk factor for heart disease is not so much the fat in the food as the fat on the person. In other words, the elevated risk factor is due to carbohydrate intolerance. When groups O and B adopt low-fat, high carbohydrate, lectin-rich diets, they gain weight. This particular kind of weight gain is a major risk factor for heart disease.

For many years, heart experts have been saying that HIGH TRIGLYCERIDES are not an independent risk for heart disease, but only dangerous in combination with other factors. However, increasing evidence points to elevated triglycerides as a risk factor on their own, and this partially explains the anomaly of the O and B pathway to heart disease[5,6].

Triglycerides are formed by three fatty chains linked to one another. Most fat in food and the human body exist in this form. Diabetics often have high triglyceride levels, and diabetes is believed to be the leading cause of hypertriglyceridemia. In other words, insulin resistance, caused by carbohydrate intolerance, leads to high triglycerides. By current standards, borderline high triglyceride levels are between 200 and 400 mg/dL; high triglyceride levels are between 400 and 1,000 mg/dL; and very high levels are over 1,000 mg/dL.

One study found that men with the highest fasting triglyceride concentrations were more than twice as likely to have heart attacks than men with the lowest levels—even after diabetes, smoking, and sedentary living were factored in. People with triglyceride levels as low as 142 mg/dL were still at risk for heart attacks, which was surprising, because levels below 200 mg/dL were considered normal.

A classic sign of insulin resistance is the "apple-shaped figure," characterized by a broad girth at the midsection. Fat cells located in the abdomen release fat into the blood more easily than fat cells found elsewhere. For example, "pear-shaped" individuals, with fat located in the hips and thighs, do not have the same health risks. The release of fat from the abdomen begins within 3 to 4 hours after a meal is consumed, compared to many more hours for other fat cells. This easy release shows up as higher triglycerides and free fatty acid levels. Free fatty acids themselves cause insulin resistance, and elevated triglycerides usually coincide with low HDL, or good cholesterol. Overproduction of insulin as a result of insulin resistance syndrome has also been shown to increase the production of very bad cholesterol, VLDL[7].

The link between obesity, triglycerides, and bad lipoproteins has been shown for blood group O. In a French study screening blood donors for cardiovascular or cerebrovascular disease, serum triglycerides and lipoproteins were shown to correlate with both obesity and group O. There is also a connection between non-secretors and high triglyceride levels, as well as insulin resistance.

At long last the medical establishment is beginning to recognize the need to step outside of its narrow box and expand its thinking regarding cardiovascular risk factors. Although there is ample evidence that cholesterol plays an important role in ATHEROSCLEROSIS and HEART DISEASE for some people, a large number of people do not fit this limited profile.

O and B: Cholesterol Protection

There is a physiological explanation for the relative protection blood groups O and B enjoy from high-protein diets. Intestinal alkaline phosphatase, an enzyme manufactured in the small intestine, has the primary function of splitting dietary cholesterol and fats, and is naturally high in blood groups O and B—especially among secretors. Conversely, blood groups A and AB have lower levels of this enzyme. Recent studies suggest that it is the inability to break down dietary fat that in part predisposes groups A and AB to higher cholesterol and more heart attacks; the opposite is true for blood groups O and B, who are aided in the breakdown of dietary fat by high amounts of intestinal alkaline phosphatase[8,9,10].

Intestinal alkaline phosphatase activity rises following the ingestion of a fat-containing meal, especially if the triglycerides in the meal are long-chain fatty acids. In a study of volunteers given different test meals, the after-meal rise in serum intestinal alkaline phosphatase activity was significantly greater following the long-chain fatty acid meal than following the medium-chain fatty acid meal, and was significantly higher in blood groups O and B over A and AB.

Paradoxically, it appears that intestinal alkaline phosphatase gives groups O and B metabolic advantages when they eat high-protein meals. In fact, consumption of protein further increases the levels of alkaline phosphatase in their intestines. Without protein in their diets, they do not gain the benefits of the specialized fat-busting enzymes in their intestines. This explains why these blood groups can lower their cholesterol by adopting high-protein diets[11].

An intriguing study helped to cast some light on why blood groups A and AB have such low levels of alkaline phosphatase activity. Researchers presented evidence that the blood group A antigen may itself inactivate alkaline phosphatase. It may be the case that the lower levels of this enzyme, and the subsequent inability to break down dietary fats, may actually be a physical expression of the A antigen. They found that the red cells of blood groups A and AB bind almost all intestinal alkaline phosphatase, while the red cells of groups O and B do so to a much lesser degree[12].

Additional Risk Factors for Cardiovascular Disease

ORAL CONTRACEPTIVES

Birth control pills can worsen cardiovascular risk factors. They raise blood cholesterol levels and increase blood pressure, so women who already have these problems should not take oral contraceptives. Smokers who use oral contraceptives run the risk of developing dangerous BLOOD CLOTS (THROMBOSIS). There is some evidence that group A and AB woman are more at risk for blood clots resulting from oral contraceptive use than groups O or B[13].

PHYSICAL INACTIVITY

Researchers have found that people who seldom exercise don't recover as well from heart attacks as physically active people. Although it is not clear if lack of exercise alone is a risk factor for developing heart disease, in combination with other factors, such as obesity, the risk is higher. Physical activity considerably decreases the bad LDL cholesterol and increases the good HDL cholesterol.

STRESS

Excessive emotional stress over a prolonged period appears to increase the risk of heart disease. STRESS can exacerbate other risk factors, such as overeating, smoking, and high blood pressure. Stress can trigger the release of hormones that promote blood clots. Stress releases fatty acids and glucose into the bloodstream. These can be converted into natural fat and cholesterol and deposited on arterial walls. Such deposits create resistance to the blood flow through the arteries, and contribute to high blood pressure.

Differences between ABO blood groups with regard to stress chemistry may account for some of the observed differences among heart disease victims that appear to be linked to blood group. In one study, blood group O heart attack patients scored significantly higher than blood group A in characteristics associated with "type A" behavior, including behavior scales and anger indexes. Blood group B subjects, as expected, were in the middle[14].

Therapies, Cardiovascular Disease

BLOOD GROUP A:

1. Cardiovascular Protocol

2. Metabolic Enhancement Protocol

3. Antistress Protocol

Specifics:

Beware of extra iron: A survey of over 1,900 Finnish men between the ages of 42 and 60 revealed a 4% increase in heart attack risk with each 1% increase in serum ferritin. Ferritin is the protein the body uses to store iron. High iron levels are believed to catalyze the formation of free radicals, which damage the artery wall.

BLOOD GROUP B:

1. Cardiovascular Protocol

2. Metabolic Enhancement Protocol

BLOOD GROUP AB:

1. Cardiovascular Protocol

2. Metabolic Enhancement Protocol

3. Antistress Protocol

BLOOD GROUP O:

1. Cardiovascular Protocol

2. Metabolic Enhancement Protocol

Related Topics

Angina pectoris

Atherosclerosis

Blood clotting disorders

Diabetes mellitus

Heart attack

Hypercholesterolemia

Hypertension

Hypertriglyceridemia

Insulin resistance

Obesity

Stress

Syndrome X

REFERENCES

1. Wong FL, Kodama K, Sasaki H, Yamada M, Hamilton HB. Longitudinal study of the association between ABO phenotype and total serum cholesterol level in a Japanese cohort. *Genet Epidemiol.* 1992;9:405–418.

2. George VT, Elston RC, Amos CI, Ward LJ, Berenson GS. Association between polymorphic blood markers and risk factors for cardiovascular disease in a large pedigree. *Genet Epidemiol.* 1987;4:267–275.

3. Tarjan Z, Tonelli M, Duba J, Zorandi A. [Correlation between ABO and Rh blood groups, serum cholesterol and ischemic heart disease in patients undergoing coronarography]. *Orv Hetil.* 1995;136:767–769.

4. Kipschidse NN, Schawgulidse NA. [Arteriosclerosis and blood lipids]. *Z Gesamte Inn Med.* 1989;44:175–176.

5. Contiero E, Chinello GE, Folin M. Serum lipids and lipoproteins associations with ABO blood groups. *Anthropol Anz.* 1994;52:221–230.

6. Borecki IB, Elston RC, Rosenbaum PA, Srinivasan SR, Berenson GS. ABO associations with blood pressure, serum lipids and lipoproteins, and anthropometric measures. *Hum Hered.* 1985;35:161–170.

7. Lewis GF, Steiner G. Acute effects of insulin in the control of VLDL production in humans. Implications for the insulin-resistant state. *Diabetes Care.* 1996;19:390–393.

8. Domar U, Hirano K, Stigbrand T. Serum levels of human alkaline phosphatase isozymes in relation to blood groups. *Clin Chim Acta.* 1991;203:305–313.

9. Nakata N, Tozawa T. [The ABO blood groups-dependent reference intervals for serum alkaline phosphatase isozymes and total activity in individuals 20–39 years of age]. *Rinsho Byori.* 1995;43:508–512.

10. Day AP, Feher MD, Chopra R, Mayne PD. Triglyceride fatty acid chain length influences the post prandial rise in serum intestinal alkaline phosphatase activity. *Ann Clin Biochem.* 1992;29:287–291.

11. Stepan J, Graubaum HJ, Meurer W, Wagenknecht C. [Isoenzymes of alkaline phosphatase—reference values in young people and effects of protein diet]. *Experientia.* 1976;32:832–834.

12. Bayer PM, Hotschek H, Knoth E. Intestinal alkaline phosphatase and the ABO blood group system—a new aspect. *Clin Chim Acta.* 1980;108:81–87.

13. Jick H, Slone D, Westerholm B. Venous thromboembolic disease and ABO blood type. A cooperative study. *Lancet.* 1969;1:539–542. No abstract available.

14. Neumann JK, Chi DS, Arbogast BW, Kostrzewa RM, Harvill LM. Relationship between blood groups and behavior patterns in men who have had myocardial infarction. *South Med J.* 1991;84:214–218.

CAVITIES–_See Dental caries_

CELIAC DISEASE–_Also known as celiac sprue; an immune reaction to gliadin, a protein found in wheat, rye, oats, and barley._

Celiac disease	RISK		
	LOW	AVERAGE	HIGH
GROUP A			
GROUP B			
GROUP AB			
GROUP O			
NON-SECRETOR			

Symptoms

- Chronic diarrhea
- Weight loss
- Iron deficiency
- General nutrient malabsorption

About Celiac Disease

Celiac disease is thought to be an immune reaction to gliadin, a protein found in the four cereal grains: wheat, rye, oats, and barley. About four out of five people with celiac disease have antibodies to gliadin in their blood. It has also been found that, in general, half the patients with gastrointestinal disorders have raised antibodies to gliadin as well. People with celiac disease have a lack of IgA, the protective antibody found in mucus, making their intestinal lining more fragile.

Blood Group Connections

There is a strong association between being a non-secretor and having overt celiac disease. Non-secretors are about 200% more likely to have celiac disease than secretors[1,2]. This would make sense, since it has been noted for over 20 years that non-secretors had lower levels of IgA than secretors[3,4].

There is some evidence that the improvement in celiac among non-secretors may be linked to the health of their Lewis (a) blood type antigen. The Lewis (a) substance in the gut of non-secretors is a large molecule. Evidence suggests that this large form of Lewis (a) is converted by the intestinal cells into a small form, which can enter the bloodstream and pass through the kidneys. Non-secretor celiac patients who have not regenerated normal mucosa after treatment have significantly higher levels of small Lewis (a) in their urine when compared with healthy individuals[5]. Another study showed that special cells of the intestines called M cells preferentially display the Lewis (a) antigen, and probably provide the material for other cells to metabolize in healthy systems. M cells are important: They are part of the Peyer's patches of the gut—the place where immune tolerance to foods is built.

Celiac disease predisposes patients to the eventual development of LYMPHOMA, illustrating the intimacy between the immune system and the gut, and how it can be deranged by dietary difficulties.

The Lectin Connection

Lectins have been extensively studied in celiac disease, but the results are inconclusive. Celiac disease seems to effect all blood groups about equally, though perhaps for different reasons. Part of the reason seems to be that gliadin, the perpetrator here, is different from wheat germ lectin, the major everyday problem for blood group O[6]. For example, studies have reported no ability to bind gliadin or gluten with N-acetyl-glucosamine (NAG), the sugar that so handily binds wheat germ lectin[7].

This is not to say that gluten doesn't appear to be somewhat lectin-like in its own right: Gluten has been shown to bind to carbohydrate-rich tissues much like a lectin. Gluten can even be inhibited by a specific sugar, alpha-D-mannose. Many intestinal influenza viruses bind to alpha-D-mannose as well. This may explain the traditional naturopathic wisdom, noted by lectinologist David Freed, which recommends that a patient fast during gastrointestinal flus[8]. In addition to bacteria, the lectin from the plant Snowdrop (*Galanthus nivalis*), which is being used to genetically alter foods, also binds alpha-D-mannose.

Therapies, Celiac Disease

BLOOD GROUP A:

1. Stomach Health Protocol
2. Intestinal Health Protocol

BLOOD GROUP B:

1. Stomach Health Protocol
2. Intestinal Health Protocol

BLOOD GROUP AB:

1. Stomach Health Protocol
2. Intestinal Health Protocol

BLOOD GROUP O:

1. Stomach Health Protocol
2. Intestinal Health Protocol

Related Topics

Cancer, lymphoma

Digestion

Immunity

Lectins

REFERENCES

1. Dickey W, Wylie JD, Collins JS, Porter KG, Watson RG, McLoughlin JC. Lewis phenotype, secretor status, and coeliac disease. *Gut.* 1994;35:769–770.
2. Heneghan MA, Kearns M, Goulding J, Egan EL, Stevens FM, McCarthy CF. Secretor status and human leucocyte antigens in coeliac disease. *Scand J Gastroenterol.* 1996;31:973–976.
3. Shinebaum R. ABO blood group and secretor status in the spondyloarthropathies. *FEMS Microbiol Immunol.* 1989;1:389–395.
4. Blackwell CC, May SJ, Brettle RP, MacCallum CJ, Weir DM. Secretor state and immunoglobulin levels among women with recurrent urinary tract infections. *J Clin Lab Immunol.* 1987;22:133–137.
5. Evans DA, Donohoe WT, Hewitt S, Linaker BD. Lea blood group substance degradation in the human alimentary tract and urinary Lea in coeliac disease. *Vox Sang.* 1982;43:177–187.
6. Giannasca PJ, Giannasca KT, Leichtner AM, Neutra MR. Human intestinal M cells display the sialyl Lewis A antigen. *Infect Immun.* 1999;67:946–953.

7. Langman MJ, Banwell JG, Stewart JS, Robson EB. ABO blood groups, secretor status, and intestinal alkaline phosphatase concentrations in patients with celiac disease. *Gastroenterology.* 1969;57:19–23.

8. Ruhlmann J, Sinha P, Hansen G, Tauber R, Kottgen E. Studies on the aetiology of coeliac disease: no evidence for lectin-like components in wheat gluten. *Biochim Biophys Acta.* 1993;1181:249–256.

CEREBRAL ANEURYSM–*See Aneurysm, cerebral*

CEREBRAL VASCULAR DISEASE–*See Aneurysm, cerebral*

CEREBROVASCULAR ACCIDENT–*See Stroke*

CERVICAL CANCER–*See Cancer, gynecological tumors*

CHEST PAIN–*See Angina pectoris; Bronchitis*

CHOLERA–*See Bacterial disease, cholera*

CHOLESTEROL–*See Hypercholesterolemia*

CHRONIC FATIGUE SYNDROME–*A syndrome involving the combination of various symptoms, including headache, muscle ache, fatigue, flu-like symptoms, fever, swelling of the lymph nodes, depression, and digestive ailments.*

Chronic fatigue syndrome	RISK		
	LOW	AVERAGE	HIGH
GROUP A			
GROUP B			
GROUP AB			
GROUP O			
NON-SECRETOR			

Symptoms

Variable

About Chronic Fatigue Syndrome

What causes chronic fatigue syndrome (CFS)? Some experts think the source is a viral illness that triggers prolonged immune activity; fatigue is a secondary symptom. Others believe that altered neurochemistry associated with depression can cause sleep abnormalities, a lower pain threshold, and depressed immune function. Still other experts are convinced that all fatigue-related symptoms stem from a primary sleep disturbance that causes an alteration of the immune system, irritability, and muscle pain.

Although CFS masquerades as a virus or autoimmune disease, the root cause may be a problem of poor metabolism in the liver. In other words, the liver is unable to detoxify chemicals, and the result is immunologic problems.

Magnesium deficiency and oxidative stress have both been identified in 54% of people with CFS. A detailed review of the literature suggests a number of marginal nutritional deficiencies may have some relevance to CFS. These include deficiencies of various B vitamins, vitamin C, magnesium, sodium, zinc, L-tryptophan, L-carnitine, coenzyme Q10, and essential fatty acids. Any of these nutrients could be marginally deficient in CFS patients, a finding that appears to be primarily due to the illness process rather than to inadequate diets.

The Centers for Disease Control defines CFS by the following criteria:

MAJOR CRITERIA

- New onset of fatigue causing 50% reduction in activity for at least 6 months

- Exclusion of other illnesses that can cause fatigue

MINOR CRITERIA

(presence of 8 of 11 of the following symptoms.):

Symptoms

- Mild fever

- Recurrent sore throat

- Painful lymph nodes

- Muscle weakness

- Muscle pain

- Prolonged fatigue after exercise

- Recurrent headache

- Migratory joint pain

- Neurological or psychological complaints

- Sleep disturbances

- Sudden onset of symptom complex

The Immune Connection

Natural killer (NK) cells are a critical component of the immune system when it comes to handling viruses effectively. In a simplified sense, NK cells act like tiny armor-piercing pieces of Velcro, cruising through the immune system. When they encounter a cell infected by a virus, they stick to the cell, and destroy it by a process called lysis. Because of the importance of NK cells in combating a virus, it comes as no surprise that studies in humans consistently point toward the vital role of NK cells in the defense against CFS.

Low levels of NK cell activity are also associated with the severity of CFS. The lower the NK cell activity, the more severe are the symptoms. There may also be a familial association between NK cell activity and CFS. Researchers have discovered that NK cell activity was much lower in individuals who had several extended family members suffering from CFS—even if they themselves did not have the disease[1–6].

Blood Group Links

Overall, blood groups O and B have the greatest susceptibility to CFS. For blood group O, CFS may be linked to nutritional deficiencies and liver toxicity.

For blood group B, CFS is likely linked with viral infections and nutritional deficiencies.

The risk for blood groups A and AB heightens during conditions of weakened immunity, especially low levels of NK cells.

Therapies, Chronic Fatigue Syndrome

BLOOD GROUP A:

1. Fatigue-Fighting Protocol

2. Immune-Enhancing Protocol

3. Antistress Protocol

BLOOD GROUP B:

1. Fatigue-Fighting Protocol

2. Antiviral Protocol

3. Liver Support Protocol

BLOOD GROUP AB:

1. Fatigue-Fighting Protocol

2. Immune-Enhancing Protocol

3. Antiviral Protocol

BLOOD GROUP O:

1. Fatigue-Fighting Protocol

2. Immune-Enhancing Protocol

3. Liver Support Protocol

Related Topics

Autoimmune diseases (general)

Cancer (general)

Immunity

Viral diseases (general)

REFERENCES

1. Fulcher KY, White PD. Randomised controlled trial of graded exercise in patients with the chronic fatigue syndrome. *BMJ.* 1997;314:1647–1652.

2. McCully KK, Sisto SA, Natelson BH. Use of exercise for treatment of chronic fatigue syndrome [review]. *Sports Med.* 1996;21:35–48.

3. Sharpe M, Hawton K, Simkin S, et al. Cognitive behaviour therapy for the chronic fatigue syndrome: a randomized controlled trial. *BMJ.* 1996;312:22–26.

4. Shaw DL et al. Management of fatigue: A physiologic approach. *Am J Med Sci.* 1962;243:758.

5. Crescente FJ. Treatment of fatigue in a surgical practice. *J Abdom Surg.* 1962;4:73.

6. Cox IM, Campbell MJ, Dowson D. Red blood cell magnesium and chronic fatigue syndrome. *Lancet.* 1991;337:757–760.

CIRRHOSIS–See Liver disease

CLUSTER HEADACHES–See Headache

COLDS–See Common cold

COLITIS, ULCERATIVE–Inflammation of the innermost lining of the colon wall.

Ulcerative colitis	RISK		
	LOW	AVERAGE	HIGH
GROUP A	███	███	
GROUP B	███	███	
GROUP AB		███	
GROUP O			███
NON-SECRETOR			

Symptoms

- Bloody diarrhea
- Abdominal pain
- Fever
- Weight loss

About Ulcerative Colitis

As the name suggests, ulcerative colitis involves only the colon and rectum, although some "backwash" may occur in the last part of the small intestine. In contrast to CROHN'S DISEASE, ulcerative colitis involves the mucosa, or the innermost lining of the colon wall. Crohn's disease involves all layers of bowel, and may involve any part of the gut, from mouth to anus. Like Crohn's, ulcerative colitis increases the risk for colon cancer.

Blood Group Links

Evidence suggests that patients with ulcerative colitis have elevated antibodies to opposing blood types[1]. This probably represents the production of blood type–like substances from the mucins of the intestinal lining by bacteria in the gut. If so, it may help explain why sulfa drugs, which work by suppressing the levels of gut bacteria, are generally effective in controlling inflammation. The intestinal microflora are known to be disturbed by inflammatory bowel disease, and it has been thought that ulcerative colitis patients were mounting some sort of allergic hypersensitivity to gut bacteria[2].

Depressing the levels of bacteria reduces the immune provocation. However, specific strains of bacteria may be capable of degrading the mucin of colitis patients into antigens that mimic an opposing blood type, which are the true cause of the immune reaction in inflammatory bowel disease. For example, bacteria producing the B antigen in the mucus of a colitis patient who is blood group A will cause the immune system of the patient to mistake the body's colon lining for a bad blood transfusion, and attack it as foreign. This has been reported in the literature, and several strains of bacteria, including species of *Proteus vulgaris,* a common gut bacteria, are capable of synthesizing a blood group B antigen (pseudo-B) out of colon mucus.

Gut bacteria are capable of manufacturing large amounts of both A and B blood group antigens by degrading colon mucin. Because of this, it might be hypothesized that blood group O, the only blood group to manufacture both anti-A and anti-B, would have a greater incidence of ulcerative colitis. The literature is mildly supportive of this, although larger and more inclusive studies need to be done[3]. However, it is true that blood group O, especially non-secretors, does mount a more intensive immune reaction than the other blood groups[4]. In my own practice, I have found that individuals with blood group O who have inflammatory bowel disease tend to develop a more aggressive form than the other blood groups, but do well when they follow the appropriate diet for their type.

Therapies, Ulcerative Colitis

ALL BLOOD GROUPS:

Conventional treatment involves the use of aminosalicylates (ASA) and corticosteroids. The old sulfa antibiotics and newer 5-ASA preparations such as Asacol (mesalamine), Pentasa (mesalamine), and Dipentum (olsalazine sodium) are still the mainstay of treatment. Acute relapses are often treated with corticosteroids, though their long-term use has substantial toxicity. In patients requiring long-term steroids, immunosuppressive agents such as Imuran (azathioprine) and 6-MP (6-mercaptopurine) are helpful in reducing the required dose of steroids. However, several months may pass before any positive reaction manifests to these drugs.

Although many gastroenterologists continue to ignore food as a provocative factor, it is doubtful that drug therapy alone can successfully cure inflammatory bowel disease.

Many gums found in commercially processed foods can intensify the effects of dietary lectins. One gum in particular, carrageenan, is used to induce ulcerative colitis–like symptoms in test animals. Because carrageenan is effective at stabilizing milk proteins, it is often used in milk and diary products. However, the studies on humans are conflicting: Given large doses, no inflammatory lesions were noticed in healthy human volunteers[5]. However, it should be noted that milk proteins as well as gums intensify the effects of dietary lectins. So, giving large doses of carrageenan, independent of milk products and lectin-containing foods, may not be sufficient to induce problems in healthy individuals.

Blood group O tends to develop the more ulcerative form of colitis that causes bleeding with elimination. This is probably due to the lack of adequate clotting factors in group O blood. Blood groups A, B, and AB tend to develop more of a mucous colitis, which is not as bloody.

In either case, follow the diet for your blood type. You will be able to avoid many of the food lectins that can aggravate the condition, and you may find your symptoms easing.

BLOOD GROUP A:

1. Intestinal Health Protocol
2. Stomach Health Protocol
3. Antistress Protocol

BLOOD GROUP B:

1. Intestinal Health Protocol
2. Anti-Inflammation Protocol
3. Antistress Protocol

BLOOD GROUP AB:

1. Intestinal Health Protocol
2. Stomach Health Protocol
3. Antistress Protocol

BLOOD GROUP O:

1. Intestinal Health Protocol
2. Anti-Inflammation Protocol
3. Yeast/Fungus Resistance Protocol

Specifics:

Avoid gums, such as carrageenan, ghatti, and acacia, which are often used as food stabilizers. Look for foods that are stabilized by other methods.

Related Topics

Crohn's disease

Digestion

Immunity

REFERENCES

1. Chiba M, Nakajima K, Arakawa H, Masamune O, Narisawa T. Anti-erythrocyte antibodies in ulcerative colitis: case report and discussion on the pathophysiology of anti-erythrocyte antibody. *Gastroenterol Jpn.* 1988;23:564–569.

2. Hentges DJ ed. *Human Intestinal Microflora in Health and Disease.* New York: Academic Press, 1983.

3. Vesely KT. Frequency of blood groups of the ABC and Rho(D) system in patients with viral hepatitis, cirrhosis of the liver, bile stones, pancreatitis, urolithiasis, and ulcerative colitis. *Rev Czech Med.* 1970;16:60–71.

4. Tandon OP, Bhatia S, Tripathi RL, Sharma KN. Phagocytic response of leucocytes in secretors and non-secretors of ABH (O) blood group substances. *Indian J Physiol Pharmacol.* 1979;23:321–324.

5. Bonfils S. Carrageenan in the human gut. *Lancet.* 1970;ii:414.

COLON CANCER—*See Cancer, colon*

COLON POLYPS—*See Polyps, colon*

COMMON COLD—*A general term describing a number of common viruses that infect the upper respiratory tract.*

Symptoms

- General malaise
- Fever
- Congestion
- Sneezing
- Sore throat

Blood Group Links

There are hundreds of different strains of cold virus, and it would be impossible to see a blood type specificity in all of them. However, studies of British military recruits showed a slightly lower overall incidence of cold viruses in recruits who were blood group A, which is consistent with our findings that blood group A was developed to be resistant to these common viruses. Viruses also have less impact on blood group AB. The A antigen, carried by both blood group A and AB, blocks the attachment of various strains of flu to the membranes of the throat and respiratory passages.

INFLUENZA, a more serious virus, also strikes blood groups O and B in preference to groups A and AB. In its early stages, influenza may have many of the symptoms of a common cold. However, the flu causes dehydration, muscle pains, and serious weakness.

The symptoms of a common cold or flu are miserable, but they are actually a sign that your immune system is trying hard to fight off the offending virus.

Therapies, Common Cold

ALL BLOOD GROUPS:

1. Maintain general good health with adequate rest and exercise, along with learning to cope with the stresses of life. Stress is a major factor in the depletion of immune system resources. This may protect you from frequent infections and may even shorten the duration of the colds and flu you do get.

2. Follow the basic dietary guidelines for your blood type. This will optimize your immune response and help shorten the course of your cold or flu.

3. Take a bit of extra vitamin C, or increase the sources of vitamin C in your diet. Small doses of the herb echinacea (*Echinacea purpurea*) helps prevent colds, or at least helps to shorten their duration.

4. Increase the humidity in your room with a vaporizer or humidifier to prevent a dry throat and nasal tissue.

5. If your throat is sore, gargle with salt water. One-half teaspoon of ordinary table salt and a tall glass of comfortably warm water provides a soothing and cleansing rinse. Another good gargle, especially if you are prone to tonsillitis, is a tea of equal parts goldenseal root (*Hydrastis canadensis*) and sage. Gargle with this mixture every few hours.

6. If your nose is runny or stuffy, use an antihistamine to reduce the reaction of tissues to the infecting virus and relieve nasal congestion. Be especially careful with ephedra-type antihistamines, such as those found in health food stores and in some over-the-counter decongestants. These can raise the blood pressure, keep you awake at night, and complicate prostate problems in men.

7. Antibiotics are not effective against viruses.

BLOOD GROUP A:

1. Immune-Enhancing Protocol

2. Antiviral Protocol

BLOOD GROUP B:

1. Immune-Enhancing Protocol

2. Antiviral Protocol

BLOOD GROUP AB:

1. Immune-Enhancing Protocol

2. Antiviral Protocol

BLOOD GROUP O:

1. Immune-Enhancing Protocol

2. Antiviral Protocol

Related Topics

Immunity

Infectious disease

Influenza

Viral disease

Constipation

COMMON CAUSES	BLOOD GROUP O	BLOOD GROUP A	BLOOD GROUP B	BLOOD GROUP AB
Acute rectal condition—i.e., hemorrhoids	*******	****	***	***
Inadequate dietary fiber	*****	*	****	*
Stress	*	******	****	**
Disruption of regular rhythm	*	******	****	**
Disease	*****	***	***	***

* = degree of risk

Constipation occurs when the stools are unusually hard or a person's bowel patterns have changed and become less frequent. Most chronic constipation is caused by poor bowel habits and irregular meals, with a diet low in bulk and water content. Some other causes are a habitual use of laxatives, a rushed and stressful daily schedule, and travel that requires abrupt adjustments of eating and sleeping patterns. Lack of physical exercise, acute illness, painful rectal conditions, and some medications may also cause constipation.

Every blood group is susceptible to constipation under the proper circumstances. Constipation is not so much a disease as a warning that something is not right with your digestive system. You'll find most of the clues in your diet:

- Are you eating enough foods in your diet that are high in fiber content?
- Are you drinking enough fluids—in particular, water and juices?
- Are you exercising regularly?

Many people simply take a laxative when they're constipated. But that doesn't solve the natural systemic causes of constipation. The long-term solution is in the diet. Blood groups A, B, and AB can supplement their diets with fibrous, unprocessed bran. Group O, in addition to eating plenty of the fibrous fruits and vegetables on their diets, can take a supplement of butyrate, a natural bulk-forming agent, as a substitute for bran (because bran is not advised for them).

Related Protocols

BLOOD GROUP A:

1. Intestinal Health Protocol
2. Liver Support Protocol
3. Detoxification Protocol

BLOOD GROUP B:

1. Intestinal Health Protocol
2. Liver Support Protocol
3. Detoxification Protocol

BLOOD GROUP AB:

1. Intestinal Health Protocol
2. Liver Support Protocol
3. Detoxification Protocol

BLOOD GROUP O:

1. Intestinal Health Protocol
2. Liver Support Protocol
3. Detoxification Protocol

Related Topics

Cancer, colon

Colitis, ulcerative

Crohn's disease

Digestion

Hemorrhoids

Lectins

Polyps, colon

Stress

CORONARY ARTERY DISEASE (CAD)–

Arterial plaque build-up producing blockages in the arteries serving the heart.

Coronary artery disease	RISK		
	LOW	AVERAGE	HIGH
GROUP A			
GROUP B			
GROUP AB			
GROUP O			
NON-SECRETOR			

Symptoms

Coronary artery disease (CAD) results from arterial plaque build-up, which produces blockages in the arteries serving the heart. It is characteristically insidious in onset, is often irregularly distributed in different vessels, and can abruptly interfere with blood flow to segments of the heart, most often when the arterial blockages rupture and spread. The major complications of CAD are angina pectoris, unstable angina, heart attack, and sudden cardiac death due to arrhythmias.

About Coronary Artery Disease

Heart disease is the leading cause of death for people over the age of 45 living in the United States. Each day, 4,100 Americans suffer a heart attack; while hundreds of thousands survive, they are left with a damaged heart. Some 7 million Americans suffer from CAD, the most common form of heart disease. This particular disease is caused by a narrowing of the coronary arteries that feed the heart. CAD is the number one killer of both men and women in the United States. Each year, more than 500,000 Americans die of heart attacks caused by CAD.

Like any other tissue in the body, the heart needs its own supply of oxygen and nutrients, which are supplied by coronary arteries. The word *coronary* comes from the Greek word meaning "wreath." And like a wreath, the three coronary arteries radiate from the heart's main artery and cover the heart. These arteries provide the constant supply of fresh, oxygenated blood to the heart muscle. If this supply is restricted or cut off for any reason, the heart muscle literally begins to starve, and can die. When heart muscle begins to die, it is called a heart attack, or MYOCARDIAL INFARCTION. If enough tissue dies, the heart no longer has the strength to pump, and it will falter or stop.

General Risk Factors and Causes

Risk factors are conditions that increase your chances of developing heart disease. Some can be changed, and some cannot. Although each of these factors raise the risk of CAD, they do not clearly define all the causes of the disease. Even with an absence of these risk factors present, some people still develop CAD.

Most risk factors for CAD are preventable with lifestyle changes. They include HIGH BLOOD PRESSURE, HIGH CHOLESTEROL, smoking, OBESITY, and physical inactivity—all of which can be controlled. Problems arise when we try to portray risk factors as being identical for entirely different groups of people. It is here that many of the recent assertions about the connections between lifestyle and cardiovascular disease begin to break down; while large numbers of people do fit the risk profile for heart disease, equally large numbers do not. It is the extra level of interpretation that genetic information such as blood type provides that adds the needed "biomarkers" to accurately pinpoint who will suffer from cardiovascular disease from one risk factor, and who may develop it for a completely different reason.

Homocysteine has recently been identified as a risk factor for coronary, peripheral, and cerebral vascular disease. Patients with homocystinuria, a rare recessive disease, have plasma homocysteine levels 10 to 20 times above normal (hyperhomocystinemia) and accelerated, premature vascular disease. Homocysteine has a direct toxic effect on endothelium and promotes THROMBOSIS (clotting) and oxidation of LDL. Modest elevations of total plasma homocysteine have multiple causes, including low levels of folic acid and vitamins B_6 and B_{12}, renal insufficiency, use of certain drugs, and genetically determined variations in homocysteine metabolic enzymes. Patients with homocysteine values in the top 5% have a 3.4 greater risk of myocardial infarctions or cardiac death than those in the lower 90% after adjustment for other risk factors. Increased homocysteine levels are associated with increased risk of a heart condition, regardless of its cause. Recent studies suggest a graded risk even for those who have the normal of range homocysteine; thus, a reduction in the normal plasma levels may be advantageous as well.

Blood Group Links

In a study of 191 coronary artery bypass candidates, investigators paradoxically found an excess of blood group O over blood group A. When they examined the data more closely, they concluded that that the tendency of blood group A individuals to develop blood clots more readily ("thrombotic proneness") caused a poorer prognosis. In essence, the individuals from blood group A were missing from the study because they had already died in greater numbers, leaving a disproportionate number of blood group O patiens among the long-term survivors[1].

ABO non-secretors have a higher incidence of heart disease, but paradoxically with the subtypes' higher incidence of alcoholism, the effects of alcohol are most protective in this group as well.

Therapies, Coronary Artery Disease

ALL BLOOD GROUPS:

The most simple and effective way to reduce plasma homocysteine is administration of folic acid 1 to 2 mg/day, which has essentially no side effects except in untreated vitamin B_{12} deficiency.

BLOOD GROUP A:

1. Cardiovascular Protocol
2. Metabolic Enhancement Protocol
3. Antistress Protocol

BLOOD GROUP B:

1. Cardiovascular Protocol
2. Metabolic Enhancement Protocol
3. Antistress Protocol

BLOOD GROUP AB:

1. Cardiovascular Protocol
2. Metabolic Enhancement Protocol
3. Antistress Protocol

BLOOD GROUP O:

1. Cardiovascular Protocol
2. Metabolic Enhancement Protocol
3. Antistress Protocol

Related Topics

Atherosclerosis

Cardiovascular disease

Diabetes mellitus, type II

Heart attack

Hypercholesterolemia

Hypotension

Insulin resistance

Stress

REFERENCES

1. Erikssen J, Thaulow E, Stormorken H, Brendemoen O, Hellem A. ABO blood groups and coronary heart disease (CHD). A study in subjects with severe and latent CHD. *Thromb Haemost.* 1980;43:137–140.

■ Cough

COMMON CAUSES	BLOOD GROUP O	BLOOD GROUP A	BLOOD GROUP B	BLOOD GROUP AB
Common cold	**	****	**	****
Bronchial diseases	*	****	********	****
Allergy	***	*****	********	*****
Autoimmune, rheumatoid arthritis	*********	****	**********	****

* = degree of risk

Cough is a symptom of many diseases. Most coughs come from simple viral infections, such as the common cold or bronchitis. Sometimes mucus is produced with the cough and sometimes not. If the color is green or yellow, it may be a hint of a more serious bacterial infection, although this is not a reliable indicator. If the color is red, there may be bleeding in the lungs.

Cough can also occur in some autoimmune diseases, such as rheumatoid arthritis.

Any cough that produces blood or blood-stained mucus, as well as any cough that lasts more that 2 weeks, requires a visit to a medical professional for an examination.

Related Protocols

BLOOD GROUP A:

1. Pulmonary Support Protocol
2. Antibacterial Protocol
3. Allergy Control Protocol

BLOOD GROUP B:

1. Pulmonary Support Protocol
2. Antibacterial Protocol
3. Allergy Control Protocol

BLOOD GROUP AB:

1. Pulmonary Support Protocol
2. Antibacterial Protocol
3. Allergy Control Protocol

BLOOD GROUP O:

1. Pulmonary Support Protocol
2. Antibacterial Protocol
3. Allergy Control Protocol

Related Topics

Allergies, environmental/hay fever

Arthritis, rheumatoid

Bacterial disease (general)

Bronchitis

Cancer, lung

Common cold

Influenza

CROHN'S DISEASE–*Inflammation and ulceration in deep layers of the intestinal wall.*

Crohn's disease	RISK		
	LOW	AVERAGE	HIGH
GROUP A	▨	▨	
GROUP B	▨		
GROUP AB	▨	▨	
GROUP O	▨		▨
NON-SECRETOR			

Symptoms

- Cramps and discomfort upon eating
- Watery to loose stools with rectal bleeding
- Weight loss
- Anorexia
- Recurrent fevers
- Growth failure in younger patients
- Urinary tract infections
- Aphthous ulcers

About Crohn's Disease

Crohn's disease is a chronic inflammatory and ulceration process that occurs in the deep layers of the intestinal wall. It has periods of remission and relapse. The most common area affected is the lower part of the small intestine, called the ileum, and the first part of the colon. This type of Crohn's disease is called ileocolitis[1].

The cause of Crohn's disease is unknown, although alterations in intestinal permeability may play a primary role. Increased intestinal permeability in Crohn's disease may promote the local disease, and also provide the route for food antigen entry[2].

The Lectin Connection

There is ample evidence that dietary LECTINS can induce increased permeability of the gut. Intestinal permeability has been theorized to account for much of the FOOD INTOLERANCE found in people today. The intestines are very selective as to the size and quality of what is normally absorbed through their lining. In one study, rats fed on diets containing kidney beans showed increased intestinal permeability to serum proteins that had been injected into their bloodstream. Afterward, kidney bean proteins injected into their bloodstream were detected in both the lumen (open space) and the walls of the small intestine. It was suggested that dietary lectins may, at least in part, be responsible for loss of serum proteins, and may contribute to other food intolerance secondary to the loss of gut integrity.

Blood Group Links

Crohn's disease, like ulcerative colitis, shows a preference to blood group O. Groups A, B, and AB

often develop inflammatory bowel conditions when there is a stress component.

Therapies, Crohn's Disease

BLOOD GROUP A

1. Intestinal Health Protocol

2. Anti-Inflammation Protocol

BLOOD GROUP B:

1. Intestinal Health Protocol

2. Anti-Inflammation Protocol

BLOOD GROUP AB:

1. Intestinal Health Protocol

2. Anti-Inflammation Protocol

BLOOD GROUP O:

1. Intestinal Health Protocol

2. Anti-Inflammation Protocol

Related Topics

Colitis, ulcerative

Digestion

Immunity

REFERENCES

1. Mayberry JF, Rhodes J. Epidemiological aspects of Crohn's disease: a review of the literature. *Gut.* 1984;25:886–899.

2. Hollander D, Vadheim CM, Brettholz E, et al. Increased intestinal permeability in patients with Crohn's disease and their relatives. A possible etiologic factor. *Ann Intern Med.* 1986;105:883–885.

CYSTIC FIBROSIS—*See Birth defects*

CYSTITIS—*Chronic bladder infections.*

Cystitis	RISK		
	LOW	AVERAGE	HIGH
GROUP A	▓		
GROUP B	▓	▓	▓
GROUP AB	▓	▓	▓
GROUP O	▓		
NON-SECRETOR	▓	▓	▓

Symptoms

- Painful, frequent urination of small amounts

- Pelvic pull or pressure

- Lower back pain (accompanied by other symptoms)

- Low-grade fever (accompanied by other symptoms)

About Cystitis

Cystitis is the result of bacteria in the bladder. The primary causes seem to be sexual activity and poor hygiene. Cystitis often follows the beginning of sexual activity, a change in partners, or unusually frequent intercourse. In fact, one study showed that cystitis was 12.8 times more common in the general population than it was among nuns (who were assumed to be celibate).

Cystitis can also occur when the normal bacteria that live in the bowel and the vagina invade the bladder. This happens if fecal matter gets into the vagina. The issue here is hygiene, although it can happen to even the most scrupulous person. In fact, *Escherichia coli* bacteria, the most common in the bowel, are said to be the cause of most bladder infections.

Cystitis can be recurrent—the same bacteria from a previous episode, incompletely treated. Or it can be a reinfection—a new episode with a new bacteria. Risk factors include previous urinary tract infections; DIABETES; pregnancy; more frequent or vigorous sexual activity than usual; use of a spermicide or diaphragm; and underlying abnormalities of the urinary tract such as tumors, strictures, and incomplete bladder emptying.

A more severe form of cystitis, called interstitial cystitis, is poorly understood. Causes are unknown but some possible causes are subclinical urinary infection, and increased bladder wall permeability to irritants such as urea.

Blood Group Links

There is good evidence that blood groups B and AB are more susceptible to cystitis. That's because the most common bacteria that produce infections, such as *E. coli*, *Pseudomonas*, and *Klebsiella*, possess a B-like appearance, and groups B and AB produce no anti-B antibodies. A form of synergy also appears to exist between urinary tract infection risk, secretor status, and the lack of ability to create anti-B isohemagglutinin. Essentially, blood groups B and AB and the non-secretor phenotype seem to work together to increase the relative risk of recurrent urinary tract infections among these women[1].

Evidence also indicates that women and children with renal scarring subsequent to recurrent urinary tract infection and pyelonephritis are more likely to be ABO non-secretors[2–4]. As many as 55% to 60% of all non-secretors have been found to develop renal scars, even with the regular use of an antibiotic treatment for urinary tract infections whereas as few as 16% of ABH secretors will develop similar renal scarring[5].

This tendency to scarring does not seem to be dictated as much by the aggressiveness of the bacterial infection, but by the more aggressive inflammatory response created by ABH non-secretors against the bacterial infection. The levels of C-reactive protein, erythrocyte sedimentation rate, and body temperature are significantly higher in non-secretors than in secretors with recurrent urinary tract infection. As a consequence, non-secretors seem to self-inflict to a degree the renal scarring occurs secondary to their acute phase inflammatory response[6].

ABO non-secretors appear to be at extra risk for recurrent urinary tract infections. In one study of women with recurrent urinary tract infections, 29% were the Lewis (a+b−) non-secretor phenotype, while another 26% were Lewis (a−b−) recessive phenotype. When the women with non-secretor and recessive phenotypes were combined and considered collectively, the odds ratio (an estimate of relative risk of recurrent urinary tract infection) for those without the secretor phenotype (Lewis (a−b+)) was 3[7–11].

When women with urinary tract infections were evaluated, the profile of ABO antigen expression was generally consistent with the ABO phenotype of the individual and appeared to be influenced by the secretor status. Secretors expressed higher levels of A, B, and O determinants than non-secretors. In addition, Lewis antigens were detected on vaginal cells and in mucus. Samples from non-secretors expressed higher levels of Le(a) and Le(x) antigens, whereas secretors expressed higher levels of Le(b) and Le(y) antigens. The levels of antigen expression varied widely among individuals with the same blood type and secretor status. Comparisons between patient and control groups showed no significant differences in ABO or Lewis antigen expression overall, or when controlling for ABO or secretor phenotypes, respectively. These findings confirm our previous observations on healthy women, and document the heterogeneity of blood group antigen expression on vaginal wall cells and mucus from women with a history of urinary tract infections[12].

Blood groups of 137 patients with acute pyelonephritis and chronic upper tract infection, cystitis, and asymptomatic bacteriuria were compared with those of a normal uninfected control population. The identified uropathogens were categorized according to the patient's blood group. There was a significant association between the diagnosis of chronic upper tract infection and blood group B as compared with controls. Analysis of the bacterial isolates showed that more patients with blood group B had infections with *Pseudomonas* sp organisms, *Klebsiella pneumoniae*, and *Proteus* sp bacteria than was expected; and fewer patients with blood group A had infections with *Pseudomonas* than predicted[13].

There was an increased number of patients in blood group AB with infections caused by *Escherichia coli* and *Klebsiella pneumoniae*. These results suggest that an individual's blood group may be a significant factor in the host-response to bacterial invasion and may influence the development of infection with certain gram-negative bacilli.

The ABO and rhesus blood groups of 280 patients of a center of nephrology were compared with a control group consisting of 4,089 blood donors. Female patients with pyelonephritis showed with a probability of error of less than 5% more frequently the blood group A (56.7 vs 41.8%) and more infrequently the blood group O (20.0% versus 39.9%). The increase of frequency of female patients of the blood group B with cystic kidneys (30.0% versus 12.6%) reached the significance level.

Early studies confirmed these findings. Robinson and co-workers[15] reported that individuals of blood groups B and AB had a significantly greater susceptibility to gram-negative enteric pathogens (other than *Shigella*). This was especially true for *Escherichia coli* and *Salmonella* bacteria in populations of African and Puerto Rican ancestry. Individuals in blood groups B and AB, regardless of ethnic background, had a 55% greater chance of developing *E. coli* infections than did individuals of blood groups A and O. They found increased risk (not statistically significant) of *E. coli* pyelonephritis in patients in groups B and AB, compared with patients in groups A and O. Cruz-Cooke and co-workers[16] found that patients in blood group B had a 50% greater probability of having urinary tract infections caused by *E. coli* compared with non-B subjects. Kinane and co-workers[1] reported that women who lacked anti-B (blood group B and AB) and were non-secretors

were at higher risk of recurrent urinary tract infections than women who lacked either anti-B or secretor substance.

Therapies, Cystitis

BLOOD GROUP A:
1. Antibacterial Protocol
2. Urinary Tract Health Protocol

BLOOD GROUP B:
1. Antibacterial Protocol
2. Urinary Tract Health Protocol

BLOOD GROUP AB:
1. Antibacterial Protocol
2. Urinary Tract Health Protocol

BLOOD GROUP O:
1. Antibacterial Protocol
2. Urinary Tract Health Protocol

Related Topics

Bacterial disease (general)

Cancer, bladder

Immunity

Lectins

REFERENCES

1. Kinane DF, Blackwell CC, Brettle RP, Weir DM, Winstanley FP, Elton RA. ABO blood group, secretor state, and susceptibility to recurrent urinary tract infection in women. *Br Med J (Clin Res Ed)*. 1982;285(6334):7–9.

2. May SJ, Blackwell CC, Brettle RP, MacCallum CJ, Weir DM. Non-secretion of ABO blood group antigens: a host factor predisposing to recurrent urinary tract infections and renal scarring. *FEMS Microbiol Immunol.* 1989;1:383–387.

3. Lomberg H, Hellstrom M, Jodal U, Svanborg Eden C. Secretor state and renal scarring in girls with recurrent pyelonephritis. *FEMS Microbiol Immunol.* 1989;1:371–375.

4. Lomberg H, de Man P, Svanborg Eden C. Bacterial and host determinants of renal scarring. *APMIS.* 1989;97:193–199.

5. Jacobson SH, Lomberg H. Overrepresentation of blood group non-secretors in adults with renal scarring. *Scand J Urol Nephrol.* 1990;24:145–150.

6. Lomberg H, Jodal U, Leffler H, De Man P, Svanborg C. Blood group non-secretors have an increased inflammatory response to urinary tract infection. *Scand J Infect Dis.* 1992;24:77–83.

7. Sheinfeld J, Schaeffer AJ, Cordon-Cardo C, Rogatko A, Fair WR. Association of the Lewis blood-group phenotype with recurrent urinary tract infections in women. *N Engl J Med.* 1989;320:773–777.

8. Similar findings by other researchers support this over representation of recurrent UTI among non-secretors both in women and children.

9. May SJ, Blackwell CC, Brettle RP, MacCallum CJ, Weir DM. Non-secretion of ABO blood group antigens: a host factor predisposing to recurrent urinary tract infections and renal scarring. *FEMS Microbiol Immunol.* 1989;1:383–387.

10. Stapleton A, Nudelman E, Clausen H, Hakomon S, Stamm WE. Binding of uropathogenic Escherichia coli R45 to glycolipids extracted from vaginal epithelial cells is dependent on histo-blood group secretor status. *J Clin Invest.* 1992;90:965–972.

11. Jantausch BA, Criss VR, O'Donnell R, et al. Association of Lewis blood group phenotypes with urinary tract infection in children. *J Pediatr.* 1994;124:863–868.

12. Lavas EL, Venegas MF, Duncan JL, et al. Blood group antigen expression on vaginal cells and mucus in women with and without a history of urinary tract infections. *J Urol.* 1994;152(pt1):345–349.

13. Ratner JJ, Thomas VL, Forland M. Relationships between human blood groups, bacterial pathogens, and urinary tract infections. *Am J Med Sci.* 1986;292:87–91.

14. Voigtmann B, Burchardt U. ABO blood groups in patients with nephropathies [in German]. *Z Gesamte Inn Med.* 1991;46:156–159.

15. Robinson MG, Tolchin D, Halpern C. Enteric bacterial agents and the ABO blood groups. *Am J Hum Genet.* 1971;23:135–145.

16. Cruz-Cooke R. Blood groups and urinary microorganisms. *J Med Genet.* 1965;(2):185–188.

D

DENTAL CARIES (TOOTH CAVITIES)–

Tooth decay, also known as cavities, caused by acidic erosion of the tooth enamel.

Dental caries	RISK		
	LOW	AVERAGE	HIGH
GROUP A	░░		
GROUP B	░░	░░	
GROUP AB	░░		
GROUP O	░░		░░
NON-SECRETOR	░░		░░

Symptoms

Tooth decay is largely asymptomatic until it becomes advanced. Signs of severe decay include:

- tooth sensitivity to heat, cold, and sweets
- gum inflammation
- pain, aching, and throbbing in jaw

About Dental Caries

Like most areas of the body exposed to the environment, the mouth is far from sterile. Bacteria linger around the gums and in between the teeth. In general these bacteria do little harm, and ac-tually in a properly balanced system have the effect of crowding out more damaging varieties.

Even a newly cleaned tooth surface is rapidly covered with a glycoprotein deposit referred to as pellicle. The pellicle is derived from components of the saliva, which adhere to the tooth surface. Components of dental pellicle include proteins, enzymes, antibodies, and mucins. The formation of pellicle is the first step in plaque formation, as pellicle soon becomes a target for the adherence of many bacteria, which subsequently induce tooth decay and GINGIVITIS.

Tooth decay is largely asymptomatic until it becomes advanced.

Blood Group Links

By embedding ABO blood group antigens in saliva and mucus, the body is in essence sending out an anchor to certain bacteria that possess the ability to attach to that particular blood type. Studies have conclusively demonstrated that these organisms use the blood group antigens embedded in the mucus and saliva as a way to dock onto the tissues. Copious amounts of blood type antigens are secreted into the saliva, and probably serve as a growth medium for certain bacterial strains.[1]

From several studies conducted on the relationship between blood groups and dental caries, blood group O appears to have the greatest risk, especially non-secretors. The group with the lowest incidence of dental caries is blood group A, especially secretors.

Non-secretors of all blood groups have a higher risk of cavities. That's because the secretion of blood group antigens in saliva tends to inhibit the ability of bacteria to attach to the tooth surface. Also, non-secretors tend to have lower levels of the IgA class antibodies in their saliva, which also compromises their ability to fight bacteria[2].

Therapies, Dental Caries

ALL BLOOD GROUPS:

1. Practice good oral hygiene: brush after every meal and floss once a day.

2. Schedule regular visits to the dentist for checkups and cleaning.

3. Pain relief for toothaches: massage gums with oil of cloves or crushed garlic.

4. Choose the safest fillings.

The most common filling used by dentists is silver amalgam, which contains high amounts of mercury. Speak with your dentist about less toxic choices, including gold and ceramic-based materials. Of course, new cements and resins are being introduced all of the time, and are quickly replacing the use of the older materials such as silver amalgam.

BLOOD GROUP A:

1. Antibacterial Protocol

BLOOD GROUP B:

1. Antibacterial Protocol

BLOOD GROUP AB:

1. Antibacterial Protocol

BLOOD GROUP O:

1. Antibacterial Protocol
2. Yeast/Fungus Resistance Protocol

Related Topics

Bacterial disease (general)

Digestion

REFERENCES

1. Tabak LA, et al. Role of salivary mucins in the protection of the digestive tract. *J Oral Pathology.* 1982;11:1–17.
2. Arneberg P, Kornstad L, Nordbo H, Gjermo P. Less dental caries among secretors than among non-secretors of blood group substance. *Scand J Dent Res* 1976;84:362–366.

DENTURE STOMATITIS—*An inflammatory condition affecting denture wearers.*

Denture stomatitis	RISK		
	LOW	AVERAGE	HIGH
GROUP A			
GROUP B			
GROUP AB			
GROUP O			
NON-SECRETOR			

Symptoms

- Infection and inflammation between the denture and the gum.

About Denture Stomatitis

Denture stomatitis is the result of an infection in the space between the denture and the gum that can inflame the entire mouth. The infection can be bacterial or fungal. Its cause can be improper hygiene or the constituents of denture adhesives.

Blood Group Links:

Denture stomatitis has been found to be much more prevalent and severe in group O. One of the more common causes of denture stomatitis is infection with *Candida albicans*, and in general group O is more susceptible to this infection than the other blood groups. It has also been reported that group O is a more frequent carrier of a *Candida* infection of the mouth known as thrush. Non-secretors are also susceptible to *Candida* infections[1,2].

Often denture adhesives are gums made from algae. Many of these gums are composed of polysaccharide sugars, which are themselves blood group specific. Perhaps these adhesives are viewed as foreign and are rejected by group O, who carry both anti-A and B antibodies in their saliva.

Therapies, Denture Stomatitis

ALL BLOOD GROUPS:

For inflammation:

1. Apply the ash of charcoaled eggplant to mouth sores.
2. Mouthwash #1: One or two fresh pomegranates. Discard the skin and save the seeds; crush them, add water, and simmer; strain the mixture to obtain the liquid, and let it cool; use the liquid as a mouthwash.
3. Mouthwash #2: Two pieces of pickled plum (plums that were soaked in vinegar with pits included). Crush the fruit, add about a tablespoon of salt and 1 cup of boiling water, and mix; when the mixture is cool, use it as a mouthwash to gargle.

BLOOD GROUP A:

1. Antibacterial Protocol

BLOOD GROUP B:

1. Antibacterial Protocol

BLOOD GROUP AB:

1. Antibacterial Protocol

BLOOD GROUP O:

1. Antibacterial Protocol
2. Yeast/Fungus Resistance Protocol

Related Topics

Bacterial disease (general)

Candidiasis

Digestion

Immunity

REFERENCES

1. Tosh FD, Douglas LJ. Characterization of a fucoside-binding adhesin of Candida albicans. *Infect Immun.* 1992; 60:4734–4739.

2. Thom SM, et al. Non-secretion of blood group antigens and susceptibility to infection by Candida species. *FEMS Microbiol Immunol.* 1989;1:401–405.

DEPRESSION, BIPOLAR (MANIC DEPRESSIVE DISORDER)–*Pathological mood swings, alternating between states of mania and depression.*

Bipolar depression	RISK		
	LOW	AVERAGE	HIGH
GROUP A			
GROUP B			
GROUP AB			
GROUP O			
NON-SECRETOR			

Symptoms

The manic phase, which normally lasts up to 3 months, is characterized by the following symptoms:

- Euphoria
- Grandiosity
- Distractibility
- Insomnia
- Racing thoughts
- Excessive talking
- High-risk behaviors

The depressive phase, which is normally longer than the manic phase (six months or more), is characterized by the following symptoms:

- Sadness
- Fatigue
- Heaviness in the body
- Excessive sleeping
- Feelings of pessimism
- Weight gain or loss

About Bipolar Depression

Individuals with bipolar disorder can be difficult to diagnose, as the length and intensity of depression and mania vary among people. Typically, episodes begin with depression, shifting to mania without warning. Initially, the manic phase might seem like a positive shift, accompanied by high energy and enthusiasm. But these positive attributes rapidly spin out of control, manifesting as wild delusions, dangerous behavior, intense emotional swings, and hyperactivity. In time, the emotional pendulum swings back, and the afflicted person "crashes" into a deep depression.

Most investigators emphasize the importance of neurotransmitter substances, such as the catecholamines noradrenaline and adrenaline, in the pathogenesis of unipolar and bipolar depressive states. According to this hypothesis, depression is associated with a deficit in brain catecholamines, while mania may be due to an excess of catecholamines. High catecholamines in the manic state are in large part the result of high levels of activity of the dopamine beta hydroxylase. Conversely, the low levels of catecholamines in the depressed state are the result of lower levels of dopamine beta hydroxylase activity.

An important aspect of the action of catecholamines is the role of the enzyme monoamine oxidase, or MAO. MAO comes in two forms— MAO-A and MAO-B. MAO-A is found throughout the body, but especially in the gastrointestinal tract, while MAO-B is found primarily in the brain. Both MAO-A and MAO-B metabolize dopamine into a variety of other compounds, and blocking this enzyme has the effect of increasing dopamine concentrations.

Platelet MAO is believed to be the peripheral marker for the central serotonin system. Low concentrations of this genetically determined marker may indicate vulnerability to psychopathology and certain behavioral disorders. Variations in both platelet MAO and dopamine beta hydroxylase have been associated with bipolar illness.

Blood Group Links

Blood group O has been shown to have difficulty breaking down catecholamines, in part due to naturally low levels of MAO[1]. There also appears to be a genetic link between blood group O and the gene for dopamine beta hydroxylase[2]. Both low platelet MAO and DBH variations are associated with bipolar illness.

These associations between blood group O and bipolar disorder have been verified by several independent research studies. Family studies have also demonstrated a higher incidence of genetically transmitted bipolar disease. Research has also shown a strong association between blood group O and UNIPOLAR DEPRESSION, which is characterized by deep depression without mania[3].

Genetic transmission in manic depressive illness has been explored in twins, adoption, association, and gene linkage studies. The hypothesis of genetic transmission has been tested by association studies with the O blood group located on chromosome 9 and other chromosomes[4].

Research was undertaken as a prerequisite for psychopharmacological studies, analyzing ABO blood groups in 66 manic-depressive patients. A significantly higher percentage of bipolar patients (70%) than unipolar patients (22%) had blood group O, while a significantly higher percentage of unipolar patients (65%) than bipolar patients (23%) had blood group A. Researchers suggested that these data had importance for the selection of subgroups of patients for psychopharmacological studies. ABO non-secretors have a higher incidence of psychiatric disorders in general[5].

Therapies, Bipolar Depression

BLOOD GROUP A:

1. Antistress Protocol
2. Nerve Health Protocol

BLOOD GROUP B:

1. Antistress Protocol

2. Nerve Health Protocol

BLOOD GROUP AB:

1. Antistress Protocol

2. Nerve Health Protocol

BLOOD GROUP O:

1. Antistress Protocol

2. Nerve Health Protocol

Specifics:

Avoid MAO inhibitors and St. John's wort.

Avoid kava-kava.

Related Topics

Depression, unipolar

Stress

REFERENCES

1. Arato M, Bagdy G, Rihmer Z, Kulcsar Z. Reduced platelet MAO activity in healthy male students with blood group O. *Acta Psychiatr Scand.* 1983;67:130–134.

2. Wilson AF, Elston RC, Siervogel RM, Tran LD. Linkage of a gene regulating dopamine-beta-hydroxylase activity and the ABO blood group locus. *Am J Hum Genet.* 1988;42:160–166.

3. Rinieris PM, Stefanis CN, Lykouras EP, Varsou EK. Affective disorders and ABO blood types. *Acta Psychiatr Scand.* 1979;60:272–278.

4. Takazawa N, Kimura T, Nanko S. Blood groups and affective disorders. *Jpn J Psychiatry Neurol.* 1988;42:753–758.

5. Rafaelsen OJ, Shapiro RW. Psychopharmacological studies in genetically determined subgroups of psychiatric patients. *Prog Neuropsychopharmacol.* 1979;3:147–154.

DEPRESSION, UNIPOLAR–*Persistent, overwhelming sadness, with a marked degree of inexplicable ennui and numbing disaffection.*

Unipolar depression	RISK		
	LOW	AVERAGE	HIGH
GROUP A			
GROUP B			
GROUP AB			
GROUP O			
NON-SECRETOR			

Symptoms

The American Psychiatric Association defines depression by the following criteria. A person with four to eight of these symptoms is considered clinically depressed.

- Low self-esteem or lack of self-confidence
- Pessimism, hopelessness, or despair
- Lack of interest in ordinary pleasures or activities
- Withdrawal from social activities
- Fatigue or lethargy
- Guilt or ruminating about the past
- Irritability or excessive anger
- Lessened productivity
- Difficulty concentrating or making decisions

About Unipolar Depression

It is estimated that about 17 million Americans experience clinical depression.

Long-term depression can be a crippling societal inhibitor, leading to increased isolation and despondency. Sometimes it is called unipolar disease to distinguish it from bipolar or manic depressive illness. Unipolar depression is more likely to develop in persons who are introverted and have anxious tendencies. Such persons often lack the requisite social skills to adjust to significant life pressures and have difficulty recovering from a depressive episode.

Most investigators emphasize the importance of neurotransmitter substances, such as the catecholamines noradrenaline and adrenaline, in the pathogenesis of unipolar and bipolar depressive states. According to this hypothesis, depression is associated with a deficit in brain catecholamines, while mania may be due to an excess of catecholamines.

Blood Group Links

While blood group O has been consistently shown to have more incidents of bipolar disorder, blood group A has been shown to have a higher incidence of unipolar disorder. In one study, undertaken as a prerequisite for psychopharmacological studies, ABO blood groups were analyzed in 66 manic-depressive patients. A significantly higher percentage of bipolar patients (70%) than unipolar patients (22%) had blood group O, while a significantly higher percentage of unipolar patients (65%) than bipolar patients (23%) had blood group A[1].

There is also a strong association between ANXIETY DISORDERS and depression. In one report, over half of patients with depression met the criteria for anxiety disorders. The combination of depression and anxiety is a major risk factor for both substance abuse and suicide. It is well documented in a number of studies that blood group A is more prone to anxiety disorders than the other blood groups. This is most likely related to higher levels of cortisol, and lower levels of melatonin[2], which are known to be factors in such disorders.

Blood group O, by virtue of a strong association with bipolar or manic depressive disorder, is prone to depression when catecholamine levels are low.

ABO non-secretors have a higher incidence of psychiatric disorders in general.

Therapies, Unipolar Depression

BLOOD GROUP A:

1. Antistress Protocol

2. Nerve Health Protocol

Specifics:

Treatments for anxiety disorders often focus on serotonin imbalances and are treated with drugs such as Luvox (fluvoxamine maleate). A more effective treatment focuses on the cortisol imbalance. A melatonin deficit is also common.

Methylcobalamin: 1–3 mg per day, taken in the morning

Melatonin: Melatonin is a hormone, and as such it is best used under a health professional's direction.

BLOOD GROUP B:

1. Antistress Protocol

2. Nerve Health Protocol

Specifics:

Treatments for anxiety disorders often focus on serotonin imbalances and are treated with drugs such as Luvox (fluvoxamine maleate). A more effective treatment focuses on the cortisol imbalance. A melatonin deficit is also common.

Methylcobalamin: 1–3 mg per day, taken in the morning

Melatonin: Melatonin is a hormone, and as such it is best used under a health professional's direction.

BLOOD GROUP AB:

1. Antistress Protocol

2. Nerve Health Protocol

BLOOD GROUP O:

1. Antistress Protocol

2. Nerve Health Protocol

Specifics:

Avoid MAO inhibitors and St. John's wort.

Avoid kava-kava.

Related Topics

Anxiety disorders

Depression, bipolar

Obsessive-compulsive disorder

Stress

REFERENCES

1. Rafaelsen OJ, Shapiro RW. Psychopharmacological studies in genetically determined subgroups of psychiatric patients. *Prog Neuropsychopharmacol.* 1979;3:147–154.

2. Catapano F, Monteleone P, Fuschino A, Maj M, Kemali D. Melatonin and cortisol secretion in patients with primary obsessive-compulsive disorder. *Psychiatry Res.* 1992;44:217–225.

DETOXIFICATION–*See Toxicity, bowel (indicanuria); Toxicity, bowel (polyamines)*

DIABETES MELLITUS, TYPE I (JUVENILE)–*A chronic metabolic disorder, caused by inadequate or irregular insulin production and release.*

Diabetes mellitus, type I	RISK		
	LOW	AVERAGE	HIGH
GROUP A			
GROUP B			
GROUP AB			
GROUP O			
NON-SECRETOR			
MN BLOOD GROUP			

Symptoms

- Hyperglycemia (high blood sugar)

- Increased thirst and hunger

- Frequent urination

- Unexplained weight loss

- Blurred vision

About Type I Diabetes Mellitus

Type I diabetes, also known as juvenile or insulin-dependent diabetes, occurs when the pancreas is unable to produce insulin. Type I diabetes usually begins in childhood and lasts throughout a diabetic's life. It can only be controlled by the use of injected insulin and daily food monitoring.

Type I diabetes is characterized by destruction of the cells that are responsible for the secretion of insulin. There is growing evidence that, though there is a considerable genetic link, type I diabetes may be—at least initially—an autoimmune disease. Type I diabetes accounts for only about 10% of all cases.

The Dynamics of Insulin Production and Metabolism

When you eat, your pancreas releases insulin into the bloodstream, which helps to absorb and use glucose, fatty acids, and amino acids. If your pancreas does not produce insulin, or if your body can't properly employ it, the foods you eat can't be metabolized. Instead of being used for energy or stored, glucose collects in the blood—which is why diabetics are said to have high blood sugar. If there is too much glucose in the blood, it can't be processed by the kidneys, and glucose is excreted in the urine. The proper term for the disease, diabetes mellitus, means literally "flowing with honey," referring to the amount of sugar excreted in the urine.

Blood Group Links

Associations between diabetes and blood groups are among some of the oldest that we have[1,2]. In general, type I diabetes has a highly significant overall association with blood groups A and AB, and this is particularly strong in males versus females. What is especially interesting is that the percentage of blood group A over blood group O in diabetes appears to increase with age. This association has been confirmed in several large independent studies, looking at literally thousands of people.

It may be that the link between group A and diabetes results from the ability of certain serum lectins to bind to both the A antigen and the insulin-producing Langerhans cells of the pancreas. This complex has been shown to stimulate the activation of the antibody IgE at the site, thereby resulting in inflammation and cell death. This would explain why both blood groups that carry an A antigen are at risk.

One of the strongest risk factors for juvenile diabetes, almost the same risk as having a mother with diabetes, is a mother–child blood group incompatibility. As we have seen, the immune consequences of maternal–fetal incompatibility are worse if the mother is blood group O and the child is blood group A. This association was particularly strong for children of ABO incompatible mothers, who went on to develop diabetes within the first 5 years of life. A matched case-control study was carried out analyzing about 20 perinatal variables affecting the mother and child. A total of 2,757 infants who became diabetic during the period 1978 to 1988 were analyzed. When each risk factor was analyzed after standardization for all other risk factors, the odds ratios of blood group incompatibility as a factor for juvenile diabetes remained significantly increased. Scrutiny of medical records for diabetic and nondiabetic children with a diagnosis of blood group incompatibility verified the connection in close to 90% of children[3].

Blood Groups and Diabetes—The Anthropological Context

Diabetes may have exerted a powerful environmental effect on the delayed occurrence of blood group A. To understand why, let's first begin by asking ourselves the question: if diabetes is a fairly deadly disease without insulin replacement, how could it have persisted genetically through the earlier times when there was no effective life-saving therapy? Several theories have been advanced, including the observation that women who have a hereditary tendency toward diabetes tend to be more fertile than normal women, and apparently begin to menstruate at a younger age.

In the late 1950s, diabetes was placed in a broader anthropological context. In Paleolithic times, when humankind lived on a low-carbohydrate, low-calorie diet, diabetes would have only rarely developed to the point that the greater fertility would have maintained the frequency of the gene. In effect, the gene should have died out long ago. However, researchers have identified the gene for diabetes as a "thrifty gene"—that is, it had a survival advantage for those who possessed it, especially during times of starvation. In those circumstances, diabetes actually helped conserve energy and store fat.

Diabetes may have been advantageous under certain primitive conditions. But today, with the availability of adequate, or more than adequate, carbohydrate-rich diets, it now provokes a different sort of result altogether.

This is especially interesting in light of research that seems to indicate that, though the overall incidence of diabetes is higher in blood group A, the percentage of group O rises in diabetics who are below average in weight.

As with stress, high blood pressure, and myocardial disease, there are substantial differences between blood group A and blood group O diabetics with regard to the rheology (fluidity) of their blood. Group A diabetics have significantly higher levels of clotting factors in their blood when compared with group O or B diabetics. This may be an important risk factor in determining the probability of developing cardiovascular complications due to diabetes.

ABO non-secretors, and especially Lewis-negative individuals, are at a greater risk of developing diabetes (especially adult-onset diabetes); and they might be at a greater risk of developing complications from diabetes. Findings suggest that an increased proportion of non-secretors are found among patients with diabetes, particularly insulin-dependent diabetes[4,5].

The Lewis negative (Le(a−b−)) red blood cell phenotype appears to confer the greatest risk of developing diabetes. This blood type is observed three times more frequently (29%) in diabetics, irrespective of their clinical type. Non-diabetics categorized as low insulin responders to glucose are also significantly more likely to be Lewis negative[6].

Among individuals with juvenile diabetes mellitus, the prevalence of severe retinopathy (damage to the retina that is a side effect of diabetes) is lower in ABO secretors than in non-secretors[7].

The MN variation of the MN blood grouping subtype is associated with a higher incidence of diabetes

Therapies, Type I Diabetes Mellitus

ALL BLOOD GROUPS:

Although there is currently no effective natural treatment alternative for injectable insulin replacement therapy in type I diabetics, there has been improvement seen in diabetics adhering to the Blood Type Diet. In addition, I'd recommend a supplement of quercetin, an antioxidant derived from plants. Quercetin has been shown to help prevent many of the complications stemming from lifelong diabetes, such as cataracts, neuropathy, and cardiovascular problems. Consult a nutritionist who is skilled in the use of phytochemicals if you decide to employ any natural medicine for diabetes; you may have to readjust your insulin dosage.

BLOOD GROUP A:

1. Cardiovascular Protocol
2. Metabolic Enhancement Protocol
3. Liver Support Protocol

BLOOD GROUP B:

1. Metabolic Enhancement Protocol
2. Immune-Enhancing Protocol
3. Liver Support Protocol

BLOOD GROUP AB:

1. Cardiovascular Protocol
2. Metabolic Enhancement Protocol
3. Liver Support Protocol

BLOOD GROUP O:

1. Metabolic Enhancement Protocol
2. Immune-Enhancing Protocol
3. Liver Support Protocol

Related Topics

Autoimmune disease (general)

Diabetes mellitus, type II

Insulin resistance (Syndrome X)

REFERENCES

1. McConnell RB, et al. *Brit Med J.* 1956;772.
2. Craig J, Wang I. *Glasgow Med J.* 1955;261.
3. Dahlquist G, Kallen B. Maternal-child blood group incompatibility and other perinatal events increase the risk for early-onset type I (insulin-dependent) diabetes mellitus. *Diabetologia.* 1992;35:671–675.
4. Patrick AW, Collier A. An infectious aetiology of insulin-dependent diabetes mellitus? Role of the secretor status. *FEMS Microbiol Immunol.* 1989;1:411–416.
5. Peters WH, Gohler W. ABH-secretion and Lewis red cell groups in diabetic and normal subjects from Ethiopia. *Exp Clin Endocrinol.* 1986;88:64–70.
6. Melis C, Mercier P, Vague P, Vialettes B. Lewis antigen and diabetes. *Rev Fr Transfus Immunohematol.* 1978;21:965–971.
7. Eff C, Faber O, Deckert T. Persistent insulin secretion, assessed by plasma C-peptide estimation in long-term juvenile diabetics with a low insulin requirement. *Diabetologia.* 1978;15:169–72.

DIABETES MELLITUS, TYPE II (ADULT ONSET)–*A syndrome characterized by hyperglycemia resulting from absolute or relative impairment in insulin secretion and/or insulin action.*

Diabetes mellitus, type II	RISK		
	LOW	AVERAGE	HIGH
GROUP A			
GROUP B			
GROUP AB			
GROUP O			
NON-SECRETOR			
MN blood group			

Symptoms

Although people with type I diabetes almost always suspect they are ill, type II diabetes can develop gradually over a period of months or years without a person realizing there's anything seriously wrong. Typical symptoms include:

- Increased thirst and hunger
- Frequent urination
- Unexplained weight loss
- Blurred vision
- Recurrent urinary tract infections

About Type II Diabetes Mellitus

Type II, also known as adult or non-insulin-dependent diabetes, comprises about 90% of all diabetes. It is most often seen in obese people over 40. In type II diabetes, the pancreas produces insulin, but the body fails to use it properly. Type II diabetes can usually be controlled by diet, weight loss, and exercise.

Type II diabetes can be a gateway to several other life-threatening conditions. There is an elevated risk of developing CORONARY ARTERY DISEASE. CAD is the leading cause of death among people with diabetes. Diabetics have been shown to have HIGHER BLOOD PRESSURE levels.

In diabetics of African ancestry, hypertension is even more widespread, affecting between 63% and 70% of all sufferers. Elderly diabetics tend to have severe circulation problems due to impaired blood flow through small arteries. Diabetes is the direct cause of some 40,000 leg and foot amputations a year in older men and women. KIDNEY FAILURE is also a fatal complication in severe diabetes.

Type II diabetes was once viewed as an adult disease. However, it is fast becoming a serious problem for children as well. Since 1995 there has been a tenfold increase in the incidence of type II diabetes in children, primarily related to obesity, poor diet, and lack of exercise.

Although people with type I diabetes almost always suspect they are ill, type II diabetes can develop gradually over a period of months or years without a person realizing there's anything seriously wrong.

General Risk Factors and Causes

The American Diabetes Association recommends that any person over age 40 with one or more of the following risk factors undergo screening:

- Family history of diabetes (parents or siblings), especially type II

- Obesity, 20% or more above recommended body weight

- Racial or ethnic risk, especially among those of American Indian, Hispanic, or African descent

- Previous experience of glucose intolerance

- Hypertension or significant hyperlipidemia

- For women, a history of gestational diabetes, or delivery of infants weighing more than 9 pounds

Blood Group Links

Non-insulin-dependent diabetics are more often blood type A when compared with control individuals. This difference is particularly marked in male diabetics. When diabetics are compared with age-matched controls, the difference is confined to the older cases[1,2].

As with stress, high blood pressure, and myocardial disease, there are substantial differences between blood type A and blood type O diabetics with regard to the rheology (fluidity) of their blood. Blood type A diabetics have significantly higher levels of clotting factors in their blood when compared with blood type O or blood type B diabetics. This may be an important risk factor in determining the probability of developing cardiovascular complications due to diabetes.

ABO non-secretors, and especially Lewis-negative individuals, are at a greater risk of developing diabetes (especially adult-onset diabetes); and they might be at a greater risk of developing complications from diabetes. Findings suggest that an increased proportion of non-secretors are found among patients with diabetes, particularly of the insulin-dependent diabetes type[3,4].

The Lewis negative (Le (a−b−)) red blood cell phenotype appears to confer the greatest risk of developing diabetes. This blood type is observed more than three times more frequently (29%) in diabetics, irrespective of their clinical type. Non-diabetics categorized as low insulin responders to glucose are also significantly more likely to be Lewis negative[5].

Non-diabetic individuals who are non-secretors of blood group antigens are prone to superficial infections by *Candida albicans*. In this study, 216 patients with diabetes mellitus who were denture wearers were examined for the presence or absence of DENTURE STOMATITIS. There was an overall trend for non-secretors to be prone to denture stomatitis compared with secretors. Stepwise linear discriminant analysis was used to dissect the contribution of secretor status and other variables to the development of the disease. Secretor status was found to be a contributory factor among patients with non-insulin dependent diabetes but not among those with insulin-dependent diabetes[6].

Diabetes Screening

The basic screening method for diabetes is the fasting blood glucose test, which measures the amount of glucose in your blood before you have eaten. The normal range is between 70 and 100 mg per deciliter (mg/dL). A blood sample is taken in the morning before any food is eaten. If the test shows a glucose level above 140 mg/dL, it is a sure indication of diabetes. However, a reading between 115 and 140 mg/dL will require further testing in the form of a glucose tolerance test.

A glucose tolerance test should be done any time fasting blood sugar is more than 115 mg/dL, or the glucose level after a meal is over 160 mg/dL. A glucose tolerance test takes several hours. You are given a sugary liquid to swallow, which temporarily produces high blood sugar. Then blood samples are taken at intervals of 30 minutes, 1 hour, 2 hours, and 3 hours, and the glucose level is measured in each sample. This tells how quickly your body is able to bring the blood sugar level back down to normal.

Therapies, Type II Diabetes Mellitus

ALL BLOOD GROUPS:

1. Alcohol consumption can exacerbate insulin resistance by contributing metabolically to hyperglycemia. Although there may be health benefits to red wine, which is extremely high in phytochemicals, it does contain extra calories as sugar. If you drink a glass of wine, have it with a meal to offset blood sugar swings.

2. Don't smoke. If you smoke because you fear the weight gain that might come with quitting, consider this: Chronic cigarette smokers are insulin resistant and hyperinsulinemic compared with non-smokers. These pre-diabetic conditions are associated with weight gain.

BLOOD GROUP A:

1. Cardiovascular Protocol
2. Metabolic Enhancement Protocol
3. Blood-Building Protocol
4. Liver Support Protocol

BLOOD GROUP B:

1. Metabolic Enhancement Protocol
2. Liver Support Protocol

Specifics:

Magnesium: 200–300 mg day.

BLOOD GROUP AB:

1. Cardiovascular Protocol
2. Metabolic Enhancement Protocol
3. Blood-Building Protocol
4. Liver Support Protocol

BLOOD GROUP O:

1. Metabolic Enhancement Protocol
2. Liver Support Protocol

Related Topics

Cardiovascular disease

Diabetes mellitus, type I

Hypertension

Insulin resistance (Syndrome X)

Obesity

REFERENCES

1. McConnell RB, et al. *Brit Med J.* 1956;772.

2. Craig J, Wang I. *Glasgow Med J.* 1955;261.

3. Dahlquist G, Kallen B. Maternal-child blood group incompatibility and other perinatal events increase the risk for early-onset type I (insulin-dependent) diabetes mellitus. *Diabetologia.* 1992 Jul;35:671–675.

4. Patrick AW, Collier A. An infectious aetiology of insulin-dependent diabetes mellitus? Role of the secretor status. *FEMS Microbiol Immunol.* 1989;1:411–416.

5. Melis C, Mercier P, Vague P, Vialettes B. Lewis antigen and diabetes. *Rev Fr Transfus Immunohematol.* 1978;21:965–971.

6. Aly FZ, Blackwell CC, MacKenzie DA, et al. Chronic atrophic oral candidiasis among patients with diabetes mellitus—role of ABH secretor status. *Epidemiol Infect.* 1991;106:355–363.

■ Diarrhea

Common Causes	BLOOD GROUP O	BLOOD GROUP A	BLOOD GROUP B	BLOOD GROUP AB	SUBGROUPS
Bacterial infection	*****	****	**********	***********	Non-secretor = ************
Irritable bowel disease	************	****	********	****	Non-secretor ************
Poor dietary habits/ consumption of dietetic products	*All groups susceptible*	*All groups susceptible*	*All groups susceptible*	*All groups susceptible*	
Stress	**	**********	******	**	

* = degree of risk

Diarrheal diseases by infectious organisms are the number-one killers worldwide. And, while we seldom hear about it in the United States, CHOLERA is still an epidemic disease in many poorer regions of the world. Other common causes of diarrhea include *Escherichia coli* infection, dysentery, giardiasis, and shigellosis (see BACTERIAL DISEASE). All of us have suffered from a bout of diarrhea at one time or another. And most of us have our own ideas of exactly what diarrhea is. For those of us in the Western world, the usual amount of water in our stool each day is generally no more than about a cupful. When it is consistently more than that, it is considered to be diarrhea.

Diarrhea in a previously healthy person is usually the result of disease. In fact, more than one hundred different diseases may cause the condition. The following are the most common. Diarrhea can be related to infectious, drug-induced, food-related, postsurgical, inflammatory, and psychological conditions. These many causes produce diarrhea by four distinct mechanisms: increased intestinal permeability, increased secretion, inflammation, and decreased absorption time.

Related Protocols

BLOOD GROUP A:

1. Antibacterial Protocol
2. Intestinal Health Protocol

BLOOD GROUP B:

1. Antibacterial Protocol
2. Intestinal Health Protocol

BLOOD GROUP AB:

1. Antibacterial Protocol
2. Intestinal Health Protocol

BLOOD GROUP O:

1. Antibacterial Protocol

2. Intestinal Health Protocol

Related Topics

Autoimmune disease (general)

Bacterial disease (general)

Digestion

Food poisoning

Inflammation

Stress

Toxicity, bowel

Digestion

The entire microbial ecosystem of the digestive tract is under the influence of blood group. Blood type genetics not only influence the levels of digestive juices and enzymes needed to efficiently metabolize food, they program the cellular characteristics of our entire digestive tract.

Many foods contain components that can react directly with the blood group antigens, resulting in inflammation and the production of toxins. Other foods address susceptibilities and strengthen our bodies against these weaknesses.

Good digestion results not only from choosing the right foods for our bodies, but also by keeping

our digestive systems tuned and balanced so that the interplay of all important elements, such as digestive juices and hormones, are optimized for maximum nutrient absorption and regular elimination.

The following is a brief journey through the digestive process, with the influence of the blood groups clearly demonstrated.

Blood Groups, Taste, and Saliva

Foods are first processed in the mouth by the mechanical action of chewing. They are then passed on to the stomach, intestines, and colon, but never actually travel as "food" through the membrane that divides this hostile inner world from our bloodstream. What we eat is acted upon by acids, enzymes, and bacteria until it is broken down so far as to be no longer recognizable. Then, and only then, is it transported into the body proper in the form of amino acids, triglycerides, and simple sugars.

As Pavlov proved, digestion actually begins on the dinner plate, with the psychological effects of aroma, color, and presentation stimulating the brain to activate the production of the digestive juices that will be needed a bit in advance of the actual food itself. This is called the *cephalic* (Latin for "head") phase of digestion, and that's why it is so important to try to make eating a relaxed event.

Taste is a chemical sense, like smell. One theory is that we have only four taste receptors, one each for sour, sweet, salt, and bitter. More complex tastes are derived from various combinations of these four basic tastes. The various taste recep-

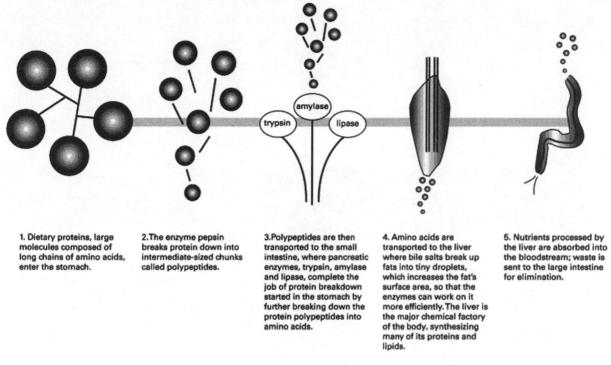

1. Dietary proteins, large molecules composed of long chains of amino acids, enter the stomach.

2. The enzyme pepsin breaks protein down into intermediate-sized chunks called polypeptides.

3. Polypeptides are then transported to the small intestine, where pancreatic enzymes, trypsin, amylase and lipase, complete the job of protein breakdown started in the stomach by further breaking down the protein polypeptides into amino acids.

4. Amino acids are transported to the liver where bile salts break up fats into tiny droplets, which increases the fat's surface area, so that the enzymes can work on it more efficiently. The liver is the major chemical factory of the body, synthesizing many of its proteins and lipids.

5. Nutrients processed by the liver are absorbed into the bloodstream; waste is sent to the large intestine for elimination.

THE DIGESTIVE ASSEMBLY LINE

tors are found in different places in the mouth. The tongue's tip is mostly sensitive to what is sweet and salty. Its sides favor what is sour. Bitter substances chiefly stimulate receptors deep in the back of the throat and up on the soft palate, above the tongue. What we perceive as flavor is actually a complex chemical interaction between the taste buds of the tongue, saliva, and the nervous system.

Saliva is a watery fluid containing a host of enzymes and hormones that help digest food as well as protect against disease and maintain a healthy digestive tract. Because saliva contains slimy glycoprotein sugars called mucins, it helps to moisten and lubricate the food we eat so that

we can swallow it. Saliva also protects the teeth and soft tissue from a variety of bacteria and viruses.

Saliva originates from several specialized glands located under the tongue and along the inside of the mouth. These are called the parotid gland and the submaxillary-sublingual glands. Since mucins are rich in glycoproteins, it should be no surprise that ABO blood group antigens are copiously produced by the submaxillary-sublingual salivary glands and extensively distributed in human saliva[1].

There is evidence that our blood group antigens have a considerable influence on our ability to

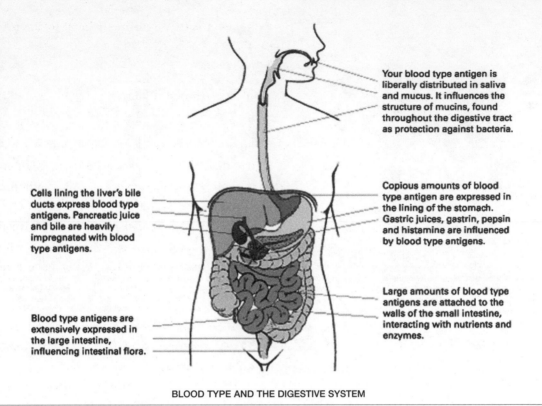

Your blood type antigen is liberally distributed in saliva and mucus. It influences the structure of mucins, found throughout the digestive tract as protection against bacteria.

Cells lining the liver's bile ducts express blood type antigens. Pancreatic juice and bile are heavily impregnated with blood type antigens.

Copious amounts of blood type antigen are expressed in the lining of the stomach. Gastric juices, gastrin, pepsin and histamine are influenced by blood type antigens.

Blood type antigens are extensively expressed in the large intestine, influencing intestinal flora.

Large amounts of blood type antigens are attached to the walls of the small intestine, interacting with nutrients and enzymes.

BLOOD TYPE AND THE DIGESTIVE SYSTEM

taste food. It may even be true that people of different blood groups may taste food differently[2]. The A, B, and O antigens in saliva are known to interact chemically with the taste buds, and blood group antigens are found in different concentrations among the different taste buds. The O antigen reacts with the majority of cells in all taste buds; the B antigen is expressed by the majority of taste cells but not by other outer layer cells. The A antigen is significantly less prominent in certain taste buds than in others[3].

Chewing breaks food down into small pieces, which actually has the effect of increasing the surface area for the digestive enzymes and acids to act on. As food is masticated, enzymes in the saliva

start the process of breaking down sugars and starches and a small amount of these are actually passed through the tissues of the mouth.

Chewing food also stimulates epidermal growth factor (EGF), a polypeptide hormone that aids the growth and repair of outer layer tissue. It is widely distributed in the body, with high concentrations detectable in saliva, the prostate gland, and in the duodenum of the small intestine. The receptor for human epidermal growth factor (EGF-R) is specific for a carbohydrate that is closely related to the human blood group A antigen. EGF-R expression plays an important role in a variety of human cancers, including oral, brain, pancreatic, breast, lung, and colorectal can-

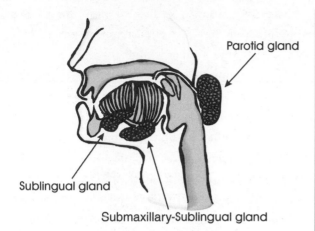

Parotid gland

Sublingual gland

Submaxillary-Sublingual gland

Saliva originates from several specialised glands located under your tongue and along the inside of your mouth. These are called the parotid gland and the submaxillary-sublingual glands. Since mucins are rich in glycoproteins, it should be no surprise that blood type antigens are copiously produced by the submaxillary-sublingual glands and are extensively distributed in human saliva.

cers. These cancers show a higher incidence in group A[4].

Like most areas of the body exposed to the environment, the mouth is far from sterile. Bacteria linger around the gums and in between the teeth. In general these bacteria do little harm; actually, in a properly balanced system, they have the effect of crowding out more destructive varieties.

By embedding your blood group antigen in saliva and mucus, the body is sending out an anchor to certain bacteria that possess the ability to attach to that particular blood group. Studies have conclusively demonstrated that these organisms use the blood group antigen embedded in the mucus and saliva as a way to dock onto the tissues. One study went so far as to state that "the amount of blood group antigens in the human ecosystem and their obvious effect in microbial systems appears to cast into doubt the idea that their primary

function is to any degree related to the red blood cell"[5].

Blood Group and Mucin

The entire lining of the gut is covered by a protective film called mucin. Mucin is widely distributed in the mucous secretions, providing a selective insulation against hostile pathogens and other foreign objects.

Mucin is composed of very large glycoprotein molecules called mucopolysaccharides, which are liberally laced with sulfur. They have a feather-like shape, which enables them to bind water, and this function gives mucous its great variability—from the thin watery mucus of a bad head cold to the thick mucus of bronchitis, the amount of water is the only difference.

Mucin also varies from one person to another. Many of the glycoproteins of mucin are in fact ABO antigens. Blood group is the single most significant influence on mucin's structure[6]. The composition of mucin can change dramatically in various disease states. By varying the amount of sulfate in mucin, the body can limit the ability of certain bacteria to consume the glycoproteins in mucus, thereby starving them.

Blood group structures embedded in mucin can act as sites for selective interaction with gut bacteria such as *H. pylori*, and viruses such as INFLUENZA. Accumulating data also suggest a very important role for mucin in what is called recognition phenomenon—the cellular homing of immune-defending lymphocytes (from areas such as the tonsils in the throat or in the intestines) toward local areas of infection[7].

Blood groups interact with these friendly bacteria in an almost symbiotic manner. Many of the end products produced by blood group–friendly bacteria help keep the cells lining the digestive tract healthy, or enhance the metabolism of other bacteria, which cannot themselves consume blood group antigens but can metabolize the resulting chemicals. Of the common flora normally seen in the digestive tract, the strains that consume blood group antigens are typically the *Bifidobacterium* (which consumes the B antigen but not A) and *Ruminococcus* species (which typically consumes both A and B).

Blood Group and Immunoglobulin A

There are five classes of antibodies made by the immune system to help protect the body. Of these, immunoglobulin A, or IgA (the words "antibody" and "immunoglobulin" are essentially interchangeable) is most involved in the health of the digestive tract. Unlike most other antibodies, which are found primarily in the bloodstream, IgA has a major presence in the digestive tract. It is the main antibody in a variety of secretions such as saliva, milk, and the mucus lining the airways and digestive tract. IgA antibodies dramatically increase during infections of the mucus lining.

IgA is liberally embedded in the mucus lining of the gut. Usually, one end of the molecule is attached to the wall, and the other projects out into the gut cavity. The IgA antibodies bind to microorganisms such as bacteria and protect us against infection by preventing them from attaching to the epithelial surface to gain entry. Once IgA binds to foreign microorganism, the combination of the antibody and the invader (now called an immune complex) triggers the release of a series of corrosive enzymes called complement, which destroys the microorganism.

IgA deficiency is the most common of all immune deficiencies, affecting upward of 9% of all Northern Europeans. Defects in IgA have been shown to predispose individuals to a celiac-like disorder of the intestines, as well as LUPUS, PERNICIOUS ANEMIA, GIARDIA INFECTION, and even INFLAMMATORY BOWEL DISEASE. In one Italian study, 8% of 56 children with low IgA had celiac disease of the small intestine, and all had antibodies to gluten and gliadin (two common proteins found in grains) in their serum[8].

Several dietary lectins have been shown to increase IgA to abnormal levels. In one study five of six individuals had increases in the IgA of their saliva after a test meal that included several lectins, including peas and peanuts. Interestingly, although two common components of wheat, gliadin and gluten, have been shown in repeated studies to increase IgA; in this study wheat germ lectin was shown to have no effect[9].

In a study of 310 people, it was found, perhaps not surprisingly, that blood group O tends to make higher amounts of IgA than other blood groups[10]. Higher levels of antibodies imply a greater risk of AUTOIMMUNE DISEASE, a situation in which the body makes antibodies that tend to inadvertently attack its own cells and tissues. Blood group O is associated with a higher rate of autoimmune diseases in general.

ABO Blood Group and Digestion

After swallowing, the food (now termed a bolus, or ball) slides down the esophagus, a stretch of tubing that connects the mouth with the stomach. The esophagus is quite muscular and can stretch out to allow the food to move downward.

Once food enters the stomach, true digestion begins. More blood group antigen is expressed in the lining of the stomach than in any other organ of the digestive tract. Also, a considerable number of hormones and secretions are directly influenced by the genetics of ABO blood groups[11]. Upon nervous stimulation, the stomach secretes a liquid known as gastric juice. Gastric juice is composed of water, hydrochloric acid, and enzymes. Abundant amounts of blood type antigens are secreted in gastric juice, more than in any other digestive secretion. The hydrochloric acid in gastric juice destroys germs in food, protecting the gut from infection. This is the acid that can reflux and cause HEARTBURN in the esophagus.

Like the rest of the digestive tract, the stomach has a protective lining called mucosa. Stomach mucosa is studded with gastric pits, similar to elongated sinkholes. These are actually glands that contain special cells that secrete acid and digestive enzymes. The shaft linings of these gastric pits are composed of cells called mucus neck cells and other prominent round cells called parietal cells. These cells manufacture mucus, which helps protect the stomach from digesting itself.

The base of the gastric glands is distinguished by other special cells called chief cells. Chief cells secrete the various protein-digesting enzymes. Recent studies have shown that a large amount of ABO blood group antigen can be found in stomach secretions. Though abundant in all stomach secretions, more blood group antigen is secreted by the enzyme-producing chief cells than by the acid-producing parietal cells[12].

Gastric juices can be stimulated by signals originating in the brain or in the stomach itself. The latter are known as stomach reflexes and often involve stretching of the stomach wall, physical stimulation of the stomach wall by the food itself, or chemical stimulation such as amino acids from protein foods and actual acid already secreted by the gastric glands. Stimulus by the nervous system activates specialized cells to produce the hormone gastrin, which in turn stimulates parietal cells to secrete even more acid.

When food enters the stomach, gastric juice becomes more alkaline as proteins buffer the existing acid in the stomach. This rise in alkalinity stimulates the release of more gastrin, and therefore the release of more acid. As proteins are digested, the acidity of the stomach contents increases, turning off gastrin release and halting the secretion of more stomach acid. The chemical histamine (well known to ALLERGY sufferers) also acts on the acid-producing cells of the stomach. This perhaps explains why chronic allergy patients have higher rates of ulcers. Although the mechanism is not completely understood, it appears that unless the acid forming cells in the stomach have their histamine receptors occupied, they will not be signaled to secrete acid, even if stimulated by gastrin. This is why conventional medicine treats ulcers with a class of drugs called histamine blockers.

Dietary proteins are large molecules composed

of long chains of amino acids, which serve as their building blocks. Protein is broken down to intermediate-sized chunks called polypeptides in the stomach by the actions of the enzyme pepsin, which is formed from its precursor, pepsinogen. Pepsin enzymatically chops up the peptide bonds by which amino acids are linked together to form proteins, releasing the individual amino acids, which can then be transported through the small intestine into the bloodstream. Although almost all breakdown of protein occurs in the stomach, only about 15% of amino acids are absorbed here; most are absorbed in the upper small intestine. Pepsin is very sensitive to the level of acidity in the stomach. In the absence of sufficient amounts of hydrochloric acid, pepsin will not become active. The amount of acid required for pepsin to do its job is quite substantial: The optimum pH level for pepsin activity in the stomach is quite sufficient to digest the stomach itself, were it not equipped with a special protective lining.

In addition to digesting proteins, the acid in the stomach serves as a barrier to most bacteria. This is an important function; the mixture of food and saliva swallowed from the mouth is not sterile, and since the upper small intestine is designed for absorption, it is undesirable for large amounts of bacteria to reach it. One of the major problems with having low stomach acidity (a condition called hypochlorhydria) is excessive bacterial overgrowth in the stomach and in the upper small intestine.

Blood Group and the Small Intestine

The small intestine requires the help of two other organs to do its job effectively. The liver makes bile, which is stored in the gallbladder and then flows out through a connection between the gallbladder and the small intestine, called the bile duct, into the duodenum. Bile salts break up fats into tiny droplets, which increases the fat's surface area, so that the enzymes can work on it more efficiently. Unlike the stomach, which requires acidity for optimum function, the small intestine requires alkalinity to do its job properly. Bile also neutralizes acid from the stomach, making the duodenum alkaline.

More than 99% of assimilation takes place in the small intestine. It is a long muscular tube measuring about 20 feet. It has three parts: the part nearest the stomach is called the duodenum; the middle part is the jejunum; and the end part is the ileum.

As the stomach contents discharge into the small intestine in the form of acidic sludge, or chyme, cells are signaled to secrete hormones into the bloodstream that turn on the next phase of digestion. Two hormones, cholecystokinin (CCK) and secretin, are involved in this process.

CCK acts on the pancreas to secrete its enzymes, and on the bile duct to secrete bile. CCK hormones help digest fat, carbohydrates, and proteins. CCK is also present in relatively high concentrations in the brain where, it is conjectured, it plays a role in appetite control. It is speculated that CCK stimulates nerve fibers in the stomach wall, causing contraction and a feeling of fullness in the stomach.

Several food lectins, including the lectins from soy beans, peanuts, kidney beans, and wheat, have been shown to influence CCK levels. Soy, peanut, and kidney bean lectins increase CCK, while wheat germ agglutinin decreases CCK. For blood groups A and AB, soy is especially good at enhancing CCK.

Secretin stimulates the liver to produce bile, and triggers the pancreas to begin secreting pancreatic juice. Pancreatic juice and bile are heavily impregnated with ABO blood group antigens[13].

Blood Group and Absorption

The pancreas helps digestion by manufacturing the enzymes trypsin, amylase, and lipase. Trypsin (and several other enzymes, including peptidase) complete the job of protein breakdown started in the stomach by further breaking down the protein polypeptides into their constituent building blocks, the amino acids. Amino acids can then be transported to the liver or elsewhere.

The liver is the major chemical factory of the body, synthesizing many of its proteins and lipids. Blood containing absorbed nutrients from the small intestine must first pass through special networks in the liver called sinusoids. Here can be found cells of the immune system called Kupffer cells, which scavenge and destroy microorganisms that may have been inadvertently absorbed with nutrients. The liver is also chemically capable of detoxifying an incredibly large inventory of poisons.

The liver aids in the absorption of fats by manufacturing bile salts, whose job it is to emulsify fats. Bile salts are steroids with detergent properties. By emulsifying fat, bile helps its digestion and absorption through the intestinal wall.

Cells lining the liver's bile ducts express blood group antigens. In addition, bile itself is a fairly rich source of blood group antigens[14]. Liver and colon cancers are known to express large amounts of blood type antigens, which is fairly unique; most cancers lose the ability to express these antigens, rather than gain it[15].

Blood Group and Intestinal Mucosa

The inside of the small intestine has a lining called the mucosa. The entire mucosa is covered in small finger-like projections, barely visible to the naked eye, called villi. The villi greatly increase the surface area of the small intestine, and to increase it more, each villi has many thousands of microvilli.

Large amounts of blood group antigens are attached to the microvilli, interacting with nutrients and enzymes to control assimilation[16].

Near each villi wall is an artery, into which food is absorbed. Within this lining very specialized cells are embedded that break food down into molecules that can then be taken up into the bloodstream and sent to the liver for further processing.

Fats, however, are handled a bit differently. In the center of villi, a lymph vessel called a lacteal helps absorb fats and send them through the lymphatic circulation and eventually into the circulatory system, where they are distributed around the body.

The enzyme amylase, made in the pancreas but used in the small intestine, completes the job originally begun with the saliva—breaking down starches to sugars such as glucose and maltose. Special enzymes called disaccharidases on the intestinal microvilli digest the respective disaccharide sugars (such as lactase, sucrase, and maltase) to simple sugars. There is some evidence to suggest that intestinal disaccharide activity is higher in blood group A over the other blood groups, which would make perfect sense since group A has a greater capacity for metabolizing complex carbohydrates than the other blood groups[17].

Blood Group and the Colon

The human colon is like a warm-blooded coral reef, rich in microbial diversity and home to vast numbers of bacterial cells. Indeed, it has been estimated that there are 10 times more bacterial cells (1,000,000,000,000,000) associated with the average human body than there are human ones (only 100,000,000,000,000). This normal bacterial flora lives on the external body surfaces and in the gut.

In the large intestine, the emphasis is on elimination, though a bit of assimilation does take place—principally electrolytes like sodium and potassium and a few vitamins. Large quantities of ABO blood group antigens are found in the gastrointestinal mucosa.

Blood group is an important influence on the growth of particular strains of bacteria in the large intestine. Many bacteria consume blood group antigens, and blood groups are extensively expressed in the human large intestine. The upper colon contains very large amounts of blood group anti-

gens, which gradually diminish to nothing at the end of the colon. This probably reflects their use as a food source by the colon bacteria; as debris passes through the colon, fewer and fewer nutrients can be found in it. The depletion of blood group antigens is just another aspect of this phenomenon.

The composition of the normal flora varies somewhat from individual to individual. Some bacterial species may be carried only transiently. Most are fairly permanent—animal experiments have shown that it can be extremely difficult to alter the composition of the normal flora of the gut in a healthy person. Many of the common bacteria choose to live in the colon of one blood group or another[18]. Sometimes this is because the bacteria can mimic the blood group of their host, and so are viewed as "self" by the host's immune system. In other circumstances, certain bacteria have a taste for one particular ABO antigen over others and prefer to nibble mucus containing that particular blood group antigen[19]. Some bacteria more easily adhere to the mucus on one blood group over others because they themselves make lectins which they use to attach to the walls of the colon, and these lectins are usually specific for one blood group[20].

Except for the transient carriage of bacteria in food, the stomach and duodenum are usually sterile as few bacteria survive the effects of gastric acid. We do know that the middle and lower portion of the small intestines are extensively colonized by a variety of bacteria, including lactobacilli. Most species of these bacteria ferment glucose into lactose, hence the name *Lactobacillus*. This genus also contains several bacteria that make up part of the natural flora of the human vagina. Because of their ability to produce lactic acid from glucose, these bacteria create an acidic environment that inhibits the growth of many of the bacterial species that lead to infections. Lactobacillus is generally harmless to humans, rarely inciting harmful infections or diseases.

Feces, the major end product of the digestive tract, is concentrated in the large intestine from waste products such as digestive mucus, bacteria, and fiber. There is little or no food left in feces; the stomach and small intestine do a very efficient job of making sure that most of the nutrients are absorbed.

Blood Group and the Colon

The colon consists of four main segments: the ascending colon, which extends upward on the right side of the abdomen; the transverse colon, which extends across the body to the left side; the descending colon, which continues downward on the left side; and the S-shaped sigmoid colon, tucked near the end of the descending colon. The appendix is a small finger-like extension from the ascending colon. The walls of the colon contain three longitudinal bands of muscle that create a purse-string appearance. These periodic indentations in the wall of the colon are called haustra.

The primary role of the colon is to reabsorb the fluid from the watery mixture that is left over after the small intestine has completed absorbing all the useful nutrients. The contents of the small intestine are quite liquid; this allows for maximum action on the part of the enzymes and acids. As the contents are dumped into the colon how-

ever, a gradual process of solidification occurs. This is accomplished by cells in the colon wall that begin to pump the water out of it. As the contents of the colon move further along, they first become semisolid. As they reach the final section of the colon, called the rectosigmoid, so much water has been pumped out that the contents are now solid and can be evacuated as stool.

The colon works best when it is moderately full. Dietary fiber fills this need, providing undigestible bulk, which acts mechanically to stimulate movement of the intestines. Although it contains no nutrients, fiber helps promote good health by providing the necessary volume to encourage timely movement of feces through the colon. Fiber also helps remove certain toxins by binding to them. Although humans cannot digest cellulose, the major component of fiber, the bacteria in the intestines can. This bacterial fermentation of fiber helps produce beneficial short-chain fatty acids, which can then be used by the cells lining the intestines for their own metabolism. Fiber also stimulates the stomach to empty and increases the speed at which food passes through the small intestine. This has been shown to improve glucose tolerance and enable digestion of starch.

People whose diets are high in refined foods (including sugar and white flour) and low in fiber content are especially susceptible to intestinal problems. In fact, colon and rectal disorders are much more common in America than in Africa, where the average diet contains seven times as much fiber.

There are two basic types of fiber: soluble and insoluble. Soluble fiber includes pectins found in fruits and certain natural gums. Fruits, vegetables, seeds, brown rice, barley, and oats are important sources of soluble fiber. Soluble fiber helps to produce a softer stool. It also chemically prevents or reduces the absorption of certain substances into the bloodstream. Insoluble fiber includes cellulose and lignin. Whole grains and the outside of seeds, fruits, legumes, and other foods are the main sources for insoluble fiber, which works like a sponge, absorbing many times its weight in water and swelling up inside the intestines. The result is more efficient elimination.

The difference in colon bacteria and the presence of blood group antigens in the colon are among the reasons that different blood groups seem to do better on different types of fiber. A sign that you are taking the wrong fiber is gas, or flatulence.

Perhaps the best sources of soluble fiber for all blood groups are the little known arabinogalactans (AG) in the Western larch tree. Larch arabinogalactan is very useful for immune support as well. In the digestive tract, larch AG has been shown to increase the concentration of short-chain fatty acids such as butyrate, which are an important energy source for the intestinal cells. Larch also helps to decrease the concentration of ammonia, a toxic byproduct of protein synthesis in the gut. The kidneys usually excrete ammonia. The ability of this fiber to increase the elimination of ammonia is so great that one study suggested its use as a supplement to dialysis in kidney patients.

Blood group antigens are the key to digestive health, forming an invisible blueprint to every aspect of the digestive process. Following the blueprint for your blood group can assure the most efficient assimilation of nutrients and an avoidance of medical conditions that plague most of the population.

Related Topics

Allergies, food

Bacterial disease (general)

Barrett's esophagus

Celiac disease

Colitis, ulcerative

Constipation

Crohn's disease

Dental caries

Denture stomatitis

Diarrhea

Gastroesophogeal reflux disease

Lectins

Liver disease

Toxicity, bowel

Ulcer (all)

REFERENCES

1. Tabak LA, et al. Role of salivary mucins in the protection of the digestive tract. *J Oral Pathology*. 1982;11:1–17.

2. Smith DV, Klevitsky R, Akeson RA, Shipley MT. Taste bud expression of human blood group antigens. *J Comp Neurol*. 1994;343:130–142.

3. Ushiyama I, Kane M, Yamamoto Y, K. Nishi. Expression of blood group related carbohydrate antigens in salivary glands and male reproductive organs from rats, cats and humans [poster EN0514]. Located at: Shiga University of Medical Science, Otsu, Shiga, Japan.

4. Ciardello F, Tortora G. Interactions between the epidermal growth factor receptor and type I protein kinase A: biological significance and therapeutic implications. *Clin Cancer Res.* 1998;4:821–828.

5. Garratty G. Blood group antigens as tumor markers, parasitic/bacterial/viral receptors, and their association with immunologically important proteins. *Clin Chim Acta.* 1988;177:147–155.

6. Lesuffleur T, Zweibaum A, Real FX. Mucins in normal and neoplastic human gastrointestinal tissues. *Crit Rev Oncol Hematol.* 1994;17:153–180.

7. Nieuw Amerongen AV, Bolscher JG, Bloemena E, Veerman EC. Sulfomucins in the human body. *Biol Chem.* 1998;379:1–18.

8. Meini A, Pillan NM, Villanacci V, Monafo V, Ugazio AG, Plebani A. Prevalence and diagnosis of celiac disease in IgA-deficient children. *Ann Allergy Asthma Immunol.* 1996;77:333–336.

9. Gibbons RJ, Dankers I. Immunosorbent assay of interactions between human parotid immunoglobulin A and dietary lectins. *Arch Oral Biol.* 1986;31:477–481.

10. Prokop O, Kohler W, Rackwitz A, Paunova R, Barthold E. [Secretory antibodies in saliva against group G streptococci]. *Immunitatsforsch Immunobiol.* 1977;153:428–434.

11. Greenwell P. Blood group antigens: molecules seeking a function? *Glyconjugate Journal.* 1997;14:159–173.

12. Li R, Zhang L, Wu M. [Distribution of ABH substances in normal secretor human tissue cells by avidin-biotin complex method]. *Hua Hsi I Ko Ta Hsueh Hsueh Pao.* 1994;25:375–379.

13. Mikkat U, Damm I, Schroder G, et al. Effect of the lectins wheat germ agglutinin (WGA) and Ulex europaeus agglutinin (UEA-I) on the alpha-amylase secretion of rat pancreas in vitro and in vivo. *Pancreas.* 1998;16:529–538.

14. Okada Y, Jinno K, Moriwaki S, et al. Blood group antigens in the intrahepatic biliary tree. I. Distribution in the normal liver. *J Hepatol.* 1988;6:63–70.

15. Greenwell P. Blood group antigens: molecules seeking a function? *Glyconjugate Journal.* 1997;14:159–173.

16. Li R, et al. Subcellular localization of blood group substances ABH in human gastrointestinal tracts [in Chinese]. *Chung Kuo I Hsueh Ko Hsueh Yuan Hsueh Pao.* 1996;18:49–53.

17. Kelly JJ, Alpers DH. Blood group antigenicity of purified human intestinal disaccharidases. *J Biol Chem.* 1973;248:8216–8221.

18. Stepan J, Graubaum HJ, Meurer W, Wagenknecht C. Isoenzymes of alkaline phosphatase-reference values in young people and effects of protein diet [in German]. *Experientia.* 1976;32:832–834.

19. Davidson BJ, MacMurray JP, Prakash V. ABO blood group differences in bone mineral density of recovering alcoholic males. *Alcohol Clin Exp. Res.* 1990;14:906–908.

20. Langman MJ, Leuthold E, Robson EB, Harris J, Luffman JE, Harris H. Influence of diet on the "intestinal" component of alkaline phosphatase in people of different ABO blood groups and secretor status. *Nature.* 1966;212:41–43.

DIPHTHERIA–*See Bacterial Disease, diphtheria*

DOPAMINE IMBALANCE–*See Stress*

DOWN SYNDROME–*See Birth defects*

DUODENAL ULCER–*See Ulcer, duodenal*

DYSMENORRHEA–*See Menstrual cycle disorders, dysmenorrhea*

E. COLI INFECTION–*See Bacterial disease, E. coli*

EAR INFECTION, OTITIS EXTERNA–*Infection or inflammation of the ear canal; also called "swimmer's ear."*

Otitis externa	RISK		
	LOW	AVERAGE	HIGH
GROUP A			
GROUP B			
GROUP AB			
GROUP O			
NON-SECRETOR			

Symptoms

- Itching

- Pain with pulling or pushing against the external ear flesh

- Offensive discharge from the ear

- Canal is swollen, and visibly full of infectious matter

About Otitis Externa

Otitis externa is an infection or inflammation of the ear canal. It's sometimes called "swimmer's ear" because one of the contributing factors is frequent wetness. Other factors include trauma to the ear canal (including hearty use of cotton swabs) or irritating substances, such as hair dye, seeping into the canal. Chronic otitis externa can be caused by eczema, dermatitis, neurodermatitis, chronic OTITIS MEDIA, and sensitivity to topical medications.

The ear infection may be localized or generalized, and is more common during the summer months. Microorganisms commonly associated with otitis externa include *Pseudomonas, Escherichia coli, Proteus vulgaris,* and *Staphylococcus aureus.*

Blood Group Links

The expression of ABO blood groups in the outer ear canal has been analyzed to determine whether there is any relationship between blood group and infections of the ear canal. In particular, the bacterium *Pseudomonas aeruginosa* was tested with different sugar solutions. It was found that this bacterium showed a specificity for the group A terminal sugar *N*-acetyl-galactosamine. The conclusion was that patients with blood group A may have a genetic predisposition to this form of otitis externa[1].

Therapies, Otitis Externa

ALL BLOOD GROUPS:

To avoid getting "swimmer's ear," the source of many bacterial infections of the ear canal:

1. Wear wax or silicone earplugs that can be softened and shaped to fit your ears. They are available at most drugstores.

2. Wear a bathing cap to help keep water from getting into the ears.

3. Don't swim in dirty water.

4. Swim on the surface of the water instead of underneath the water.

To treat a mild case of "swimmer's ear," the goal is to clean and dry the ear outer canal without doing further damage to the top layer of skin.

1. Shake your head to expel trapped water.

2. Dry the ear canal: Take a clean facial tissue, twist each corner into a tip, and gently place each tip into the ear canal for 10 seconds. Repeat with the other ear, using a new tissue.

3. Use an over-the-counter product such as Swim-Ear. Drop it into the ears to fight infection.

4. Do not remove earwax. This coats the ear canal and protects it from moisture.

BLOOD GROUP A:

1. Yeast/Fungus Resistance Protocol

2. Antibacterial Protocol

BLOOD GROUP B:

1. Yeast/Fungus Resistance Protocol

2. Antibacterial Protocol

BLOOD GROUP AB:

1. Yeast/Fungus Resistance Protocol

2. Antibacterial Protocol

BLOOD GROUP O:

1. Yeast/Fungus Resistance Protocol

2. Antibacterial Protocol

Related Topics

Bacterial disease (general)

Ear infection, otitis media

REFERENCES

1. Steuer MK, Hofstadter F, Probster L, Beuth J, Strutz J. Are ABH antigenic determinants on human outer ear canal epithelium responsible for Pseudomonas aeruginosa infections? *ORL J Otorhinolaryngol Relat Spec.* 1995;57:148–152.

EAR INFECTION, OTITIS MEDIA (CHILDHOOD EAR INFECTION)—*An infection of the inner ear, most common in young children.*

Otitis media	RISK		
	LOW	AVERAGE	HIGH
GROUP A			
GROUP B			
GROUP AB			
GROUP O			
NON-SECRETOR			

Symptoms

Symptoms of acute otitis media usually develop suddenly and can include the following:

- Pain
- Coughing
- Nasal congestion
- Fever
- Irritability
- Discharge from the ear
- Loss of appetite
- Vomiting

About Otitis Media

As many as two-thirds of all children under 6 years of age suffer from chronic ear infections, accounting for half of all visits to pediatricians. Most of these children have allergies to both environmental and food-based particles.

Several studies have shown that the ear fluids of children with a history of chronic ear infections lack specific chemicals called complement, which are needed to attack and destroy the bacteria. Another study showed that a serum lectin called mannose binding protein is missing in the ear fluid of children with chronic infections. This lectin apparently binds to mannose sugars on the surface of the bacteria and agglutinates them, allowing for their faster removal. Both of these important immune factors eventually do develop in their proper amounts, which may help explain why the frequency of ear infections gradually lessens as the child ages.

Ear infections are terribly painful for a child. Most of these infections are a backup of noxious fluids and gases into the middle ear because of an obstructed connecting pipe, the eustachian tube. This tube can become swollen because of allergic reactions, weakness in the tissues surrounding it, or infections.

Why Antibiotics Aren't the Answer

According to the American Academy of Pediatrics, the most common reason for prescribing antibiotics to children is ear infection: 20–25 million cases are diagnosed each year in the United States. But there is growing worry that the overuse of antibiotics is making the bacteria that cause ear infections—and more serious ailments—resistant to the drugs. This has doctors and parents looking for new alternatives.

Why do antibiotics stop working? A baby's first ear infection is typically treated with a mild antibiotic such as amoxicillin. With the child's next ear infection, amoxicillin is given again. Eventually, the ever more resistant infection returns, and amoxicillin is no longer effective. The escalation phenomenon—the process of using stronger and stronger drugs, and ever more invasive treatments—has begun. When antibiotics no longer work, and the painful infections continue, a myringotomy is performed. This is a process in which tiny tubes called grommets are surgically implanted through the eardrum to increase the drainage of fluid from the middle ear into the throat.

General Risk Factors and Causes

Risk factors include attending daycare centers, formula feeding, smoking in the household, male gender, and a family history of middle ear disease. Otitis media occurring in the first year life is a risk factor for recurrent otitis media. Increased risk is also correlated with a sibling history of otitis media.

Blood Group Links

Blood groups A and AB children have greater problems with mucus secretions from improper diet—a factor in ear infections. In type A children, dairy products are usually the culprit; whereas type AB children may experience sensitivities to corn in addition to milk. In general, these children are also more likely to have throat and respiratory problems that can often move into the ears. Because the immune systems of type A and type AB children are tolerant of a wider range of bacteria, some of their problems stem from the lack of an aggressive response to the infectious organism.

When the ABO blood groups of 610 patients with documented secretory otitis media were compared with those of a control group, the preponderance of group A and shortage of group O was considered statistically significant. Researchers concluded that the blood group abnormalities of otitis media patients may indicate hereditary trends[1].

In another study that supported the hereditary connection, the relative causal importance of certain established risk factors along with maternal blood group A were studied in 225 children from conception to age 7. Taken alone, maternal blood group A provided a relative risk for intervention of 2.82. Taken separately, the noted occurrence of an attack of acute otitis media before the first birthday provided a relative risk of 6.13. However, when the factors of maternal blood group A and attack before the first birthday were combined, the relative risk climbed steeply to 26.77. Researchers concluded that the influence of blood group A on otitis media was significant enough to warrant further studies[2].

Blood groups O and B children seem to develop ear infections less frequently, and when they do occur, they are usually easier to treat. More often than not, a change in diet is sufficient to eliminate the problem.

Therapies, Otitis Media

BLOOD GROUP A:

1. Immune-Enhancing Protocol

2. Antibacterial Protocol

BLOOD GROUP B:

1. Antiviral Protocol

BLOOD GROUP AB:

1. Immune-Enhancing Protocol

2. Antibacterial Protocol

BLOOD GROUP O:

1. Immune-Enhancing Protocol

2. Antibacterial Protocol

Specifics:

Most ear infections can be prevented in blood group O children simply by employing breast-feeding instead of bottle feeding. Breastfeeding for a period of a year or so allows a child's immune system and digestive tract time to develop. Blood group O children will also avoid ear infections if they are taken off wheat and dairy products. They're unusually sensitive to these foods at an early age, but their immunity is easily augmented by the use of higher-value proteins such as fish and lean red meats.

Related Topics

Bacterial disease (general)

Ear infection, otitis externa

Lectins

REFERENCES

1. Mortensen EH, Lildholdt T, Gammelgard NP, Christensen PH. Distribution of ABO blood groups in secretory otitis media and cholesteatoma. *Clin Otolaryngol.* 1983;8:263–265.
2. Gannon MM, Jagger C, Haggard MP. Maternal blood group in otitis media with effusion. *Clin Otolaryngol.* 1994;19: 327–331.

ECZEMA–*See Allergies, environmental/hay fever; Allergies, food*

EMBOLISM–*See Stroke*

EMPHYSEMA (CHRONIC OBSTRUCTIVE PULMONARY DISEASE, OR COPD)–*Permanent destruction of the bronchial walls, affecting lung capacity.*

Emphysema	RISK		
	LOW	AVERAGE	HIGH
GROUP A			
GROUP B			
GROUP AB			
GROUP O			
NON-SECRETOR			

Symptoms

- Chronic cough
- Spitting or coughing mucus (expectoration)
- Breathlessness upon exertion
- Progressive reduction in the ability to exhale

About Emphysema

The process leading to emphysema is most often triggered by cigarette smoke, which produces an imbalance in the chemicals that protect the lungs under ordinary circumstances. Enzymes called *proteases*, particularly those known as *elastase* and *trypsin*, are produced by the immune system to fight infection and injury. However, if they are overproduced, they attack normal lung cell tissues and impair the structural integrity of *elastin*, the material that is essential for the "springy" quality of lung tissue. The walls of the alveoli that join the very small airways (the bronchioles) become inflamed and damaged. (In a rare, inherited form of emphysema known as alpha-1-antitrypsin deficiency, both the walls of the bronchioles and alveoli to which they connect, usually in the lower lungs, are diseased.)

Over time the alveolar walls lose elasticity. Pockets of dead air called *bullae* form in the injured areas, impeding the ability to exhale and reducing normal respiratory function. Inhalation, however, is not impaired, and until the late stages of the disease, oxygen and carbon dioxide levels are normal.

Emphysema is a major cause of disability and death in the United States, second only to heart disease as a cause of disability. Men have been affected much more than women in the past, no doubt due to their more marked smoking; however, with the advent of increased smoking among women, the disease's prevalence in females is also increasing.

The standard measure of the progress of this disease is a test of forced expiratory volume (FEV) as a percentage of forced volume capacity (FVC).

Blood Group Links

ABO non-secretors have a higher incidence of emphysema. Studies have shown that non-secretors have significantly lower mean values of forced expiratory volume in 1 second as a percentage of forced vital capacity ($FEV_1/FVC\%$), and a significantly larger proportion of them had aberrant values, defined as $FEV_1/FVC\%$ of less than 68. These differences remained when mean values or rates of aberrancy were adjusted for other factors that have been reported to alter the risk of airway obstruction. In view of the known chronic obstructive pulmonary disease (COPD)/peptic ulcer and non-secretor/duodenal ulcer associations, these findings suggest that the ability to secrete ABO antigens into secretions of the respiratory and gastrointestinal tract may have a protective effect on the outer layer of organs in general, or on the lung and portions of the gut specifically[1].

A study of cigarette smokers as part of the Northwick Park Heart Study in Northwest London, England, found that secretors of ABO antigen had a higher mean peak expiratory flow rate than did non-secretors. The relationship was independent of other factors known to affect peak expiratory flow rate[2].

Consistently greater declines of lung function have also been noted in individuals carrying the A blood group allele, especially older Caucasian male smokers[3,4].

Therapies, Emphysema

ALL BLOOD GROUPS:

Emphysema is irreversible. Prevention is the only real way to avoid permanent damage.

1. If you smoke, find a program to help you stop smoking.

2. Avoid dust, fumes, pollutants, and other irritating inhalants.

BLOOD GROUP A:

1. Pulmonary Support Protocol

BLOOD GROUP B:

1. Pulmonary Support Protocol

BLOOD GROUP AB:

1. Pulmonary Support Protocol

BLOOD GROUP O:

1. Pulmonary Support Protocol

Related Topics

Bronchitis

Cancer, lung

REFERENCES

1. Cohen BH, Bias WB, Chase GA, et al. Is ABH nonsecretor status a risk factor for obstructive lung disease? *Am J Epidemiol.* 1980;111:285–291.
2. Haines AP, Imeson JD, Meade TW. ABH secretor status and pulmonary function. *Am J Epidemiol.* 1982;115:367–370.
3. Menkes HA, Cohen BH, Beaty TH, Newill CA, Khoury MJ. Risk factors, pulmonary function, and mortality. *Prog Clin Biol Res.* 1984;147:501–521.
4. Khoury MJ, Beaty TH, Newill CA, Bryant S, Cohen BH. Genetic-environmental interactions in chronic airways obstruction. *Int J Epidemiol.* 1986;15:65–72.

ENDOMETRIAL CANCER–*See Cancer, uterine*

ENVIRONMENTAL ALLERGIES–*See Allergies, environmental/hay fever*

EPSTEIN-BARR VIRUS–*See Viral disease, mononucleosis*

ESOPHAGEAL CANCER–*See Cancer, esophageal*

ESTROGEN DEPLETION–*See Menopausal/perimenopausal conditions*

F

FATIGUE–_See Chronic fatigue syndrome_

▉ Fever

Fever is a physiologic response to disease or trauma that causes a rise in the body's core temperature. Fever is defined as a body temperature above 100°F (37.7°C). It is usually accompanied by malaise, lethargy, and weakness. Fever is not a disease but a symptom of illness. It is an immune system attempt to rid the body of offending organisms and to promote healing.

Common Causes	BLOOD GROUP O	BLOOD GROUP A	BLOOD GROUP B	BLOOD GROUP AB	NON-SECRETORS
Infection— bacterial or viral	***	*********	********	*********	************
Injury or trauma (including surgery)	All groups suscepti-ble	All groups suscepti-ble	All groups suscepti-ble	All groups suscepti-ble	
Tumors	***	**********	***	***********	

* = degree of risk

Related Protocols

BLOOD GROUP A:

1. Chronic Illness Recovery Protocol
2. Antibacterial Protocol
3. Antiviral Protocol

BLOOD GROUP B:

1. Chronic Illness Recovery Protocol
2. Antibacterial Protocol
3. Antiviral Protocol

BLOOD GROUP AB:

1. Chronic Illness Recovery Protocol
2. Antibacterial Protocol
3. Antiviral Protocol

BLOOD GROUP O:

1. Chronic Illness Recovery Protocol
2. Antibacterial Protocol
3. Antiviral Protocol

Related Topics

Bacterial disease (general)

Cancer (general)

Trauma

Viral disease (general)

FIBROCYSTIC BREAST—*Inflammation and tenderness in the cystic tissue of a woman's breast.*

Fibrocystic breast disease	RISK		
	LOW	AVERAGE	HIGH
GROUP A			
GROUP B			
GROUP AB			
GROUP O			
NON-SECRETOR			

Symptoms

Symptoms of fibrocystic breasts usually occur in the second half of a woman's menstrual cycle. They include the following:

- Pain
- Swelling
- Extreme breast sensitivity
- Palpable cysts
- Concurrent premenstrual syndrome symptoms: bloating, craving for sweets, anxiety/mood swings

About Fibrocystic Breasts

Fibrocystic breast disease is the most common breast disease in women, occurring in about 20% of premenopausal females. The normal menstrual cycle is responsible for biphasic stimulation of the breasts, first through the proliferation of breast tissue by estrogens and then of the alveolar tissue by progesterone. Most women do not notice such changes, but in some females the breast symptoms are quite noticeable and uncomfortable. Common causes of benign breast lumps (sometimes referred to as "nodular breasts") include:

- Fluid-filled cysts, which are thought to arise from obstructed milk ducts
- Solid fibroadenomas, which are caused by an overgrowth of connective tissue within the lobules (milk-producing glands) of the breast

Under the influence of hormonal changes, benign cysts often enlarge and become painful just before the menstrual period. If a lump is unusually firm or irregular, a needle biopsy or a surgical biopsy may be needed to rule out cancer. Other benign solid breast masses include fat necrosis, a condition involving breast tissue death, and sclerosing adenosis, a fibrocystic proliferation of small ducts, which can be diagnosed only by biopsy. Possible causes of benign cysts include a luteal phase defect in progesterone, increased estrogen, hyperprolactinemia, and organ hypersensitivity to estrogen sensitivity to methylxanthines and dietary fat intake.

Aside from cysts, another prominent feature of fibrocystic breasts is fibrosis, in which fibrous tissue makes areas of the breast feel rubbery, firm, or hard to the touch. Fibrosis is not harmful. Some 90% of all women develop lumpy breasts at some phase of their lives, most commonly during the latter half of their reproductive years. With rare exceptions, having lumpy breasts does not generally raise a woman's risk for breast cancer.

Of far greater concern is a rare type of benign breast lump called atypical hyperplasia, or unusual cell enlargement. Research suggests that atypical hyperplasia increases breast cancer risk by three to five times, particularly among women with a family history of the disease. According to the American Cancer Society, about 70% of biopsies done for benign breast conditions contain no hyperplasia; about 26% have usual hyperplasia; and only 4% have atypical hyperplasia. Women with a history of atypical hyperplasia should be screened more frequently for breast cancer.

Blood Group Links

A loss of AB antigen expression in the breast appears to be a consistent marker of the benign proliferative duct lesions associated with fibrocystic disease. The early loss of AB antigen supports a possible link between fibrocystic disease and breast cancer. However, in contrast to other tissues, loss of AB antigen expression in proliferative breast lesions is not necessarily evidence of malignancy[1].

Therapies, Fibrocystic Breast

ALL BLOOD GROUPS:

1. *Maintain a healthy weight.* In some cases, being overweight can make breast tissue heavier and thus make pain and tenderness worse.

2. *Use warm compresses.* Apply to tender areas.

3. *Wear a supportive bra.* Wearing a comfortable but supportive bra can sometimes help, especially if you are large-breasted and physically active.

4. *Reduce salt intake,* especially toward the end of the menstrual cycle. The sodium in salt causes fluid retention throughout the body, including the breasts.

5. *Drain cysts.* If the pain is caused by a fluid-filled cyst, it can often be lessened in minutes by aspirating (draining) the fluid through a needle.

BLOOD GROUP A:

1. Female Balancing Protocol

BLOOD GROUP B:

1. Female Balancing Protocol

BLOOD GROUP AB:

1. Female Balancing Protocol

BLOOD GROUP O:

1. Female Balancing Protocol

Related Topics

Cancer, breast

Immunity

Menstrual cycle disorders, premenstrual syndrome

REFERENCES

1. Strauchen JA, Bergman SM, Hanson TA. Expression of A and B tissue isoantigens in benign and malignant lesions of the breast. *Cancer*. 1980;45:2149–2155.

FIBROIDS, UTERINE–*Benign tumors of the uterus.*

Fibroids, uterine	RISK		
	LOW	AVERAGE	HIGH
GROUP A			
GROUP B			
GROUP AB			
GROUP O			
NON-SECRETOR			

Symptoms

Often uterine fibroids have no accompanying symptoms, but others cause the following:

- Excessive menstrual bleeding
- Anemia
- Vaginal discharge
- Uterine pain or cramps

About Uterine Fibroids

Uterine fibroids are benign tumors of the uterus, occurring in about 25% of women over age 35. They are often asymptomatic, and are first discovered during a pelvic exam. They may, how-ever, cause excessive menstrual bleeding, and pelvic pain or bloating. Their growth is increased during pregnancy and with estrogen therapy, and they tend to atrophy after menopause. They may either grow into the lumen or into the pelvic cavity, or remain in the wall of the uterus. These benign tumors usually develop in young women. Their growth is positively correlated with estrogen stimulation and they generally regress following pregnancy and after menopause. The later reproductive and perimenopausal age groups are at risk for their development.

Blood Group Links

Uterine fibroids are most common in groups A and AB, probably because the cellular growth factors that are responsible for the proliferation of uterine tissue can be stimulated by the A antigen. It has been shown that rapidly growing endometrial tissue is heavily infiltrated with blood group antigens, whereas normal endometrial tissue is not.

Therapies, Uterine Fibroids

BLOOD GROUP A:

1. Immune-Enhancing Protocol
2. Female Balancing Protocol

Specifics:

Yoga exercises help some women relieve the sensations of heaviness and pressure.

BLOOD GROUP B:

1. Immune-Enhancing Protocol

2. Female Balancing Protocol

BLOOD GROUP AB:

1. Immune-Enhancing Protocol

2. Female Balancing Protocol

Specifics:

Yoga exercises help some women relieve the sensations of heaviness and pressure.

BLOOD GROUP O:

1. Immune-Enhancing Protocol

2. Female Balancing Protocol

Related Topics

Blood clotting disorders

Immunity

Menopausal disorders

FIBROMYALGIA–*See Autoimmune disease, fibromyalgia*

FLU–*See Viral disease, influenza*

FOOD ALLERGIES–*See Allergies, food*

FOOD INTOLERANCE–*See Allergies, food*

FOOD POISONING–*Food-related illnesses caused by bacteria, parasites, chemicals, or other toxins.*

Food poisoning	RISK		
	LOW	AVERAGE	HIGH
GROUP A (*Salmonella*)			
GROUP B (*Shigella*)			
GROUP AB (*Salmonella*)			
GROUP O			
NON-SECRETOR			

Symptoms

Different bacterial strains may present differently, but the most common symptoms of food poisoning include the following:

- Nausea
- Vomiting
- Diarrhea
- Fever
- Difficulty breathing

About Food Poisoning

As many as 80 million Americans are afflicted with some form of food poisoning every year. Most of our food supply—including meat, poultry, fish, dairy products, fruits, and vegetables—is capable of being contaminated.

Although there are many sources of food poisoning, the following are most common.

SALMONELLA

Salmonella is the bacteria responsible for about half of all food poisonings. It is generally found in raw animal products such as meat, eggs, and poultry. In particular, *Salmonella* turns up with increasing frequency in slaughtered turkey and chickens. The symptoms of *Salmonella* poisoning, which include nausea, diarrhea, and fever, occur within 12 to 48 hours of ingesting the contaminated food. Not everyone who eats contaminated food gets sick—the problem seems to occur most frequently in young children, the elderly, and the infirm. However, even in those mildly infected, the unpleasant and debilitating symptoms can linger for a few days.

STAPHYLOCOCCUS AUREUS

The microorganism *S. aureus* is responsible for a little more than 25% of all food-borne illnesses. The contamination can occur in any prepared food, meat, poultry or fish dish. It is carried in the noses and throats of most people. That's why sneezing or coughing on food—especially a protein-containing food like meat or pudding—can contaminate it. Symptoms include mild diarrhea, sometimes accompanied by nausea and vomiting. It is not the bacterium itself that brings on the symptoms, but the toxins the bacterium produces. Even though cooking kills the bacteria, it does not destroy the toxins.

CLOSTRIDIUM PERFRINGENS

Sometimes referred to as the cafeteria germ, the *C. perfringens* bacterium accounts for about 1 in 10 reported cases of food poisoning. It usually occurs in settings where large batches of meat, turkey, and other foods are prepared. Like *S. aureus,* it produces toxins, or spores, that are resistant to the heat of cooking. It causes a mild illness of short duration (12 to 24 hours) and is rarely serious enough to warrant medical attention.

ESCHERICHIA COLI

The overwhelming cause of *E. coli* infection is exposure to undercooked, contaminated ground beef. Large outbreaks of *E. coli* O157:H7 have been reported in the United States, including an outbreak in 1993 linked to undercooked hamburgers that resulted in more than 600 reported cases and four deaths. But animal products are not alone in initiating the spread of this infection. In 1996, more than 6,000 schoolchildren in Japan developed *E. coli* O157:H7 infection from eating contaminated radish sprouts. Though vegan enthusiasts tend to emphasize meat as a cause of *E. coli* infection, since 1995 raw sprouts have been associated with 13 outbreaks of food-borne disease due to *E. coli* or *Salmonella.* Contamination of the sprouts themselves, rather than improper handling, is believed to have been the source of the problem.

BOTULISM

Botulism is the most severe food-borne illness, but it is also the most rare: There are fewer than 100 cases reported during a year in the entire country. One familiar telltale sign of the presence of the bacteria that leads to botulism is a bulging food can. The toxin responsible for the bulging is produced by the bacterium *Clostridium botulinum,* commonly found in soil, water, and manure. Besides bulging cans, also be wary of cracked jars and loose lids. The symptoms of botulism can range from double vision and difficulty breathing to death for the most severe cases.

BACILLUS CEREUS

Many people believe that harmful bacteria is limited to meat, poultry, fish, and dairy products. However, the bacterium *B. cereus* is present in starchy foods such as noodles, as well as in meat and poultry. In fact, fried rice has been identified as a leading cause in the United States of a vomit-inducing food-borne illness caused by the *B. cereus* microorganism. Leftover fried rice that is not promptly refrigerated, then is reheated too briefly to kill the resulting bacteria is a primary cause of the illness.

Blood Group Links

Anyone can get food poisoning. But certain blood types are naturally more susceptible, because of their tendency toward a weakened immune system. In particular, groups A and AB are more likely to fall prey to *Salmonella* food poisoning, which is usually the result of leaving food uncovered and unrefrigerated for too long. Furthermore, these bacteria will be harder for groups A and AB to get rid of once they've found a home in their systems. Group B, who is generally more susceptible to inflammatory diseases, is more likely to be severely affected when eating food that is contaminated with the *Shigella* organism, a bacteria found on plants that causes dysentery[1]. All blood groups can contract infections from *E. coli* bacteria[2–6].

Therapies, Food Poisoning

ALL BLOOD GROUPS:

According to the Centers for Disease Control, up to 85% of the incidences of food poisoning could be avoided if people followed basic health and safety guidelines in the preparation, storage, and serving of foods.

To prevent Salmonella *poisoning:*

- Rinse meat and poultry with cold water before cooking to remove some of the bacteria.

- Cook poultry until there is no pink meat. If you use a meat thermometer, check to see that the meat reaches an internal temperature of 180° to 185°F (82.2° to 85°C). Make sure to insert the thermometer into the thickest part of the chicken—the thigh, away from the bone—to get the most accurate reading.

- Keep utensils and cutting boards used to prepare meat and poultry separate from those used to prepare fruit and vegetables. For example, if you prepare a mixed chicken and vegetable dish, use a separate knife and cutting board for the chicken, and another for the vegetables.

- Be sure to thoroughly wash all the utensils you use to prepare raw meat and poultry with hot, soapy water. Dishwasher water is hot enough.

- Keep wood cutting boards clean by washing them every few days with a diluted bleach-and-water solution. The bleach should kill any bacteria.

- Don't partially cook meat ahead of time. Partially cooking burgers and then refrigerating them for tomorrow's barbecue can be dangerous, especially if the raw meat does not become hot enough to kill bacteria. Bacteria can grow rapidly in partially cooked meat as it cools.

▪ Place raw meat on the lowest refrigerator shelf to prevent its juices from dripping onto other foods, thereby contaminating them. Put the meat on a platter, even if it's wrapped, to prevent juices from running onto the refrigerator surface.

To prevent S. aureus *and* C. perfringens *infection:*

▪ Never leave uncooked or already cooked foods at room temperature for long periods of time. A lukewarm temperature of 40° to 140°F (4.4° to 60°C) (not piping hot, but not as cold as a refrigerator) allows bacteria to grow rapidly and thereby produce more toxins.

▪ Thaw frozen foods in the refrigerator, not on the counter, to prevent them from getting too warm.

▪ Keep foods hot on the stove or in the oven until you are ready to serve them. Even a dish as seemingly harmless as a rice casserole can produce enough toxins to be potentially dangerous if it is left to sit out at room temperature for more than 2 hours.

▪ Refrigerate leftovers as soon as possible.

▪ When cooking large batches of food, such as stew, divide the leftovers into small batches so that, once in the refrigerator, they will quickly cool to temperatures that limit the growth of bacteria.

To prevent E. coli *infection:*

▪ Avoid eating undercooked hamburgers or other ground beef products in restaurants.

▪ Drink only pasteurized milk, juice, or cider.

▪ Wash fruits, sprouts, and vegetables thoroughly, especially those that will not be cooked.

▪ Keep raw meat separate from ready-to-eat foods.

▪ Wash hands, counters, and utensils with hot soapy water after contact with raw meat.

▪ Never place cooked hamburgers or ground beef on the same plate that held the raw patties.

BLOOD GROUP A:

1. Antibacterial Protocol
2. Intestinal Health Protocol

BLOOD GROUP B:

1. Antibacterial Protocol
2. Immune-Enhancing Protocol

BLOOD GROUP AB:

1. Antibacterial Protocol
2. Intestinal Health Protocol

BLOOD GROUP O:

1. Antibacterial Protocol
2. Immune-Enhancing Protocol

Related Topics

Bacterial disease, *E. coli*

Bacterial disease (general)

Immunity

Infectious disease

Toxicity, bowel (polyamines)

REFERENCES

1. Springer GF. Role of human cell surface structures in interactions between man and microbes. *Naturwissenschaften.* 1970;57:162–171.

2. Yang N, Boettcher B. Development of human ABO blood group A antigen on Escherichia coli Y1089 and Y1090. *Immunol Cell Biol.* 1992;70 (pt 6):411–416.

3. Lindstedt R, Larson G, Falk P, et al. The receptor repertoire defines the host range for attaching Escherichia coli strains that recognize globo-A. *Infect Immun.* 1991;59:1086–1092.

4. Gabr NS, Mandour AM. Relation of parasitic infection to blood group in El Minia Governorate, Egypt. *J Egypt Soc Parasitol.* 1991;21:679–683.

5. Wittels EG, Lichtman HC. Blood group incidence and Escherichia coli bacterial sepsis. *Transfusion.* 1986;26:533–535.

6. Black RE, Levine MM, Clements ML, Hughes T, O'Donnell S. Association between O blood group and occurrence and severity of diarrhoea due to Escherichia coli. *Trans R Soc Trop Med Hyg.* 1987,81:120–123.

FUNGAL DISEASE, CANDIDIASIS (DIGESTIVE, SYSTEMIC)–*An infection caused by yeast overgrowth in the gastrointestinal tract.*

Candidiasis, digestive	RISK		
	LOW	AVERAGE	HIGH
GROUP A			
GROUP B			
GROUP AB			
GROUP O			
NON-SECRETOR			

Symptoms, Digestive Candidiasis

- Bloating
- Gas, especially after eating carbohydrates and drinking yeast-containing products

Systemic *Candida* infection can cause the following:

- Fever
- Malaise
- Hypotension
- Altered mental state

About Digestive Candidiasis

The yeast *Candida albicans* is present in the digestive tract of many otherwise healthy individuals. Ironically, one of the primary factors in recurrent yeast infections is long-term overuse of antibiotics. This can develop into acute systemic candidiasis, one of the most serious manifestations of systemic colonization. The organism potentially can hematogenously disseminate systemically. This disseminated form of candidiasis affects at least 120,000 patients annually in the United States.

Blood Group Links

In general, blood group O is more inclined to *Candida* hypersensitivity than other blood groups[1], and group O non-secretors have the greatest susceptibility.

Overall, non-secretors have a much higher rate of candidiasis. The protective effect afforded by the secretor gene might be due to the ability of glycocompounds in the body fluids of secretors to inhibit adhesins on the surface of the yeast. Non-secretor saliva may not only fail to prevent attachment of *Candida* sp but may actually promote the binding of *Candida* sp to tissue. In one study, among individuals with non-insulin-dependent diabetes mellitus, 44% of non-secretors were found to be oral carriers of this yeast[2].

Although non-secretors are only about 15% to 20% of the population, they are significantly over-represented among individuals with either oral or vaginal *Candida* infections, making up almost 50% of affected individuals[2]. The inability to secrete blood group antigens in saliva also appears to be a risk factor in the development or persistence of chronic hyperplastic candidiasis. In one study, the proportion of non-secretors of blood group antigens among patients with chronic hyperplastic candidiasis was 68%. Women with recurrent vaginal yeast infections are also much more likely to be non-secretors[3,4].

Therapies, Candidiasis (Digestive, Systemic)

BLOOD GROUP A:

1. Yeast/Fungus Resistance Protocol
2. Immune-Enhancing Protocol
3. Stomach Health Protocol

BLOOD GROUP B:

1. Yeast/Fungus Resistance Protocol
2. Immune-Enhancing Protocol
3. Intestinal Health Protocol

BLOOD GROUP AB:

1. Yeast/Fungus Resistance Protocol
2. Immune-Enhancing Protocol
3. Intestinal Health Protocol

BLOOD GROUP O:

1. Yeast/Fungus Resistance Protocol
2. Allergy Control Protocol
3. Intestinal Health Protocol

Related Topics

Digestion

Immunity

Infectious disease

Toxicity, bowel

REFERENCES

1. Tosh FD, Douglas LJ. Characterization of a fucoside-binding adhesin of Candida albicans. *Infect Immun.* 1992; 60:4734–4739.

2. Aly FZ, Blackwell CC, MacKenzie DA, et al. Chronic atrophic oral candidiasis among patients with diabetes mellitus—role of ABH secretor status. *Epidemiol Infect.* 1991; 106:355–363.

3. Thom SM, Blackwell CC, MacCallum CJ, et al. Non-secretion of blood group antigens and susceptibility to infection by Candida species. *FEMS Microbiol Immunol.* 1989;1:401–405.

4. Lamey PJ, Darwazeh AM, Muirhead J, Rennie JS, Samaranayake LP, MacFanane TW. Chronic hyperplastic candidosis and secretor status. *J Oral Pathol Med.* 1991;20:64–67.

FUNGAL DISEASE, CANDIDIASIS (ORAL "THRUSH")–*Infection of the oral tissues with* Candida albicans; *often an opportunistic infection in people with AIDS or other conditions that depress the immune system.*

Candidiasis (oral/"thrush")	RISK		
	LOW	AVERAGE	HIGH
GROUP A			
GROUP B			
GROUP AB			
GROUP O			
NON-SECRETOR			

Symptoms

- Oral lesions
- Creamy white plaques on the tongue or buccal mucosa

About Oral Candidiasis

Oral candidiasis, or thrush, commonly affects people with AIDS or other conditions that compromise the T-cell-mediated immune defense mechanisms. It will occasionally affect others as well. Certain risk factors are immunosuppression, antibacterial therapy, dentures, chronic use of oral or inhaled steroids, use of birth control pills, or hyperglycemia.

Blood Group Links

ABO non-secretors have a higher incidence of oral candidiasis, Lewis (a+b−) more than Lewis (a−b−). Oral carriage of *Candida* is also significantly associated with blood group O; among non-secretors of blood group antigens, group O non-secretors are most likely to carry *Candida*[1].

Although non-secretors are only about 15% to 20% of the population, they are significantly over-represented among individuals with either oral or vaginal *Candida* infections, making up almost 50% of affected individuals[2]. The inability to secrete blood group antigens in saliva also appears to be a risk factor in the development or persistence of chronic hyperplastic candidiasis. In one study, the proportion of non-secretors of blood group antigens among patients with chronic hyperplastic candidiasis was 68%[3].

Non-diabetic individuals who are non-secretors of blood group antigens are prone to superficial infections by *Candida albicans*. In one study, 216 patients with DIABETES MELLITUS who were denture wearers were examined for the presence or absence of DENTURE STOMATITIS. There was an overall trend for non-secretors to be prone to denture stomatitis compared with secretors. When a stepwise linear discriminant analysis was used to dissect the contribution of secretor status and other variables to the development of the disease, secretor status was found to be a contributory factor among patients with non-insulin-dependent diabetes but not among those with insulin-dependent diabetes[4].

Oral candidiasis shows a higher incidence of group O over other ABO groups.

Therapies, Candidiasis (Oral "Thrush")

ALL BLOOD GROUPS:

1. Nystatin or amphotericin B are available as mouthwashes and lozenges.

2. Dentures should be soaked in nystatin solution.

3. Miconazole 2% or nystatin cream, twice daily for 1 week, usually produces rapid improvement.

BLOOD GROUP A:

1. Yeast/Fungus Resistance Protocol

2. Immune-Enhancing Protocol

BLOOD GROUP B:

1. Yeast/Fungus Resistance Protocol

2. Immune-Enhancing Protocol

BLOOD GROUP AB:

1. Yeast/Fungus Resistance Protocol

2. Immune-Enhancing Protocol

BLOOD GROUP O:

1. Yeast/Fungus Resistance Protocol

2. Immune-Enhancing Protocol

Related Topics

Denture stomatitis

Immunity

Viral disease, AIDS

REFERENCES

1. Burford-Mason AP, Weber JC, Willoughby JM. Oral carriage of Candida albicans, ABO blood group and secretor status in healthy subjects. *J Med Vet Mycol.* 1988;26:49–56.
2. Thom SM, Blackwell CC, MacCallum CJ, et al. Non-secretion of blood group antigens and susceptibility to infection by Candida species. *FEMS Microbiol Immunol.* 1989;1:401–405.
3. Lamey PJ, Darwazeh AM, Muirhead J, Rennie JS, Samaranayaka LP, MacFanane TW. Chronic hyperplastic candidosis and secretor status. *J Oral Pathol Med.* 1991;20:64–67.
4. Aly FZ, Blackwell CC, MacKenzie DA, et al. Chronic atrophic oral candidiasis among patients with diabetes mellitus—role of ABH secretor status. *Epidemiol Infect.* 1991; 106:355–363.

FUNGAL DISEASE, CANDIDIASIS (VAGINAL)–*Vaginal yeast infection.*

Candidiasis (vaginal)	RISK		
	LOW	AVERAGE	HIGH
GROUP A	▓▓		
GROUP B	▓▓		
GROUP AB	▓▓▓		
GROUP O		▓▓	
NON-SECRETOR			▓▓

Symptoms

- Edema
- Vaginal burning

- Pain on urination
- Creamy vaginal discharge

About Vaginal Candidiasis

Vaginal candidiasis is an infection caused by the yeast *Candida albicans,* which thrives in warm, moist areas such as the groin, the armpit (axilla), and the submammary region. DIABETIC and immunosuppressed patients, as well as those receiving systemic antibiotic therapy, are at increased risk. The organism may be carried asymptomatically in the bowel, mouth, and vagina, so treated sites may become reinfected.

Blood Group Links

ABO non-secretors have a higher incidence of vaginal yeast infections. Women with recurrent vaginal yeast infections are much more likely to be non-secretors. Combining both ABO non-secretor phenotype and absence of the Lewis gene (a−b−), studies have determined that the relative risk of chronic recurring vaginal yeast infections is between 2.41 and 4.39, depending on the analysis technique and control group[1].

Therapies, Candidiasis (Vaginal)

ALL BLOOD GROUPS:

Clotrimazole: a 100-mg vaginal insert can be applied once a day for 7 days. Nystatin vaginal suppositories can also be used.

BLOOD GROUP A:

1. Yeast/Fungus Resistance Protocol
2. Immune-Enhancing Protocol
3. Antibiotic Support Protocol

BLOOD GROUP B:

1. Yeast/Fungus Resistance Protocol
2. Immune-Enhancing Protocol
3. Antibiotic Support Protocol

BLOOD GROUP AB:

1. Yeast/Fungus Resistance Protocol
2. Immune-Enhancing Protocol
3. Antibiotic Support Protocol

BLOOD GROUP O:

1. Yeast/Fungus Resistance Protocol
2. Immune-Enhancing Protocol
3. Antibiotic Support Protocol

Related Topics

Diabetes

Immunity

Viral disease, AIDS

REFERENCES

1. Thom SM, Blackwell CC, MacCallum CJ, et al. Nonsecretion of blood group antigens and susceptibility to infection by Candida species. *FEMS Microbiol Immunol.* 1989;1:401–405.

G

GALLBLADDER CANCER—*See Cancer, gall-bladder*

GALLSTONES—*Pieces of solid matter, usually composed of cholesterol and bilirubin, that form in the gallbladder.*

Gallstones	RISK		
	LOW	AVERAGE	HIGH
GROUP A			
GROUP B			
GROUP AB			
GROUP O			
NON-SECRETOR			

Symptoms

Most patients remain asymptomatic for long periods, frequently for life. When stones cause obstructions the following symptoms may occur:

- Colicky pain, growing in intensity
- Inflammation of the liver and gallbladder
- Nausea and vomiting

About Gallstones

The gallbladder is a small sac that sits just beneath the liver. It serves as a sort of storage room for bile. It is the job of the gallbladder to concentrate bile and then release it to aid digestion when food is passing through the small intestine. Sometimes components of bile—especially cholesterol and bilirubin—come out of solution and form crystals in the gallbladder, much as sugar crystallizes when we make rock candy. These pieces of hard matter are called gallstones. Most patients remain asymptomatic for long periods, frequently for life. When stones cause obstructions, symptoms may occur.

In the United States, almost 80% of patients with gallstones have stones made of hardened cholesterol. Gallstones may be as small as a grain of sand or as large as a golf ball, and the gallbladder may contain anywhere from one stone to hundreds. Sometimes the gallbladder contains only crystals and stones too small to see with the naked eye. This condition is called biliary sludge.

When gallstones simply exist in the gallbladder and don't cause any problems, there is really no cause for concern. But once they form, there's a small but real likelihood they can cause illness.

General Causes and Risk Factors

It has been estimated that about a third of all women over 50 will have gallstones. They are about half as prevalent in men. About 5% of patients with gallstones will have symptoms within a year of their formation. As the body ages we tend to have higher cholesterol and lower bile salts in the gallbladder fluid, increasing the risk for gallstones. Obesity is also a very strong risk factor.

Some drugs, such as oral contraceptives, will predispose a person to gallstones.

Blood Group Links

Blood group A seems more prone to gallstones over the other blood groups. In one study 321 gallstone patients were compared to 688 healthy control individuals; patients with group A showed more likelihood of contracting gallstones than groups O and B[1]. Group A also seems to have a greater risk of CANCER OF THE GALLBLADDER over the other blood types[2].

Therapies, Gallstones

BLOOD GROUP A:

1. Liver Support Protocol
2. Metabolic Enhancement Protocol
3. Detoxification Protocol

BLOOD GROUP B:

1. Liver Support Protocol
2. Metabolic Enhancement Protocol
3. Detoxification Protocol

BLOOD GROUP AB:

1. Liver Support Protocol
2. Metabolic Enhancement Protocol
3. Detoxification Protocol

BLOOD GROUP O:

1. Liver Support Protocol
2. Metabolic Enhancement Protocol
3. Detoxification Protocol

Related Topics

Crohn's disease

Digestion

Liver disease

Obesity

REFERENCES

1. Chakravartti MR, Chakravartti R. ABO bloodgroups in cholelithiasis. *Ann Genet* 1979;22:171–172.
2. Villalobos JJ, Vargas F, Villareal HA, et al. A 10-year protective study on cancer of the digestive system [in Spanish]. *Rev Gastroenterol Mex.* 1990;55:17–24.

GASTRITIS– *A chronic inflammation of the stomach lining.*

Gastritis	RISK		
	LOW	AVERAGE	HIGH
GROUP A			
GROUP B			
GROUP AB			
GROUP O			
NON-SECRETOR			

Symptoms

- Nausea
- Vomiting
- Discomfort in the upper abdomen
- In severe cases, gastric bleeding, bloody vomit, and dark bloody stools

About Gastritis

Gastritis is an inflammatory reaction in the stomach. It typically involves the mucosa; seldom will the full thickness of the stomach wall be involved. There can be erosive gastritis, which is generally a reaction to injury by noxious chemical agents, especially something like non-steroidal anti-inflammatory agents (NSAIDs) or alcohol. Reflux gastritis is a reaction to exposure to bile and pancreatic juice usually associated with a defective pylorus—the sphincter that connects the esophagus to the stomach. Infectious gastritis is commonly associated with the microbe *Helicobac-*

ter pylori. Viruses may also be associated with infectious gastritis. Many people confuse gastritis with ulcers, but it is exactly the opposite. Ulcers are produced by hyperacidity. Gastritis is caused by very low stomach acid content. Gastritis occurs when the stomach acid gets so low that it no longer functions as a microbial barrier. Without adequate levels of acid, microbes will live in the stomach and cause serious inflammation.

General Causes and Risk Factors

Causes of gastritis include excessive alcohol intake, overuse of nonsteroidal anti-inflammatory drugs (NSAIDs), bile reflux, pancreatic enzyme reflux, stress, radiation, infections with *Staphylococcus aureus* exotoxins and *H. pylori*, viral infection, and pernicious anemia.

Blood Group Links

It has long been known that hyperacidity is more common to blood groups O and B; low stomach acid is typical for blood groups A and AB. In a 1955 study published in the British medical journal *The Lancet*, researchers reported on the pattern of stomach acid secretion in patients with peptic ulcer, pernicious anemia, and stomach cancer. Of the 111 patients examined, in the group experiencing both stomach cancer and a complete lack of stomach acid production, the ratios of group A to group O were almost 2 to 1.

In 1959, the production of both stomach acid and pepsin was studied in both Caucasians and people of African ancestry, and analyzed according to ABO blood group. While the secretion of both gastric acid and pepsin was about the same for both races, substantial differences were found among the blood groups. Impairment of stomach acid production was much more common in group A than group O, and the level of plasma pepsinogen was also higher in group O over group A. In a separate study, the same researcher also found that a lack of stomach acid was significantly more common among blood group A individuals reporting digestive problems. Other studies done around the same time in India also showed differences in stomach acid production between blood groups O and A in response to a standardized test meal.

One reason that low stomach acid is linked to blood group A may have to do with the role of epidermal growth factor (EGF). EGF is a polypeptide hormone that stimulates the growth and repair of outer layer protective tissue. EGF is widely distributed in the body, with high concentrations detectable in saliva, the prostate gland, and in the duodenum of the small intestine. EGF also has the effect of decreasing gastric acid secretion. The receptor for EGF shares a similarity with the A antigen—so much so that, in tests, antibodies directed against the EGF receptor also bind to the A antigen. This could play a role in the increased incidence of certain cancers in blood group A individuals, and also might explain why stomach acid secretions are lower in blood group A than the other blood groups.

Therapies, Gastritis

BLOOD GROUP A:

1. Stomach Health Protocol
2. Antibacterial Protocol
3. Detoxification Protocol

Specifics:

Avoid corticosteroid drugs, which can cause gastric distress.

Don't smoke. Smoking exacerbates inflammation of the stomach lining.

BLOOD GROUP B:

1. Stomach Health Protocol
2. Antibacterial Protocol
3. Detoxification Protocol

BLOOD GROUP AB:

1. Stomach Health Protocol
2. Antibacterial Protocol
3. Intestinal Health Protocol

BLOOD GROUP O:

1. Stomach Health Protocol
2. Antibacterial Protocol
3. Intestinal Health Protocol

Related Topics

Bacterial disease (general)

Digestion

Immunity

Viral disease (general)

GASTROESOPHAGEAL REFLUX DISEASE (GERD)–*A chronic condition involving the backup of hydrochloric acid from the stomach into the esophagus.*

GERD	RISK		
	LOW	AVERAGE	HIGH
GROUP A	███	███	
GROUP B	███	███	
GROUP AB	███	██	
GROUP O	███	███	███
NON-SECRETOR	███	██	

Symptoms

- Burning sensation in upper abdomen and chest (heartburn)
- Regurgitation of the stomach contents all or part way back into the mouth
- Acidic, sour taste
- Bloating, gas, nausea

About GERD

Gastroesophageal reflux disease (GERD), or chronic heartburn, affects more than 20 million Americans on a daily basis. Heartburn has nothing directly to do with the heart. The name is derived from the symptomatic burning in the upper abdomen and chest. GERD can be caused by a number of conditions, including a hiatal hernia. However, the more common reason so many people are afflicted with chronic heartburn is poor dietary habits. When the acidic balance is disrupted, acid backs up through the sensitive opening that connects your esophagus with your stomach.

Between 10% and 20% of people with chronic GERD will develop BARRETT'S ESOPHAGUS (a precancerous change in the cells lining the esophagus) and 5% to 10% of these people have an increased risk of developing ESOPHAGEAL CANCER or STOMACH CANCER.

In the past, reflux was solely attributed to hiatal hernias; however, this is now known to be incorrect, as there are many asymptomatic hiatal hernia patients and many symptomatic reflux patients who do not show hiatal hernia on x-ray.

Several factors may be involved:

- Incompetent lower esophageal sphincter
- Reduced sphincter pressure from alcohol, drugs, smoking, etc.
- From lying down, bending over, or from a hiatal hernia when the stomach contents are situated near to the gastroesophageal junction
- When the gastric pressure is increased, such as from pregnancy or general obesity

Additionally, esophagitis may be caused by infections like herpes or CANDIDIASIS, and by mucosal damage from burns or chemicals.

Blood Group Links

Blood group O, with naturally high stomach acid production, is much more prone to develop GERD. However, when blood group A contracts GERD, it is more likely to advance to the precancerous condition, Barrett's esophagus, and even esophageal cancer. ABO non-secretors have a higher incidence of GERD[1,2].

Therapies, Gastroesophageal Reflux Disease (GERD)

BLOOD GROUP A:

1. Stomach Health Protocol

2. Immune-Enhancing Protocol

3. Sinus Health Protocol

BLOOD GROUP B:

1. Stomach Health Protocol

2. Antistress Protocol

BLOOD GROUP AB:

1. Stomach Health Protocol

2. Immune-Enhancing Protocol

3. Sinus Health Protocol

BLOOD GROUP O:

1. Stomach Health Protocol

2. Anti-Inflammation Protocol

Related Topics

Barrett's esophagus

Digestion

Immunity

REFERENCES

1. Torrado J, Ruiz B, Garay J, et al. Blood-group phenotypes, sulfomucins, and Helicobacter pylori in Barrett's esophagus. *Am J Surg Pathol.* 1997;21:1023–1029.

2. Mufti SI, Zirvi KA, Garewal HS. Precancerous lesions and biologic markers in esophageal cancer. *Cancer Detect Prev.* 1991;15:291–301.

GENERALIZED ANXIETY DISORDERS (GAD)–*See Anxiety disorders*

GENETICS–*See Part 1*

GERD–*See Gastroesophageal reflux disease (GERD)*

GERMAN MEASLES–*See Rubella*

GESTATIONAL TROPHOBLASTIC DISEASE–*See Birth defects*

GIARDIA–*See Parasitic disease,* Giardia

GINGIVITIS–*See Periodontal disease*

GLAUCOMA–*A problem of gradually increasing intraocular pressure causing at first a slow loss of peripheral vision, but leading to late loss of central vision and complete blindness if uncontrolled.*

Glaucoma	RISK		
	LOW	AVERAGE	HIGH
GROUP A			
GROUP B			
GROUP AB			
GROUP O			
NON-SECRETOR			
RH NEGATIVE			

Symptoms

- Frequent need to change prescription for glasses or contact lenses

- Impaired nighttime vision
- Seeing halos around lights
- Gradual loss of vision, starting with peripheral vision

About Glaucoma

Glaucoma is a specific pattern of optic nerve damage and visual field loss caused by a number of different eye diseases. Most, but not all of these diseases, are characterized by elevated intraocular pressure, which is not the disease itself, but the most important risk factor for the development of glaucoma.

Generally, there are no early symptoms. By the time the patient is aware of visual field loss, the degree of optic nerve atrophy is generally quite marked. Central vision is generally last to be affected; peripheral vision is lost first and is usually asymptomatic.

There are three types of glaucoma:

Primary open-angle glaucoma (POAG). Approximately 1% of all Americans have this form of glaucoma, making it the most common form of glaucoma in our country. It occurs mainly among people over 50 years of age.

There are no symptoms associated with POAG. The pressure in the eye slowly rises and the cornea adapts without swelling. Because of this, the disease often goes undetected until it has progressed to the point that the damage is irreversible.

Normal-tension glaucoma. Normal-tension glaucoma, also known as low-tension glaucoma, is characterized by progressive optic nerve damage and visual field loss with a statistically normal intraocular pressure. This form of glaucoma, which is being increasingly recognized, may ac-

count for as many as one-third of the cases of open-angle glaucoma in the United States. Normal-tension glaucoma is thought to be related, at least in part, to poor blood flow to the optic nerve, which leads to death of the cells that carry impulses from the retina to the brain.

Angle-closure glaucoma. Angle-closure glaucoma affects nearly half a million people in the United States. There is a tendency for this disease to be inherited, and often several members of a family will be afflicted. It is most common in people of Asian descent and people who are far-sighted.

General Causes and Risk Factors

Exfoliation syndrome, a common cause of glaucoma, is found everywhere in the world, but is most common among people of European descent. In about 10% of the population over age 50, a whitish material—which under a microscope looks like tiny flakes of dandruff—builds up on the lens of the eye. This exfoliation material is rubbed off the lens by movement of the iris and at the same time, pigment is rubbed off the iris. Exfoliation syndrome can lead to both open-angle glaucoma and angle-closure glaucoma, often producing both kinds of glaucoma in the same individual.

Blood Group Links

There are some blood group associations with glaucoma. A series of 474 mixed cases of glaucoma was assessed to determine whether there were any genetic differences between different types of glaucoma. Using ABO blood groups, Rhesus groups and ABO secretion or non-secretion, the researchers identified certain differences. ABO non-secretors have a higher incidence of glaucoma. Rh-negative individuals showed lower rates of chronic closed-angle glaucoma. There was a significant absence of blood group A secretors and an increase in group B secretors in both pseudoexfoliation with raised intraocular pressure compared with chronic closed-angle glaucoma[1].

Therapies, Glaucoma

ALL BLOOD GROUPS:

Since glaucoma is often without symptoms in the early stages, individuals over age 50 should have an annual eye exam.

BLOOD GROUP A:

1. Immune-Enhancing Protocol

BLOOD GROUP B:

1. Immune-Enhancing Protocol
2. Metabolic Enhancement Protocol

BLOOD GROUP AB:

1. Metabolic Enhancement Protocol

BLOOD GROUP O:

1. Immune-Enhancing Protocol

Related Topics

Aging diseases

Blood clotting disorders

REFERENCES

1. Brooks AM, Gillies WE. Blood groups as genetic markers in glaucoma. Br J Ophthalmol 1988 Apr;72(4):270–3

GLIOMA–See Cancer, glioma and other brain tumors

GONORRHEA–See Bacterial disease, gonorrhea

GRAVES' DISEASE–See Thyroid disease, Graves'

Growth and Maturity

Maturity begins earlier today than a century ago, probably because of improvements in nutrition, general health, and living conditions. For example, the age at menarche in the United States declined by 2 months per decade between 1850 and 1950, although it has now leveled off. Even so, the age of onset and rapidity of development vary with each person and are influenced by genetic and environmental factors. Somatic growth of males and females includes attainment of adult height and weight, musculoskeletal growth, and increased size of all organs (except the lymphatics, which decrease in size) and the brain, which reaches maximum weight during adolescence.

The growth spurt in boys occurs between ages 13 and 15½; a gain of about 4 inches can be expected in the year of peak velocity. For girls, the growth spurt begins at about age 11, may reach 3½ inches in the year of peak. In terms of velocity, female growth is almost completed by age 13½.

In general, boys are heavier and taller than girls when growth is complete because they have a longer growth period. At age 18, about ¾ inch of growth remains for boys and slightly less for girls, for whom growth is 99% complete. One adolescent may develop early and another late, but both may reach the same height.

Blood Group Links

Analyses performed within ethnic groups showed that several variables, including beta-lipoprotein cholesterol and systolic blood pressure, were sufficient to discriminate between individuals possessing the B antigen (B and AB) and those not possessing the B antigen (A and O) in the Caucasian subsample. However, height in itself can account for the detected difference: B group individuals are taller than non-B individuals by a mean value of 2.4 cm. Further tests support the conclusion that the strongest association is between ABO blood type and height[1].

The age at menarche in relation to ABO blood group phenotypes and hemoglobin-E genotypes was studied among 290 girls belonging to Mongol ethnicity in the North Eastern region of India. The study showed that the age at menarche was influenced by the abnormal hemoglobin E genotype as well as ABO blood group phenotype. Hemoglobin E is an important antibody related to immune system integrity. Thus, the genetic markers play a pivotal role in the growth and development of an individual[2].

Related Topics

Autoimmune disease, general

Hypercholesterolemia

Immunity

Menstrual cycle disorders, amennorhea

REFERENCES

1. Borecki IB, Elston RC, Rosenbaum PA, Srinivasan SR, Berenson GS. ABO associations with blood pressure, serum lipids and lipoproteins, and anthropometric measures. *Hum Hered.* 1985;35:161–170.
2. Balgir RS. Menarcheal age in relation to ABO blood group phenotypes and haemoglobin-E genotypes. *J Assoc Physicians India.* 1993;41:210–211.

GUM DISEASE–*See Periodontal disease*

GYNECOLOGICAL TUMORS–*See Cancer, gynecological tumors*

◼ Halitosis (bad breath)

COMMON CAUSES	BLOOD GROUP O	BLOOD GROUP A	BLOOD GROUP B	BLOOD GROUP AB	SUB GROUPS
Gingivitis or periodontal disease	**********	**	**	***	Non-secretors *************
Systemic disease such as diabetes and esophageal tumors	**	*********	**	**********	
Poor dental hygiene	*All blood groups*	*All blood groups*	*All blood groups*	*All blood groups*	
Bowel toxicity	*All blood groups*	*All blood groups*	*All blood groups*	*All blood groups*	

* = degree of risk

Halitosis may be produced from ingested or inhaled substances that are excreted in part by the lungs; from gingival or dental disease; or from fermentation of food particles in the mouth. It may also result from systemic diseases, such as diabetes and infectious diseases.

There is a relationship between high internal polyamine levels (bowel toxicity) and bad breath.

Related Protocols

BLOOD GROUP A:

1. Antibacterial Protocol

2. Detoxification Protocol

BLOOD GROUP B:

1. Antibacterial Protocol

2. Detoxification Protocol

BLOOD GROUP AB:

1. Antibacterial Protocol

2. Immune-Enhancing Protocol

3. Detoxication Protocol

BLOOD GROUP O:

1. Antibacterial Protocol

2. Anti-Inflammation Protocol

3. Detoxication Protocol

Related Topics

Dental caries

Denture stomatitis

Diabetes

Infectious disease

Periodontal disease

Toxicity, bowel (polyamines)

HASHIMOTO'S THYROIDITIS–_See Thyroid disease, Hashimoto's thyroiditis_

HAY FEVER–_See Allergies, environmental/hay fever_

▓ Headache

COMMON TYPES	BLOOD GROUP O	BLOOD GROUP A	BLOOD GROUP B	BLOOD GROUP AB	SUB GROUPS
Migraine	**	*********	**	***********	Non-secretors **************
Tension	All blood groups	All blood groups	All blood groups	All blood groups	
Cluster	****	*********	**********	********	

* = degree of risk

Headaches are usually classified as three different types: migraine, tension, and cluster.

Migraines are the most severe, chronic type of headache, occurring when the blood vessels of the head and neck spasm or constrict, which decreases blood flow. A migraine commonly lasts from 6 to 48 hours and is characterized by a throbbing, which is usually worse on one side of the head.

Tension headaches are quite common and may occur as the result of any number of circumstances. The most common include close work under poor lighting conditions; cramps from assuming an unnatural head or neck position for long periods of time; arthritis; abnormalities in neck muscles, bones or discs; eye strain; misalignment of teeth or jaws; noise; or poor lighting. They may also be brought on by emotional factors.

Cluster headaches are a common form of recurrent, chronic headache, characterized by sudden sharp pain that disappears within an hour. Cluster headaches appear to be related to the release of histamine and serotonin.

Related Protocols:

BLOOD GROUP A:

1. Antistress Protocol

2. Allergy Control Protocol

3. Detoxification Protocol

Specifics:

Feverfew (Tanacetum parthenicum) 250 mg: 1 capsule twice daily

BLOOD GROUP B:

1. Antistress Protocol

2. Nerve Health Protocol

3. Detoxification Protocol

Specifics:

Riboflavin (B vitamin) 50 mg: 1 capsule twice daily

BLOOD GROUP AB:

1. Antistress Protocol
2. Allergy Control Protocol
3. Detoxification Protocol

Specifics:

Atractylodis Macrocephalae 250 mg: 1–2 capsules daily

BLOOD GROUP O:

1. Antistress Protocol
2. Allergy Control Protocol
3. Anti-Inflammation Protocol
4. Detoxification Protocol

Related Topics

Allergies (general)

Cardiovascular disease

Inflammation

Stress

HEART ATTACK–_See Myocardial infarction_

HEART DISEASE–_See Cardiovascular disease_

HEARTBURN–_See Gastroesophageal reflux disease_

HEMOLYTIC DISEASE OF NEWBORNS–_See Birth defects_

■ Hemorrhoids

COMMON CAUSES	BLOOD GROUP O	BLOOD GROUP A	BLOOD GROUP B	BLOOD GROUP AB	SUB GROUPS
Constipation and straining to pass stools	*******	****	***	***	Non-secretors *************
Obesity	All blood groups	All blood groups	All blood groups	All blood groups	
Pregnancy and childbirth	All blood groups	All blood groups	All blood groups	All blood groups	

* = degree of risk

Hemorrhoids (often called "piles") are clusters of veins in the anus, just under the membrane that lines the lowest part of the rectum and anus. They occur when veins in the rectum enlarge from straining or pressure. The most common causes are constipation and the accompanying extra straining to pass stools, obesity, and pregnancy and childbirth—all of which place a strain on the anus.

Related Protocols

BLOOD GROUP A:

1. Liver Support Protocol
2. Detoxification Protocol
3. Surgical Recovery Protocol

Specifics:

Collinsonia Canadensis (stone root) 100–200 mg twice daily.

BLOOD GROUP B:

1. Intestinal Health Protocol

2. Liver Support Protocol

3. Stomach Health Protocol

4. Surgical Recovery Protocol

Specifics:

Bupleurum falcatum 150 mg: 1–2 capsules daily

BLOOD GROUP AB:

1. Intestinal Health Protocol

2. Liver Support Protocol

3. Detoxification Protocol

4. Surgical Recovery Protocol

BLOOD GROUP O:

1. Intestinal Health Protocol

2. Liver Support Protocol

3. Detoxification Protocol

4. Surgical Recovery Protocol

Related Topics

Cancer, colon

Colitis, ulcerative

Crohn's disease

Digestion

Lectins

Polyps, colon

Stress

HEPATITIS–See Viral Disease, hepatitis B and C

HIGH BLOOD PRESSURE–See Hypertension

HIGH CHOLESTEROL–See Hypercholesterolemia

HIGH TRIGLYCERIDES–See Hypertriglyceridemia

HIVES–See Allergies

HODGKIN'S DISEASE–See Cancer, lymphoma

HOOKWORM–See Parasitic disease, hookworm

H. PYLORI ULCER–See Ulcer, Helicobacter pylori

HYPERACTIVITY–See Attention deficit disorders

HYPERCHOLESTEROLEMIA–High cholesterol.

Hypercholesterolemia	RISK		
	LOW	AVERAGE	HIGH
GROUP A			
GROUP B			
GROUP AB			
GROUP O			
NON-SECRETOR			

Symptoms

There are no symptoms of high cholesterol. It must be detected with a blood test.

About Cholesterol

Cholesterol is an essential nutrient necessary for many functions, including repairing cell membranes, manufacturing vitamin D on the skin's surface, and creating hormones such as estrogen and testosterone. Although the body acquires some cholesterol through diet, about two-thirds is manufactured in the liver, its production stimulated by saturated fat. Saturated fats are those found in animal products, such as meat and dairy.

Cholesterol is a rather strange molecule. Most people think of it as a fat or grease, but cholesterol is actually an alcohol, although it doesn't behave much like alcohol. Its numerous carbon and hydrogen atoms are put together in an intricate three-dimensional network, impossible to dissolve in water. All living creatures use this indissolubility cleverly, incorporating cholesterol into their cell walls to make cells waterproof, much like a commercial water sealant waterproofs a backyard deck. Having waterproof cells is especially critical for the normal functioning of the nerves, since this helps with their ability to conduct electricity. So, not surprisingly, the highest concentration of cholesterol in the body is found in the brain and other parts of the nervous system. Because cholesterol is insoluble in water and thus also in blood, it is transported in our circulation inside particles composed of fats and proteins called lipoproteins.

Lipoproteins are easily dissolved because their outside is composed mainly of proteins that are water soluble. The inside of the lipoproteins is composed of fats, which have the space to carry molecules such as cholesterol. Lipoproteins have various names according to how dense they are. The best known are high density lipoprotein (HDL) and low density lipoprotein (LDL).

The main task of HDL is to carry cholesterol from the tissues, including the artery walls, to the liver. Here it is excreted with the bile, or used for other purposes such as providing a starting point for the manufacture of hormones, such as estrogen, progesterone and testosterone. Only 15% to 20% of cholesterol is transported by HDL, called "good" cholesterol.

LDL, called "bad" cholesterol, transports cholesterol from the liver, where most of our body's cholesterol is produced, to the tissues such as the walls of the blood vessels. When a cell needs cholesterol, it calls for LDLs, which then deliver the cholesterol to the inside of the cells. LDL transports most of the cholesterol in the blood, between 60% and 80%.

The difference between "good" and "bad" is essentially determined by which direction the cholesterol is going. A number of follow-up studies have shown that a lower-than-normal level of HDL cholesterol and a higher-than-normal level of LDL cholesterol are associated with a greater risk of having a heart attack. This is sometimes expressed as a ratio between HDL/LDL; a low HDL/LDL ratio is a risk factor for coronary heart disease, and a high ratio is considered protective. However, in reality, without factoring in the genetics of blood type, your cholesterol level tells very little about your future health.

Blood Group Links

A growing body of research demonstrates that elevated cholesterol as a risk factor for cardiovascular disease is a far more significant factor for blood groups A and AB than for groups O and B.

The relationship between ABO blood groups and total serum cholesterol level was examined in a Japanese population to determine whether elevated cholesterol levels are associated with blood group A, as has been demonstrated in many West European populations. Their results showed that cholesterol levels were very significantly elevated in the blood group A compared to non-A groups[1].

A study examining a total of 380 marker/risk factor combinations found positive associations between blood group A and both serum total cholesterol and low-density lipoprotein cholesterol, while a negative association was found between blood group B and serum total cholesterol[2].

A Hungarian study measured the cholesterol of 653 patients who underwent coronary angiography between 1980 and 1985 in the Hungarian Institute of Cardiology. Their results showed that blood group A was more frequent and blood group O was less frequent among cardiac patients than normally found in the Hungarian population, and that there were differences between the blood groups as to the areas of the vessels where the narrowing of the coronary arteries had occurred[3].

In a nationwide sample of more than 6,000 adolescents aged 12 to 17 years who were Caucasian and of African ancestry, ABO blood group and coronary risk factor levels were measured. Blood group A1 was associated with significantly higher serum total cholesterol levels in Caucasian females independent of all other risk factors, in Caucasian males independent of age and weight, and in southern females of African ancestry independent of age and weight[4]. A separate study (the Bogalusa Heart Study) looked at 656 Caucasian adolescents and 371 adolescents of African ancestry and found the same results with regard to cholesterol (group A being higher than others). Higher levels of LDL lipoproteins were also in group A adolescents over the other blood types.

A survey of 600 men in the city of Edinburgh Scotland showed a significantly higher level of serum cholesterol in men who were blood group A versus all others. No association between Rh groups and cholesterol was found[5].

An 8-year study of 7,662 men published in the prestigious *British Medical Journal* found that blood group A is linked to a higher incidence of ISCHEMIC HEART DISEASE, as well as to higher total serum cholesterol concentrations[6].

Several forms of elevated lipoproteins are inherited. One of the more common forms of hyperlipoproteinemia is called type IIB, and it is characterized by increased LDL ("bad cholesterol") and VLDL ("very bad cholesterol"). Type IIB hyperlipoproteinemia is characterized by premature hardening of the arteries, obstruction of the carotid artery (the artery which supplies the head and brain), PERIPHERAL ARTERY DISEASE, HEART ATTACK, and STROKE. Since all of these disorders show higher rates of occurrence in blood group A, it is not surprising that studies have found a significant connection between a hyper-lipoproteinemia IIb and blood group A in both newborns and in patients after MYOCARDIAL INFARCTION[7].

Therapies, Hypercholesterolemia

BLOOD GROUP A:

1. Cardiovascular Protocol

2. Detoxification Protocol

3. Liver Support Protocol

BLOOD GROUP B:

1. Cardiovascular Protocol

2. Detoxification Protocol

3. Liver Support Protocol

BLOOD GROUP AB:

1. Cardiovascular Protocol

2. Detoxification Protocol

3. Liver Support Protocol

BLOOD GROUP O:

1. Cardiovascular Protocol

2. Detoxification Protocol

3. Liver Support Protocol

Related Topics

Cardiovascular disease

Coronary artery disease

Digestion

Hypertriglyceridemia

REFERENCES

1. Tarjan Z, Tonelli M, Duba J, Zorandi A. [Correlation between ABO and Rh blood groups, serum cholesterol and ischemic heart disease in patients undergoing coronarography]. *Orv Hetil.* 1995;136:767–769.

2. Wong FL, Kodama K, Sasaki H, Yamada M, Hamilton HB. Longitudinal study of the association between ABO phenotype and total serum cholesterol level in a Japanese cohort. *Genet Epidemiol.* 1992;9:405–418.

3. George VT, Elston RC, Amos CI, Ward LJ, Berenson GS. Association between polymorphic blood markers and risk factors for cardiovascular disease in a large pedigree. *Genet Epidemiol.* 1987;4:267–275.

4. Gillum RF. Blood groups, serum cholesterol, serum uric acid, blood pressure, and obesity in adolescents. *J Natl Med Assoc.* 1991;83:682–688.

5. Whincup PH, Cook DG, Phillips AN, Shaper AG. ABO blood group and ischaemic heart disease in British men. *BMJ.* 1990;300:1679–1682.

6. Magnus P, Berg K, Boressen AL. Apparent influence of marker genotypes on variation in serum cholesterol in monozygotic twins. *Clin Genet.* 1981;(19):67–70.

7. Oliver MF, Geizerova H, Cumming RA, Heady JA. Serum-cholesterol and ABO and rhesus blood-groups. *Lancet.* 1969;2:605–606.

HYPERIMMUNITY–*See Autoimmune disease (general)*

HYPERTENSION (HIGH BLOOD PRESSURE)—*Elevation of systolic and/or diastolic blood pressure.*

Hypertension	RISK		
	LOW	AVERAGE	HIGH
GROUP A			
GROUP B			
GROUP AB			
GROUP O			
NON-SECRETOR			
NN			

Symptoms

Hypertension is a "silent" disease, with no noticeable symptoms.

About Hypertension

When blood pressure is taken, two numbers are recorded. The systolic reading (the number on top) measures the pressure within the arteries as your heart beats out blood. The diastolic reading (the number on the bottom) measures the pressure present within the arteries as your heart rests between beats.

- Normal systolic pressure is 120 and normal diastolic pressure is 80, or 120 over 80 (120/80).
- Hypertension is 140/90 under age 40, and 160/95 over age 40.

Hypertension increases the frequency of illness and the death rate. This is related to the severity and the duration of hypertension as well as to other risk factors such as smoking, obesity, and high serum cholesterol. Severe illness and death due to hypertension is much more likely once the heart is enlarged. The incidence of HEART ATTACK increases 30-fold in patients with hypertension and an enlarged heart. In the latter condition, approximately 16% of such patients will have a heart attack per year. Hypertension affects the cerebral artery, impairing blood flow to the brain and eventually leading to STROKE.

General Causes and Risk Factors

Factors involved in the development of high blood pressure include the following:

- Excess salt intake
- Potassium deficiency
- Inadequate fiber in diet
- Excess sucrose intake
- Food sensitivities or allergies
- Thyroid problems, both hyper (overactive) and hypo (underactive)
- Obesity
- Calcium and magnesium deficiency
- Toxic heavy metals found in acid rain (Cadmium and lead, the two most common toxicities, can be detected via hair analysis.)
- Smoking (Cadmium is also present in cigarette smoke.)

Blood Group Links

Blood group B seems to have a lower incidence of hypertension over the other blood groups and group A the highest.

Blood viscosity (thickness) among patients with hypertension has been shown to vary by ABO blood group, with hypertensive blood groups A and AB showing greater blood viscosity than hypertensive blood groups B or O[1].

Although the MN blood type system is not as important as the ABO and secretor systems, it has some importance in two aspects of cardiovascular disease: blood pressure and sensitivity to dietary fat intake.

In 1964, researchers in England showed that there was a consistently higher incidence in elevated systolic blood pressure (the top number in a blood pressure reading that denotes the pressure in the arteries between heartbeats) in people who have the NN blood type than those with either the MN or MM blood type. This was done with a study population of 179 residents of Easter Island, who had migrated off the island and were subject to mainland influences[2].

Therapies, Hypertension

ALL BLOOD GROUPS:

Primary hypertension has no cure, but treatment can modify its course. It is estimated that only 24% of hypertensive patients in the United States have their blood pressure controlled to less than 140/90 mm Hg, and 30% are unaware that they have hypertension. Most authorities would agree that patients with systolic blood pressure averaging 140 to 159 mm Hg and/or diastolic blood pressure of 90 to 94 mm Hg should receive antihypertensive drugs if lifestyle modifications do not normalize their blood pressure.

BLOOD GROUP A:

1. Cardiovascular Protocol
2. Antistress Protocol

BLOOD GROUP B:

1. Cardiovascular Protocol
2. Antistress Protocol

BLOOD GROUP AB:

1. Cardiovascular Protocol
2. Antistress Protocol

BLOOD GROUP O:

1. Cardiovascular Protocol
2. Antistress Protocol

Related Topics

Blood clotting disorders

Cardiovascular disease

Coronary artery disease

Stress

Stroke

REFERENCES

1. Dintenfass L, Bauer GE. Dynamic blood coagulation and viscosity and degradation of artificial thrombi in patients with hypertension. *Cardiovascular Research.* 1970;(4):50–60.

2. Cruz-Coke R, Nagel R, Etcheverry R. Effects of locus MN on diastolic blood pressure in a human population. *Ann Hum Genet Lond.* 1964;(28):39–47.

HYPERTHYROIDISM–See *Thyroid disease, hyperthyroidism*

HYPERTRIGLYCERIDEMIA (HIGH TRI-GLYCERIDES)–*Elevated triglyceride concentration in the blood.*

Hypertriglyceridemia	RISK		
	LOW	AVERAGE	HIGH
GROUP A			
GROUP B			
GROUP AB			
GROUP O			
NON-SECRETOR			

Symptoms

There are no specific symptoms that are related to high triglycerides, but they often occur in the presence of the following:

- Diabetes
- Obesity
- Coronary artery disease

About Triglycerides

Triglycerides are formed by three fatty chains linked to each other. Most fat in food and the human body exists in this form. Diabetics often have high triglyceride levels. DIABETES is believed to be the leading cause of hypertriglyceridemia. Treating diabetes successfully will sometimes normalize triglycerides.

Increasing evidence points to elevated triglycerides as a risk factor for HEART DISEASE. For some individuals elevated triglycerides may be a more important risk factor than elevated CHOLESTEROL. The reasons triglycerides increase a person's risk of heart disease remain unclear. High triglycerides are associated with low levels of HDL ("good") cholesterol and with increased amounts of small dense LDL, the worst form of cholesterol. In one recent study, men with the highest fasting triglyceride concentrations were more than twice as likely to have a heart attack than men with the lowest levels, even after the study adjusted for such risk factors as smoking, sedentary lifestyle, and diabetes.

The most common forms of hypertriglyceridemia seen in clinical practice are not the primary (familial) types, but those secondary to other disorders such as OBESITY, excess alcohol consumption, and chronic severe uncontrolled diabetes mellitus.

Blood Group Links

Elevated triglycerides seem to be a primary pathway to cardiovascular disease for groups O and B. Two separate studies have shown that individuals who had a B antigen had higher triglyceride levels than expected[1].

Obesity is a major cardiovascular risk factor for blood group O. It is associated with a lessened sensitivity to insulin, so many overweight individuals eventually go on to develop diabetes. It is a well-known fact that people with diabetes are much more likely to have a heart attack than people without diabetes. This is because the diabetic process tends to accelerate the damage to their arteries, which leads to the arteries hardening and narrowing. Excess weight forces the heart to work harder. On average, weight reduction lowers cholesterol by about 10%, depending on the degree of the weight lost. Interestingly, it is only cholesterol transported by bad LDL that goes down; the small part transported by good HDL goes up.

The trio of obesity, triglycerides, and "bad" lipoproteins has been linked to heart disease in blood group O. In a French study of blood donors, serum triglycerides and lipoproteins were shown to correlate with both obesity and blood group O in a study screening for cardiovascular or cerebrovascular disease[2].

Therapies, Hypertriglyceridemia

ALL BLOOD GROUPS:

1. In most overweight patients, including those with primary and familial hypertriglyceridemia, triglyceride levels drop sharply with only modest weight loss. A person usually does not need to reach ideal body weight or even to lose more than 10 to 15 pounds to bring triglycerides within normal range.

2. Reduce your alcohol intake to three or fewer drinks per week. If your triglyceride levels are above 500 mg/dL, alcohol consumption should be discontinued.

BLOOD GROUP A:

1. Cardiovascular Protocol
2. Metabolic Enhancement Protocol

BLOOD GROUP B:

1. Cardiovascular Protocol
2. Metabolic Enhancement Protocol

BLOOD GROUP AB:

1. Cardiovascular Protocol
2. Metabolic Enhancement Protocol

BLOOD GROUP O:

1. Cardiovascular Protocol
2. Metabolic Enhancement Protocol

Related Topics

Cardiovascular disease

Coronary artery disease

Digestion

Hypercholesterolemia

REFERENCES

1. Contiero E, Chinello GE, Folin M. Serum lipids and lipo-proteins associations with ABO blood groups. *Anthropol Anz.* 1994;52:221–230.

2. Terrier E, Baillet M, Jaulmes B. [Detection of lipid abnormalities in blood donors]. *Rev Fr Transfus Immunohematol.* 1979;22:147–158.

HYPOTHYROIDISM–*See Thyroid disease, hypothyroidism*

I

Immunity

The acquired immune system is made up of cells that will react with only a specific antigen displayed either on the surface of the invading organism or on the surface of an antigen-presenting cell. B- and T-lymphocyte cells are the sole members of this group. Precursors to lymphocytes, called stem cells, can differentiate into either T-cells or B-cells. T-cells differentiate in the thymus and B-cells differentiate in the bone marrow. Each lymphocyte will recognize and become activated by only one antigen. If, for example a *Streptococcus* bacteria enters the body, a lymphocyte that is specific for the bacteria's antigen must encounter it for an effective immune response to be initiated. The lymphocytes that participate in the recognition process, antibody production, and killing process are permanently committed to respond only to that particular antigen on every subsequent exposure, and are therefore said to have "memory."

Cell-Mediated Immunity

Various white blood cells have specific kinds of immune responses. Granulocytes are the most numerous type of white blood cells in the body. They are classified by their ability to accept different types of dyes in the laboratory, based on the pH of the dye. Neutrophils are stained by neutral dyes, eosinophils by acid dyes, and basophils by basic dyes. In the bloodstream, each class has very distinct functions.

Neutrophils. Neutrophils are the workhorse of the body's defense against bacterial infections. Neutrophils, which are also known as polymorphonuclear leukocytes (PMN), constitute the first line of defense against infectious agents or "nonself" substances that penetrate the body's physical barriers. Normally, a serious bacterial infection causes the body to produce an increased number of neutrophils. Neutrophils can move out of the blood vessels into the infected tissue to attack the bacteria. The pus in a boil (abscess) is made up mostly of neutrophils.

Neutrophils are made in the bone marrow and circulate in the bloodstream. Neutrophils can migrate toward sites of infections and destroy invaders by engulfing them (a process called phagocytosis) or by liberating powerful inflammatory free radical chemicals to destroy them externally.

Neutrophils can increase in response to normal stresses such as exercise, pregnancy, excessive cold

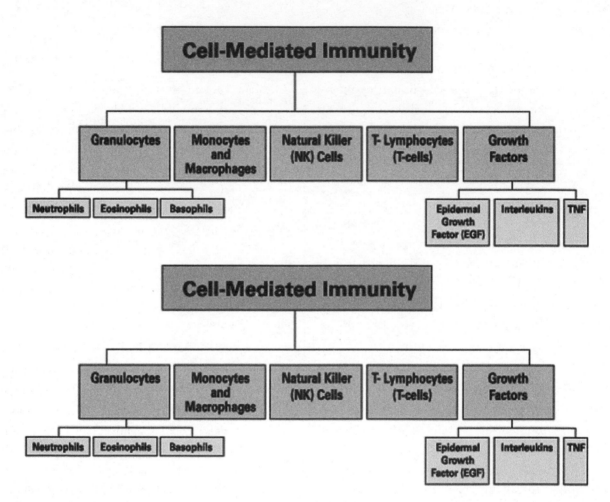

THE IMMUNE SYSTEM

or heat, or emotional states. Neutrophils can also activate and contribute to inflammatory conditions, causing AUTOIMMUNE problems. However, the most common cause of neutrophil activation is a bacterial infection. When the white blood count is low, there may not be enough neutrophils to defend against bacterial infections.

Eosinophils. Both eosinophils and neutrophils attach or "tether" to microbial invaders by the use of lectin-like molecules called selectins. These selectin molecules, like their lectin cousins in nature, attach to glycoproteins on the surface of bacteria, allowing the neutrophils and eosinophils the opportunity to kill them with their free radical chemicals. Normal adult blood contains 0 to 4% eosinophils. Eosinophils can migrate between the blood vessel cells into tissue or into an area of inflammation in the same manner as neutrophils.

The most common causes of increased levels of eosinophils are drug reactions, ALLERGIES, or parasites. Many people with allergies such as ASTHMA and HAY FEVER have elevated eosinophils. Many foreign substances that are capable of stimulating allergic activity by activating eosinophils also appear to simultaneously stimulate the production of anti-blood type antibodies.

Basophils. Basophil cells make up about 0 to 2% of normal blood cells, and are characterized by abundant packets or "granules" inside their bodies. Basophils are found in low numbers in the blood. Their functions are not well understood but they are known to be involved in allergic hypersensitivity responses. These cells have high affinity for an antibody called IgE. Attaching to IgE causes the basophils to release heparin and his-

tamine. Basophils are often increased in ULCERATIVE COLITIS, certain LEUKEMIAS, and certain forms of ANEMIA. Unlike neutrophils and eosinophils, which have a lifespan measured in hours, basophils can apparently live for years.

Monocytes and Macrophages: The Scavengers

Monocytes and macrophages are sort of the Department of Sanitation for the immune system. They are intimately related to each other, as they assume one type of shape (the monocyte) in the blood and another (the macrophage) in the tissues.

Monocytes. Monocytes account for 2% to 9% of normal blood leukocytes. Monocytes leave the marrow when they mature, and they enter the bloodstream, where they circulate for about 14 hours before entering tissue to transform into macrophages. Monocytes are processors of antigen for T-cells, and like neutrophils, they can engulf bacteria.

One not uncommon occurrence in pregnancy is ABO HEMOLYTIC DISEASE, caused by sensitization of the mother's immune system to the blood type antigens of the fetus she is carrying. In most cases the mother's antibodies against blood group antigens A or B of the fetus are able to sensitize its red blood cells for destruction by monocytes.

Macrophages. Macrophages are an example of antigen-presenting cells that take in the invading organism, break it down, and present it to T-cells. If the T-cell is specific for the antigens found in the bacterium (there are many potential antigens in each organism), it becomes activated. One of the most important molecules used by macrophages to kill microorganisms is nitric oxide.

When macrophages encounter bacteria and interferon, the gene responsible for the production of nitric oxide is made in large numbers. When a macrophage encounters a site of infection or inflammation, the gene encoding inducible nitric oxide synthase is activated and the amino acid arginine is converted to citrulline, releasing free nitric oxide.

There is evidence indicating that those who carry a B antigen (blood groups AB and B) may have some difficulty in controlling the activity of nitric oxide. This may help explain why blood group B has been associated with chronic, lingering viral infections.

NK Cells: The "Pac Men"

Natural killer (NK) cells are a subset of T-cells that function as a first line of defense against cancer cells and viral infection. Their primary function is to cause the spontaneous destruction of either a cancer or viral-infected cell. NK cells do not kill indiscriminately. They have several very specialized, lectin-like receptors that recognize major histocompatibility complex molecules expressed on normal cells.

Higher NK activity may be associated with blood group AB, when compared with blood groups A, B, and O. In general, the lowest NK cell activity has been associated with blood group A. Rh blood type might also influence NK cell activity. While some studies found no association, other researchers have observed a higher NK activity against target cells in individuals with Rh negative blood.

Growth Factors

Growth factors are proteins that bind to receptors on the cell surface, with the primary result of activating cellular proliferation and/or differentiation. Many growth factors are quite versatile, stimulating cellular division in numerous different cell types; others are specific to a particular cell type. Here are some of the more commonly known factors and their principal activities.

Epidermal growth factor (EGF), like all growth factors, binds to very specialized receptors on the surface of responsive cells. EGF inhibits certain carcinomas as well as hair follicle cells. EGF also has the effect of decreasing gastric acid secretion. The receptor for EGF shares a similarity with the blood group A antigen; in tests, antibodies directed against the EGF receptor also bound to the A antigen. This could play a role in the increased incidence of certain cancers in group A. No doubt it is also one of the reasons stomach acid secretions are lower in blood group A than in the other groups.

Interleukin-1 (IL-1) is one of the most important immune-modifying interleukins. The main function of IL-1 is to enhance the activation of T-cells in response to antigen.

Interleukin-2 (IL-2) is produced and secreted by activated T-cells and is the major interleukin responsible for T-cell proliferation. IL-2 also exerts effects on B-cells, macrophages, and NK cells. The production of IL-2 occurs primarily by CD4[+] T-helper cells.

Interleukin-4 (IL-4) induces B-cell proliferation, eosinophil and mast cell growth and function, and IgE expression on B-cells. Allergic individuals have a greater propensity to produce IL-4. Many dietary lectins induce the activation of IL-4, which implies that for many people the allergic reaction to dietary lectins may be more important than their agglutinating abilities.

Interleukin-8 (IL-8) acts as a chemo-attractant for leukocytes and connective tissue cells. IL-8 is produced by monocytes, neutrophils, and NK cells and acts as a homing device for neutrophils, basophils, and T-cells.

Tumor necrosis factor (TNF) comes in two varieties, alpha and beta. TNF-alpha is part of a major immune response, increasing cellular responsiveness to growth factors and inducing signaling pathways that lead to proliferation. TNF-alpha is a critical part of the rejection process that occurs when someone is transfused with the wrong blood type. TNF-beta is characterized by its ability to kill a number of different cell types and induce others to differentiate into other forms that result in their death.

Antibodies

There are four classes of antibodies.

- *Immunoglobulin G (IgG)* is the most abundant form of antibody in the blood. IgG antibodies are considered the long-term or memory antibodies. For example, once we have been exposed to the measles virus, our body fights off the original infection over time, and further reinfection is prevented because the B lymphocytes now have a memory of the original measles virus antigen, and have flexed their muscles a bit. For now on, your bloodstream contains traces of anti-measles IgG antibody which serves to protect against reinfection.

IgG is the only class of antibody to pass the placental barrier. Therefore, the mother's IgG provides the only antibody protection for newborns until their own immune system is able to contribute to antibody production. Only blood group O individuals produce anti-A or anti-B in the IgG class. This is why occasionally a case of maternal–fetal incompatibility can result when a blood group O mother is carrying an A or B fetus. The anti-A or anti-B IgG antibodies of the group O mother cross the placenta and react with the fetus.

Blood group O not only carries anti-A and anti-B antibodies, but also a third antibody called anti-AB, which is also an IgG class antibody and can react with either A or B antigens.

- *Immunoglobulin M (IgM)* accounts for about 10% of the total antibody pool in the body and is the predominant antibody of the early immune response. IgM antibodies are the anti-blood type antibodies. IgM is the first antibody to be produced in response to infection since it does not require "class switch" to another antibody class. IgM is the only class produced by the fetus. It is also the largest of the antibodies. IgM binds to antigens on the surface of a bacteria like a spider. Because of its shape and size, IgM is particularly good at causing agglutination. It is the only antibody that is capable of destroying antigen-containing cells without the assistance of any other cells of the immune system. By far the greater majority of the antibodies we make to an opposing blood type (isoagglutinins) are IgM class antibodies. The power of these antibodies to agglutinate red blood cells is amply demonstrated during a blood typing session. When a slide of red cells is mixed with the opposing antibody, the agglutination produced is so strongly reactive that the results can be seen with the unaided eye.

■ *Immunoglobulin A (IgA)* class antibodies are not found in very high concentrations in the blood. Rather, they are primarily found on the mucosal surfaces of the body. IgA is found abundantly in saliva, tears, and breast milk (especially colostrum) and is the primary defense at mucosal surfaces such as bronchioles of the lungs, and the nasal passages, prostate, vagina, and intestine. It normally guards against bacterial and viral infections.

IgA deficiency is the most commonly seen immune deficiency. The deficiency is lifelong and precautions need to be taken to prevent infections. In general, IgA deficiency occurs once in every 400 to 2,000 individuals. However, its incidence varies across racial and ethnic lines. Many IgA-deficient patients are healthy, with no more than the usual number of infections. Others may typically suffer with recurrent ear, sinus, or lung infections that may not respond to standard courses of antibiotics. These patients can have an increased frequency of ALLERGIES, ASTHMA, chronic DIARRHEA (often due to parasites), and autoimmune diseases.

IgA levels have been found to be significantly lower in non-secretors than in secretors. This probably helps to explain why non-secretors have higher incidences of RHEUMATIC HEART DISEASE and chronic KIDNEY DISEASE (glomerulonephritis) over non-secretors: The lower levels of IgA cannot prevent microorganisms from gaining access to the bloodstream from the oral cavity and digestive tract.

■ *Immunoglobulin E (IgE)* is the antibody of allergy. It is produced by B-cells in response to particular allergens. IgE molecules can readily bind to the allergen that causes their production because they are "specific" for the original allergen. Specific IgE molecules travel through the blood and attach to receptors on the surface of mast cells. Different IgE antibodies are produced for each type of allergen, whether it's latex, pet dander, oak pollen, or ragweed pollen. Once on the mast cell surface, allergen-specific IgE can remain for weeks or even months, always ready to bind to the original allergen. The next time the allergen enters the body, the allergic cascade begins and eventually results in the release of histamines from the mast cell. Different chemicals are produced and released, depending on the allergen. These chemicals target certain areas of the body, producing a wide range of symptoms in just minutes or up to an hour.

Dietary lectins have been shown to induce the production of interleukin-4, which in turn activates IgE. This perhaps explains why one of the more common benefits reported by those who follow the blood type food plans is an improvement in allergic manifestations, SINUSITIS, and asthma.

Complement: Chemical Weapons of the Immune System

Though many of the defense mechanisms that are part of our normal immune response are the result of specific cells, such as lymphocytes or neutrophils, there is one very important chemical mechanism without which neither the cellular or humoral part of our defenses would work. One of the most important is a cascade of enzymes made by the liver. The term "complement" was coined by Paul Ehrlich to describe the activity in serum that could heighten the ability of specific antibodies to destroy bacteria.

Visualize complement as a collection of chemicals held in suspended animation in the serum of our blood. If a series of provocations occurs, complement begins to appear, activated by a cascade of enzyme reactions. This cascade is much like a phone tree that parents might use to alert each other of a canceled school day. If Ms. Smith talks to the school and finds out that school is canceled, she might then called Ms. Brown and Mr. Jones. They in turn would each call two other parents, and so on. Complement works the same way. A foreign antigen, or the attachment of an antibody, activates the first enzyme in the complement cascade, which activates the next, and the next— each amplifying the effect of the previous. The final product is the liberation of a very nasty series of enzymes. Complement's role is diverse and essential. It includes:

• *Controlling inflammation through immune garbage removal.* Although the complement system is very much involved in killing things, one of its other major functions is the removal of immune complexes, the insoluble gunk that results from the interaction of an antibody with its antigen. When an antibody attaches to a foreign antigen, the resultant combination very often comes out of solution, or precipitates, much like sugar crystals will precipitate on a string to make rock candy. These precipitates are called immune complexes. Immune complexes can cause problems if they build up in the blood or tissues; part of the job of complement is to help clear them and make them soluble, allowing them to bind to red blood cells which then pass them on to scavenger cells for their ultimate removal. In several autoimmune diseases, including LUPUS, it was found that complement deficiencies can predispose individuals to developing the disease. The build-up of immune complexes play a role in autoimmunity.

• *Coating invaders so they can be seen.* Some complement proteins can coat the microorganism to allow its ingestion by white blood cells (a process called opsonization). Many white blood cells have selectins for certain complement proteins on their surfaces, such as neutrophils, monocytes, and macrophages. When one of the complement proteins binds to a bacteria, these white blood cells can now bind to it as well.

• *Killing invaders single-handedly.* Still others go ahead and just kill the invader itself, by attaching to its surface and drilling holes into it. This is done by attacking the membrane of the bacteria through the production of something called the membrane attack complex—in essence, a molecular tube that is assembled through the surface of the bacteria, causing it to deflate.

• *Acting as a homing beacon.* Others attach to the interloper and act like a homing beacon to other cells of the immune system such as NK cells. On B-lymphocyte cells several complement proteins interact with immune complexes containing complement components and activate, producing antibodies to the foreign substance.

- *Controlling inflammation.* Complement activation results in the production of pro-inflammatory chemicals. One of the more potent complement proteins, C5a, helps to localize the elements of the inflammatory response to the site of inflammation. It causes neutrophils to degranulate, releasing oxygen free radicals, prostaglandins, and eicosanoids. It induces FEVER by stimulating interleukin production, and it causes mast cells and basophils to degranulate, releasing histamine. Histamine released from the mast cells causes the tiny capillaries in our body to become more permeable, allowing white blood cells to migrate into the tissues. The effect of complement on inflammation is one of the main reasons low density lipoprotein (LDL) cholesterol is so bad for us. LDL cholesterol stimulates complement to increase inflammation at the site of the artery wall, one of the first phases of the damage that will in time become artery plaque.

There are three pathways by which complement can be activated:

- The classic pathway is triggered primarily by immune complexes containing an antigen and antibody. This is the most common manner in which complement can be activated.

- The alternative pathway is activated principally by repeating polysaccharide structures such as those found on bacteria. This is probably an older mechanism, which has the advantage of working without the need for outside help by antibodies.

- The lectin pathway was first uncovered by immunologists in the 1980s. The lectin pathway is similar to the classic pathway except it is initiated by a lectin found in our serum called mannan-binding lectin or mannan-binding protein (MBP). MBP binds to the sugar mannose, which is very common on the surface of bacteria. MBP is a member of the serum lectins class, a special class of lectins that are part of the immune system of many higher animals, including humans. Leeks apparently have the same lectin, or one very similar. One of the most important functions of MBP is protection against repeated ear infection in children.

Not surprisingly, many dietary lectins bind mannose, including the lectin from the common garlic bulb (*Allium sativa*). Since in this function the garlic bulb lectin is identical to MBP, it is feasible that some of the antibacterial effects from garlic consumption may result not from the well-known antibacterial component allicin, but rather from the lectin in the plant stimulating the formation of complement. The actions of mistletoe (*Viscum album*), a popular Christmas ornamental and very well-known alternative therapy for certain types of cancer in Europe, are apparently the result of a lectin contained in the plant. Studies have shown that mistletoe lectin has the effect of increasing complement in addition to several antibodies.

There is evidence that lectins may be involved in the recognition between cells, or between cells and various carbohydrate-containing molecules. This suggests that they may be involved in the regulation of physiological functions. They seem to play an important role in the defense mechanisms of plants against the attack of microorganisms, pests, and insects. Fungal infection or wounding of the plant seems to increase lectins. Lectins are believed to be nature's own insecticides; because of this, they have attracted the attention of scientists who are genetically engineering food plants to contain specific lectins. The result will not only have an insecticide effect, but will also be hostile to harmful bacteria in the human and animal gut.

It has increasingly been shown that the body uses lectins (or lectin-like molecules) to accomplish many of its most basic functions, including cell-to-cell adherence, the control of inflammation, the spread of cancer cells, and even the programmed death of certain specific cells of the immune system.

Non-Secretor Status and the Immune System

In general, ABO non-secretors are far more likely to suffer from an immune disease than secretors, especially when it is provoked by an infectious organism. Non-secretors also have genetically induced difficulties removing immune complexes from their tissues, which increases the risk of their systems attacking tissue that contains these complexes. In other words, non-secretors are a bit more predisposed to view their own tissue as unfriendly.

Non-secretors are predominantly affected by virtually every immune system disorder:

- Non-secretors are more prone to generalized inflammation than secretors.

- Non-secretors are more prone to both TYPE I AND TYPE II DIABETES than are secretors.

- Non-secretors who are type I diabetics have much more consistent problems with the yeast *Candida albicans,* especially in their mouths and upper gastrointestinal tracts.

- Non-secretors account for 80% of all FIBROMYALGIA sufferers, irrespective of blood type.

- Non-secretors have an increased prevalence of a variety of autoimmune diseases including ANKYLOSING SPONDYLITIS, reactive ARTHRITIS, psoriatic arthropathy, SJÖGREN'S SYNDROME, MULTIPLE SCLEROSIS, and GRAVES' DISEASE.

- Non-secretors have an extra risk for recurrent URINARY TRACT INFECTIONS, and between 55% and 60% of non-secretors have been found to develop renal scars even with the regular use of antibiotic treatment for urinary tract infections.

INDIGESTION–*See Gastroesophageal reflux disease; Nausea*

Infectious Diseases

Infectious diseases still kill about 13 million people a year worldwide. Even in the United States, 180,000 people died of infectious diseases in 1998. Six infectious diseases killed about 90% of all persons who died before the age of 44: AIDS, TUBERCULOSIS, malaria, measles, DIARRHEA, and PNEUMONIA.

Infection has two factors: susceptibility and survivability. You may be susceptible to a particular infectious disease, but have a high level of survivability against it. You may have a natural resistance to a certain type of infectious disease, but if you contract it, your system breaks down and your survivability becomes questionable.

Blood Group Links

Your blood group dictates the severity of an infection. It also has the ability to adapt to an onslaught, build defenses against it, and to repel it the next time it attempts to attack. Blood group antigens allow the body to fend off some infectious diseases, and impair and limit its response against other infectious diseases.

Many of the most problematic infectious diseases of both the past and present create more problems for some blood groups, while other blood groups are relatively protected. Many experts have made strong arguments that the pressure applied by infectious diseases along blood group lines has been one of the primary factors influencing natural selection and blood group distributions.

Today, if blood groups A and AB feel more vulnerable with their higher rates of CANCER and CARDIOVASCULAR DISEASE, blood group O was certainly more vulnerable 100 to 200 years ago with its susceptibility to infectious diseases such as tuberculosis. Depending upon the place and the time in our history, different blood groups have offered significant advantages. These advantages are a direct result of the relative degree of protection blood group antigens can offer against severe forms of infectious diseases, which over the course of human history have been among the single largest challenge to human health and survival.

The Black Death (YERSINIA) in the Middle Ages killed a third of the entire population of Europe. Those who fled spread the plague to Africa and Asia, where untold millions died. This specific infectious disease, *Yersinia pestis,* produced an O-like antigen. Many of those who died in the sweeping plagues of medieval times were blood group O. In another epidemic redress, survival of the fittest tipped the scales toward a higher relative population of blood group As than there had previously been. Consider this: The single greatest challenge to human survival may also have been the greatest single motivator of diversity and change, leading to an increase in the numbers of survivors of other blood groups.

A century ago, more Europeans died from CHOLERA, an infection of the digestive tract causing extreme fluid loss often leading to death, than from any other illness. Again and again, studies have shown that this disease has a great preference for blood group O over the other blood groups.

At one point in time, smallpox was among the most feared diseases in Europe. We rarely hear of smallpox today, because it has been virtually eradicated. Blood groups O and B always had a greater resistance to and better outcomes with this disease. However, smallpox showed a marked selective effect on groups A and AB. Some researchers have even suggested that, because of this selective pressure to eliminate groups A and AB, certain regions of the world such as Iceland, which were somewhat isolated and exposed to repeated small-pox epidemics, still have a low frequency of group A and a high frequency of group O genes. This is an example of blood group interacting with an infectious agent to promote natural selection.

These are not isolated examples, nor are they remote. Infectious diseases still act selectively, applying genetic pressure for adaptation along blood group lines. And, while group O may have an advantage in modern civilized societies, the wild-card public health factor of infectious disease could at some point shift this advantage to another blood group.

Strong proof for the theory that blood group was an extremely critical influence on the survival of early humanity is the fact that virtually every infectious disease known to influence population demographics (malaria, cholera, typhus, influenza, and tuberculosis) has a preferred blood group that is especially susceptible, and an opposing blood group that is resistant.

Related Topics

Bacterial disease (general)

Bacterial disease, cholera

Bacterial disease, diphtheria

Bacterial disease, *E. coli*

Bacterial disease, gonorrhea

Bacterial disease, *Klebsiella pneumoniae*

Bacterial disease, meningitis

Bacterial disease, pneumonia

Bacterial disease, *Shigella*

Bacterial disease, staphylococcal infection

Bacterial disease, tuberculosis

Bacterial disease, typhoid

Bacterial disease, *Yersinia* (plague)

Viral disease (general)

Viral disease, AIDS

Viral disease, hepatitis

Viral disease, influenza

Viral disease, mononucleosis

Viral disease, mumps

INFERTILITY—*The inability to conceive a child.*

Infertility	RISK		
	LOW	AVERAGE	HIGH
GROUP A			
GROUP B			
GROUP AB			
GROUP O			

Symptoms

- Inability to conceive after a period of 12 months of regular sexual activity

About Infertility

It is estimated that about 15% to 20% of all American couples have trouble conceiving a child. The most common causes include the following:

Male:

- Inadequate production of sperm

Female:

- Blocked fallopian tubes
- Menstrual irregularities

Both:

- Sexually transmitted diseases
- Incomplete intercourse

Contraceptives and Fertility

Several studies have been conducted on natural killer (NK) cell (IMMUNITY) activity in women using oral contraceptives. In one study, the researchers found a significantly reduced NK cell activity after 3 months. After 6 months on the oral contraceptives, levels were still generally lower than normal.

In another study female medical students using oral contraceptives had lower NK function and were also found to have increased frequency of sneezing, gastrointestinal distress, runny nose, sore throat, coughing, and total illness symptoms, relative to nonusers of oral contraceptives.

Blood Group Links

Increasingly, we are learning that blood group incompatibility may be a critical factor in infertility. ABO incompatible couples (a blood group A male fertilizing a blood group O female) are frequently seen when miscarriages occur, especially very early in the gestational term. One study of 288 miscarriages showed that there was an excess of blood groups A and B in otherwise normal fetuses that spontaneously aborted. It was concluded that ABO incompatibility between mother and fetus was almost exclusively the cause of miscarriage of chromosomally normal fetuses, and is a likely cause of all early miscarriages[1].

A study of 102 infertile couples showed that 87% were blood group incompatible. The same study also found that, in seven couples with markedly delayed fertility, the nine children that did result were all blood group O, which made them compatible with the mother. The investigators suggested that the infertility was due to the presence of antibodies in the secretions of the mother's genital tract, or incompatible sperm from the father[2].

In another study, a total of 589 compatible mating couples were compared with 432 incompatible mating couples. The mean number of living children presented a significant difference. There was a 21% deficiency of blood group A children in the two groups. Similarly, there was a 16% deficiency of blood group B children in the two groups. There was a 31.9% rate of miscarriage associated with incompatible matings, as compared with 17.15% in compatible matings. This led researchers to theorize that ABO incompatibility results in "cervical hostility" between the man's blood group antigen, which is present in his sperm, and the woman's opposing antibodies (isoagglutinins), present in her cervical mucus[3].

In general, levels of isoagglutinins are higher

in individuals of African ancestry. Caucasians had higher anti-A than anti-B levels, and those levels were higher in females than in males. In those of African ancestry, the anti-B levels were almost as high as anti-A levels, and little sex difference was found[4].

Therapies, Infertility

ALL BLOOD GROUPS:

Opposing blood group antibodies can be induced by foods that contain opposing blood group antigens. It is not unreasonable to conclude that the many case histories of previously infertile women conceiving and producing healthy offspring by simply eating correctly for their blood type is the result of the lowering of these opposing blood group antibodies. How? By avoiding continued reinoculation with the problematic foods.

BLOOD GROUP A:

1. Female Balancing Protocol
2. Male Health Protocol
3. Detoxification Protocol

BLOOD GROUP B:

1. Female Balancing Protocol
2. Male Health Protocol
3. Detoxification Protocol

BLOOD GROUP AB:

1. Female Balancing Protocol
2. Male Health Protocol
3. Detoxification Protocol

BLOOD GROUP O:

1. Female Balancing Protocol
2. Male Health Protocol
3. Detoxification Protocol

Related Topics

Immunity

Menstrual cycle disorders

REFERENCES

1. Lauritsen JG, Grunnet N, Jensen OM. Materno-fetal ABO incompatibility as a cause of spontaneous abortion. *Clin Genet.* 1975;7:308–316.
2. Solish GI. Distribution of ABO isohaemagglutinins among fertile and infertile women. *J Reprod Fertil.* 1969;18:459–474.
3. Cantuaria AA. Blood group incompatibility and cervical hostility in relation to sterility. *Obstet Gynecol.* 1978;51:193–197.
4. Kulkarni AG, Ibazebe R, Fleming AF. High frequency of anti-A and anti-B haemolysins in certain ethnic groups of Nigeria. *Vox Sang.* 1985;48:39–41.

Inflammation

The word *inflammation* literally means "a burning," and has been in the medical literature since the first century AD when the Roman physician Celsus formulated his famous cardinal signs of inflammation: *calor* (heat), *ruber* (redness), *tumor* (swelling), and *dolor* (pain). To this list, the noted German pathologist Rudolf Virchow added *functio laesa* (loss of function).

In and of itself, inflammation serves a positive function. Without an adequate inflammatory response to fight infection and promote healing of damaged tissue, we would not survive for long. The types of damage that induce inflammation include tissue damage, bone fracture, and injuries due to cuts, burns, infections, and ALLERGIES. At the same time, however, the inflammatory response exists within every living cell as a biochemical and cellular time bomb. More people die from inflammatory diseases than all other disease processes combined; just ponder for a moment the huge number of medical conditions with the ending "-itis."

Inflammation is closely integrated with the immune responses that constitute healing and repair of damaged tissue. Virtually all of the white blood cells (neutrophils, lymphocytes, eosinophils, basophils, and monocytes), as well as the blood clotting platelets and mast cells, are involved in the inflammatory response. The cells involved either contain or can produce more than 100 chemical mediators of the inflammatory response. (See IMMUNITY.)

Inflammation directs the protective molecules of the immune system into damaged tissues by increasing the blood supply to the infected area and increasing capillary permeability, processes that allow larger molecules to pass through the outer layer than would normally be allowed so that new recruits can migrate into the affected area.

The cytokines that play important roles in inflammation include interleukin-1 (IL-1) and IL-6, which induce the release of acute phase proteins such as complement, and act as fever producers or pyrogens. Tumor necrosis factor causes leukocytes to adhere to the walls of the blood vessels by promoting the expression of adhesion molecules, such as the selectins. Once the leukocytes adhere, they are stimulated to migrate farther by other chemical attractants that are being produced by cells already at the injury site. If the inflammation is due to infection, the initial response will be the phagocytic cells of innate immunity, which will attach to the microbes nonspecifically, or through receptors for complement or antibody if these have already coated the interloper. Once attached, the phagocytic cells extend long arms of the cell bodies around the virus or bacteria until they connect, forming a sac inside the cell filled with the microbe. At that point the white blood cell begins to pump in powerful enzymes to kill the microbe. These enzymes are a class called lysozymes or peroxidases; they work by producing a highly reactive species of oxygen that can fuse with the outer membranes of bacteria, or directly destroy the genetic material of bacteria and viruses.

If the infection persists, the phagocytic response will be supplemented by the elements of acquired immunity, such as antibodies and mast cells with their packets of histamine granules. Histamine is a prominent player in many types of inflammation, including allergy. The antihistamine drugs that many depend on during an allergy season are acting effectively as anti-inflammatory agents by reducing the production of histamine.

The protracted process of inflammation can often be more harmful than the event that originally stimulated it. A system of such complexity with so many different players can be difficult to control. Many chemicals involved in the immune response are very caustic, as their main purpose is to kill the invader. If the inflammatory reaction is too intense, there can be a spillover of these chemicals, resulting in damage to the tissue in the area as well.

One of the reasons that blood group O is more prone to inflammatory problems in general may have to do with the fucose sugar that forms its blood group antigen. Fucose sugars serve as adhesion molecules for lectin-like molecules found on white blood cells (selectins), which allow for migration of white blood cells from the bloodstream into the areas of inflammation[1].

Inflammation also results when tissue injury activates blood clotting factors that promote the clotting or coagulation cascade. Through a multi-step process, the cascade results in the production of plasmin, which controls the dissolution of the clot and activates complement and inflammatory kinins, which cause smooth muscle contraction, increase vascular permeability, induce adhesion molecule expression on endothelial cells, and cause pain and itching sensations.

Factor VII, one of the important clotting factors and typically elevated in blood group A, is elevated instead in blood group B individuals when they are in the acute stage of inflammation[2]. Therefore, blood group B is more susceptible to severe inflammatory response in trauma and injury.

One of the more important inflammatory molecules of the immune response is fibrinogen, an acute-phase reactant (like complement) that increases in concentration in response to trauma,

tissue inflammation, and pregnancy as well as the introduction of biological stimulators as growth hormone, inflammatory prostaglandins, and certain bacterial toxins. Fibrinogen is produced by the liver and taken up by the platelets. Fibrinogen is a tenacious molecule that rapidly finds its way to a variety of surfaces, including foreign materials and the underlayment of the blood vessels. During inflammation, fibrinogen escapes into the tissues where it is converted into fibrin.

As with STRESS, MYOCARDIAL INFARCTION, DIABETES, and certain malignancies, THYROID DISEASE is characterized by viscosity (thickness) differences among the blood groups, especially when group A is compared to group O. Blood group A individuals with thyroid disease have been found to have higher levels of fibrinogen and a lower albumin/fibrinogen ratio when compared to blood group O. The inflammatory processes of the body use fibrinogen, von Willebrand factor, and factor VIII as "adhesive glues" to form a matrix of collagen, platelets, and fibrin[3].

Related Topics

Ankylosing spondylitis

Arthritis, rheumatoid

Autoimmune disease (general)

Colitis, ulcerative

Crohn's disease

Immunity

Lectins

Thyroid disease

REFERENCES

1. Listinsky JJ, Siegal GP, Listinsky CM. Alpha-L-fucose: a potentially critical molecule in pathologic processes including neoplasia. *Am J Clin Pathol.* 1998;110:425–440.

2. O'Donnell J, Tuddenham EG, Manning R, et al. High prevalence of elevated factor VIII levels in patients referred for thrombophilia screening: role of increased synthesis and relationship to the acute phase reaction. *Thromb Haemost.* 1997;77:825–828.

3. Dintenfass L, Forbes CD. Effect of fibrinogen on aggregation of red cells and on apparent viscosity of artificial thrombi in haemophilia, myocardial infarction, thyroid disease, cancer and control systems: effect of ABO blood groups. *Microvasc Res.* 1975;9:107–118.

INFLAMMATORY BOWEL DISEASE–*See*

Colitis, ulcerative; Crohn's disease

INFLUENZA–*See Viral disease, influenza*

INSOMNIA–*The inability to sleep.*

Insomnia	RISK		
	LOW	AVERAGE	HIGH
GROUP A			
GROUP B			
GROUP AB			
GROUP O			
NON-SECRETOR			

Symptoms

- Inability to sleep enough at night
- Difficulty falling asleep at night
- Waking up during the night
- Daytime fatigue or sleepiness
- Loss of concentration and mental alertness

About Insomnia

Insomnia is the most common of all sleep disorders. Almost everyone has occasional sleepless nights, perhaps due to STRESS, indigestion, or drinking caffeinated beverages. Insomnia is a lack of sleep that occurs on a regular or frequent basis, often for no apparent reason. Insomnia is often accompanied by unwanted daytime naps. Many persons spend 10 to 12 hours in bed at night trying to sleep.

Sleep can be adversely affected by an erratic sleep–wake schedule, an unpleasant bedroom environment (extreme temperature, uncomfortable bed, excessive noise, inappropriate lighting, or a restless or snoring bed partner), poor timing of meals, lack of regular exercise, DEPRESSION, and inappropriate or excessive use of caffeine, alcohol, or medications.

Insomnia is relatively common in the elderly, because as we grow older our sleep patterns and lifestyles change. Complaints of insomnia among the elderly often center on sleep maintenance or early morning awakening (common with depression). Social isolation and daytime inactivity contribute to insomnia, as do alcohol and over-the-counter sleep preparations.

The Circadian Rhythm

A regulated sleep cycle is essential to well-being and the health of the immune system.

Many of our bodily systems function on 24-hour clocks. Bone growth has a 24-hour clock. Skin regeneration has a 24-hour clock. The IMMUNE SYSTEM has a 24-hour clock. And our sleep–wake cycle functions on a 24-hour clock. In fact, our bodies have more than 100 circadian rhythms. Each unique 24-hour cycle influences an aspect of our body's function, including body temperature, hormone levels, heart rate, blood pressure, and even pain threshold. Almost no area is unaffected by circadian rhythms. Scientists can't explain precisely how the brain keeps this 24-hour time schedule, but they do know that the brain relies on outside influences such as sunlight and darkness to help with the regulation.

The stress hormone cortisol is also released on a 24-hour cycle, so adherence to the circadian rhythm has a tremendous influence on stress levels. Under ideal circumstances, cortisol's schedule results in the highest levels being produced between 6 and 8 A.M., with a gradual decline throughout the day.

Researchers have proposed that the 24-hour secretion of cortisol helps cue many of the other 24-hour rhythms. For example, a midnight cortisol value above 3 nanomoles will disrupt bone regeneration on the following day by shifting the relative balance of bone metabolism away from making new bone and toward bone turnover. A similar process occurs with skin regeneration. By raising cortisol at night, the ability of skin to regenerate declines. Skin literally ages before its time. The immune system will be disrupted if the cortisol level is high during sleep. High cortisol levels disrupt REM sleep.

A study was conducted on military cadets to determine the effect of multiple stresses in addition to a circadian disruption. The study was conducted during a 5-day training course of heavy physical exercise, food deprivation, and sleep deprivation. The 24-hour levels of the hormones DHEA, testosterone, and thyroid-stimulating hormone decreased substantially. After the first 12 hours, all of the other lab measures of thyroid function showed a consistent and constant decline. Not surprisingly, cortisol went up. Of course performance began to trail off, but what about the circadian rhythm? The researchers found in their own words "the circadian rhythm was extinguished." Fortunately, the training course ended after 5 days, but even after another 5 days of rest, the circadian rhythms of the cadets had not completely normalized[1].

Blood Group Links

With higher than normal levels of cortisol, blood groups A and B have a greater tendency to experience sleep disturbances, especially in conditions of stress. This is a vicious cycle, since sleep disturbances themselves produce higher levels of cortisol.[2]

Therapies, Insomnia

ALL BLOOD GROUPS:

1. *Avoid over-the-counter sleep aids.* Over-the-counter sleep aids contain antihistamines to induce drowsiness. Over time they lose their effectiveness and actually have a reverse effect.

2. *Exercise.* Exercise according to your blood group's recommendation not only reduces stress levels but also promotes a regulated sleep cycle.

3. *Avoid or limit caffeine, alcohol and nicotine.* Caffeine and nicotine can keep you from falling asleep. Alcohol can cause unrestful sleep and frequent awakenings.

4. *Reset your body's clock.* If you fall asleep too early, use light to push back your internal clock. In the evenings, go outside in the sun or sit near a bright light.

5. *Avoid or limit naps.* Naps can make it harder to fall asleep at night. If you can't get by without one, try to limit a nap to 45 minutes.

BLOOD GROUP A:

1. Antistress Protocol
2. Liver Support Protocol
3. Detoxification Protocol

Specifics:

Methylcobalamin: 1–3 mg per day, taken in the morning

Melatonin: 200 mg per day, taken in the evening

BLOOD GROUP B:

1. Antistress Protocol
2. Liver Support Protocol
3. Detoxification Protocol

Specifics:

Methylcobalamin: 1–3 mg per day, taken in the morning

Melatonin: 200 mg per day, taken in the evening

BLOOD GROUP AB:

1. Antistress Protocol
2. Liver Support Protocol
3. Detoxification Protocol

BLOOD GROUP O:

1. Antistress Protocol
2. Liver Support Protocol
3. Detoxification Protocol

Related Topics

Aging diseases

Anxiety disorders

Depression, bipolar

Depression, unipolar

Stress

REFERENCES

1. Opstad K. Circadian rhythm of hormones is extinguished during prolonged physical stress, sleep and energy deficiency in young men. *Eur J Endocrinol.* 1994;131:56–66.
2. von Treuer K, Norman TR, Armstrong SM. Overnight human plasma melatonin, cortisol, prolactin, TSH, under conditions of normal sleep, sleep deprivation, and sleep recovery. *J Pineal Res.* 1996;20:7–14.

INSULIN RESISTANCE (SYNDROME X)–

A cluster of metabolic disorders viewed as a pathway to diabetes and cardiovascular disease.

Insulin resistance	RISK		
	LOW	AVERAGE	HIGH
GROUP A			
GROUP B			
GROUP AB			
GROUP O			
NON-SECRETOR			

Symptoms

- Insulin resistance
- High blood sugar
- Hypertension
- High cholesterol
- High triglycerides
- Obesity

About Syndrome X

It is often the case that certain metabolic conditions occur simultaneously. That is, a person with DIABETES may also be overweight and have HIGH BLOOD PRESSURE; or someone with HEART DISEASE may also have HIGH TRIGLYCERIDES, OBESITY, and diabetic symptoms. In recent years, medical researchers have given increasing attention to a condition they've named Syndrome X. Syndrome X is a clustering of metabolic problems. The factors are the following:

- Insulin resistance (cells do not respond effectively to the insulin that the body creates)
- Elevated plasma glucose (high blood sugar)
- Lipid regulation problems (elevated triglycerides, increased small low density lipoproteins, and decreased high density lipoproteins)
- High blood pressure
- A prothrombic state (prothrombin is a plasma protein produced in the liver in the presence of vitamin K, and converted into thrombin in the clotting of blood)
- Obesity (especially central obesity, a predisposition to carrying gained weight in the abdomen)

These factors combine to form Syndrome X. This cluster of metabolic disorders interacts and promotes the development of adult-onset type II diabetes, atherosclerosis, and cardiovascular disease.

Blood Group Links

Syndrome X is most common for blood group A, followed by blood group B. This often includes elevated fasting blood sugar levels, impaired glucose tolerance, hypertension, and high cholesterol and triglycerides. Higher than average cortisol levels, which are typical for group A and group B individuals, add to the severity of the syndrome, because they produce a very similar carbohydrate and lipid metabolism profile as that found in individuals impaired by Syndrome X[1].

Although blood groups O and AB are less likely

to have Syndrome X, certain foods will set in motion a pattern of insulin resistance for them. In effect, all blood groups are vulnerable to Syndrome X, given a regular diet rich in the wrong kind of foods for one's blood type.

Because of the associations with non-secretor status and both diabetes and heart disease, many different researchers have explored the connection between Syndrome X and Lewis and non-secretor blood types. Just as is the case with diabetes and heart disease, individuals with Lewis (a−b−) phenotype are most predisposed to Syndrome X. It has even been hypothesized that Lewis (a−b−) men and Syndrome X share a close genetic relationship on chromosome 19 and that the Lewis (a−b−) phenotype is a genetic marker of the insulin resistance syndrome[2,3].

Another reason non-secretors have higher incidences of Syndrome X is because they form clots more readily and have slower bleeding times. Non-secretors, and especially Lewis negative individuals, are at a greater risk of developing adult-onset diabetes, according to studies. They also are at greater risk of developing complications from diabetes. In addition, data show that non-secretors and Lewis negative individuals are more at risk for heart attacks.

Therapies, Insulin Resistance (Syndrome X)

ALL BLOOD GROUPS:

Most people with a weight problem have the entire cluster of symptoms associated with Syndrome X, or at least a few of them. Weight loss can be crucial to the repair of all of the metabolically impaired functions of Syndrome X. Re-

ducing overall body fat can eradicate potentially debilitating long-term effects.

BLOOD GROUP A:

1. Metabolic Enhancement Protocol
2. Cardiovascular Protocol
3. Liver Support Protocol

BLOOD GROUP B:

1. Metabolic Enhancement Protocol
2. Cardiovascular Protocol
3. Liver Support Protocol

BLOOD GROUP AB:

1. Metabolic Enhancement Protocol
2. Cardiovascular Protocol
3. Liver Suppport Protocol

BLOOD GROUP O:

1. Metabolic Enhancement Protocol
2. Cardiovascular Protocol
3. Liver Support Protocol

Related Topics

Cardiovascular disease

Coronary artery disease

Diabetes metllitus, type II

Hypercholesterolemia

Hypertension

Hypertriglyceridemia

Obesity

REFERENCES

1. Petit JM, Morvan Y, Mansuy-Collignon S, et al. Hypertrig-lyceridaemia and Lewis (A-B-) phenotype in non-insulin-dependent diabetic patients. *Diabetes Metab.* 1997;23:202–204.

2. Petit JM, Morvan Y, Viviani V, et al. Insulin resistance syndrome and Lewis phenotype in healthy men and women. *Horm Metab Res.* 1997;29:193–195.

3. Clausen JO, Hein HO, Suadicani P, Winther K, Gyntelberg F, Pedersen O. Lewis phenotypes and the insulin resistance syndrome in young healthy white men and women. *Am J Hypertens.* 1995;8:1060–1066.

INTERMITTENT CLAUDICATION–*See Peripheral artery disease*

INTERSTITIAL CYSTITIS–*See Cystitis*

IRON DEFICIENCY ANEMIA–*See Anemia, iron deficiency*

IRREGULAR PERIODS–*See Menstrual cycle disorders*

ISCHEMIC HEART DISEASE–*Condition affecting the supply of oxygen to the heart muscle itself.*

Ischemic heart disease	RISK		
	LOW	AVERAGE	HIGH
GROUP A			
GROUP B			
GROUP AB			
GROUP O			
NON-SECRETOR			

Symptoms

- Squeezing pressure, heaviness, or mild ache in the chest (usually behind the breastbone)
- Aching in a tooth with or without squeezing pressure or heaviness in the chest
- Aching into the neck muscles or jaw
- Aching into one or both arms
- Aching into the back
- A feeling of gas in the upper abdomen and lower chest
- A feeling that you're choking or shortness of breath
- Paleness and sweating

About Ischemic Heart Disease

Ischemic heart disease can occur when an artery bringing blood to the heart is narrowed by spasm or disease, causing a loss of oxygen. It is a sign of CORONARY ARTERY DISEASE.

As many as 3 to 4 million Americans may have ischemic episodes without knowing it. These people, who have ischemia without pain, have silent ischemia. They may have a heart attack with no prior warning. In addition, people with ANGINA (chest pain) also may have undiagnosed episodes of silent ischemia. Various tests, such as an exercise test or a 24-hour portable monitor for an electrocardiogram (Holter monitor), are used to diagnose silent ischemia.

Blood Group Links

The relationship of factor VIII (see BLOOD CLOT-TING DISORDERS) activity, FVIIIC, and von Willebrand factor antigen (vWF:Ag), with ischemic heart disease were examined in 1,393 men who were aged 40 to 64 years old at their entry to the Northwick Park Heart Study (NPHS). These men had experienced 178 first major episodes of ischemic heart disease during an average follow-up period of 16.1 years. The incidence of ischemic heart disease was significantly higher in those of blood group AB than in those of groups O or B, particularly for fatal events. There was no evidence that the FVIIIC and vWF:Ag associations with ischemic heart disease are determined by ABO group. Thus, the factor VIII and ABO blood group effects appeared to be independent. Group AB may be a genetic marker of characteristics influencing other indices of ischemic heart disease risk such as short stature; the Northwick Park Heart Study found that the men (though not women) of group AB were about 2 cm shorter than those of other groups[1].

An 8-year study of 7,662 men published in the prestigious *British Medical Journal* found blood type A was linked to a higher incidence of ischemic heart disease, as well as to higher total serum cholesterol concentrations[2].

Results from the NHLBI Family Heart Study also showed a higher risk of coronary heart disease (odds ratio was 2.0 [95% confidence interval = 1.2 to 3.1]) for Lewis (a−b−) versus other Lewis groups. TRIGLYCERIDES were significantly higher in the Lewis (a−b−) individuals. Among women, there was also a trend toward increased risk of coronary heart disease among Lewis negative phenotypes; however, the trend was dramatically weaker than among the men[3].

Additional research has duplicated these results, supporting and adding to the evidence that the Lewis negative phenotype Lewis (a−b−) is a marker of high risk for the development of ischemic heart disease. Even excluding the Lewis negative phenotype, the secretor phenotype Lewis (a−b+) was found to be a genetic marker of resistance against the development of ischemic heart disease, whereas ABH non-secretor status is a risk factor predisposing individuals toward heart disease[4].

Therapies, Ischemic Heart Disease

BLOOD GROUP A:

1. Cardiovascular Protocol

2. Metabolic Enhancement Protocol

3. Antistress Protocol

BLOOD GROUP B:

1. Cardiovascular Protocol

2. Metabolic Enhancement Protocol

3. Antistress Protocol

BLOOD GROUP AB:

1. Cardiovascular Protocol

2. Metabolic Enhancement Protocol

3. Antistress Protocol

BLOOD GROUP O:

1. Cardiovascular Protocol
2. Metabolic Enhancement Protocol
3. Antistress Protocol

Related Topics

Angina pectoris

Cardiovascular disease

Coronary artery disease

Diabetes mellitus

Hypertension

Insulin resistance

Myocardial infarction

Obesity

Stress

J

JAUNDICE (YELLOWING OF THE SKIN)–*See Liver disease*

K

KIDNEY FAILURE–*See Aging diseases*

KIDNEY INFECTION–*See Cystitis*

KIDNEY STONES–*Formation of calcified urine stones in the urinary tract.*

Kidney stones	RISK		
	LOW	AVERAGE	HIGH
GROUP A			
GROUP B			
GROUP AB			
GROUP O			

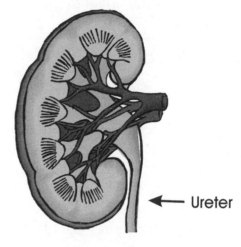

THE KIDNEY

Urine flows from the kidney through the ureter into the bladder.

Symptoms

Kidney stones are asymptomatic unless the stone is large or causes a blockage or infection. Then, the most common symptoms include:

- Intense, cramping pain (abdominal spasms) radiating from the lower back down to the groin
- Bloody, cloudy, or foul-smelling urine
- Nausea and vomiting
- Persistent urge to urinate
- Fever and chills if an infection is present

About Kidney Stones

Kidney stones occur when urine becomes too concentrated. This causes minerals and other substances in the urine to form crystals on the inner surfaces of the kidneys. Over time these crystals may combine to form a small, hard, stone-like mass. Sometimes this mass, or stone, breaks off and passes into the ureter, one of the two thin tubes that leads from the kidneys to the bladder. Kidney stones are asymptomatic unless the stone is large or causes a blockage or infection.

There's evidence these stones have plagued humans for millennia—scientists have found traces of kidney stones in mummies more than 7,000 years old. Today, more than 1 million cases are reported each year in the United States, and that number is steadily increasing, perhaps related to poor dietary practices.

General Causes and Risk Factors

There is a strong familial risk factor in the development of kidney stones. Other possible causes include frequent urinary tract infections, poor dietary habits, inadequate fluid consumption, and limited physical activity. Some thyroid medications and calcium-based antacids may increase the risk of developing kidney stones.

Blood Group Links

Blood group A individuals tend to have higher levels of calcium in their urine when compared to the other ABO groups. In one study, stone-formers underwent a metabolic investigation and ABO blood group determination. The incidence of blood groups in patients was similar to the ABO phenotype distribution in the general population. Patients with blood group A displayed hypercalciuria in 54% of the cases. Among these, group A patients with positive family history showed higher mean values of calcium excretion and lower ones of GAGs. These results indicated a link to ABO phenotypes as well as a familial risk factor[1].

Therapies, Kidney Stones

ALL BLOOD GROUPS:

Reduce your intake of oxalate from food as a way to reduce urinary oxalate. Although many foods contain oxalate, only a few appear to increase urinary oxalate. These foods are spinach, rhubarb, beet greens, nuts, chocolate, tea, bran, almonds, peanuts, and strawberries.

BLOOD GROUP A:

1. Urinary Tract Health Protocol

BLOOD GROUP B:

1. Urinary Tract Health Protocol

BLOOD GROUP AB:

1. Urinary Tract Health Protocol

BLOOD GROUP O:

1. Urinary Tract Health Protocol

Related Topics

Bacterial disease (general)

Cystitis

REFERENCES

1. Caudarella R, Malavolta N, Rizzoli E, Stefani F, D'Antuono G. Idiopathic calcium urolithiasis: genetic aspects. *Ann Med Interne (Paris)*. 1986;137:200–202.

KLEBSIELLA PNEUMONIAE—*See Bacterial disease*, Klebsiella pneumoniae

L

LEARNING DISABILITIES–*See Attention deficit disorders*

Lectins

All living things manufacture sugars on their surfaces, and sometimes these sugars are also secreted in free form as a type of protective coating. A good example of these free sugars are the algae slimes found on top of stagnant water and our own mucus secretions. Among the tens of thousands of different complex sugars produced by the cell for use in signaling and recognition is one that determines ABO blood group.

Like the other surface sugars, blood group antigens telescope out from the cell wall, and are found principally in the bloodstream and digestive tract. While they are attached to the cell wall, they are not fixed in place—rather, they move around the cell's surface. Sticking out the way they do, in a world of things reacting with one blood group or another, it would seem inevitable that they would get tangled up with things. Most of the time these are agglutination-type reactions.

This is a handy attribute for a bacteria that is trying to stick to the mucus lining of your bladder. Mucus is a rich depository of blood group antigens, especially in secretors, and it serves to protect the delicate mucus membranes, which, unlike skin, are soft and vulnerable. Bacteria, viruses, yeast, and fungi have developed this agglutination ability to gain a beachhead in their continual battle. Mucus is best described as an insulating flypaper. If the bacteria attaches to the mucus instead of the actual tissue, it will be carried away when the mucus separates from the tissue.

Unlike microbes, which use agglutination as an offensive weapon, plants often use agglutinins as a sort of chemical minefield, lacing their tissues with agglutinins against bacteria and fungi to protect against invasion. This is especially important in germinating seeds and early shoots, where they glue up any predatory fungi or bacteria. The actions of these plant agglutinins have been likened to primitive immune systems—functioning in a manner akin to our own antibodies. The appearance of agglutinins in common foods has an additional significance. Many of them are specific for one blood group or another.

Living things manufacture agglutinins in a great variety of shapes and forms, and they don't share any real characteristics other than the ability to clump sugars together.

Lectins are similar to a selective Velcro, a powerful way for organisms in nature to attach themselves to other organisms in nature. This natural Velcro comes in two varieties, one-sided and two-sided. The one-sided variety just gets stuck on things. Lots of germs, and even our own immune systems, use the one-sided variety all the time. Cells in the bile ducts of the liver have lectins on their surfaces to help them snatch up bacteria and parasites. Bacteria and other microbes have lectins on their surfaces that work rather like suction cups so that they can attach to the slippery mucus linings of the body. Sometimes the lectins that viruses or bacteria use can be blood group specific, making the microbe a stickier pest for a person of the favored blood group.

Two-sided lectins stick other cells together, like two tennis balls stuck together by a piece of two-sided Velcro. Think of the fuzz on the tennis ball as the assortment of sugars (including one that determines blood group) that line the surface of the cell.

The degree that lectins stick to cells is mostly determined by the amount of glycoconjugates (or degree of glycosylation) that a particular tissue has. The cells lining the small intestine wall, for example, are typically very glycosylated, and thus less able to bind lectins. Yet it is not just the amount of glycoconjugates that determines the reactivity of dietary lectins. Remember that lectins are very choosy about what they deign to attach to, and their criteria are highly individualized.

Factors influencing glycosylation in the intestines, and hence the activity of dietary lectins, include:

- *Animal species:* Many lectins react with the glycoconjugates of one species and not another. Soybean agglutinin, for example, tends to react with the intestinal cells of rodents more aggressively than with humans.

- *Blood group specificity:* Many lectins are blood group specific.

- *Age:* In some animals, glycoconjugate synthesis drops with age; this is generally not true of humans.

- *Particular area of the small intestine:* The upper intestine (where most absorption occurs, hence the place you would least likely want to have lectin interactions) is more glycosylated than the lower.

- *Position along the villi:* Certain lectins prefer different areas of the finger-like projections of the intestinal wall, called villi.

- *State of cell maturation:* Immature cells that rush in to fill a gap in the defenses of the intestines are much more glycosylated than mature cells, hence they are less able to bind lectins.

- *Diet:* Certain dietary components, such as gums, can enhance the binding of food lectins. On the other hand, certain sugars are specific for a particular lectin and can block its attachment.

- *Bacterial status:* Bacteria in the lower intestine can interact with glycoproteins such as the

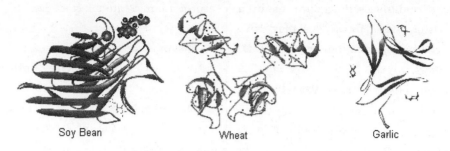

Soy Bean   Wheat   Garlic

DIVERSE STRUCTURAL NATURE OF LECTINS

As can be seen from these 3-dimensional representations, the lectins from different food sources show no similarity with each other. For example, the lectin from soy is a large molecule, while the lectin from wheat germs is a rather small molecule.

blood group antigens, and influence a lectin's ability to attach to them.

- *Sickness or pathology:* Crohn's disease or other inflammatory diseases of the intestines can increase glycosylation. Thus, these tissues are more liable to interact with food lectins.

Effects of Lectins

Lectins are always specific to the species from which they are derived. For example, the lectin found in wheat is different from the lectin found in soy; it has a different shape and it attaches to a different combination of sugars. Lectins are most widely distributed in plants. Particularly abundant in legumes, they account for between 2% and 3% of the total protein content of soybeans, lentils, and peanuts. The second most common source of lectins is seafood, particularly eel, shellfish, snails, halibut, and flounder.

Because they are commonly found in grains, seafood, legumes, and vegetables, lectins are widely abundant in the typical diet. Even tiny amounts of a lectin will suffice to clump huge numbers of cells.

Although many lectins are destroyed by normal cooking, which is why grains and beans are edible, many are not. The lectin found in wheat germ will resist heating at 110°C (230°F) for 30 minutes. Other food lectins known to resist destruction by cooking include apples, carrots, wheat brans, canned corns, pumpkin seeds, bananas, and wheat flour. The clumping abilities of banana agglutinin are actually enhanced by heating. Researchers have also noted high levels of lectin activity in dry roasted peanuts, and certain processed breakfast cereals[1]. Lectins from kidney beans can resist mild cooking and retain their activity, even at 90°C (194°F) for 3 hours. Presoaking the beans, however, results in complete loss of lectin activity.

Many foods showed agglutinating activity so substantial that the extracts could be diluted several-fold. Crude extracts of various foods (tomato, lettuce, cucumber, wheat bran and whole wheat, sesame and sunflower seeds, vanilla yogurt, coconut, banana and baby food banana, carrot, onion, apple, alfalfa, and soy protein) have also been found to bind to human saliva. This may have some significance in the development of dental cavities. Conversely, a lectin found in avocados actually inhibits the binding of bacteria to tooth plaque.

Many lectin-containing foods evade cooking because they are normally eaten raw, such as tomatoes, now the primary vegetable source of vitamins and minerals in the U.S. diet. Unlike most lectins, which usually react with only one blood group or another, tomato lectin is a panagglutinin; it is able to attach itself with equal ease to the cells of all blood groups. The average American consumes around 200 milligrams of lectins per year from tomatoes alone, and many other salad ingredients are rich in lectins.

Studies show that up to 5% of the ingested dietary lectins are absorbed into the bloodstream. Here they can clump and bind to red and white blood cells, destroying them. It has been proposed that much of the low-grade anemia seen in Third World countries may be caused by the destruction of red blood cells from lectin-rich grain and bean diets. However, the actions of food lectins on the digestive tract are probably much more potent. Here they can cause inflammation of the mucus linings, and mimic many of the symptoms of food allergies.

Effects on Digestion

Many people are known to be intolerant to gluten, the most common lectin found in wheat and other grains. The gluten lectin binds to the lining of their small intestine, causing irritation and in-

flammation. Peanut lectin also appears to have a great affinity for certain cells lining the stomach.

A syndrome that is indistinguishable from CELIAC DISEASE, a disorder characterized by abdominal cramps and severe DIARRHEA, can be produced in some people by soybeans. It has been noted that the intestinal tissues of most people with inflammatory bowel diseases such as COLITIS and CROHN'S DISEASE are highly sensitive to the effects of food lectins. This is probably because the digestive tracts of people with these disorders are lined with large numbers of immature cells, the result of the constant need to replace destroyed tissue. Immature cells have more sugar receptors on the surfaces, to which lectins can more easily bind. These sugar receptors disappear as the cells age.

Food lectins interacting with the digestive tract have been known to stimulate the release of histamine, a chemical capable of producing very powerful allergic symptoms. This has led several researchers to ascribe a role to dietary lectins as a cause of FOOD ALLERGY. Laboratory rats treated with jack bean or wheat germ lectin developed a gut membrane that was impermeable to small food molecules, but very permeable to the large, highly allergenic food molecules, a situation common in food allergy[2].

Lectins interfere with protein digestion. Researchers observed that wheat germ agglutinin (WGA) dramatically enhanced the activity of membrane–bound maltase, the enzyme that breaks down complex sugars into simple sugars in the small intestine. Under the same conditions, aminopeptidase activity—the enzyme that breaks down polypeptides into amino acids—was inhibited by wheat germ lectin[3].

Dietary lectins can cause growth in the size of the digestive organs. They do this by amplifying other growth stimulants through the release of a class of chemicals called polyamines. A number of studies have shown that increases in the size of the intestines, liver, and pancreas can occur as a result of feeding tests to animals of dietary lectins[4].

Lectins impair absorption. Test animals fed a diet composed mostly of raw navy bean flour were smaller, and had 50% less ability to absorb glucose and use dietary protein than did a control group that was fed navy beans with inactivated lectin. Lectins from wheat germ (*Triticum aestivum*), thorn apple (*Datura stramonium*), or nettle root (*Urtica dioica*) added to the diet of test animals reduced the digestibility and utilization of dietary proteins, and stunted the animals' growth. Wheat germ lectin did the most damage. The researchers were quite certain that the lectins had been bound and actively transported across the intestinal membrane. The three lectins acted as growth factors for the gut, and interfered with its metabolism and function to varying degrees. The study also found that "an appreciable portion of the absorbed wheat germ lectin was transported across the gut wall into the systemic circulation, where it was deposited in the walls of the blood and lymphatic vessels." Wheat germ lectin also stimulated the growth of the pancreas, while causing the thymus, a gland linked to immune system function, to shrink. The study concluded, "Although the transfer of the gene of wheat germ lectin into crop plants has been advocated to increase their insect resistance, the presence of this lectin in the diet may harm higher animals at the concentrations required to be effective against most pests. Its use in plants as natural insecticide is not without health risks for man"[5].

Lectins block digestive hormones. Cholecystokinin (CCK), a hormone that helps digest fat, protein, and carbohydrates by stimulating the secretion of digestive enzymes, is affected by several dietary lectins, especially wheat germ[6]. The lectins bind to CCK receptors and inhibit its action. Since CCK is also present in the brain in relatively high concentrations, it is thought to play a role in appetite control, so these lectins also may contribute to weight problems. Thus, when CCK is suppressed, appetite is increased. According to a working hypothesis, when lectins block the CCK receptor they inhibit the secretion of amylase, an enzyme necessary for the digestion of carbohydrates. The activity of amylase is naturally higher in blood group A, which makes perfect sense as group A is more suited to metabolizing complex carbohydrates than the other blood groups.

Lectins influence gut permeability. Our intestines are very selective about the size and quality of what is absorbed through their lining. Food lectins have been shown to increase gut permeability, which may exacerbate the condition of those who are already on their way to developing an allergy or intolerance to other proteins[7].

In one study, animals fed diets containing kidney beans showed increased intestinal permeability to serum proteins that had been injected into their bloodstreams. Then they were given an even bigger dose of kidney bean protein. The protein, again injected into the animals' bloodstreams, leaked into the open space of the inner body and was also detected in the walls of the small intestine. This showed that dietary lectins may be at least partially responsible for the loss of serum proteins, and they may also contribute to other food intolerances as a consequence of the loss of gut integrity.

Dietary lectins damage the intestinal lining. It has been known for over 15 years that several legume lectins damage the delicate microvilli of intestinal absorptive cells in the small intestine. In one study, test animals were given red kidney bean lectin. Within 2 to 4 hours, the microvilli of test animals showed extensive vesiculation—bubbling—along the length of the villi, which returned to near normal within 20 hours. The individual length of the microvilli were also reduced significantly, but again returned to normal within 20 hours. The investigators speculated that "microvilli may be repeatedly damaged and repaired after ingestion of specific dietary lectins."

Lectins and Blood Groups

As mentioned earlier, lectins can be blood group specific—that is, able to agglutinate the cells of one ABO type but not those of another. Lima bean lectin agglutinates cells of human group A but not those of O or B. The seeds of *Lotus tetragonobolus* can agglutinate group O specifically, and *Bandeiraea simplicifolia* can agglutinate group B. The specificity of lectins is so sharply defined that they can even differentiate among blood subgroups. In fact, until *Dolichos biflorens* lectin was shown to react more vigorously with some A cells than others, we did not know that there were two varieties of A: A1 and A2.

Other blood groups can be distinguished by lectins, such as M and N types, and lectins can help distinguish secretor status.

Group O–Specific Lectins

Given that blood group O developed far earlier than the other blood groups, it is not surprising that many of the later agricultural foods, such as common grains, react negatively with this blood group. Probably the most problematic lectin for group O is found in wheat germ and whole wheat products. Wheat germ lectin can slow group O metabolism, causing an insulin-resistant obesity problem. To a lesser degree, this is also true of corn and corn byproducts.

Blood group O should also avoid catfish, eels, caviar, walnuts, eggplants, white potatoes, alfalfa sprouts, and blackberries. Rh-positive group O individuals should avoid blueberries, bananas, and papayas.

Group A–Specific Lectins

A large number of foods contain lectins capable of clumping the blood and tissues of blood group A. These foods include lima beans, string beans, pinto beans, navy beans, commercial mushrooms, most commercial breakfast cereals, tomatoes, cinnamon, flounder, swordfish, cantaloupe, bananas, apples, eggplant, anchovies, cauliflower, oranges, shrimp, trout, and clams.

Soy is a special circumstance: It possesses the ability to clump small numbers of normal group A cells, but it also has a great ability to detect and clump many forms of cancers that group A is prone to develop.

Group B–Specific Lectins

Blood group B should avoid chicken, peanuts, pomegranates, persimmons, sunflower seeds, sesame seeds, beets, salmon, radishes, apples, trout, black-eyed peas, mung bean sprouts, corn, and buckwheat.

Group AB–Specific Lectins

Blood group AB should avoid any of the foods that contain lectins capable of reacting with groups A or B.

Effects on Other Bodily Systems

Many lectins, including those found in wheat germ, lentils, and green peas, can bind to the body's insulin receptors and mimic the effects of insulin. Wheat germ and lentil lectins are as effective as insulin at enhancing glucose metabolism, and have been shown to enhance the effectiveness of insulin itself[8].

This has significant implications for people who must watch their weight. By enhancing the effectiveness of insulin, these lectins may stimulate greater deposits of fat and inhibit fat burnoff. I have found this to be particularly true of type O when they consume a diet high in complex carbohydrates; when they switch to a high-protein diet, they usually have an easier time losing weight.

Cranberry juice is a well-known home remedy for simple BLADDER INFECTIONS. It works by inhibiting the ability of bacteria to adhere to the bladder wall, because cranberry juice is rich in the same sugar found on the bladder walls that are bacteria's source of attachment, an effect not unlike running a piece of adhesive tape through the dustbin.

Nervous tissue, as a rule, is very sensitive to the agglutinating effect of food lectins. This may explain why certain researchers feel that allergy-avoidance diets may be of benefit in certain types of nervous disorders such as HYPERACTIVITY. Russian researchers have noted that the brains of SCHIZOPHRENICS were more sensitive to the attachment of certain common food lectins.

Injections of lentil lectin into the knee joint cavities of non-sensitized rabbits resulted in the development of ARTHRITIS that was indistinguishable from RHEUMATOID ARTHRITIS. Many people with arthritis feel that avoiding the "nightshade vegetables," such as tomatoes and white potatoes, seems to help their arthritis. Not a surprising conclusion, since most nightshades are very high in lectins.

Food lectins can also interact with the surface receptors of the body's white cells, often programming them to multiply rapidly. These lectins are called mitogens because they cause the white cells to enter mitosis, the process of reproduction.

Lectins activate autoantibodies in inflammatory and AUTOIMMUNE DISEASES. Almost everyone has antibodies to dietary lectins in their bloodstream. Some of these have been linked to immune damage to the kidneys in nephropathy (kidney disease) patients. It has been suggested that the antibody produced in rheumatoid arthritis may in fact require activation by wheat germ lectin[9].

The Cancer–Lectin Connection

Under normal circumstances, the production of surface sugars by the cell is highly specific and controlled. In a CANCER cell this is not true. Because their genetic material is scrambled, cancer cells lose much of the control over the production of their surface sugars, and usually manufacture them in greater amounts than a normal cell would. In effect, cancer cells are "fuzzier" than normal cells on their outside, which make them more liable to tangle up if they come in contact with the appropriate lectin. In fact, malignant cells are as much as 100 times more sensitive to the agglutinating effects of lectins than are normal cells. If two slide preparations are prepared, one containing normal cells and the other malignant, an equal dose of the appropriate lectin will convert the slide with malignant cells into a huge entangled clump, whereas the slide of normal cells will only show little, if any, change[10–12].

When cancer cells become agglutinated into huge tangles of hundreds, thousands, or millions, the immune system becomes reactivated. Now the antibodies can target the clumps of cancer cells, identifying them for destruction. This is usually performed by powerful scavenger cells found in the liver.

REFERENCES

1. Nachbar MS, Oppenheim JD. Lectins in the United States diet: a survey of lectins in commonly consumed foods and a review of the literature. *Am J Clin Nutr.* 1980;33:2338–2345.

2. Pusztai A. *Proc Int Symp Control Rel Bioact Mater.* 1995;22:161–162.

3. Erickson RH, Kim J, Sleisenger MH, Kim YS. Effect of lectins on the activity of brush border membrane-bound enzymes of rat small intestine. *J Pediatr Gastroenterol Nutr.* 1985;4:984–991.

4. Grant G. Anti-nutritional effects of soyabean: a review. *J Anim Sci.* 1982;55:1087–1098.

5. Tchernychev B, et al. Natural human antibodies to dietary lectins. *FEBS Lett.* 1996;397:139–142.

6. Jordinson M, Playford RJ, Calam J. Effects of a panel of dietary lectins on cholecystokinin release in rats. *Am J Physiol.* 1997;273(1):G946–G950.

7. Greer F, Pusztai A. Toxicity of kidney bean (Phaseolus vulgaris) in rats: changes in intestinal permeability. *Digestion.* 1985;32:42–46.

8. Weinman MD, Allan CH, Trier JS, Hagen SJ. Repair of microvilli in the rat small intestine after damage with lectins contained in the red kidney bean. *Gastroenterology.* 1989;97:1193–1204.

9. Coppo R, Amore A, Roccatello D, et al. IgA antibodies to dietary antigens and lectin-binding IgA in sera from Italian, Australian, and Japanese IgA nephropathy patients. *American Journal of Kidney Diseases.* 1991;17:480–487.

10. Gan RL. [Peanut lectin-binding sites in gastric carcinoma and the adjacent mucosa]. *Chung-hua Ping Li Hsueh Tsa Chih.* 1990;19:109–111.

11. Lin M, Hanai J, Gui L. Peanut lectin-binding sites and mucins in benign and malignant colorectal tissues associated with schistomatosis. *Histol Histopathol.* 1998;13:961–966.

12. Melato M, Mustac E, Valkovic T, Bottin C, Sasso F, Jonjic N. The lectin-binding sites for peanut agglutinin in invasive breast ductal carcinomas and their metastasis. *Pathol Res Pract.* 1998;194:603–608.

LEUKEMIA–*See Cancer, leukemia*

LIVER CANCER–*See Cancer, liver*

LIVER DISEASE–*Alterations in the functioning of the liver.*

Liver disease	RISK		
	LOW	AVERAGE	HIGH
GROUP A			
GROUP B			
GROUP AB			
GROUP O			

Symptoms

The onset of cirrhosis is often silent, with few specific symptoms to identify what is happening in the liver. As continued scarring and destruction occur, the following signs and symptoms may appear:

- Loss of appetite
- Nausea and vomiting
- Weight loss
- Enlargement of the liver
- Jaundice (yellow discoloration of the whites of the eyes and skin, because bile pigment can no longer be removed by the liver)
- Itching due to the retention of bile products in the skin
- Abdominal swelling due to an accumulation of fluid caused by the obstruction of blood flow through the liver
- Vomiting of blood
- Increased sensitivity to drugs due to inability of the liver to inactivate them

About the Liver

The liver is an organ of truly titanic function. It contributes to the health of the body through its profound effects on several systems, including digestion.

- *The liver is the major chemical factory of the body.* The liver synthesizes many of the body's proteins and lipids.
- *The liver is the great filter of the body.* Blood, containing absorbed nutrients from the small intestine, must first pass through special networks in the liver called sinusoids. Within the sinusoids are found cells of the immune system called Kupffer cells, which scavenge and destroy microorganisms that may have been inadvertently absorbed with nutrients. The liver is also chemically capable of detoxifying an incredibly large inventory of poisons.
- *The liver aids in the absorption of fats.* The liver manufactures bile salts that allow fats to be emulsified (allowing them to mix with water). Bile salts are steroids with detergent properties. By emulsifying fat bile, the salts help its digestion and absorption through the intestinal wall.

Bile is a sticky green fluid produced by the liver. The bile is released into a network of bile ducts that all come together to form the common hepatic duct. Synthesis of bile represents the major use of cholesterol by the body, and accounts for more than half of the 800 mg per day of cholesterol that the average adult uses in his or her metabolic processes. By comparison, the second most common use of cholesterol, the synthesis of steroid hormones, consumes only about 50 mg of cholesterol per day. Since digestion requires more than the actual 400 mg of bile salts produced and secreted into the intestine each day, the body actually recycles bile salts again and again.

About Liver Disease

There are a number of severe problems that can develop in the liver. Alcohol, hepatitis, and drug use tax the functioning of the liver severely, and may lead to cirrhosis. Cirrhosis is a term that refers to a group of chronic liver diseases in which normal liver cells are damaged and replaced by scar tissue. The distortion of the normal liver structure by the scar tissue interferes with the flow of blood through the liver. It also compromises liver function: The loss of normal liver tissue compromises the liver's ability to perform some of its critically important functions. Cirrhosis and other liver diseases take the lives of over 25,000 Americans each year and rank eighth as a cause of death.

Primary biliary cirrhosis (PBC) is a chronic liver disease that causes slow, progressive destruction of bile ducts in the liver. This destruction interferes with the excretion of bile. Continued liver inflammation causes scarring and eventually leads to cirrhosis. Cirrhosis is present only in the later stage of the disease. In the early stages of the illness, the main problem is the build up of substances (like acids and cholesterol) in the blood that are normally excreted into the bile.

The onset of cirrhosis is often silent, with few specific symptoms to identify what is happening in the liver. As continued scarring and destruction occur, the signs and symptoms listed previously may appear.

Blood Group Links

Alcohol, hepatitis, drug use, and common tropical infections of the liver that can cause fibrosis or scarring appear to a marked degree more frequently in blood group A, and to a lesser extent in groups B and AB. Blood group O, which may have developed anti-A and anti-B antibodies as an early protection against parasites, is relatively immune to them[1,2].

Blood groups A, B, and AB tend to have higher levels of GALLSTONES, diseases of the bile ducts, jaundice, and cirrhosis of the liver, than blood group O. Group A has the highest incidence.

Therapies, Liver Disease

BLOOD GROUP A:

1. Liver Support Protocol

2. Stomach Health Protocol

3. Antiviral Protocol (if viral hepatitis)

4. Detoxification Protocol

BLOOD GROUP B:

1. Liver Support Protocol

2. Stomach Health Protocol

3. Antiviral Protocol (if viral hepatitis)

4. Detoxification Protocol

BLOOD GROUP AB:

1. Liver Support Protocol

2. Stomach Health Protocol

3. Antiviral Protocol (if viral hepatitis)

4. Detoxification Protocol

BLOOD GROUP O:

1. Liver Support Protocol

2. Stomach Health Protocol

3. Antiviral Protocol (if viral hepatitis)

4. Detoxification Protocol

Related Topics

Alcoholism

Autoimmune disease, sarcoidosis

Cancer, gallbladder

Cancer, liver

Cancer, pancreatic

Digestion

Gallstones

Viral disease, hepatitis B and C

REFERENCES

1. Feher J, Lengyel G, Blazovics A. Oxidative stress in the liver and biliary tract diseases. *Scand J Gastroenterol Suppl.* 1998; 228:38–46.

2. Billington BP. A note on the distribution of ABO blood groups in bronchiectasis and portal cirrhosis. *Aust Annal Med.* 1956;5:20–22.

LOU GEHRIG'S DISEASE–*See Amyotrophic lateral sclerosis (ALS)*

LUNG CANCER–*See Cancer, lung*

LUPUS–*See Autoimmune disease, systemic lupus erythematosis*

LYMPHOMA–*See Cancer, lymphoma*

M

MALIGNANCY–_See Cancer (general)_

MANIC DEPRESSIVE DISORDER–_See Depression, bipolar_

MELANOMA–_See Cancer, melanoma_

MENINGITIS–_See Bacterial disease, meningitis_

MENOPAUSAL/PERIMENOPAUSAL CONDITIONS–_Conditions associated with hormonal changes accompanying perimenopause and menopause._

Menopausal/ perimenopausal conditions	RISK		
	LOW	AVERAGE	HIGH
GROUP A			
GROUP B			
GROUP AB			
GROUP O			

Symptoms

The symptoms and degree of symptoms vary greatly among menopausal and perimenopausal women. Except for the cessation of menses, some women are relatively free of symptoms, while others suffer a variety of complaints, including:

- Hot flashes
- Insomnia
- Vaginal dryness
- Urinary leakage
- Dry skin
- Mood swings
- Weight gain

About Menopause

Menopause is a process that takes place over a period of years—typically, between the ages of 47 and 55, although the exact time frame varies for each individual. This time frame is referred to as perimenopause, meaning, literally, "around menopause."

Although the decline in female hormones is normal, marking the passage from childbearing years, it can also increase the risk of certain conditions. For example, OSTEOPOROSIS, a thinning of the bones that eventually leads to frailty and even death, is a negative result of estrogen deficiency.

The symptoms and degree of symptoms vary

greatly among menopausal and perimenopausal women. Except for the cessation of menses, some women are relatively free of symptoms, while others suffer a variety of complaints.

Blood Group Links

Although no studies specifically link blood groups and menopausal conditions, blood groups A and AB have a high susceptibility for BREAST CANCER, making them poor candidates for traditional hormone replacement therapy because elevated levels of estrogen are also associated with breast cancer.

Therapies, Menopausal/Perimenopausal Conditions

ALL BLOOD GROUPS:

An effective alternative to conventional hormone replacement therapy may be the newly available phytoestrogens, which are estrogen-like and progesterone-like preparations derived from plants, principally soybeans, alfalfa, and yams. Many of these preparations are available as a cream that can be applied to the skin several times a day. Plant phytoestrogens are typically high in the estrogen fraction called estriol, whereas chemical estrogens are based on estradiol. The medical literature conclusively shows that supplementation with estriol inhibits the occurrence of breast cancer. Phytoestrogens lack the potency of the chemical estrogens, but they are definitely effective against many of the troubling symptoms of menopause, including hot flashes and vaginal dryness. Because they are only weak

estrogens, they will not suppress any estrogen production by the body, unlike the chemical estrogen. It is interesting that in Japan, where the typical diet is high in phytoestrogens, there is no concise Japanese word for menopause. Undoubtedly the widespread use of soy products, which contain the phytoestrogens genistein and daidzein, serves to modulate the severe symptoms of menopause.

Additional ways to relieve menopausal symptoms include the following:

1. Wear layered clothing so that you can remove items if you feel overheated during the day.

2. Avoid caffeine and alcohol; they can trigger hot flashes in some women.

3. Take tepid showers to help bring down a heightened body temperature.

4. Use a lubricating cream such as K-Y Jelly, Replens, or Astroglide for vaginal dryness or itching. Nonabsorbable or minimally absorbable estrogen cream can add lubrication to the vagina without systemic effect.

BLOOD GROUP A:

1. Menopause Support Protocol
2. Female Balancing Protocol
3. Metabolic Enhancement Protocol

BLOOD GROUP B:

1. Menopause Support Protocol
2. Female Balancing Protocol
3. Metabolic Enhancement Protocol

BLOOD GROUP AB:

1. Menopause Support Protocol

2. Female Balancing Protocol

3. Metabolic Enhancement Protocol

BLOOD GROUP O:

1. Menopause Support Protocol

2. Female Balancing Protocol

3. Metabolic Enhancement Protocol

Related Topics

Cancer, breast

Immunity

Osteoporosis

MENORRHAGIA–*See Menstrual cycle disorders, menorrhagia*

MENSTRUAL CYCLE DISORDERS, AMENORRHEA–*Failure to menstruate.*

Amenorrhea	RISK		
	LOW	AVERAGE	HIGH
GROUP A	▓		
GROUP B	▓	▓	
GROUP AB	▓	▓	
GROUP O	▓	▓	

Symptoms

- Failure to begin menstruating by age 14

- Lack of maturation (development of breast and pubic hair) at puberty

- Absence of menstruation for a period of 6 months prior to perimenopause

About the Menstrual Cycle

The average menstrual cycle lasts approximately 28 days, and can be divided into four stages.

Stage 1, the initial onset, is menstruation, lasting about 5 days. Menstruation is the shedding of the endometrium (the lining of the uterus), which signals that an egg has not been fertilized during the last cycle. At the time of menstruation, the female hormones estrogen and progesterone are at their lowest levels, a signal to the hypothalamus and pituitary glands to start secreting follicle-stimulating hormone (FSH) and luteinizing hormone (LH). FSH is the hormone that stimulates the development of the ovarian follicle, prompting the maturation of a new egg to be released at ovulation. LH is the hormone that stimulates the production of estrogen by the ovaries, and is responsible for the release of the egg (ovulation).

Stage 2 takes place from approximately days 6 through 11, during which time the LH and estrogen levels continue to rise.

Stage 3 begins about day 12, with a surge of estrogen and LH, followed by a decline in estrogen production and a rise in FSH. On about day 14, or within 36 hours of the LH surge, the follicle releases the mature egg and ovulation takes place. This is the time when fertilization occurs if a sperm unites with a mature egg.

Stage 4 comprises the second half of the cycle. The ruptured follicle, which has produced the mature egg, undergoes a change called luteinization,

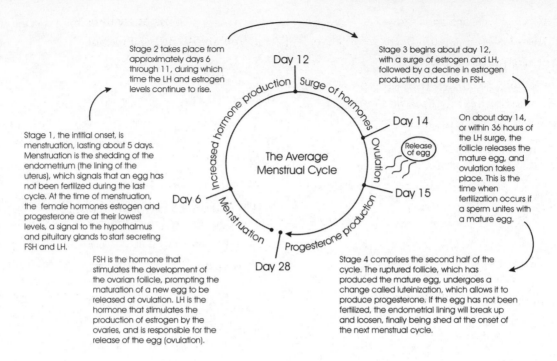

Stage 1, the intitial onset, is menstruation, lasting about 5 days. Menstruation is the shedding of the endometrium (the lining of the uterus), which signals that an egg has not been fertilized during the last cycle. At the time of menstruation, the female hormones estrogen and progesterone are at their lowest levels, a signal to the hypothalmus and pituitary glands to start secreting FSH and LH.

Stage 2 takes place from approximately days 6 through 11, during which time the LH and estrogen levels continue to rise.

Stage 3 begins about day 12, with a surge of estrogen and LH, followed by a decline in estrogen production and a rise in FSH.

On about day 14, or within 36 hours of the LH surge, the follicle releases the mature egg, and ovulation takes place. This is the time when fertilization occurs if a sperm unites with a mature egg.

FSH is the hormone that stimulates the development of the ovarian follicle, prompting the maturation of a new egg to be released at ovulation. LH is the hormone that stimulates the production of estrogen by the ovaries, and is responsible for the release of the egg (ovulation).

Stage 4 comprises the second half of the cycle. The ruptured follicle, which has produced the mature egg, undergoes a change called luteinization, which allows it to produce progesterone. If the egg has not been fertilized, the endometrial lining will break up and loosen, finally being shed at the onset of the next menstrual cycle.

which allows it to produce progesterone. Progesterone is the hormone that prepares the uterine lining for pregnancy. During this stage of the cycle, LH and FSH levels drop, while progesterone continues to rise, thickening the outer layer of the endometrium in preparation for pregnancy. If the egg has not been fertilized, the endometrial lining will break up and loosen, finally being shed at the onset of the next menstrual cycle.

About Amenorrhea

Primary amenorrhea is defined as the failure to menstruate by age 14, and the absence of secondary characteristics, like breast and hair development. Even when breast and pubic hair have developed, it refers to the failure to menstruate by age 16. Menstrual patterns run in families; if a mother got her period late, her daughter may have the same experience.

In addition to pregnancy and MENOPAUSE, which should always be ruled out, other causes of amenorrhea are normal. For instance, following childbirth, menstruation may not begin again for several months. Some women fail to regain normal menses after stopping oral contraceptives, but most return to normal within 6 months.

STRESS can affect menstruation. Overwork, personal crises, poor sleep, and poor eating habits may all contribute to a missed period.

Amenorrhea can also be a sign of an endocrine system disorder such as an adrenal disorder, DIABETES, or HYPOTHYROIDISM.

Psychotropic drugs, anticonvulsants, chemotherapy, and anti-estrogens like tamoxifen can also interfere with menstruation.

Amenorrhea accompanied by hirsutism (excess facial and body hair, and sometimes acne and oily skin) implies a possible adrenal disorder causing an excess of male hormones.

Blood Group Links

The age at menarche in relation to ABO blood group phenotypes and hemoglobin-E genotypes have been studied among 290 girls belonging to Mongol ethnic stock in the northeastern region of India. The study shows that the age at menarche is influenced by the abnormal hemoglobin-E genotype as well as ABO blood group phenotype. The genetic markers play a pivotal role in the growth and development of an individual[1].

Therapies, Amenorrhea

BLOOD GROUP A:
1. Female Balancing Protocol

BLOOD GROUP B:
1. Female Balancing Protocol

BLOOD GROUP AB:
1. Female Balancing Protocol

BLOOD GROUP O:
1. Female Balancing Protocol

Related Topics

Anxiety disorders

Growth and maturity

Stress

Thyroid disease, hypothyroidism

REFERENCES

1. Balgir RS. Menarcheal age in relation to ABO blood group phenotypes and haemoglobin-E genotypes. *J Assoc Physicians India.* 1993;41:210–211.

MENSTRUAL CYCLE DISORDERS, DYSMENORRHEA–*Painful menstruation.*

Dysmenorrhea	RISK		
	LOW	AVERAGE	HIGH
GROUP A	░	░	
GROUP B	░	░	
GROUP AB	░	░	
GROUP O	░	░	

Symptoms

The discomfort begins prior to the period, or with the onset of bleeding, and usually subsides within 2 to 3 days after bleeding begins. Symptoms include:

- Low abdominal pain
- Cramping, pulling, or constrictive pangs
- Pain radiating into the back and down the legs
- Clots in menstrual blood
- Premenstrual syndrome (PMS)

About Dysmenorrhea

Dysmenorrhea can be primary (functional) or secondary (acquired). Primary dysmenorrhea occurs during ovulatory cycles, without any identified disorder in the genital tract. Very often, a woman's liver may be hypofunctioning; she is constipated (estrogens can be reabsorbed from the bowel if the stools are not evacuated frequently enough); and she is hormonally imbalanced, with too high an estrogen level in relation to her progesterone levels.

Secondary dysmenorrhea indicates painful periods due to an identifiable cause such as endometriosis, UTERINE FIBROIDS, pelvic inflammatory disease, or inflammation from an intrauterine contraceptive device (IUD). The majority of dysmenorrhea sufferers also have PMS, and the two syndromes often merge in a welter of signs and symptoms.

Blood Group Links

Although no studies have been performed linking ABO blood groups with dysmenorrhea, many of the potential underlying conditions, such as endometriosis and uterine fibroids, show a higher incidence in groups A and AB.

Therapies, Dysmenorrhea

BLOOD GROUP A:

1. Female Balancing Protocol
2. Anti-Inflammation Protocol

BLOOD GROUP B:

1. Female Balancing Protocol
2. Anti-Inflammation Protocol

BLOOD GROUP AB:

1. Female Balancing Protocol
2. Anti-Inflammation Protocol

BLOOD GROUP O:

1. Female Balancing Protocol
2. Anti-Inflammation Protocol

Related Topics

Blood clotting disorders

Cancer, gynecological tumors

MENSTRUAL CYCLE DISORDERS, MENORRHAGIA–*Heavy menses.*

Menorrhagia	RISK		
	LOW	AVERAGE	HIGH
GROUP A	▒	▒	
GROUP B	▒	▒	
GROUP AB	▒	▒	
GROUP O	▒	▒	▒

Symptoms

- Excessive bleeding during menses

About Menorrhagia

Menorrhagia falls under a broader category of "abnormal bleeding"—prolonged, excessive, or irregular with regard to time of the cycle. It is important in the diagnosis to determine that bleeding is coming from the vagina and not the urethra or the rectum.

Menorrhagia can result from many causes, which are so varied that they may be treated as separate conditions. Dysfunctional uterine bleeding (DUB) describes abnormal uterine bleeding not associated with tumor, inflammation, or pregnancy. This is commonly caused by unopposed estrogen stimulation from a tumor or disease condition, leading the endometrial tissue to hypertrophy and eventually to sloughing and bleeding.

Causes include HYPOTHYROIDISM, endometrial proliferation, hyperplasia, anovulation (lack of ovulation), polycystic ovaries, ovarian tumor, obesity, endometrial polyps, endometrial neoplasia, and FIBROIDS. Risk factors include OBESITY, anovulation, and hormone replacement therapy without progestin.

Blood Group Links

Oral contraceptives may have a blood-group related effect on blood clotting, which is especially important for blood group O.

A randomized clinical trial of oral contraceptives evaluated 67 women on a regimen of 50 mcg of ethinyl estradiol and 1.0 mg of norethindrone; 61 women on a regimen of 35 mcg of ethinyl estradiol and 1.0 mcg of norethindrone; and 64 women on a regimen of 35 mcg of ethinyl estradiol and 0.5 mg of norethindrone. The ABO blood group was determined for all of the women. An analysis of the interrelationships among antithrombin III (blood clotting factor) by activity method, oral contraceptive type, and ABO blood group showed larger declines in clotting activity for blood group O women using the highest estrogen dose preparation[1].

Therapies, Menorrhagia

BLOOD GROUP A:

1. Female Balancing Protocol

2. Blood-Building Protocol

BLOOD GROUP B:

1. Female Balancing Protocol

2. Blood-Building Protocol

BLOOD GROUP AB:

1. Female Balancing Protocol
2. Blood-Building Protocol

BLOOD GROUP O:

1. Female Balancing Protocol
2. Blood-Building Protocol

Related Topics

Blood clotting disorders

Cancer, gynecological tumors

Menopausal/perimenopausal conditions

REFERENCES

1. Burkman RT, Bell WR, Zacur HA, Kimball AW. Oral contraceptives and antithrombin III: variations by dosage and ABO blood group. *Am J Obstet Gynecol.* 1991;164(1):1453–1458.

MENSTRUAL CYCLE DISORDERS, PREMENSTRUAL SYNDROME (PMS)–

A constellation of symptoms that arise in the 7 to 14 days before menses starts.

Premenstrual syndrome	RISK		
	LOW	AVERAGE	HIGH
GROUP A			
GROUP B			
GROUP AB			
GROUP O			

Symptoms

- Nervousness
- Irritability
- Emotional instability
- Depression
- Headaches
- Edema
- Swollen, achy breasts
- Food cravings

About PMS

Although most women experience minor physical or emotional changes before menstruation, about 10% of women have symptoms severe enough to impede their daily life. More than 150 symptoms are associated with PMS, including tension, irritability, breast tenderness, bloating, and gastric distress.

Severe symptoms of PMS, including DEPRESSION, irritability, and mood swings, are referred to as premenstrual dysphoric disorder. There is a risk for other conditions such as depression. Caffeine and high fluid intake can exacerbate PMS symptoms, and STRESS may precipitate the symptoms. The severity of PMS increases with age.

Blood Group Links

Although no studies directly link premenstrual syndrome with blood groups, many of the common symptoms are more typical of blood groups A and B, especially in highly stressful conditions.

Therapies, Premenstrual Syndrome

BLOOD GROUP A:

1. Female Balancing Protocol

2. Antistress Protocol

3. Fatigue-Fighting Protocol

BLOOD GROUP B:

1. Female Balancing Protocol

2. Antistress Protocol

3. Fatigue-Fighting Protocol

BLOOD GROUP AB:

1. Female Balancing Protocol

2. Antistress Protocol

3. Fatigue-Fighting Protocol

BLOOD GROUP O:

1. Female Balancing Protocol

2. Antistress Protocol

3. Fatigue-Fighting Protocol

Related Topics

Depression, unipolar, bipolar

Digestion

Lectins

Stress

METABOLISM—*See Insulin resistance*

METASTASIS—*See Cancer, general*

MIGRAINE—*See Headache*

MISCARRIAGE—*See Infertility*

MITRAL VALVE PROLAPSE—*See Cardiovascular disease*

MONONUCLEOSIS—*See Viral disease, mononucleosis*

MOUTH SORES—*See Fungal disease, candidiasis (oral)*

MULTIPLE SCLEROSIS—*See Autoimmune disease, multiple sclerosis*

MUMPS—*See Viral disease, mumps*

MUSCULOSKELETAL INJURY—*Damage to the muscles or bone.*

Musculoskeletal Injury	RISK		
	LOW	AVERAGE	HIGH
GROUP A (peritendinitis)	░	░	
GROUP B	░		
GROUP AB	░	░	
GROUP O (tendon rupture)	░	░	

Symptoms

- Pain
- Swelling
- Stiffness
- Inability to move the affected limb

About Musculoskeletal Injury

The healing of injuries such as sprains, strains, and skin wounds requires the involvement of many body systems, including the circulatory system, the immune system, and the cellular mechanisms. All are needed to repair and grow new tissues.

Blood Group Links

There are differences among the blood groups in susceptibility to common musculoskeletal injuries.

The distribution of the ABO blood groups was studied in 917 patients with specific musculoskeletal diagnoses. The ABO blood group distribution of patients with ruptures of the Achilles tendon, and of patients with chronic Achilles peritendinitis, differed from control individuals. The ABO blood group distribution was not associated with any other musculoskeletal injuries studied. The blood group A to O ratio was 1.42 in the control population. In the group with rupture of the Achilles tendon this ratio was 1.0, and in the group with Achilles peritendinitis it was 0.70. The association between injuries of the Achilles tendon and the ABO blood group distribution was in ac-

cordance with an earlier report. There may be a genetic linkage between the ABO blood groups and the molecular structure of the tissue of Achilles tendon[1].

In a Hungarian study, 53% of the 873 cases of subcutaneous (spontaneous) tendon ruptures treated by the National Institute of Traumatology belonged to blood group O; that percentage was significantly higher than found in the healthy population (31.1%) of Hungary. The ratio of the tendon rupture patients belonging to blood group A was significantly lower (27.1%) than in the overall population (42.4%). The ratio of the cases belonging to group O among the multiple tendon rupture and re-rupture patients proved to be over 70%. On the basis of this data, the investigators suggested that there is a relation between the ABO blood group system and the tendon rupture. Blood group O individuals are more likely to experience a tendon rupture, whereas blood group A individuals appear to be more protected against tendon rupture[2].

Therapies, Musculoskeletal Injury

BLOOD GROUP A:

1. Immune Enhancing Protocol
2. [Women] Menopause Support Protocol
3. Anti-Inflammation Protocol
4. Arthritis Protocol

BLOOD GROUP B:

1. Immune-Enhancing Protocol
2. [Women] Menopause Support Protocol
3. Anti-Inflammation Health Protocol

4. Arthritis Protocol

BLOOD GROUP AB:

1. Immune-Enhancing Protocol

2. [Women] Menopause Support Protocol

3. Anti-Inflammation Protocol

4. Arthritis Protocol

BLOOD GROUP O:

1. Immune-Enhancing Protocol

2. [Women] Menopause Support Protocol

3. Anti-Inflammation Protocol

4. Arthritis Protocol

Related Topics

Arthritis, osteo-

Blood clotting disorders

Inflammation

REFERENCES

1. Kujala UM, Jarvinen M, Natri A, et al. ABO blood groups and musculoskeletal injuries. *Injury.* 1992;23:131–133.

2. Jozsa L, Barzo M, Balint JB. [Correlations between the ABO blood group system and tendon rupture.] *Magy Traumatol Orthop Helyreallito Seb.* 1990;33:101–104.

MYASTHENIA GRAVIS–*See Autoimmune disease, myasthenia gravis*

MYOCARDIAL INFARCTION–*Heart attack.*

Myocardial infarction	RISK		
	LOW	AVERAGE	HIGH
GROUP A			
GROUP B			
GROUP AB			
GROUP O			
NON-SECRETOR			

Symptoms

About two-thirds of patients experience symptoms days to weeks before a heart attack, including the following:

- Unstable or crescendo angina
- Shortness of breath
- Fatigue

Symptoms that a heart attack is occurring include the following:

- Deep, substernal, visceral chest pain described as aching or pressure, often with radiation to the back, jaw, or left arm
- Apprehension and a sense of impending doom
- Nausea and vomiting (potentially)

About Heart Attacks

Heart attacks occur when there is severe scarring or death of heart muscle due to lack of oxygen. Oxygen-rich blood is blocked by a blood clot in a coronary artery, usually due to plaque-related narrowing of the artery—this is known as CORONARY ARTERY DISEASE. Heart attacks do not always occur in cases of coronary artery disease, but individuals with arterial blockages are at great risk for heart attacks.

Blood Group Links

Numerous studies have made the connection between blood groups and all forms and signs of HEART DISEASE, including heart attacks.

A study of 255 women published in the *Journal of the American Medical Association*, originally designed to study the effects of smoking on the rates of heart attack in women, also found several other factors were significantly associated with heart attacks in this group. These factors included HYPERTENSION, ANGINA PECTORIS, family history, DIABETES MELLITUS, and blood group A. The study confirmed numerous other findings that blood group A has a higher risk of heart disease[1].

A 1985 study looked at blood groups and heart attacks in two different age groups: those 65 years old and older, and younger patients. The predominance of blood group A in patients with cardiac infarction was deemed "highly significant" in both age groups. This study was unique in that other risk factors, such as smoking, HIGH BLOOD PRESSURE, diabetes, and HIGH CHOLESTEROL levels, were excluded from the study. When the researchers looked specifically at the more elderly population, the predominance of blood group A in the older patients with cardiac infarction was even higher. The researchers concluded that the result "strongly suggests the existence of a genetic factor associated with blood group A, and independent of the other risk factors which are also responsible for a greater incidence of cardiac infarction"[2].

Data further allow the conclusion that the ABO non-secretor phenotypes are a risk factor for myocardial infarction. This is particularly true for recessive Lewis blood types and even more so among men than women. ABO secretors seem to have been given a bit of genetic resistance against heart disease, whereas Lewis negative individuals appear to be at the highest risk[3].

The relation of total serum alkaline phosphatase and serum cholesterol in convalescing patients of myocardial infarction to the patient's secretor status and blood group has been studied. Serum cholesterol and alkaline phosphatase levels showed a significant difference in secretors (98) and non-secretors (56) in myocardial groups. The total cholesterol and total serum alkaline phosphatase levels showed a significant difference in secretors when blood groups A and O were compared, with blood group O having much higher levels of serum alkaline phosphatase and much lower levels of cholesterol. In non-secretors, blood group O had higher levels of cholesterol and group A had higher levels of alkaline phosphatase[4,5].

Therapies, Myocardial Infarction

BLOOD GROUP A:

1. Cardiovascular Protocol
2. Metabolic Enhancement Protocol
3. Antistress Protocol

BLOOD GROUP B:

1. Cardiovascular Protocol
2. Metabolic Enhancement Protocol
3. Antistress Protocol

BLOOD GROUP AB:

1. Cardiovascular Protocol
2. Metabolic Enhancement Protocol
3. Antistress Protocol

BLOOD GROUP O:

1. Cardiovascular Protocol
2. Metabolic Enhancement Protocol
3. Antistress Protocol

Related Topics

Angina pectoris

Atherosclerosis

Blood clotting disorders

Diabetes mellitus, type II

Heart attack

Hypercholesterolemin

Hypertension

Obesity

REFERENCES

1. Stolley PD, Shapiro S. Myocardial infarction in women under 50 years of age. *JAMA.* 1983;250:2801–2806.
2. Platt D, Muhlberg W, Kiehl L, Schmitt-Ruth R. ABO blood group system, age, sex, risk factors and cardiac infarction. *Arch Gerontol Geriatr.* 1985;4:241–249.
3. Hein HO, Sorensen H, Suadicani P, Gyntelberg F. The Lewis blood group—a new genetic marker of ischaemic heart disease. *J Intern Med.* 1992;232:481–487.
4. Mehta NJ, Rege DV, Kulkarni MB. Total serum alkaline phosphatase (SAP) and serum cholesterol in relation to secretor status and blood groups in myocardial infarction patients. *Indian Heart J.* 1989;41:82–85.
5. Bayer PM, Hotschek H, Knoth E. Intestinal alkaline phosphatase and the ABO blood group system—a new aspect. *Clin Chim Acta.* 1980;108:81–87.

Nausea

COMMON CAUSES	BLOOD GROUP O	BLOOD GROUP A	BLOOD GROUP B	BLOOD GROUP AB	SUBGROUPS
Intestinal virus			**********	************	
Bacterial, parasitic infection		**********	**********	**********	
Food intolerance	**********		*********		
Stress		*********	*********		
Pregnancy	ALL BLOOD GROUPS	ALL BLOOD GROUPS	ALL BLOOD GROUPS	ALL BLOOD GROUPS	ALL BLOOD GROUPS
Motion sickness	ALL BLOOD GROUPS	ALL BLOOD GROUPS	ALL BLOOD GROUPS	ALL BLOOD GROUPS	ALL BLOOD GROUPS
Neurological disorders			*********		
Chemotherapy		**********		**********	
Liver disease (bloody vomit)	**********				

* = degree of risk

Therapies, Nausea

ALL BLOOD GROUPS:

Chew a 1-inch piece of raw ginger or sip ginger tea.

BLOOD GROUP A:

1. Stomach Health Protocol

BLOOD GROUP B:

1. Liver Support Protocol

BLOOD GROUP AB:

1. Stomach Health Protocol

BLOOD GROUP O:

1. Stomach Health Protocol

Related Topics

Bacterial disease (general)

Cancer (general)

Food poisoning

Liver disease

Parasitic disease

Stress

Viral disease (general)

NEUROSES, PHOBIAS—*See Anxiety disorders; Obsessive-compulsive disorder; Stress*

NEUROTRANSMITTER IMBALANCE—*See Stress*

NIGHT SWEATS—*See Menopausal/ perimenopausal conditions*

NITRIC OXIDE—*See Stress*

O

OBESITY–*The state of being more than 25 per-cent above normal weight-for-height; or having a body fat percentage greater than 30 percent for women and 25 percent for men.*

Obesity	RISK		
	LOW	AVERAGE	HIGH
GROUP A			
GROUP B			
GROUP AB			
GROUP O			

Symptoms

- Hypoglycemia/insulin resistance
- Edema
- Low muscle-to-fat ratio

About Obesity

Obesity is a relatively new phenomenon. For most of history, the human race waged a fierce battle against famine. The people who had the most meat on their bones were usually the survivors. Women with broad hips and thighs were better able to mobilize necessary fat to nourish a developing fetus and to produce sufficient milk for breastfeeding. So, weight gain was in many ways a plus, providing a source of stored energy, available for the inevitable periods of famine following periods of engorgement. This was nature's way of ensuring survival of the species.

Today, particularly in the Western world, malnutrition is not characterized by scarcity but by the inability of our systems to properly use many of the foods we eat. Obesity is ultimately a state of improper nutrition, resulting in a derangement of the hormone balance. This derangement upsets the metabolic equation, which is why people often find it impossible to lose weight, even on very low calorie diets.

The Obesity Spiral

Once an individual is overweight, it becomes even more difficult to restore a normal balance, due to the alteration of metabolic balance. Obesity is always accompanied by INSULIN RESISTANCE, resulting in hyperinsulinemia, in direct proportion to the amount of visceral body fat. More body fat equals increasing insulin resistance.

In fact, many metabolic derangements occur in proportion to the amount of body fat. METABOLISM is shifted toward normalization as body fat is shed.

371

In a review of obesity in children, investigators have reported metabolic stumbling blocks in a variety of endocrine systems, including thyroid hormone activation, stress hormone production, androgen levels, growth hormone, and insulin levels. In these children, both basal and stimulated (by sugar or starch) insulin concentrations were high. The condition most certainly exists in adults as well. The regulation of energy metabolism in obesity is different from normal conditions in several key areas.

Being overweight produces leptin resistance. Leptin (not lectin!) is a hormone associated with the obesity gene. Leptin acts on the brain's hypothalamus to regulate the extent of body fat, the ability to burn fat for energy, and satiety. When you're overweight, your leptin levels increase, but its action is stifled. In obesity, leptin levels increase in concert with insulin levels, leading some researchers to conclude that insulin resistance plays a role with this "obesity hormone."

Being overweight promotes cortisol resistance. As a general rule, when you are overweight, you will have chronically higher levels of cortisol (stress hormone) production. Fat tissue accelerates the turnover of cortisol, facilitating cortisone production, which stimulates ACTH secretion and maintains stimulation of the adrenal cortex. Furthermore, high levels of cortisol in itself promote weight gain. It's a vicious cycle. Cortisol differs from other steroid hormones, such as sex hormones, in that it is classified as a glucocorticoid. That means its primary action involves increasing blood sugar levels at the expense of muscle tissue. While this is the desired effect in a fight-or-flight

situation, on a chronic basis it will lead to insulin resistance, and an alteration in body composition from muscle to fat. Furthermore, researchers believe that high cortisol tends to increase appetite, due to an association with leptin. In animal research, it was shown that cortisol is the primary factor that prevents leptin from decreasing appetite, increasing metabolism, and decreasing body fat. Similar findings have been shown with humans. This has special relevance for blood groups A and B, whose basal levels of cortisol are high to begin with.

Being overweight decreases growth hormone. Growth hormone (GH) secretion is decreased in obesity, and even substances known to increase GH secretion work poorly in obese individuals as compared with lean individuals. The hyperinsulinism and resistance to insulin also intervene in hormonal regulation. They elevate the insulin-like growth factor 1 (IGF-1), which inhibits the production of growth hormone. Since growth hormone promotes lean body mass, enhances the peripheral conversion of thyroid hormone to T_3 (metabolically active thyroid hormone), and enhances processes aimed at fat burning, the reduction in this hormone has a negative effect on the body composition.

In addition to these consequences of obesity, long-term insulin resistance can lead to life-threatening conditions. Over time, as pancreatic beta cells continue to produce larger and larger amounts of insulin and remain unable to normalize blood sugar, they will eventually become exhausted. The progression to full-fledged DIABETES can occur over time. In a preliminary stage, blood tests will just show a tendency to higher than normal levels of blood sugar, a sign of impending or prolonged hyperglycemia. However, if this state of prolonged hyperglycemia is maintained, a deterioration to non–insulin-dependent diabetes mellitus (type II) becomes likely.

Active Tissue Mass versus Body Fat

The first aspect of metabolism to consider is muscle mass. Health and metabolism are compromised not so much from too much weight, but from too much body fat and too little muscle. As such, it is much more important to know the amount of muscle mass as well as overall weight.

A critical aspect of metabolism is known as basal metabolic rate (BMR). BMR is best thought of as the amount of calories burned during the course of a day while at rest. As a general rule, BMR tends to decrease with age, with loss of muscle mass almost solely responsible for this observed decline. While a low BMR might indicate a great deal of difficulty with losing weight, an excessively high BMR would also not be ideal from a health perspective, since it might indicate a tendency toward catabolic or overly aggressive metabolism. As with most aspects of health, a balanced BMR is probably the most ideal. But within reason, the higher this value, the better.

Metabolically active tissue is defined as muscle tissue and organ tissues such as liver, brain, and heart, which actively burn fuel. It is often referred to as active tissue mass. Some of the advantages of an increased active tissue mass include more strength, which is associated with better health

and lower biological age, increased BMR, increased aerobic capacity, improved cardiovascular system health, better utilization of sugar, improved maintenance of good cholesterol, improved bone density, and greater resistance to gaining fat.

A greater body percentage of active tissue mass translates into a more aggressive anti-fat metabolism, because more muscle tissue actually increases the rate and amount of fat used for fuel while at rest.

While body composition is a measure of the percentage of muscle to fat, under many weight loss circumstances the body composition can improve, but at the same time muscle tissue can be lost. This is the major flaw with drastic semi-starvation, calorie-restricted diets. These diets can drop the percentage of fat well enough, but they do nothing to increase the percentage of active tissue mass. The metabolic rate of dieters is left unchanged, which predisposes them to regain the weight they've lost as soon as they begin eating normally again.

Another key factor is the ratio of intracellular to extracellular water in the body. This provides a measurement of the hydration of cells. In a healthy state, there is a tendency to maintain greater quantities of fluid inside cells. A value of about 57% to 60% intracelluar water is excellent. Edema is fluid build-up outside of cells. Many obese individuals have very high levels of extracellular water, usually the result of eating "avoid" foods, sedentary lifestyle habits, high amounts of cellular toxicity, and high stress. Many obese individuals have concentrations of extracellular water in their bodies in excess of 60% to 70%, and concentrations of intracellular water as low as 35%.

Blood Group Links

Blood groups have a significant influence on metabolic balance. There are several factors:

1. The effect of dietary lectins. LECTINS, many of which are blood group specific, have insulin-like effects on fat cell receptors. However, unlike insulin, which has a temporary effect on these receptors, once these lectins bind to the receptor they signal fat cells to stop burning fat and to store extra calories as fat. In effect, eating these lectins results in the body scavenging any extra sugars/carbohydrates and converting them to unwanted fat. Consuming large amounts of insulin-mimicking lectins specific to your blood group increases your body fat and decreases your active tissue mass.

2. The influence of genetically programmed insulin resistance on metabolic efficiency. Many non-secretors have insulin-resistance syndrome, which can cause impairment of triglyceride conversion, resulting in a lowered metabolic rate. Low metabolism also promotes the storage of excess fluid as extracellular water, leading to edema.

3. Improper utilization of energy, through stress and exercising inappropriately. High levels of cortisol, often produced in high amounts by blood groups A and B when under STRESS, can have a significant effect on metabolism.

4. ABO genetics: High-stress conditions can increase cortisol production in blood groups A and B, impairing conversion of thyroid hormone. Stud-

ies have also shown a lower level of thyroid metabolism in group A individuals.

Therapies, Obesity

ALL BLOOD GROUPS:

The individualized protocols are supplementary to following the recommended Blood Type Diet and exercise regimens.

BLOOD GROUP A:

1. Metabolic Enhancement Protocol
2. Antistress Protocol
3. Detoxification Protocol

BLOOD GROUP B:

1. Metabolic Enhancement Protocol
2. Antistress Protocol
3. Liver Support Protocol

BLOOD GROUP AB:

1. Metabolic Enhancement Protocol
2. Detoxification Protocol
3. Immune-Enhancing Protocol

BLOOD GROUP O:

1. Metabolic Enhancement Protocol
2. Detoxification Protocol
3. Immune-Enhancing Protocol

Related Topics

Diabetes

Hypertriglyceridemia

Insulin resistance

Thyroid disease

OBSESSIVE-COMPULSIVE DISORDER (OCD)–*Uncontrolled mental activity, provoking a compulsion to act in a repetitive and ritualistic manner.*

Obsessive-compulsive disorder	RISK		
	LOW	AVERAGE	HIGH
GROUP A			
GROUP B			
GROUP AB			
GROUP O			

Symptoms

Obsession:

- Fear of dirt or contamination
- Concern with order, symmetry, and exactness
- Constantly thinking about certain sounds, images, words, or numbers
- Fear of harming a family member or friend
- Fear of thinking evil or sinful thoughts

Compulsion:

- Excessive hand washing
- Checking repeatedly that doors are locked and appliances turned off
- Arranging items in a precise order
- Counting over and over to a certain number
- Touching certain objects several times

About Obsessive-Compulsive Disorder

Approximately 5 million people in the United States, or about 1 in every 50 Americans, suffer from obsessive-compulsive disorder (OCD). It affects men, women, and children, as well as people of all races, religions, and socioeconomic backgrounds. There are two features to this disorder. *Obsession* is recurrent and persistent thoughts, ideas, or images that involuntarily invade the conscious awareness. Common obsessive thoughts may be about violence, contamination, or worry about a tragic event. *Compulsion* is an act the individual feels compelled to take in response to an obsession, even though it is senseless and tends to be repetitive. A great deal of ANXIETY is created if this compulsion is not acted on. An example of compulsion is repetitive hand washing in an individual with obsessions about cleanliness or contamination. Usually the compulsive action temporarily relieves the anxiety; but the relief is short-lived and the compulsion soon returns.

OCD patients have higher levels of cortisol and lower levels of melatonin than normal individuals, and have higher levels of free cortisol in their urine. Indeed, it appears that the effect of using serotonin modulators to treat OCD may actually work in part by lowering cortisol levels.

Blood Group Links

Several independent studies clearly document an association between blood group A and obsessive-compulsive disorder. In one large study of normal volunteers using a questionnaire called the Leyton Obsessional Inventory, blood group O was noticeably absent, which verified previous studies showing a high rate of OCD in blood group A as compared to blood group O. Interestingly, the catecholamines, which have such an important role in the stress response of group O, have no role in OCD[1].

In a large 1983 study of OCD sufferers, blood group A was again shown to be associated with a higher incidence of OCD over other groups, in addition to a higher incidence of hysteria. Blood group O was found to have a higher incidence of PHOBIAS than the other blood groups[2].

In a 1986 study, two groups of psychiatric outpatients of group O and group A completed a questionnaire called the Brief Symptom Inventory. In both groups, blood group A patients scored significantly higher than blood group O patients on the "Obsessive-Compulsive" and "Psychoticism" factors. The investigators concluded that "these findings are not attributable to differences in age, sex or diagnosis, and are consistent with several previous studies. The influence of blood type on symptom expression may be mediated by cell membrane characteristics, influenced in part by blood type"[3].

Therapies, Obsessive-Compulsive Disorder

BLOOD GROUP A:

1. Antistress Protocol
2. Cognitive Improvement Protocol

BLOOD GROUP B:

1. Antistress Protocol
2. Cognitive Improvement Protocol

BLOOD GROUP AB:

1. Antistress Protocol
2. Cognitive Improvement Protocol

BLOOD GROUP O:

1. Antistress Protocol
2. Cognitive Improvement Protocol

Related Topics

Anxiety disorders

Stress

REFERENCES

1. Rinieris PM, Stefanis CN, Rabavilas AD, Vaidakis NM. Obsessive-compulsive neurosis, anancastic symptomatology and ABO blood types. *Acta Psychiatr Scand.* 1978;57:377–381.

2. Boyer WF. Influence of ABO blood type on symptomatology among outpatients: study and replication. *Neuropsychobiology.* 1986;16:43–46.

3. Rinieris PM, Stefanis CN, Rabavilas AD. Obsessional personality traits and ABO blood types. *Neuropsychobiology.* 1980;6:128–131.

OCULAR LESIONS–*See Glaucoma*

OSTEOARTHRITIS–*See Arthritis, osteo*

OSTEOPOROSIS–*Fragile, brittle bones, caused by a depletion of calcium, most typical in dedicated athletes and the elderly.*

Osteoporosis	RISK		
	LOW	AVERAGE	HIGH
GROUP A	██	██	
GROUP B	██		
GROUP AB	██		
GROUP O	██		██

Symptoms

- Back pain
- Loss of height
- Curving spine
- Easily broken bones
- Rib pain
- Abdominal pain
- Tooth loss

About Osteoporosis

The process of bone breakdown and repair occurs throughout life. With osteoporosis, the calcium that keeps bones strong is lost, and new bone formation stops occurring to repair bone loss. The result is that the skeleton becomes fragile, and the bones grow thin and brittle.

Bone loss happens over time, accelerating with age and menopause. To some extent, every person, male and female, experiences a degree of bone loss with age. But it's a far less severe problem for men, since they start out with about 30% more bone mass than women and tend to lose it more slowly. It's also less severe in women of African ancestry or who have darker skin, because they have about 10% more bone mass than women of European or Asian ancestry or who have fair skin.

Hip fractures among elderly women are a costly and devastating epidemic in this country. Osteoporosis carries a $7 billion annual medical price tag, and $5 billion of that is due to hip fractures. Aside from the cost, hip fractures are associated with high morbidity and mortality. Falling down is the leading cause of death among people over age 75, mainly among women. All patients with hip fractures require hospitalization, and between 12% and 20% die during the first year. Of those who survive, 50% will never walk independently again.

General Risk Factors and Causes

- Family history—especially a mother with osteoporosis
- A thin and small frame
- Light skin
- A sedentary lifestyle
- Excessive consumption of alcohol and caffeine
- Low muscle mass

- Taking calcium-depleting medications, such as cortisone

- Premenopause hysterectomy or early menopause

- Smoking

- Eating disorders

The Calcium Connection

Calcium is a mineral essential for building bones and teeth and for maintaining bone strength. Bones and teeth contain 99% of the body's calcium stores. When bones don't contain enough calcium, they weaken. The body's ability to absorb calcium is influenced by the form in which it is taken, its interaction with other nutrients, and the way it is absorbed into and eliminated from the body.

Certain nutrients have a direct affect on calcium absorption. Vitamin D, which is converted to a hormone called calcitriol, regulates the transport of calcium from the digestive tract to the bloodstream and into the bones. Normal amounts of vitamin D (5 to 10 micrograms a day), primarily received from the sun and by consuming fortified foods, are sufficient. Those not regularly exposed to sunlight might need a little more dietary vitamin D.

Phosphorous is another mineral that has an effect on bone density. Too much or too little phosphorous in the body can harm bone formation. Magnesium is important for the body's utilization of calcium and vitamin D. Protein is vital to the formation of bones, but too much protein can increase the amount of calcium lost in the urine.

When protein breaks down in the body, it produces organic acids, and the body pulls calcium carbonate out of the bones to act as a buffer. So, although too little protein can damage bones, too much can weaken them.

Certain medications can also leach calcium from the system. For example, thyroid hormone encourages bone loss. Other medical treatments that can deplete calcium include cortisone, chemotherapy, long-term lithium therapy, anticonvulsants, and long-term use of phosphate-binding antacids. Endocrine disorders can also contribute to osteoporosis. These include HYPERTHYROIDISM, hyperparathyroidism, Cushing's syndrome, and TYPE I DIABETES.

Blood Group Links

Blood group A has the highest incidence of osteoporosis for two reasons. First, evidence suggests that intestinal alkaline phosphatase enzyme, in addition to enhancing fat breakdown, also enhances the absorption of calcium. Groups A and AB are known to have lower levels of intestinal alkaline phosphatase. On the other hand, groups O and B, with higher levels, are less susceptible to osteoporosis[1].

In a study of recovering male alcoholics, who almost always have experienced long periods of sub-par nutrition, blood group O patients had significantly higher bone densities. The patients with other blood groups lost a significant amount of bone with advancing age, while group O did not. The investigators noted that "although alcoholism is a factor in the development of osteopenia, in males the ABO blood type status plays a significant role in the maximal mineralization of the skeleton, and the amount of bone reabsorption during aging, independent of alcohol abuse"[2].

In addition, people with higher stomach acid tend to absorb calcium more efficiently, giving groups A and AB, with naturally low stomach acid levels, a disadvantage.

Therapies, Osteoporosis

BLOOD GROUP A:

1. Menopause Support Protocol
2. Metabolic Enhancement Protocol

BLOOD GROUP B:

1. Menopause Support Protocol
2. Metabolic Enhancement Protocol

BLOOD GROUP AB:

1. Menopause Support Protocol
2. Metabolic Enhancement Protocol

BLOOD GROUP O:

1. Menopause Support Protocol
2. Metabolic Enhancement Protocol

Related Topics

Diabetes

Menopausal/perimenopausal conditions

Obesity

REFERENCES

1. Kolodchenko VP. [ABO, rhesus and MN system blood groups and spinal osteochondrosis.] *Tsitol Genet.* 1979;13: 232–233.
2. Davidson BJ, MacMurray JP, Prakash V. ABO blood group differences in bone mineral density of recovering alcoholic males. *Alcohol Clin Exp Res.* 1990;14:906–908.

OTITIS EXTERNA–*See Ear infection, otitis externa*

OTITIS MEDIA–*See Ear infection, otitis media*

OVARIAN CANCER–*See Cancer, ovarian*

P

PANCREATIC CANCER–*See Cancer, pancreatic*

PANIC DISORDER–*See Anxiety disorders*

PARASITIC DISEASE, AMOEBA–*Infection of the colon with* Entamoeba histolytica.

Parasitic disease, amoeba	RISK		
	LOW	AVERAGE	HIGH
GROUP A			
GROUP B			
GROUP AB			
GROUP O			

Symptoms

- Intermittent diarrhea and constipation
- Flatulence and cramping
- Abdominal pain
- Tenderness over the liver and ascending colon
- Stools containing mucus and blood

About Amoebic Dysentery

Amoebic dysentery, common in the tropics but uncommon in temperate climates, is characterized by episodes of frequent semi-liquid stools that often contain blood, mucus, and live *Entamoeba histolytica* trophozoites (parasites). Abdominal findings range from mild tenderness to frank abdominal pain, with high fevers and systemic toxic symptoms. Between relapses, symptoms diminish to recurrent cramps and loose or very soft stools, but emaciation and ANEMIA continue. Symptoms of subacute appendicitis may occur. Surgery in such cases may result in peritonitis. Chronic infection commonly mimics INFLAMMATORY BOWEL DISEASE, and presents as intermittent nondysenteric DIARRHEA with abdominal pain, mucus, flatulence, and weight loss. Chronic infection may also present as amebomas, tender, palpable masses or ring-shaped lesions in the upper intestine (cecum) and ascending colon that resemble carcinomas.

The worldwide distribution of parasites is determined by geographic factors, socioeconomic strata, age, and crowding, with poor food preparation and a lapse in the standard of water and personal sanitation being the major factors. Genetic factors also play a minor role in the acquisition, pathogenesis, and clearance of these infections.

Blood Group Links

Though one study showed that amoeba did not seem to adhere to the red blood cells of any particular blood type over another[1,2], a separate study showed that the percentage of amoeba scavenged by the immune system was higher if the amoebas were attached to group A or group AB red blood cells, as opposed to groups O and B[3]. Though no particular blood group seemed to contract the parasite more than the others, groups A and AB seemed to mount a better immune response to it. One study suggested this might explain why amoebic infection was associated with blood group B.

Therapies, Amoebic Dysentery

ALL BLOOD GROUPS:

Adhere to safe travel guidelines. If you are traveling to an underdeveloped country adhere to the following guidelines:

- Avoid raw or undercooked meat and seafood.

- Avoid raw vegetables and fruit, unless peeled.

- Avoid tap water and ice made from tap water.

- Avoid buying food from street vendors.

- Take along water-purifying tablets (available in pharmacies and sporting goods stores) if you're hiking or backpacking through undeveloped areas.

- Check travel guides for restaurants that have high food safety standards.

- Use bottled water for drinking and brushing your teeth, even in hotels. Carbonated water may be the safest, since carbonation appears to kill some of the microorganisms. Be sure that the bottles have been properly sealed.

BLOOD GROUP A:

1. Antibacterial Protocol
2. Antibiotic Support Protocol
3. Intestinal Health Protocol

BLOOD GROUP B:

1. Antibacterial Protocol
2. Antibiotic Support Protocol
3. Intestinal Health Protocol

BLOOD GROUP AB:

1. Antibacterial Protocol
2. Antibiotic Support Protocol
3. Intestinal Health Protocol

BLOOD GROUP O:

1. Antibacterial Protocol
2. Antibiotic Support Protocol
3. Intestinal Health Protocol

Related Topics

Bacterial disease (general)

Immunity

Infectious diseases

REFERENCES

1. Gabr NS, Mandour AM. Relation of parasitic infection to blood group in El Minia Governorate, Egypt. *J Egypt Soc Parasitol.* 1991;21:679–683.
2. Lopez-Revilla R, Cano-Mancera R. Adhesion of Entamoeba histolytica trophozoites to human erythrocytes. *Infect Immun.* 1982;37:281–285.

3. Alonso P, Zubiaur E. Phagocytic activity of three Naegleria strains in the presence of erythrocytes of various types. *J Protozool.* 1985;32:661–664.

PARASITIC DISEASE, *GIARDIA*–*Infection of the small intestine with the flagellated protozoan* Giardia lamblia.

Parasitic disease, *Giardia*	RISK		
	LOW	AVERAGE	HIGH
GROUP A			
GROUP B			
GROUP AB			
GROUP O			

Symptoms

- Watery, malodorous diarrhea
- Abdominal cramps and distention
- Flatulence
- Intermittent nausea
- Low-grade fever
- Chills, malaise, and headaches
- Weight loss
- Failure to thrive (in children)

About *Giardia*

Giardia infection (sometimes called "Montezuma's Revenge") usually results from consuming tainted water supplies. *Giardia* may be found in wild animals, contaminated streams, and well water. Giardiasis outbreaks can occur in communities where water supplies are contaminated with raw sewage. It can be contracted by drinking water from lakes or streams inhabited by water-dwelling animals, such as beavers and muskrats, or where domestic animals, such as sheep, have caused contamination. It's also spread by direct contact, which has caused outbreaks among the children and the workers in daycare centers. The most common symptom is DIARRHEA, which by itself can be serious and debilitating.

Blood Group Links

A number of studies have shown that *Giardia* has a surface antigen that mimics the A antigen. So it more frequently infects those who are blood group A and to some extent blood group AB, and the infections are more severe and threatening than for groups O and B[1,2].

Therapies, *Giardia*

ALL BLOOD GROUPS:

Scrupulous personal hygiene may prevent person-to-person transmission. Treatment of asymptomatic cyst passers reduces the spread of infection, but whether treatment of asymptomatic infected children in daycare centers is cost-effective remains unclear. Water can be decontaminated by boiling or heating it to at least 70°C (158°F) for 10 minutes. *Giardia* cysts resist routine levels of chlorination; iodine-based disinfection must be carried out for at least 8 hours to be effective. Some filtration devices can remove *Giardia* cysts from contaminated water.

BLOOD GROUP A:

1. Antibacterial Protocol

2. Antibiotic Support Protocol

3. Intestinal Health Protocol

BLOOD GROUP B:

1. Antibacterial Protocol

2. Antibiotic Support Protocol

3. Intestinal Health Protocol

BLOOD GROUP AB:

1. Antibacterial Protocol

2. Antibiotic Support Protocol

3. Intestinal Health Protocol

BLOOD GROUP O:

1. Antibacterial protocol

2. Antibiotic Support Protocol

3. Intestinal Health Protocol

Related Topics

Bacterial disease (general)

Immunity

Infectious diseases

REFERENCES

1. Barnes GL, Kay R. Blood-groups in giardiasis. *Lancet.* 1977; 1:808.

2. Bouree P, Bonnot G. Study of relationship of ABO and Rh blood group, and HLA antigens with parasitic diseases. *J Egypt Soc Parasitol.* 1989;19:67–73.

PARASITIC DISEASE, HOOKWORM—*Infection with* Ancylostoma duodenale *or* Necator americanus *causing abdominal pain and iron-deficiency anemia.*

Parasitic disease, hookworm	RISK		
	LOW	AVERAGE	HIGH
GROUP A	███	███	
GROUP B	███		
GROUP AB	███	███	
GROUP O	███	███	

Symptoms

Hookworm infection is asymptomatic in most cases. However, during the acute phase, symptoms may include the following:

- Spasmodic gastric pain
- Anorexia
- Flatulence
- Diarrhea
- Weight loss

Chronic infection may lead to the following symptoms:

- Iron-deficiency anemia
- Pallor and weakness
- Tachycardia
- Lassitude

- Impotence
- Edema

About Hookworm

Hookworm infection occurs upon contact with an infected person or animal. It begins when the worm is in the larval stage. It penetrates the skin and migrates during its life cycle through the liver and the lungs, and it attaches to the mucosa of the small intestine where it matures. Hookworms deplete the body of nutrients, and a major effect is severe chronic iron-deficiency anemia. About 25% of the world's population is infected with hookworms.

Blood Group Links

Hookworm shows a higher incidence of group O over other ABO groups[1].

Therapies, Hookworm

ALL BLOOD GROUPS:

1. Mebendazole is the drug of choice in the United States. A cure rate of 99% has been reported after a course of 100 mg for 3 days.

2. General support and correction of anemia may be needed first if the infection is heavy and the anemia is severe. Anemia usually responds well to oral iron, but parenteral iron or blood transfusions may be required in very severe cases. An anthelmintic may be given as soon as the patient's condition is stable.

BLOOD GROUP A:

1. Antibacterial Protocol
2. Antibiotic Support Protocol
3. Blood-Building Protocol
4. Intestinal Health Protocol

BLOOD GROUP B:

1. Antibacterial Protocol
2. Antibiotic Support Protocol
3. Intestinal Health Protocol

BLOOD GROUP AB:

1. Antibacterial Protocol
2. Antibiotic Support Protocol
3. Blood-Building Protocol
4. Intestinal Health Protocol

BLOOD GROUP O:

1. Antibacterial Protocol
2. Antibiotic Support Protocol
3. Intestinal Health Protocol

Related Topics

Anemia

Bacterial disease (general)

Immunity

Infectious diseases

REFERENCES

1. Bouree P, Bonnot G. Study of relationship of ABO and Rh blood group, and HLA antigens with parasitic diseases. *J Egypt Soc Parasitol.* 1989;19:67–73.

PARKINSON'S DISEASE–*A chronic progressive disorder characterized by slowness of purposeful movement, resting tremor, and muscle rigidity.*

Parkinson's disease	RISK		
	LOW	AVERAGE	HIGH
GROUP A	▓		
GROUP B	▓	▓	
GROUP AB	▓	▓	
GROUP O	▓	▓	▓

Symptoms

Variable

About Parkinson's Disease

Parkinson's disease usually afflicts middle-aged or elderly individuals, and it is extremely gradual in progression. In the majority of patients, it is not a familial disorder, but occurs randomly. Although the syndrome is well-represented in a worldwide distribution, the manifestations often are clearly marked, and the disease is easily diagnosed, the pathophysiology is poorly understood.

There is no cure for Parkinson's, only treatment of the symptoms. The course is progressive and very gradual, and patients may live their normal lifespan with the disease. Others may become increasingly incapacitated, and eventually wind up in wheelchairs, or dependent upon others for normal daily activities such as dressing and food preparation.

Symptoms include the following:

Cogwheel rigidity: The arm makes ratchet-like catches when it is put through passive movements. This is a result of hypertonia of the muscles, which equally affects opposing muscles. There may be pain, cramping, and decreased strength, although the patient retains normal sensation and reflexes in the limbs. The patient's writing will become small and hard to read.

Lead-pipe rigidity: The arm generally resists any movement. There may be pain, cramping, and decreased strength, although the patient retains normal sensation and reflexes in the limbs. The patient's writing will become small and hard to read.

Bradykinesia: All voluntary movements exhibit general slowing.

Akinesia: There is a lack, or even an absence, of the spontaneous movements associated with the typical animation of a normal individual.

Festinating gait: An individual had difficulty initiating walking from a standing position. He or she will take several small, awkward steps, and then break into a jog or run to keep from falling. The typical pose during walking includes small, shuffling steps, often dragging the feet, a slightly bent-over posture, and the arms held flexed at 90 degrees and tightly at the sides.

Propulsion or retropulsion: This describes the patient who easily falls forward or backward, respectively, upon being lightly pushed.

Fixed facial mien: The typical facial expression of a Parkinson's patient is fixed and immobile, and the voice is monotonous. There may be drooling at the corners of the mouth. The eyes stare and do not blink as often as normal.

Resting tremor: The classic tremor of Parkinson's patients occurs during rest, and resembles pill-rolling between the fingers, with the hand bent. It often occurs only on one side of the body, but may eventually affect both sides. Although it is most pronounced in the hands, similar tremors are also seen in the legs, lips, tongue, and eyelids (when they are firmly closed). The tremor disappears during voluntary movements and during sleep. It worsens with fatigue, emotional STRESS, and embarrassment; many patients will try to hide their affected hand in their pocket or cover it with their unaffected hand.

Depression: About half of Parkinson's patients present with, or will develop, depression.

Blood Group Links

Parkinson's disease is associated with low levels of dopamine, which is why MAO inhibitors are often used for treatment. Inhibiting MAO has the effect of raising dopamine levels. Blood group O is associated with dopamine imbalances. It is possible that group O is more susceptible. Parkinson's disease appears to be less common in blood group A, and appears to take a milder clinical course[1].

Therapies, Parkinson's Disease

BLOOD GROUP A:

1. Cognitive Improvement Protocol
2. Nerve Health Protocol

BLOOD GROUP B:

1. Cognitive Improvement Protocol
2. Nerve Health Protocol

BLOOD GROUP AB:

1. Antistress Protocol
2. Cognitive Improvement Protocol
3. Nerve Health Protocol

BLOOD GROUP O:

1. Cognitive Improvement Protocol
2. Antistress Protocol
3. Nerve Health Protocol

Related Topics

Aging diseases

Stress

REFERENCES

1. Sherrington R, Curtis D, Brynjolfsson J, et al. A linkage study of affective disorder with DNA markers for the ABO-AK1-ORM linkage group near the dopamine beta hydroxylase gene. *Biol Psychiatry.* 1994;36:434–442.

PEPTIC ULCER–*See Ulcer, peptic*

PERIODONTAL DISEASE–*Also called gum disease, a chronic inflammation of the gums, accompanied by a decline of the support structure to the teeth.*

Periodontal disease	RISK		
	LOW	AVERAGE	HIGH
GROUP A			
GROUP B			
GROUP AB			
GROUP O			

Symptoms

- *Gingivitis* (inflammation of the gums, with redness and bleeding)

- *Periodontia* (dental pockets and loose teeth, with redness, swelling, and pain)

About Periodontal Disease

Although proper care of the teeth and gums is an important factor in preventing periodontal disease, it is far from the entire story. Periodontal disease is caused by an immune deficiency, making it a systemic, not a localized, disease.

Blood Group Links

Studies repeatedly show distinct differences among the blood groups for the rates of occurrence of periodontal disease and gingivitis. Blood groups A, B, and AB are more often affected than blood group O.

One study looked at 238 Caucasians, divided into four groups: normal, ulcerative gingivitis, chronic gingivitis, and periodontosis. The results showed that the chronic gingivitis group was significantly different in ABO typing than the control group, with the gingivitis patients having a larger percentage of blood group AB, and a smaller percentage of blood group O. The periodontosis group showed more blood group A and B sufferers and a smaller percentage of blood group O than the healthy controls[1].

Therapies, Periodontal Disease

BLOOD GROUP A:

1. Antibacterial Protocol

BLOOD GROUP B:

1. Antibacterial Protocol

BLOOD GROUP AB:

1. Antibacterial Protocol

BLOOD GROUP O:

1. Antibacterial Protocol

2. Yeast/Fungus Resistance Protocol

Related Topics

Bacterial disease

Dental caries

Digestion

REFERENCES

1. Kaslick RS, West TL, Chasens AI. Association between ABO blood groups, HL-A antigens and periodontal diseases in young adults: a follow-up study. *J Periodontol.* 1980;51:339–342.

PERIPHERAL ARTERY DISEASE–*Lack of blood flow to the extremities.*

Peripheral artery disease	RISK		
	LOW	AVERAGE	HIGH
GROUP A	▓	▓	
GROUP B	▓		
GROUP AB	▓	▓	
GROUP O	▓	▓	

Symptoms

- Persistent leg pain and cramps when walking

About Peripheral Artery Disease

It is estimated that peripheral artery disease occurs in approximately 12% of the adult population, or approximately 22 million Americans. The prevalence of peripheral artery disease increases with advancing age, so much so that almost 20% of people over 70 years of age have the disease.

The most common symptom of mild to moderate peripheral artery disease is intermittent claudication. The classic sign of intermittent claudication is leg pain in the calves after walking for five or more minutes, due to a partial obstruction of the blood flow to the legs. At rest, the leg muscles do not require much blood, so most people feel comfortable, even with severe obstruction of the arteries leading to their legs. However, when they walk, their leg muscles require a large amount of blood, and a partial obstruction of the arteries can prevent extra blood from getting through. Once their leg muscles suffer from a lack of oxygen, they begin to cramp and hurt.

General Risk Factors and Causes

People with elevated cholesterol levels are much more likely to have atherosclerosis than people with low cholesterol levels. Many important nutritional approaches to protecting against ATHEROSCLEROSIS are aimed at lowering serum cholesterol levels.

People with DIABETES are also at very high risk for atherosclerosis.

People with elevated TRIGLYCERIDES may also be at a high risk for atherosclerosis.

Blood Group Links

In one study, serum lipoprotein and lipid levels in patients with intermittent claudication were examined according to ABO blood group. A predominance of blood group A (61%) was found[1].

An excess of blood group A was also found in a group of 125 patients suffering from venous thrombosis in a Brazilian population. There is a clear gender effect on the disease incidence, women being more frequently affected. However, the mean age was not different, regardless of gender. No differences were found in the disease incidence when those of Caucasian and African ancestry were compared. An excess of group A and a scarcity of group O was observed among the patients. The analysis of the combined data from 10 different published series showed a group A to group O relative incidence that was significantly higher than the norm[2].

Therapies, Peripheral Artery Disease

BLOOD GROUP A:

1. Cardiovascular Protocol

2. Blood-Building Protocol

3. Metabolic Enhancement Protocol

BLOOD GROUP B:

1. Cardiovascular Protocol

2. Blood-Building Protocol

3. Metabolic Enhancement Protocol

BLOOD GROUP AB:

1. Cardiovascular Protocol

2. Blood-Building Protocol

3. Metabolic Enhancement Protocol

BLOOD GROUP O:

1. Cardiovascular Protocol

2. Blood-Building Protocol

3. Metabolic Enhancement Protocol

Related Topics

Blood clotting disorders

Cardiovascular disease

Stroke

REFERENCES

1. Horby J, Gyrtrup HJ, Grande P, Vestergaard A. Relation of serum lipoproteins and lipids to the ABO blood groups in patients with intermittent claudication. *J Cardiovasc Surg (Torino).* 1989;30:533–537.

2. Robinson WM, Roisenberg I. Venous thromboembolism and ABO blood groups in a Brazilian population. *Hum Genet.* 1980;55:129–131.

PERNICIOUS ANEMIA–*See Anemia, pernicious*

PHOBIAS–*See Anxiety disorders; Obsessive-compulsive disorder; Stress*

PHYSICAL EXERCISE–*See Stress*

PLAGUE–*See Bacterial disease,* Yersinia *(plague)*

PMS–*See Menstrual cycle disorders, premenstrual syndrome*

PNEUMONIA–*See Bacterial disease, pneumonia*

POLYAMINES–*See Toxicity, bowel (polyamines)*

POLYCYSTIC OVARY SYNDROME–*A multisystem syndrome that involves insulin resistance and excessive production of androgens.*

Polycystic ovary syndrome	RISK		
	LOW	AVERAGE	HIGH
GROUP A			
GROUP B			
GROUP AB			
GROUP O			

Symptoms

- Hirsutism
- Obesity
- Diabetes
- Insulin resistance

About Polycystic Ovary Syndrome

Polycystic ovary syndrome (PCOS) is caused by an overproduction of hormones by the ovary, and can be manifested by either AMENORRHEA or irregular bleeding. PCOS leads to a steady production of estrogen, and an unopposed stimulation of the endometrium that raises the risk of endometrial and breast cancer. Oral contraceptives can sometimes be used to establish regularity.

INSULIN RESISTANCE, a common phenomenon in women with polycystic ovaries, is often a cause of HEART DISEASE, OBESITY, and other hormonal problems later on in life.

Another factor in PCOS may be inadequate deposits of lutein, which is shown to reduce cystic formation. The female ovary is a very metabolically active organ, and the follicles must cut their way out when a woman ovulates by secreting an enzyme to bore a hole to the exterior. Normally there is quite a bit of lutein in the ovarian tissue to snuff out the inflammation that results. If not, the tissue becomes cystic. Lutein is the yellow pigment in plants (*lutea* is Latin for "yellow").

Blood Group Links

Although no studies directly link blood groups and PCOS, blood groups A and AB are highly susceptible to the primary risk factors, which include insulin resistance and obesity.

Therapies, Polycystic Ovary Syndrome

BLOOD GROUP A:

1. Female Balancing Protocol
2. Metabolic Enhancement Protocol

BLOOD GROUP B:

1. Female Balancing Protocol
2. Metabolic Enhancement Protocol

BLOOD GROUP AB:

1. Female Balancing Protocol
2. Metabolic Enhancement Protocol

1. Female Balancing Protocol

2. Metabolic Enhancement Protocol

Related Topics

Insulin resistance

Menstrual cycle disorders

Obesity

POLYPS, COLON–*Normally benign growths in the colon.*

Colon polyps	RISK		
	LOW	AVERAGE	HIGH
GROUP A			
GROUP B			
GROUP AB			
GROUP O			

Symptoms

- Rectal bleeding
- Cramps, abdominal pain, or obstruction
- Prolapse
- Diarrhea

About Colon Polyps

Polyps are growths that develop in the colon. They vary in size and appearance; some look like a wart when small, and a cherry on a stem or fig when they grow. Polyps of the colon and rectum are almost always benign and usually produce no symptoms. However, polyps should be taken seriously because they can with time turn into cancer.

The incidence of polyps increases with age. The cumulative risk of cancer developing in an unremoved polyp is 2.5% at 5 years. Polyps larger than 1 centimeter have a greater cancer risk associated with them than smaller polyps. It has been shown that the removal of polyps by colonoscopy reduces the risk of getting colon cancer significantly. Both polyps as well as colon cancer occur much more frequently in industrialized, Western societies.

Polyps tend to cluster in families. Having a first-degree relative such as a sibling, parent, or child with colon polyps raises one's chances of having polyps. People with first-degree relatives with INFLAMMATORY BOWEL DISEASE are at increased risk, and those who have a first-degree relative with COLON CANCER have a fourfold increase in risk over the general population.

Blood Group Links

Colon polyps express large amounts of ABO antigens[1]. Blood groups A and AB are more susceptible to colon polyps that eventually progress to COLON CANCER. This progression is marked by a decline in the amount of ABO antigen. As the disease progresses, the antigen may disappear altogether[2].

Therapies, Colon Polyps

1. Maintain regular screening habits. Rectal polyps may be palpable by digital examination

but usually are discovered by endoscopy. Because rectal polyps are often multiple and may coexist with cancer, a complete colonoscopy is mandatory even if a lesion is found by flexible sigmoidoscopy. On barium enema x-rays, a polyp appears as a rounded filling defect. Double-contrast (pneumocolon) examination is valuable, but fiberoptic colonoscopy is more reliable. Polyps are more common in the colon than in the small bowel.

2. Don't smoke. Persons smoking more than 20 cigarettes a day are 250% more likely to have polyps as opposed to nonsmokers who otherwise have the same risks.

3. Limit alcohol. Persons who drink have an 87% increased likelihood of having polyps compared to nondrinkers. Those who both smoke and drink are 400% more likely to develop polyps compared to their peers who neither smoke nor drink.

4. Eat a lot of fava beans (groups O and B) and mushrooms (groups A and AB). Standard domestic mushrooms (*Agaricus bisporus*) and fava beans (*Vicia faba*) have been shown to contain lectins that can inhibit the progression of normal colon cells to cancer cells[3].

BLOOD GROUP A:

1. Intestinal Health Protocol

2. Cancer Prevention Protocol

BLOOD GROUP B:

1. Intestinal Health Protocol

2. Cancer Prevention Protocol

BLOOD GROUP AB:

1. Intestinal Health Protocol

2. Cancer Prevention Protocol

BLOOD GROUP O:

1. Intestinal Health Protocol

2. Cancer Prevention Protocol

Related Topics

Cancer, colon

Digestion

Immunity

REFERENCES

1. Itzkowitz SH. Blood group-related carbohydrate antigen expression in malignant and premalignant colonic neoplasms. *J Cell Biochem Suppl.* 1992;16G:97–101.

2. Schoentag R, Primus FJ, Kuhns W. ABH and Lewis blood group expression in colorectal carcinoma. *Cancer Res.* 1987; 47:1695–1700.

3. Jordinson M, El-Hariry I, Calnan D, Calam J, Pignatelli M. Vicia faba agglutinin, the lectin present in broad beans, stimulates differentiation of undifferentiated colon cancer cells. *Gut.* 1999;44:709–714.

POST TRAUMATIC STRESS DISORDER (PTSD)–*See Anxiety disorders*

PREMENSTRUAL SYNDROME–*See Menstrual cycle disorders, premenstrual syndrome*

Probiotics

In 1910, a Russian biologist named Élie Metchnikoff proposed that the best way to improve health and prolong life was to eliminate gastrointestinal toxicity. Many in the medical establishment regarded him as a quack. Intestinal "cleansing" was something of a fad at the time; restorative clinics and spas were a favorite upper-crust getaway, and dubious elixirs flooded the market. The medical establishment, pathologically suspicious of any theory that did not bear its imprimatur, discounted Metchnikoff's idea along with all the rest—a real shame, since it happened to be valid.

Metchnikoff coined the word *probiotic*, meaning "in favor of life," to explain his premise that aging is a process mediated by chronic exposure to putrefactive intoxication caused by imbalances in intestinal bacteria. This process, he suggested, could be halted by the routine ingestion of lactic acid bacteria and their "cultured" food products.

Today, nearly a century later, it is widely accepted that "friendly" intestinal bacteria protect cells, improve immune function, and have a positive effect on our ability to fully use the nutrients in foods. Blood group antigens orchestrate the proper balance of friendly bacteria.

Blood group antigens are complex sugars, which are consumed by bacteria. Different blood group antigens are composed of different combinations of sugars, and bacteria are choosy. Many of the friendly bacteria, in effect, eat right for their type all of the time, by using blood group antigens as their preferred food supply. When there are enough of them, they will compete for food much more effectively than the more harmful forms and will eventually crowd bad bacteria out. Proper strains of colon bacteria, matched to blood group, will metabolize the blood group antigens into short-chain fatty acids, which are very beneficial for the health of the colon.

Where does this "preference" come from? It is based on a concept known as adherence. Much like a key will only click into its preferred lock, bacteria will only adhere to certain configurations of sugars that form complementary attachment sites. While not all of the attachment sites for bacteria in the intestines and digestive tract are blood-type specific, the process of attachment for many friendly (and unfriendly) bacteria is dictated by blood group. In fact, almost 50% of all bacterial strains tested show some blood-group specificity.

Another aspect of blood-group preference is the LECTIN-like activity associated with bacteria— making them friendly to one blood group and unfriendly to another. Some strains of beneficial bacteria can agglutinate red blood cells, an activity that is dictated by blood group.

In general, however, all blood groups will benefit from the overall effects of specific, friendly bacteria and cultured foods. Probiotics provide a lifeline to the ailing system, promoting detoxification and healing.

Health Benefits of Probiotics

Regular consumption of the right cultured foods (foods teeming with probiotic bacteria, such as yogurt) according to blood group promotes significant health benefits.

Friendly bacteria restore intestinal balance, which results in:

- The prevention of adherence of unwanted microorganisms
- The production of a wide array of antibacterial and antifungal compounds
- Improved resistance against bacteria such as *Escherichia coli*, *Salmonella*, *Shigella*, *Helicobacter pylori*

Friendly bacteria enhance immunity by:

- Promoting improved antiviral immune system function
- Increasing natural killer cell activity
- Increasing S-IgA
- Producing nitric oxide
- Modulating cell-mediated immune response
- Preventing some autoimmune diseases
- Evoking anti-Tn antibodies
- Decreasing IgE response
- Enhancing immune system response to administered vaccines

- Mediating against radiation-induced leukopenia

In many respects, friendly bacteria can be thought of as having "adaptogenic" effects on the immune system. They appear to modulate the nonspecific immune response differently in healthy and hypersensitive people. This is seen as an immuno-stimulatory effect in healthy individuals, and as a down-regulation of immuno-inflammatory responses in hypersensitive individuals.

Friendly bacteria promote detoxification by:

- Inactivating and eliminating carcinogens
- Decreasing mutagenic compounds
- Decreasing activity of ornithine decarboxylase
- Decreasing activity of tryptophanase
- Decreasing activity of neuraminidase
- Decreasing levels of polyamines, cresols, and indoles
- Decreasing ammonia
- Decreasing levels of nitrates and nitrites
- Enhancing liver function and promoting elimination of bile acids
- Enhancing cholesterol METABOLISM

Friendly bacteria promote healthy digestion by:

- Normalizing stool volume and regularity
- Producing digestive enzymes that help digest proteins, carbohydrates, and fibers

- Decreasing intestinal permeability

- Decreasing food sensitivities

- Decreasing lactose intolerance

- Decreasing intestinal INFLAMMATION

Friendly bacteria enhance bioavailability of nutrients by:

- Alleviating symptoms of malabsorption

- Increasing the absorption of zinc, calcium, iron, copper, manganese, and phosphorous

- Increasing the production of vitamins B_1, B_2, B_3, B_5, B_6, B_{12}, A, K, folic acid, biotin, and tocopherols

Health Benefits of Cultured Foods

- Cultured foods contain a vast array of health promoting vitamins, minerals, and accessory phytochemicals.

- Culturing is a method to ease the DIGESTION and improved bioavailability of nutrients.

- Culturing increases the bioavailability of health-benefiting compounds like isoflavones and bioflavonoids.

- Culturing actually improves the amino acid and protein efficiency ratios of foods.

- Cultured foods contain high levels of vitamin K, tocopherols, and vitamin B_{12}.

- Culturing improved stability and retention of vitamin C levels in the foods.

- Culturing augments some of the metabolic benefits of these foods.

- Cultured foods are tremendous antioxidants.

- Cultured foods possess substantial anti-CANCER properties.

- Cultured foods can actually improve the metabolism and elimination of substances like alcohol.

- Cultured foods promote heart health through a number of blood type–specific mechanisms.

- Cultured foods provide excellent growth promoting substrates (e.g., act as probiotics for the continued growth of good bacteria within the digestive tract).

Related Topics

Autoimmune disease (general)

Bacterial disease (general)

Cancer (general)

Digestion

Food poisoning

Immunity

Inflammatory bowel disease

Parasitic disease

Toxicity, bowel

Ulcer (general)

PROSTATE CANCER–*See Cancer, prostate*

PROSTATIC HYPERPLASIA, BENIGN–*A gradual enlargement of the prostate gland, common in men over age 50.*

Benign prostatic hyperplasia	RISK		
	LOW	AVERAGE	HIGH
GROUP A	███	███	
GROUP B	███		
GROUP AB	███	███	
GROUP O	███		
SECRETORS	███	███	

Symptoms

- Frequent need to urinate, especially at night
- Incomplete bladder emptying
- Pressure on the bladder
- Lower urinary tract infections
- Pain and burning with urination

About Benign Prostatic Hyperplasia

The prostate is a small organ about the size of a walnut. It is located below the bladder and surrounds the urethra. The role of the prostate is to manufacture the fluid that becomes semen. Enlargement of the prostate, or benign prostatic hyperplasia (BPH), occurs primarily due to hormonal changes that come with aging. It is estimated that more than 50% of men will experience BPH in their lifetime. Some suggest that BPH typically indicates low levels of male hormones.

Blood Group Links

Blood groups A and AB men have a higher risk of developing prostate cancer. Secretors tend to have a greater incidence of prostate cancer than non-secretors. Since BPH may be an initial sign of the eventual development of prostate cancer, groups A and B, especially secretors, need to be especially vigilant.

Therapies, Benign Prostatic Hyperplasia

BLOOD GROUP A:

1. Male Health Protocol
2. Immune-Enhancing Protocol
3. Cancer Prevention Protocol

BLOOD GROUP B:

1. Male Health Protocol
2. Immune-Enhancing Protocol
3. Cancer Prevention Protocol

BLOOD GROUP AB:

1. Male Health Protocol
2. Immune-Enhancing Protocol
3. Cancer Prevention Protocol

BLOOD GROUP O:

1. Male Health Protocol

2. Immune-Enhancing Protocol

3. Cancer Prevention Protocol

Related Topics

Cancer, prostate

Immunity

RHEUMATIC FEVER/HEART DISEASE–

An acute inflammatory complication of group A streptococcal infection.

Rheumatic fever	RISK		
	LOW	AVERAGE	HIGH
GROUP A			
GROUP B			
GROUP AB			
GROUP O			
NON-SECRETOR			

Symptoms

In diagnosing rheumatic fever, doctors generally look for either the presence of two of the following major criteria or the presence of one major plus two minor criteria. In all cases, evidence of a preceding strep throat is key to making a diagnosis of rheumatic fever.

Major Criteria:

- Inflammation of the heart, sometimes indicated by weakness and shortness of breath or chest pain

- Painful ARTHRITIS, most often affecting the ankles, wrists, knees, and elbows, and migrating from joint to joint

- Involuntary jerky movement of the limbs and face, or more subtle movement difficulties, such as marked deterioration in handwriting

- Broad, pink or faint-red, non-itching patches on the skin (uncommon)

- Lumps under the skin (uncommon)

Minor Criteria:

- Joint pain without inflammation

- FEVER

- Previous rheumatic fever or evidence of rheumatic heart disease

- Abnormal heartbeat on an electrocardiogram

- Blood test indicating inflammation

- New heart murmurs

About Rheumatic Fever/Heart Disease

Rheumatic fever is a serious inflammatory condition that can affect many parts of the body—heart, joints, nervous system, and skin. Although rheumatic fever can occur at any age, the most frequent incidence is in young people between the ages of 5 and 15 years. Rheumatic fever is precipitated by an overactive immune response to a STREPTOCOCCAL INFECTION.

Blood Group Links

ABO non-secretors have a higher incidence of rheumatic fever and rheumatic heart disease, and are more susceptible to the overactive immune response to the streptococcal infection[1].

Streptococcal infections occur more often in blood group B individuals than in the other blood groups, increasing their susceptibility to rheumatic fever[2]. There is also a connection between blood group B and neonatal group B streptococci infections. This association is strong enough to be evident even based on the mother's blood group—that is, a blood group B infant with a blood group B mother has double the risk of infection[3].

Therapies, Rheumatic Fever/Heart Disease

BLOOD GROUP A:

1. Immune-Enhancing Protocol

2. Antibacterial Protocol

BLOOD GROUP B:

1. Immune-Enhancing Protocol

2. Antibacterial Protocol

BLOOD GROUP AB:

1. Immune-Enhancing Protocol

2. Antibacterial Protocol

BLOOD GROUP O:

1. Immune-Enhancing Protocol

2. Antibacterial Protocol

Related Topics

Autoimmune disease (general)

Inflammation

Streptococcus infection

REFERENCES

1. Glynn AA, Glynn LE, Holborrow EJ. Secretion of blood group substances in rheumatic fever: a genetic requirement for susceptibility? *Brit Med J.* ii:266–270.
2. Ligtenberg AJ, Veerman EC, de Graaff J, Nieuw Amerongen AV. Saliva-induced aggregation of oral streptococci and the influence of blood group reactive substances. *Arch Oral Biol.* 1990;35 suppl:141S–143S.
3. Regan JA, Chao S, James LS. Maternal ABO blood group type B: a risk factor in the development of neonatal group B streptococcal disease. *Pediatrics.* 1978;62:504–509.

RHEUMATOID ARTHRITIS–*See Arthritis, rheumatoid*

RHINITIS–*See Allergies, environmental/hay fever*

RICKETS–*Bone formation resulting from inadequate calcium in bones.*

Rickets	RISK		
	LOW	AVERAGE	HIGH
GROUP A			
GROUP B			
GROUP AB			
GROUP O			

Symptoms

- Skeletal deformities

- Growth disturbances

- Hypocalcemia (abnormally low levels of calcium in the blood)

- Muscular weakness

- Irritability

About Rickets

Children with rickets have abnormal bone formation resulting from inadequate calcium in bones. This lack of calcium can result from inadequate exposure to sunshine or from lack of vitamin D in the diet. Vitamin D is essential for calcium absorption. Rickets is worsened by a lack of dietary calcium.

Rickets can also be caused by conditions that impair absorption of vitamin D and/or calcium, even when these nutrients are consumed in appropriate amounts. Activation of vitamin D in the body requires normal liver and kidney function. Damage to either organ can cause rickets.

Blood Group Links

In an effort to study the role of genetics in vitamin D deficiency rickets, 400 infants with rickets, aged from 6 months to 2 years, were randomly chosen and were examined for sex differences and ABO typing. A significant predominance of the male sex was found: the sex ratio was 1:43. Blood group A was significantly associated with rickets, both among males or females. The alkaline phos-phatase values were significantly higher in male infants: 91% of them had levels above 30 alkaline phosphatase units, whereas the corresponding percentage of females was 72%. This indicates that the disease is more severe among males. The study gives added support for the belief that there is a genetic factor in nutritional rickets[1].

Therapies, Rickets

ALL BLOOD GROUPS:

Sun exposure, required by the body to make vitamin D, must involve at least some direct exposure to skin (hands, face, arms, etc.). The ultraviolet light that triggers vitamin D formation is blocked by clothing. Depending on latitude, sunlight during the winter may not provide enough ultraviolet light to help the body make vitamin D. At other times during the year, even 30 minutes of exposure per day will usually lead to large increases in the amount of vitamin D made. If it is difficult to get sunlight exposure, full-spectrum lighting can be used to stimulate vitamin D production.

BLOOD GROUP A:

1. Liver Support Protocol

2. Stomach Health Protocol

3. Intestinal Health Protocol

BLOOD GROUP B:

1. Liver Support Protocol

2. Stomach Health Protocol

3. Intestinal Support Protocol

BLOOD GROUP AB:

1. Liver Support Protocol

2. Stomach Health Protocol

3. Intestinal Health Protocol

BLOOD GROUP O:

1. Liver Support Protocol

2. Stomach Health Protocol

3. Intestinal Health Protocol

Related Topics

Digestion

Musculoskeletal injury

REFERENCES

1. el-Kholy MS, Abdel Mageed FY, Farid FA. A genetic study of vitamin D deficiency rickets: 2-sex differences and ABO typing. *J Egypt Public Health Assoc.* 1992;67:213–222.

RUBELLA (GERMAN MEASLES)–*Three-day measles.*

Rubella	RISK		
	LOW	AVERAGE	HIGH
GROUP A	▓		
GROUP B	▓		
GROUP AB	▓		
GROUP O	▓	▓	

Symptoms

- Malaise
- Swollen glands
- Rash

About Rubella

Rubella is a contagious viral infection, usually with mild constitutional symptoms, that may result in abortion, stillbirth, or congenital defects in infants born to mothers infected during the early months of pregnancy. Since rubella often goes undiagnosed in mild cases, it is impossible to know the exact percentage of those infected, but it is estimated that 10% to 15% of young women are not infected in childhood—which makes them vulnerable during pregnancy.

Epidemics occur at irregular intervals during the spring; major epidemics occur at about 6- to 9-year intervals. In the United States incidence is now at its lowest point in history. However, outbreaks continue to occur and rubella must still be identified and susceptible populations immunized. IMMUNITY appears to be lifelong after natural infection.

Blood Group Links

A case study noted that an infant with probable congenital rubella infection developed altered blood group expression. This was noted at 4 months of age. The child's blood was tested on seven separate occasions during the first 8 weeks of life and identified as blood group A. However, on repeat testing, her cells failed to agglutinate with anti-A and anti-AB typing serum. The A antigen was present, however. Altered expression of blood group A (loss of agglutinability) has occurred previously only in association with hematologic (blood) malignancy[1].

Therapies, Rubella

ALL BLOOD GROUPS:

The rubella vaccine should not be given to any person with a defective or altered immune system (such as those with LEUKEMIA, LYMPHOMA, or other malignancies), or to people who have a serious febrile illness, or during prolonged therapy with corticosteroids or radiation, or during chemotherapy.

BLOOD GROUP A:

1. Antiviral Protocol

2. Immune-Enhancing Protocol

BLOOD GROUP B:

1. Antiviral Protocol

2. Immune-Enhancing Protocol

BLOOD GROUP AB:

1. Antiviral Protocol

2. Immune-Enhancing Protocol

BLOOD GROUP O:

1. Antiviral Protocol

2. Immune-Enhancing Protocol

Related Topics

Immunity

Viral disease (general)

REFERENCES

1. Sherman LA, Silberstein LE, Berkman EM. Altered blood group expression in a patient with congenital rubella infection. *Transfusion.* 1984;24:267–269.

SALMONELLA–*See Bacterial disease (general)*

SARCOIDOSIS–*See Autoimmune disease, sarcoidosis*

SCHIZOPHRENIA–*A Mental disorder involving psychosis.*

Schizophrenia	RISK		
	LOW	AVERAGE	HIGH
GROUP A			
GROUP B			
GROUP AB			
GROUP O			

Symptoms

- Loss of contact with reality (psychosis)
- Hallucinations (false perceptions)
- Delusions (false beliefs)
- Abnormal thinking
- Flattened affect (restricted range of emotions)
- Diminished motivation
- Disturbed work and social functioning

About Schizophrenia

Worldwide, the prevalence of schizophrenia appears to be about 1%, although pockets of higher or lower prevalence exist. In the United States patients with schizophrenia occupy about 25% of all hospital beds and account for about 20% of all social security disability days. Schizophrenia is more prevalent than ALZHEIMER'S DISEASE, DIABETES, or MULTIPLE SCLEROSIS. Prevalence of schizophrenia appears to be greater among lower socioeconomic classes in urban areas, perhaps because its disabling effects lead to unemployment and poverty. Similarly, a greater prevalence among single persons may reflect the effect of illness or illness precursors on social functioning. Typically, the peak age of onset is 18 to 25 years in men and 26 to 45 years in women. However, onset in childhood, early adolescence, or late life is not uncommon.

Vulnerability to schizophrenia may include genetic predisposition; intrauterine, birth, or postnatal complications; or viral infections. Maternal exposure to influenza in the second trimester of pregnancy, and Rh incompatibility in a second or subsequent pregnancy are associated with an increased risk of schizophrenia in offspring.

Blood Group Links

Researchers studied the ABO blood groups and the secretor status of 210 schizophrenic patients born in Budapest. The patients were classified according to three forms of process—continuous, shift-like, and recurrent. In continuous schizophrenia there was a greater number of blood group A patients and a smaller number of blood group O. A greater number of blood group O and a smaller number of blood group A individuals experienced the shift-like form. For the recurrent form, there was an increase of group O non-secretors[1].

In a study that may provide important clues to the genesis of schizophrenia, patients were divided according to ABO blood groups. Significant differences were found between groups A and O in the albumin–fibrinogen ratio, fibrinogen level, and blood viscosity of patients. The general level of abnormalities of blood viscosity factors (plasma and blood viscosity, aggregation of red cells, apparent viscosity of artificial thrombi) and biochemical factors (fibrinogen level, albumin–fibrinogen ratio, albumin–globulin ratio) observed in the patients studied suggested that depressive and schizoid anxiety, but in particular the depressive anxiety, might show a concurrent pathology of blood rheology and coagulation. A difference of significance is observed in a number of factors between patients and normal values. Also, a significant difference is observed in some of the blood viscosity factors and functions between the groups of DEPRESSIVE and schizoid ANXIETY patients. These results open a new line of inquiry: primarily, that there is a physiological difference between normal individuals and patients suffering from chronic anxiety; and secondarily, that there are some physiological differences between the depressive and the schizoid anxiety. It is not possible to state whether an elevation of the blood viscosity factors is the cause or result of the mental condition, but by its very presence an elevation of blood viscosity might affect the cardiovascular system and thus cause a secondary deterioration of different organic functions. This correlation seems to be a link to explain the role of anxiety in the causation of cardiovascular and cerebral conditions by means of biological parameters. While the study did not state a conclusion regarding risk factors, it is clear that groups A and O have very different blood viscosity patterns[2].

Therapies, Schizophrenia

BLOOD GROUP A:

1. Nerve Health Protocol

2. Antistress Protocol

3. Cognitive Improvement Protocol

BLOOD GROUP B:

1. Nerve Health Protocol

2. Antistress Protocol

3. Cognitive Improvement Protocol

BLOOD GROUP AB:

1. Nerve Health Protocol

2. Antistress Protocol

3. Cognitive Improvement Protocol

BLOOD GROUP O:

1. Nerve Health Protocol

2. Antistress Protocol

3. Cognitive Improvement Protocol

Related Topics

Anxiety disorders

Blood clotting disorders

Depression, bipolar

Depression, unipolar

Stress

REFERENCES

1. Faludi G. [Relationship between schizophrenia, ABO system and secretory system]. *Encephale*. 1981;7:143–152.
2. Dintendast L, Zador I. Blood rheology in patients with depressive and schizoid anxiety. *Biorheology*. 1976;(13):33–36.

SCLEROSING CHOLANGITIS–*An autoimmune disease of the bile ducts, often accompanied by inflammation of the colon.*

Sclerosing cholangitis	RISK		
	LOW	AVERAGE	HIGH
GROUP A			
GROUP B			
GROUP AB			
GROUP O			
NON-SECRETOR			

Symptoms

- Dry eyes and dry mouth
- Fever
- Pain (upper right quadrant)
- Jaundice
- Colitis

About Sclerosing Cholangitis

Sclerosing cholangitis is an autoimmune disease of the bile ducts often accompanied by inflammation of the colon. It is found more commonly in men, typically developing around the age of 35 to 40. It has been theorized that the actual cause of sclerosing cholangitis may initially be an infection of the bile ducts, with a subsequent misguided attack by the immune system on healthy cells as well. Conventional treatment of sclerosing cholangitis is not very effective, and, in many cases, patients must undergo liver transplants to survive.

Blood Group Links

The distribution of carbohydrate antigens of the ABO, Lewis, and Kell (a minor blood group) systems was examined in biliary and colonic cells of 11 patients with primary sclerosing cholangitis (PSC). There was inappropriate staining with anti-A and anti-B in biliary epithelium of PSC patients compared with normal individuals and control patients with inflammatory bowel disease. Expression of Lewis antigens was increased in patients with cholestatic liver disease. Ninety-one percent of PSC patients showed a similar pattern of inappropriate staining by anti-A and anti-B antibodies in colonic epithelium compared with 33% of normal and 42% of inflammatory bowel disease control patients[1]. This result implied a higher risk for contracting PSC among groups A, B and AB.

Therapies, Sclerosing Cholangitis

BLOOD GROUP A:

1. Liver Support Protocol
2. Immune-Enhancing Protocol
3. Anti-Inflammation Protocol
4. Detoxification Protocol

BLOOD GROUP B:

1. Liver Support Protocol
2. Immune-Enhancing Protocol
3. Anti-Inflammation Protocol
4. Detoxification Protocol

BLOOD GROUP AB:

1. Liver Support Protocol
2. Immune-Enhancing Protocol
3. Anti-Inflammation Protocol
4. Detoxification Protocol

BLOOD GROUP O:

1. Liver Support Protocol
2. Immune-Enhancing Protocol
3. Anti-Inflammation Protocol
4. Detoxification Protocol

Related Topics

Autoimmune disease (general)

Colitis, ulcerative

Inflammation

Liver disease

REFERENCES

1. Bloom S, Heryet A, Fleming K, Chapman RW. Inappropriate expression of blood group antigens on biliary and colonic epithelia in primary sclerosing cholangitis. *Gut.* 1993;34: 977–983.

SHIGELLA–*See Bacterial disease,* Shigella

SINUSITIS–*An acute or chronic inflammation of the nasal sinuses.*

Sinusitis	RISK		
	LOW	AVERAGE	HIGH
GROUP A			
GROUP B			
GROUP AB			
GROUP O			

Symptoms

- Profuse, thick, colored nasal drainage
- Bad-tasting post-nasal drip
- Cough
- Head congestion
- Headache
- Plugged-up nose
- Feeling of facial swelling
- Toothache

About Sinusitis

The primary function of the sinuses is to warm, moisten, and filter the air in the nasal cavity. They also play a role in our ability to vocalize certain sounds. Sinusitis, which is common in the winter, may last for months or years if inadequately treated. Although COLDS are the most common cause of acute sinusitis, people with allergies may also be predisposed to developing sinusitis. ALLERGIES can trigger inflammation of the sinuses and nasal mucous linings. This INFLAMMATION prevents the sinus cavities from clearing out bacteria, and increases the chance of developing secondary bacterial sinusitis.

Structural problems in the nose—such as narrow drainage passages, tumors or polyps, or a deviated nasal septum (the wall between the left and right sides of the nose)—may be another cause of sinusitis. Surgery is sometimes needed to correct these problems. Many patients with recurring or chronic sinusitis have more than one factor that predisposes them to infection.

Blood Group Links

Blood group B and to a somewhat lesser extent blood group O are most susceptible to sinusitis that is provoked by allergies.

Therapies, Sinusitis

BLOOD GROUP A:

1. Sinus Health Protocol
2. Allergy Control Protocol
3. Antibacterial Protocol

BLOOD GROUP B:

1. Sinus Health Protocol
2. Allergy Control Protocol
3. Antibacterial Protocol

BLOOD GROUP AB:

1. Sinus Health Protocol
2. Allergy Control Protocol
3. Antibacterial Protocol

BLOOD GROUP O:

1. Sinus Health Protocol
2. Allergy Control Protocol
3. Antibacterial Protocol

Related Topics

Allergies (general)

Bacterial disease (general)

Immunity

SJÖGREN'S SYNDROME–*See Autoimmune disease, Sjögren's syndrome*

SKIN LESIONS–*See Cancer, melanoma*

SKIN RASH–*See Allergies, environmental/hay fever*

SLEEP APNEA–*See Snoring*

SNORING—*Noisy sleep.*

Snoring	RISK		
	LOW	AVERAGE	HIGH
GROUP A			
GROUP B			
GROUP AB			
GROUP O			
NON-SECRETOR			

Symptoms

- Noisy sleep

About Snoring

Snoring affects about half of men and 25% of women, most age 50 or older. It occurs when air flows past relaxed tissues in the throat, causing the tissues to vibrate with breathing. Having a low, thick soft palate or enlarged tonsils or adenoids can narrow the airway. Likewise, an elongated uvula—triangular piece of tissue hanging from the soft palate—obstructs airflow and increases vibration. Being significantly overweight contributes to narrowing of the throat tissues. With age, the throat muscles also naturally weaken and sag.

Snoring may also be associated with sleep apnea. In this condition, excessive sagging of throat tissues causes the airway to collapse, preventing normal breathing. Sleep apnea generally breaks up loud snoring with 10 seconds to a half-minute of silence. Eventually, the lack of oxygen and an increase in carbon dioxide wake up the snorer, forcing the airway open with a loud snort.

Blood Group Links

Individuals from every blood group may be susceptible to snoring, depending on the related condition. However, ABO non-secretor status offers a slightly increased risk for habitual snoring[1].

Therapies, Snoring

ALL BLOOD GROUPS:

1. Avoid alcoholic beverages, tranquilizers, sleeping pills, and antihistamines before retiring.
2. Sleep prone or on your side.
3. Raise the head of the bed.

BLOOD GROUP A:

1. Pulmonary Support Protocol
2. Allergy Control Protocol
3. Sinus Health Protocol

BLOOD GROUP B:

1. Pulmonary Support Protocol
2. Allergy Control Protocol
3. Sinus Health Protocol

BLOOD GROUP AB:

1. Pulmonary Support Protocol
2. Allergy Control Protocol
3. Sinus Health Protocol

BLOOD GROUP O:

1. Pulmonary Support Protocol
2. Allergy Control Protocol
3. Sinus Health Protocol

Related Topics

Allergies (general)

Asthma

Cardiovascular disease

Obesity

REFERENCES

1. Jennum P, Hein HO, Suadicani P, Sorenson H, Gyntelberg F. Snoring, family history, and genetic markers in men. The Copenhagen Male Study. *Chest.* 1995;107:1289–1293.

SPINA BIFIDA–*See Birth defects*

SQUAMOUS CELL CANCER–*See Cancer, melanoma*

STAPH INFECTION–*See Bacterial disease, staphylococcal infection*

STOMACH CANCER–*See Cancer, stomach*

STREP THROAT–*See Bacterial disease, pneumonia;* Streptococcus *infection*

STREPTOCOCCUS **INFECTION**–*Infection with the* **streptococcus** *bacterium.*

Strep infection	RISK		
	LOW	AVERAGE	HIGH
GROUP A			
GROUP B			
GROUP AB			
GROUP O			

Symptoms

- Strep throat
- Scarlet fever
- Skin infections (impetigo, cellulitis/erysipelas)
- Pneumonia, septic arthritis

About *Streptococcus* Infection

The Group A *Streptococcus* bacterium is responsible for most cases of streptococcal illness. Other types (B, C, D, and G) may also cause infection. Group B *Streptococcus* (GBS) is a bacterium that causes life-threatening infections in newborns. GBS can also cause disease in pregnant women, the elderly, and adults with other illnesses. Pregnant women can transmit GBS to their newborns at birth. GBS is the most common cause of blood infections and meningitis in newborns.

Blood Group Links

An aggregation of strains of *Streptococcus rattus, S. mutans,* and *S. salivarius* taken by saliva from individuals of blood groups A, B, and O was investigated. Blood group A saliva had a significantly higher aggregation activity with *S. rattus* than blood group B saliva. However, *S. mutans* and *S. salivarius* were better aggregated by blood group B saliva—and aggregation was most significant with *S. mutans*[1].

The blood group A–specific carbohydrate, *N*-acetyl-D-galactosamine, inhibited aggregation of

S. rattus, but not of the other strains. The blood group B–specific carbohydrate, D-galactose, inhibited aggregation of *S. mutans* but not of *S. rattus* or *S. salivarius.* L-Fucose, specific for blood group O, failed to inhibit aggregation of any of the three strains. These findings suggest that blood group–specific substances may be involved in bacterial aggregation[2].

In a prospective study of maternal genital colonization with GBS at the time of delivery, epidemiological data, including ABO blood group, were recorded for 1,062 patients. Blood group B was found in a statistically significant higher proportion of patients colonized with GBS compared with the total population. Blood group B women were twice as likely to be colonized as blood groups O and A. Researchers suggested that GBS may possess a B-like antigen. One may speculate that a mutation toward an affinity for the human ABO blood group type B accounts for the advent of the GBS as a significant perinatal pathogen[3].

Therapies, *Streptococcus* Infection

BLOOD GROUP A:

1. Antibacterial Protocol
2. Antibiotic Support Protocol
3. Immune-Enhancing Protocol

BLOOD GROUP B:

1. Antibacterial Protocol
2. Antibiotic Support Protocol
3. Immune-Enhancing Protocol

BLOOD GROUP AB:

1. Antibacterial Protocol
2. Antibiotic Support Protocol
3. Immune-Enhancing Protocol

BLOOD GROUP O:

1. Antibacterial Protocol
2. Antibiotic Support Protocol
3. Immune-Enhancing Protocol

Related Topics

Bacterial disease (general)

Rheumatic fever/heart disease

REFERENCES

1. Haverkorn MJ, Goslings WR. Streptococci, ABO blood groups, and secretor status. *Am J Hum Genet.* 1969;21:360–375.
2. Ligtenberg AJ, Veerman EC, de Graaff J, Nieuw Amerongen AV. Saliva-induced aggregation of oral streptococci and the influence of blood group reactive substances. *Arch Oral Biol.* 1990;35 (suppl):141S–143S.
3. Regan JA, Chao S, James LS. Maternal ABO blood group type B: a risk factor in the development of neonatal group B streptococcal disease. *Pediatrics.* 1978;62:504–509.

STRESS–*Conditions resulting from imbalances in stress hormones.*

Stress	RISK		
	LOW	AVERAGE	HIGH
GROUP A			
GROUP B			
GROUP AB			
GROUP O			

Symptoms

- Indigestion
- Disrupted or restless sleep
- Failure to remember dreams
- Sleep apnea
- Poor tolerance to heat or severe climates
- Muscle tension
- Predictable drops in energy during the day
- Cold hands

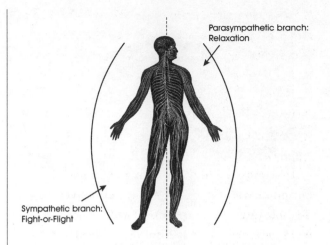

The automatic nervous system depends on the balance of the sympathetic and parasympathetic.

About Stress

Under circumstances of physiological or emotional stress, the body protects itself by reversing its polarities, shifting the relative balance of the autonomic (automatic) nervous system, which is actually two systems. The sympathetic nervous system is responsible for the initial "fight or flight" response. The parasympathetic branch is responsible for relaxing the nervous system after whatever set off the alarms indicating danger has passed. The proper functioning of both systems is a critical component of good health. Together, the two branches of the nervous system communicate with the endocrine system and internal organs to help maintain proper function and to respond to a wide range of potential challenges.

For the most part, the two branches of the nervous system are antagonists. They tend to work best in balanced opposition to one another. For example, sympathetic activity causes the heart to beat faster and more forcefully, whereas parasympathetic activity slows down the heart rate and unclenches the arterial muscle walls, allowing freer blood flow and oxygenation of the heart muscle.

The key to the proper functioning of the nervous system is balance. Problems occur when one of the two parts of this system has a continued dominance over the other for prolonged periods of time. Chronic stress acts like a weight on a scale—it tilts the scale in favor of the sympathetic branch at the expense of the parasympathetic branch. Since many of the body's activities associated with health and healing are driven by parasympathetic activity, prolonged time intervals with the scales out of balance will inevitably lead to a breakdown. The mechanics of a normal stress response involve the synchronized action of three endocrine glands: the hypothalamus, pituitary, and adrenal. We refer to this interplay as the HPA axis.

In a situation of stress, the hypothalamus gland

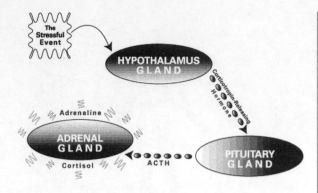

STRESS RESPONSE
The HPA Axis

At the moment of stress, the hypothalamus gland in the brain activates a messenger molecule called corticotropin-releasing hormone. Corticotropin-releasing hormone alerts the pituitary gland to release adrenocortropic hormone (ACTH). ACTH signals the adrenal gland to release its supply of stress hormones—adrenaline and cortisol.

in the brain, often called the master gland, releases a messenger molecule called corticotropin-releasing hormone. This messenger hormone alerts the pituitary gland to release adrenocorticotropic hormone (ACTH). ACTH signals the adrenal gland to release its supply of stress hormones—adrenaline and cortisol. When the stress has ended, the hypothalamus gland is signaled to stop producing the messenger hormone. Homeostasis—balance—is restored.

The two types of stress hormones are catecholamines and cortisol, and these are the hormones that are most closely linked to the blood groups.

Two catecholamines are released from the adrenal gland in response to stress: epinephrine, more commonly recognized as adrenaline, and norepinephrine, also called noradrenaline. When these powerful chemicals are released into the bloodstream, there is an increase in heart rate, an increase in blood pressure, a decrease in digestive capability, an increase in arousal or alertness, and an overall shifting of resources toward fight, flight, exercise, or some form of physical activity. The catecholamines can be thought of as the shock troops of the nervous system, acting as the immediate, short-term response to stress.

Cortisol, on the other hand, is more like an occupying army—in for the long haul. Cortisol is a catabolic hormone; it will function to break down muscle tissue and convert the proteins from the tissue into energy. (It will leave fat for the body to use later.) The adrenal glands will flood the system with cortisol in any traumatic situation. Exposure to cold, starvation, bleeding, SURGERY, infections, injuries, pain, and excessive amounts of exercise will be met by cortisol. Emotional and mental stress also influence the increase of this hormone. But cortisol also stimulates and marshals the powerful forces within our systems, all geared to survival.

Cortisol is essential for life. Since it enables us to get out of the way of danger, we would quickly die when exposed to stress if our adrenal glands stopped making this key hormone. However, cortisol is a double-edged sword. Excessive or prolonged release of cortisol disrupts the balance of a number of our internal systems. While the proper levels of cortisol will reduce inflammation, decrease our tendency to allergies, and help to heal tissue and wounds, inappropriate levels will create the opposite effect. ULCERS, HIGH BLOOD PRESSURE, HEART DISEASE, muscle loss, AGING of the skin, increased risk of bone fractures, and insomnia are just some of the costs of cortisol intoxication. Chronic overproduction of cortisol also severely compromises the immune system, making us susceptible to viral infections. High cortisol levels can produce the daytime "brain fog" known as diurnal cognitive dysfunction. As a matter of fact, people with ALZHEIMER'S DISEASE and senile dementia have chronically high cortisol levels.

Stress and Immune Performance

Research is clear that acute stress in virtually any form will cause a temporary lowering of immune system defenses; chronic stress will result in long-term effects on the immune system. For example, natural killer (NK) cells, responsible for destroying cells infected with viruses and cancer cells, are significantly affected by stress. Chronic stress—whether due to external challenges such as heavy metal exposure, pollution, white noise, loss of sleep, overwork, emotional challenges, stressful life events, daily hassles, bad self-image, poor mood, lack of exercise, poor nutrition, or any other negative component—will always result in decreased NK activity[1].

A severe life stress is associated with up to a 50% reduction of NK cell activity. In fact, the impact of stress on NK cell activity is much more severe than some of the worst lifestyle habits, such as alcohol consumption and tobacco smoking[2]. In addition, the production of IgA—probably the single most important aspect of humoral (antibody) immunity found in the mucus secretions of the DIGESTIVE SYSTEM, mouth, lungs, urinary tract, and other body cavities—shows a substantial decline under stress[3].

Stress and Cardiovascular Health

Stress and the emotions associated with stress are important risk factors for cardiovascular disease. The Mayo Clinic has reported that psychological stress is the strongest predictor of future cardiac events, such as cardiac death, arrest, and attacks. During the 6 months after release from the initial hospitalization, distressed patients had significantly higher rates of cardiovascular re-hospitalization, recurrent health events, and recurrent "hard events" (cardiac death, MYOCARDIAL INFARCTION, or cardiac arrest and resuscitation) in comparison with nondistressed patients. Adjustment for other factors associated with a risk of early re-hospitalization and recurrent events did not reduce the strength or significance of the association between psychological distress and early cardiovascular re-hospitalization or recurrent heart events. Emotional stress has been found to be more predictive of death from cancer and heart disease than smoking. People who were unable to manage their stress effectively had a 40% higher death rate than nonstressed individuals[4,5].

Blood Group Links

While all of the blood types respond to stress by secreting more cortisol, blood group A and to a somewhat lesser extent group B start with a higher basal level in their blood all the time. In addition, blood group A produces more adrenaline in response to stress than the other blood groups, although group A also has the greatest ability to break down or eliminate catecholamine hormones, like adrenaline[6]—restoring to normal levels more rapidly after the stress has passed.

In times of stress, blood group O individuals and to a somewhat lesser extent group AB individuals tend to secrete higher levels of the catecholamines noradrenaline and adrenaline. This facility enables them to respond quickly and efficiently to danger. Their recovery is more difficult because it takes them longer to break down catecholamines. An enzyme called monoamine oxidase (MAO) is responsible for, among other things, the breakdown or inactivation of adrenaline and noradrenaline. When measuring the activity of MAO in platelets, research has shown that blood group O has the lowest activity of this enzyme. This may explain their difficulty breaking down the catecholamines noradrenaline and adrenaline[7], and maintaining a normal balance in the absence of stress.

Therapies, Stress

BLOOD GROUP A:

1. Antistress Protocol

BLOOD GROUP B:

1. Antistress Protocol

BLOOD GROUP AB:

1. Antistress Protocol

BLOOD GROUP O:

1. Antistress Protocol

Related Topics

Cancer (general)

Cardiovascular disease

Immunity

REFERENCES

1. Glaser R, Kiecolt-Glaser JK, Malarkey WB, Sheridan JF. The influence of psychological stress on the immune response to vaccines. *Ann N Y Acad Sci.* 1998;840:649–655.
2. Kusaka Y, Morimoto K. Does lifestyle modulate natural killer cell activities [review, in Japanese]? *Nippon Eiseigaku Zasshi.* 1992;46:1035–1042.
3. Irwin M, Patterson T, Smith TL, et al. Reduction of immune function in life stress and depression. *Biol Psychiatry.* 1990;27:22–30.
4. Allison TG, Williams DE, Miller TD, et al. Medical and economic costs of psychologic distress in patients with coronary artery disease. *Mayo Clin Proc.* 1995;70:734–42.
5. Eysenck HJ. Personality, stress and cancer: prediction and prophylaxis. *Br J Med Psychol.* 1988;61(pt 1):57–75.
6. Goldin LR, Gershon ES, Targum SD, Sparkes RS, McGinniss M. Segregation and linkage studies of plasma dopamine-beta-hydroxylase (DBH), erythrocyte catechol-O-methyltransferase (COMT), and platelet monoamine oxidase (MAO): possible linkage between the ABO locus and a gene controlling DBH activity. *Am J Hum Genet.* 1982;34:250–262.
7. Locong AH, Roberge AG. Cortisol and catecholamines response to venisection by humans with different blood groups. *Clin Biochem.* 1985;18:67–69.

STROKE (CEREBROVASCULAR ACCIDENT)—*A critical cerebral event, such as a hemorrhage or blood clot, that cuts off the blood supply to the brain.*

Stroke	RISK		
	LOW	AVERAGE	HIGH
GROUP A (clots)			
GROUP B			
GROUP AB			
GROUP O (bleeding)			

Symptoms

- Sudden numbness, weakness, or paralysis of the face, arm, or leg—usually on one side of the body

- Loss of speech, or trouble talking or understanding speech

- Sudden blurred, double, or decreased vision

- Dizziness, loss of balance, or loss of coordination

- Sudden, severe headache with no apparent cause

- Difficulty swallowing

About Stroke

Stroke is the third leading cause of death and the leading cause of adult disability in the United States. The death rate from stroke is decreasing, but the incidence of stroke is rising. This means that more people are surviving strokes, but also that more people are having them.

After age 55, the risk of having a stroke doubles in each successive decade. Almost 35% of strokes occur in those between 75 to 84 years of age. The incidence of stroke is 30% higher for men than women. Individuals of African ancestry are 60% more likely to suffer a stroke than Caucasians, and are two and a half times more likely to die of a stroke. HYPERTENSION, ATHEROSCLEROSIS, HEART DISEASE, atrial fibrillation, and DIABETES MELLITUS are risk factors for stroke.

Blood Group Links

The term "stroke" has been largely applied to blood clots in the brain. However, bleeding or hemorrhaging are also common causes. Together, these are often referred to as cerebrovascular accidents, or CVAs. Blood groups A and AB have a general tendency toward problems associated with blood clotting, whereas with blood groups O and B the problems appear to be more linked to excessive bleeding and poor clotting.

These tendencies have been verified in several studies, the largest being performed on over 1,460 stroke patients, and reported in the British medical journal the *Lancet*. In 329 cases, the cause of death was certified as cerebral THROMBOSIS (brain clot). In the thrombosis cases, there was an excess of blood groups A and AB, and fewer patients of blood groups O and B. In the 482 strokes that were the result of cranial bleeding, the reverse was true: a significantly higher number of patients were blood groups O and B, rather than blood groups A and AB[1–6].

Therapies, Stroke

BLOOD GROUP A:

1. Antistress Protocol

2. Cardiovascular Protocol

3. Metabolic Enhancement Protocol

BLOOD GROUP B:

1. Antistress Protocol

2. Cardiovascular Protocol

3. Metabolic Enhancement Protocol

BLOOD GROUP AB:

1. Antistress Protocol

2. Cardiovascular Protocol

3. Metabolic Enhancement Protocol

BLOOD GROUP O:

1. Antistress Protocol

2. Cardiovascular Protocol

3. Metabolic Enhancement Protocol

Related Topics

Blood clotting disorders

Cardiovascular disease

Coronary artery disease

Ischemic heart disease

Peripheral artery disease

REFERENCES

1. Sostaric V, Bozicevic D, Brinar V, Grbavac Z. Hereditary antigen characteristics of blood in ischemic cerebrovascular accident. *Neurol Croat.* 1991;40:3–11.

2. Ionescu DA, Ghitescu M, Marcu I, Xenakis A. Erythrocyte rheology in acute cerebral thrombosis. Effects of ABO blood groups. *Blut.* 1979;39:351–357.

3. Ionescu DA, Marcu I, Bicescu E. Cerebral thrombosis, cerebral haemorrhage, and ABO blood-groups. *Lancet.* 1976; 1:278–280.

4. Strang RR. Age, sex, and ABO blood group distributions of 150 patients with cerebral arteriovenous aneurysms. *J Med Genet.* 1967;4:29–30.

5. Ismagilov MF, Petrova SE. [ABO blood group system and vegetative-vascular disorders in children]. *Zh Nevropatol Psikhiatr.* 1981;81:1487–1488.

6. Colonia VJ, Roisenberg I. Investigation of associations between ABO blood groups and coagulation, fibrinolysis, total lipids, cholesterol, and triglycerides. *Hum Genet.* 1979;48: 221–230.

SUDDEN INFANT DEATH SYNDROME (SIDS)–*Unexplained sudden death of a healthy infant.*

Sids	RISK		
	LOW	AVERAGE	HIGH
GROUP A			
GROUP B			
GROUP AB			
GROUP O			
NON-SECRETORS (bacterial cause)			

Symptoms

Babies who die of SIDS appear healthy with no complaints, but may have had a minor upper respiratory or gastrointestinal infection in the last 2 weeks of life.

About SIDS

SIDS is the sudden death of an infant under 1 year of age that remains unexplained after a thorough case investigation, including performance of a complete autopsy, examination of the death scene, and review of the clinical history. SIDS was first defined in 1969 and the definition was revised again in 1989. Possible causes are abnormalities in respiratory control and arousal responsiveness, central intervertebral nervous system abnormalities, and cardiac arrhythmias.

SIDS may occur when a combination of factors coincide, such that infectious agents, climactic changes, or environmental factors may act as a trigger. The highest incidence of SIDS is found among infants of Native American or African ancestry. The time of year—the late fall and winter months—may be a factor. The time of day—between midnight and 6 A.M.—is also related statistically. Other factors may include low birth weight and intrauterine growth retardation.

Certain maternal factors increase the risk of SIDS. These include use of cigarettes, use of drugs such as cocaine or opiates during pregnancy, and a maternal anemia during pregnancy.

There are conflicting reports that some toxigenic bacteria (*Clostridium botulinum*, *Clostridium difficile*, enterotoxigenic *Escherichia coli*, and *Staphylococcus aureus*) might be implicated in SIDS. *S. aureus* is a common microorganism and its toxins are very powerful. The pyrogenic toxic shock syndrome toxin of *S. aureus* can kill a previously healthy adult, so it might easily kill a small infant.

Blood Group Links

Based on studies of the susceptibility of infants to other infections, researchers speculate that colonization of infants by toxin-producing *S. aureus* may be related to blood group. The Lewis blood group antigen appears to act as a receptor for some microorganisms. Epithelial cells expressing high concentrations of Lewis bound appreciably more toxin-producing *S. aureus* than did cells expressing low concentrations of the antigen. Lewis is expressed in secretions of nearly 90% of infants aged 3 months, the peak age for SIDS[1].

Researchers believe that *S. aureus* fits the mathematical model for SIDS. Both staphylococci and/or their toxins were identified in a significant proportion of SIDS cases. Isolation of staphylococci from healthy infants was associated with the 2- to 4-month age range, a risk factor consistently found in all epidemiological studies of SIDS. This might reflect the developmental stage in which 80% to 90% of infants express the Lewis(a) antigen, which has been shown to be one of the receptors for *S. aureus*[2].

Therapies, SIDS

(Maternal—before, during, and after pregnancy)

BLOOD GROUP A

1. Immune-Enhancing Protocol
2. Nerve Health Protocol

BLOOD GROUP B:

1. Immune-Enhancing Protocol
2. Nerve Health Protocol

BLOOD GROUP AB:

1. Immune-Enhancing Protocol
2. Nerve Health Protocol

BLOOD GROUP O:

1. Immune-Enhancing Protocol
2. Nerve Health

Related Topics

Bacterial disease (general)

Immunity

REFERENCES

1. Grzeszczuk J. Lewis antigens as a possible cause of sudden death of previously healthy adults and infants and of diseases and phenomena linked to tissue ischemia. *Med Hypotheses.* 1997;49:525–527.
2. Saadi AT, Weir DM, Poxton IR, et al. Isolation of an adhesin from Staphylococcus aureus that binds Lewis a blood group antigen and its relevance to sudden infant death syndrome. *FEMS Immunol Med Microbiol.* 1994;8:315–320.

SYNDROME X–*See Insulin resistance*

SYSTEMIC LUPUS ERYTHEMATOSUS–

See Autoimmune disease, systemic lupus erythematosus

TENSION HEADACHE–*See Headache*

THOMSEN-FRIEDENREICH (T) ANTI-GEN–*See Cancer (general)*

THROMBOSIS–*See Stroke*

THYROID CANCER–*See Cancer, thyroid*

THYROID DISEASE (general)–*An abnormal functioning of the thyroid, either hyper or hypo.*

Thyroid disease	RISK		
	LOW	AVERAGE	HIGH
GROUP A (HYPOTHYROIDISM)	▓	▓	
GROUP B	▓		
GROUP AB	▓		
GROUP O (AUTOIMMUNE/ HYPERTHYROIDISM)	▓	▓	
NON-SECRETORS (HYPERTHYROIDISM)	▓	▓	

Symptoms

Hyperthyroidism:

- Weight loss
- Excessive hunger
- Heavy sweating
- Palpitations
- Racing heart
- Hyperdefecation
- Bulging eyeballs
- Goiter

Hypothyroidism:

- Hair loss
- Dry skin
- Fluid retention
- Muscle weakness
- Gait problems
- Cold intolerance
- Constipation
- Sluggishness
- Fatigue

About Thyroid Disease

The thyroid gland sits above the windpipe, and works with the pituitary gland to regulate the body's METABOLISM. It does this through the hormone thyroxine. Thyroxine synthesis depends on an adequate amount of iodine in the diet (found mostly in seafoods and iodized salt). When iodine is low, a goiter is formed, and thyroxin production may fail. Before iodine was readily available in the diet, goiters were quite common.

When there is a deficiency of thyroxine, the pituitary gland senses the deficit and produces a stimulating hormone called thyroid-stimulating hormone (TSH), which makes the thyroid grow and work harder to keep up with thyroxine production.

When it is stimulated by TSH, the thyroid makes two primary hormones called T_4 and T_3. It makes a lot of T_4, which is not very active; conversely, it makes only a small amount of T_3, which is very active. For T_4 to have any real impact as a hormone, it is metabolized in peripheral tissues by a series of biochemical reactions called phenolic conjugation, deamination, decarboxylation, and a cascade of monodeiodinations, resulting eventually in either the formation of T_3 or reverse T_3 (rT_3). About 80% of the T_3 produced in the body is actually produced in this manner in the peripheral tissues and is not at all related to production by the thyroid. The production of rT_3, on the other hand, is hormonally inactive. If more rT_3 is produced than T_3 in peripheral tissues, the cells will function as if the thyroid is underactive, when it is, in fact, working normally. This is referred to as low T_3 syndrome, and it is an important factor in the body's adjustment to STRESS.

Hyperthyroidism, the most common thyroid disease, is the result of too much thyroxine being produced, and loss of control by the pituitary. Rarely, it is caused by an excess of TSH made by the pituitary. Hyperthyroidism can be caused by an overactive area of the gland, or it can be caused by the autoimmune condition known as Graves' disease.

The opposite of hyperthyroidism is hypothyroidism, which is an underproduction of thyroxine. Hypothyroidism is almost always an autoimmune disease, in which the body makes antibodies to its own thyroid gland. The most common form of hypothyroidism is an autoimmune condition called Hashimoto's thyroiditis.

Stress and Thyroid Disease

A clear link has been found between thyroid disease and stress. The most dramatic example was a study of the Danish population during the 1941 to 1945 German occupation. There was a very high incidence of hyperthyroidism in the population, compared to the previous 100 years. A recent study of 116 women with Graves' disease found that most of them experienced stressful events immediately prior to their diagnoses. We can also see a relationship between thyroid disease and DEPRESSION. Lithium, a drug used to treat manic depression, often causes hypothyroidism. Somehow, lithium, a heavy salt, stimulates the production of antibodies that didn't exist before, and these antibodies attack the thyroid. This effect is 10 times more common in women using lithium than in men using lithium. Depression itself is associated with hypothyroidism.

Thyroid function will also be compromised by eating an extremely low-calorie diet. Since the role of thyroid hormones is to govern energy expenditure, the effect of too few calories on the hormone will be to slow down the metabolism.

This biological instinct has been responsible for our survival during periods of scarcity.

Blood Group Links

Blood group O tends to have more autoimmune thyroid disease—both Graves' and Hashimoto's. While a normal thyroid doesn't express large amounts of blood group antigens, a sick one can generate enormous amounts. Inflamed thyroid tissue generates large amounts of the A antigen. Blood group O carries anti-A antibodies in its serum.

While blood group A has been shown to have more hypothyroidism, it is possible that high cortisol levels might mimic low thyroid production, causing a misdiagnosis (see Hypothyroidism)[1].

ABO non-secretors have a higher incidence of Graves' disease. The inability to secrete the water-soluble glycoprotein form of the ABO blood group antigens into saliva is significantly more common in patients with Graves' disease than control individuals (40% versus 27%) but not among those with Hashimoto's thyroiditis or spontaneous primary atrophic hypothyroidism. ABH non-secretors with Graves' disease were found to produce higher levels of antitubulin antibodies, while levels of other antibodies were similar to secretors[2].

Therapies, Thyroid Disease

ALL BLOOD GROUPS:

1. Hypothyroidism is often controlled with replacement thyroid hormone pills. Side effects and complications from overreplacement (or underreplacement) replacement of this pow-

erful hormone can occur. Treatment of hyperthyroidism requires long-term anti-thyroid drug therapy, or destruction of the thyroid gland with radioactive iodine or surgery. Both of these treatment approaches carry certain risks and long-term side effects.

2. Hyperactive thyroid tissue is much more sensitive to the agglutinating effects of lectins found in wheat and soybeans than is healthy thyroid tissue, so a low-lectin diet is indicated.

BLOOD GROUP A:

1. Metabolic Enhancement Protocol

2. Detoxification Protocol

BLOOD GROUP B:

1. Metabolic Enhancement Protocol

2. Detoxification Protocol

BLOOD GROUP AB:

1. Metabolic Enhancement Protocol

2. Detoxification Protocol

BLOOD GROUP O:

1. Metabolic Enhancement Protocol

2. Detoxification Protocol

Related Topics

Autoimmune disease (general)

Graves' disease

Hashimoto's thyroiditis

Hyperthyroidism

Hypothyroidism

Obesity

Stress

REFERENCES

1. Carmel R, Spencer CA. Clinical and subclinical thyroid disorders associated with pernicious anemia. Observations on abnormal thyroid-stimulating hormone levels and on a possible association of blood group O with hyperthyroidism. *Arch Intern Med.* 1982;142:1465–1469.

2. Toft AD, Blackwell CC, Saadi AT, et al. Secretor status and infection in patients with Graves' disease. *Autoimmunity.* 1990;7:279–289.

THYROID DISEASE, GRAVES'– *The autoimmune stimulation of thyroid tissue.*

Graves' disease	RISK		
	LOW	AVERAGE	HIGH
GROUP A			
GROUP B			
GROUP AB			
GROUP O			
NON-SECRETORS			

Symptoms

- Weight loss
- Excessive hunger
- Heavy sweating
- Palpitations

- Racing heart
- Hyperdefecation
- Bulging eyeballs
- Goiter

About Graves' Disease

Graves' disease is the most common form of hyperthyroidism. It is an autoimmune condition in which the body produces antibodies that overstimulate the thyroid gland, so it produces too much thyroid hormone. The cause of Graves' disease is unknown but may be related to a genetic or immune system disorder. Other disorders of the endocrine system may be present in people with Graves' disease.

Blood Group Links

Blood group O tends to have more autoimmune thyroid disease—both Graves' and Hashimoto's. While a normal thyroid doesn't express large amounts of blood group antigens, a sick one can generate enormous amounts. Inflamed thyroid tissue generates large amounts of the A antigen. Blood group O carries anti-A antibodies in its serum[1].

ABO non-secretors have a higher incidence of Graves' disease. The inability to secrete the water-soluble glycoprotein form of the ABO blood group antigens into saliva is significantly more common in patients with Graves' disease than control individuals (40% versus 27%) but not among those with HASHIMOTO'S THYROIDITIS or spontaneous primary atrophic hypothyroidism. ABH non-secretors with Graves' disease were found to produce higher levels of antitubulin antibodies, while levels of other antibodies were similar to secretors[2].

Therapies, Graves' Disease

ALL BLOOD GROUPS:

Hyperactive thyroid tissue is much more sensitive to the agglutinating effects of lectins found in wheat and soybeans than is healthy thyroid tissue, so a low-lectin diet is indicated.

BLOOD GROUP A:

1. Metabolic Enhancement Protocol
2. Detoxification Protocol

BLOOD GROUP B:

1. Metabolic Enhancement Protocol
2. Detoxification Protocol

BLOOD GROUP AB:

1. Metabolic Enhancement Protocol
2. Detoxification Protocol

BLOOD GROUP O:

1. Metabolic Enhancement Protocol
2. Detoxification Protocol

Related Topics

Autoimmune disease (general)

Hashimoto's thyroiditis

Hyperthyroidism

Hypothyroidism

Obesity

Stress

REFERENCES

1. Carmel R, Spencer CA. Clinical and subclinical thyroid disorders associated with pernicious anemia. Observations on abnormal thyroid-stimulating hormone levels and on a possible association of blood group O with hyperthyroidism. *Arch Intern Med.* 1982;142:1465–1469.
2. Toft AD, Blackwell CC, Saadi AT, et al. Secretor status and infection in patients with Graves' disease. *Autoimmunity.* 1990;7:279–289.

THYROID DISEASE, HASHIMOTO'S THYROIDITIS–*The autoimmune destruction of thyroid tissue.*

Hashimoto's thyroiditis	RISK		
	LOW	AVERAGE	HIGH
GROUP A			
GROUP B			
GROUP AB			
GROUP O			

Symptoms

- Hair loss
- Dry skin
- Fluid retention
- Muscle weakness

- Gait problems
- Cold intolerance
- Constipation
- Sluggishness
- Fatigue

About Hashimoto's Thyroiditis

Hashimoto's thyroiditis is the result of an immune system destruction of thyroid tissue. It is believed to be the most common cause of primary hypothyroidism in North America; the condition is eight times more prevalent in women than in men, and its incidence increases with age. A family history of thyroid disorders is common, and incidence is increased in patients with chromosomal disorders, including Turner, Down, and Klinefelter syndromes. Histologic studies reveal extensive infiltration of lymphocytes in the thyroid with lymphoid follicles. Other forms of autoimmune disease may coexist with Hashimoto's thyroiditis, including PERNICIOUS ANEMIA, RHEUMATOID ARTHRITIS, LUPUS, and SJÖGREN'S SYNDROME. Other autoimmune endocrine disorders may also be present, including Addison's disease and insulin-dependent DIABETES MELLITUS.

Blood Group Links

Blood group O tends to have more autoimmune thyroid disease—both Graves' and Hashimoto's. While a normal thyroid doesn't express large amounts of blood group antigens, a sick one can generate enormous amounts. Inflamed thyroid tissue generates large amounts of the A antigen.

Blood group O carries anti-A antibodies in its serum[1], making O more susceptible.

Therapies, Hashimoto's Thyroiditis

ALL BLOOD GROUPS:

Treatment of Hashimoto's thyroiditis usually requires lifelong replacement therapy with thyroid hormone to decrease goiter size and treat the hypothyroidism. Occasionally, the hypothyroidism is transient. The average oral replacement dose with L-thyroxine is 75 to 150 mg/day.

BLOOD GROUP A:

1. Metabolic Enhancement Protocol
2. Detoxification Protocol

BLOOD GROUP B:

1. Metabolic Enhancement Protocol
2. Detoxification Protocol

BLOOD GROUP AB:

1. Metabolic Enhancement Protocol
2. Detoxification Protocol

BLOOD GROUP O:

1. Metabolic Enhancement Protocol
2. Detoxification Protocol

Related Topics

Autoimmune disease (general)

Graves' disease

Obesity

REFERENCES

1. Carmel R, Spencer CA. Clinical and subclinical thyroid disorders associated with pernicious anemia. Observations on abnormal thyroid-stimulating hormone levels and on a possible association of blood group O with hyperthyroidism. *Arch Intern Med*. 1982;142:1465–1469.

THYROID DISEASE, HYPERTHYROIDISM–*Excessive release of thyroid hormone.*

Hyperthyroidism	RISK		
	LOW	AVERAGE	HIGH
GROUP A			
GROUP B			
GROUP AB			
GROUP O			
NON-SECRETOR			

Symptoms

- Weight loss
- Excessive hunger
- Heavy sweating
- Palpitations
- Racing heart
- Hyperdefecation
- Bulging eyeballs
- Goiter

About Hyperthyroidism

Hyperthyroidism, the most common thyroid disease, is the result of too much thyroxine being produced, and loss of control by the pituitary. Rarely, it is caused by an excess of thyroid-stimulating hormone (TSH) made by the pituitary. Hyperthyroidism can be caused by an overactive area of the gland, or it can be caused by the autoimmune condition known as Graves' disease.

Blood Group Links

Blood group O has a higher incidence of hyperthyroidism compared to the other ABO groups. In one study of 162 patients with PERNICIOUS ANEMIA, 24.1% had clinical thyroid disease. Eight of nine hyperthyroid patients and all seven patients with low TSH levels were blood group O, contrasting significantly with hypothyroid subjects, who were more often blood group A[1].

ABO non-secretors have a higher incidence of hyperthyroidism. The inability to secrete the water-soluble glycoprotein form of the ABO blood group antigens into saliva is significantly more common in patients with GRAVES' DISEASE than control individuals (40% versus 27%) but not among those with HASHIMOTO'S THYROIDITIS or spontaneous primary atrophic hypothyroidism. ABH non-secretors with hyperthyroidism were found to produce higher levels of antitubulin antibodies, while levels of other antibodies were similar to secretors[2].

Therapies, Hyperthyroidism

ALL BLOOD GROUPS:

Hyperactive thyroid tissue is much more sensitive to the agglutinating effects of lectins found in wheat and soybeans than is healthy thyroid tissue, so a low-lectin diet is indicated.

BLOOD GROUP A:

1. Metabolic Enhancement Protocol

2. Detoxification Protocol

BLOOD GROUP B:

1. Metabolic Enhancement Protocol

2. Detoxification Protocol

BLOOD GROUP AB:

1. Metabolic Enhancement Protocol

2. Detoxification Protocol

BLOOD GROUP O:

1. Metabolic Enhancement Protocol

2. Detoxification Protocol

Related Topics

Autoimmune disease (general)

Graves' disease

Hashimoto's thyroiditis

Hypothyroidism

Obesity

REFERENCES

1. Carmel R, Spencer CA. Clinical and subclinical thyroid disorders associated with pernicious anemia. Observations on abnormal thyroid-stimulating hormone levels and on a possible association of blood group O with hyperthyroidism. *Arch Intern Med.* 1982;142:1465–1469.

2. Toft AD, Blackwell CC, Saadi AT, et al. Secretor status and infection in patients with Graves' disease. *Autoimmunity.* 1990;7:279–289.

THYROID DISEASE, HYPOTHYROID-ISM–*Inadequate release of thyroid hormone.*

Hypothyroidism	RISK		
	LOW	AVERAGE	HIGH
GROUP A			
GROUP B			
GROUP AB			
GROUP O Autoimmune			

Symptoms

- Hair loss
- Dry skin
- Fluid retention
- Muscle weakness
- Gait problems
- Cold intolerance
- Low body temperature
- Constipation

- Sluggishness
- Fatigue

About Hypothyroidism

Hypothyroidism is an underproduction of thyroxine. Hypothyroidism is almost always an autoimmune disease, in which the body makes antibodies to its own thyroid gland. The most common form of hypothyroidism is an autoimmune condition called Hashimoto's thyroiditis.

The Stress Factor

In the mid-1960s, Dr. John Tintera postulated that 60% of people with low basal metabolism/temperature, a symptom of hypothyroidism, did not actually have any thyroid problem—rather, that it was a stress-related reaction at the level of the adrenals and cortisol. The 60% misdiagnosed patients were predominantly blood groups A, B, and AB.

Thyroid hormone secretion, unlike many of the body's rhythmic systems, doesn't have a 24-hour rhythm of its own. The thyroid's rhythm is basal: Left to its own devices, it just keeps on ticking. However, this basal activity can be influenced by changes in the levels of cortisol and DHEA. Evidence quite clearly shows that high cortisol will cause thyroid-stimulating hormone (TSH) production to drop, reducing the conversion of T_4 to T_3 (the active form of the hormone). Lower T_3 levels mean lower metabolic activity, and a rise in the conversion of T_4 to the inactive rT_3. This in turn can stimulate a chain of events leading to the body's own destruction of the thyroid.

After a bout of stress, high levels of rT_3 often persist. The control valve in this peripheral conversion process appears to be cortisol, and perhaps the cortisol to DHEA ratio. When cortisol is high, more rT_3 is converted from T_4. When cortisol is low, more T_3 is converted from T_4.

When an individual who has maladapted to stress is placed on thyroid support, whether Synthroid (T_4) or Armour (natural extract), it can create long-term problems. Initially, thyroid therapy will boost the metabolic rate and improve the condition. However, by increasing energy and placing more stress on an already over-stressed system, eventually, misprescribed thyroid therapy will leave the individual in a worse state.

Blood Group Links

It's easy to see why blood group A might symptomatically appear to suffer from hypothyroid. Blood group A has a more severe response to stress, which might initially seem like low thyroid hormone levels.

Independent studies have shown that blood group A has a greater tendency toward hypothyroidism than the other blood groups[1].

Therapies, Hypothyroidism

ALL BLOOD GROUPS:

Hypothyroidism is controlled with replacement thyroid hormone pills. Side effects and complications from overreplacement (or underreplacement) of this powerful hormone can occur. Overreplacement can lead to hyperthyroidism; underreplacement can exacerbate the symptoms of hypothyroidism.

BLOOD GROUP A:

1. Metabolic Enhancement Protocol

2. Detoxification Protocol

BLOOD GROUP B:

1. Metabolic Enhancement Protocol

2. Detoxification Protocol

BLOOD GROUP AB:

1. Metabolic Enhancement Protocol

2. Detoxification Protocol

BLOOD GROUP O:

1. Metabolic Enhancement Protocol

2. Detoxification Protocol

Related Topics

Autoimmune disease (general)

Graves' disease

Hashimoto's thyroiditis

Hyperthyroidism

Obesity

REFERENCES

1. Carmel R, Spencer CA. Clinical and subclinical thyroid disorders associated with pernicious anemia. Observations on abnormal thyroid-stimulating hormone levels and on a pos- sible association of blood group O with hyperthyroidism. *Arch Intern Med*. 1982;142:1465–1469.

TOOTH DECAY–*See Dental caries*

TOXEMIA, PREGNANCY–*Dangerous hypertension during the final weeks of pregnancy.*

Toxemia of pregnancy	RISK		
	LOW	AVERAGE	HIGH
GROUP A	▓	▓	
GROUP B	▓	▓	
GROUP AB	▓	▓	
GROUP O	▓	▓	▓

Symptoms

- Elevated blood pressure on two blood pressure readings, 6 hours apart
- Edema
- Rapid excessive weight gain
- Gastric pain
- Headache
- Visual disturbance
- Apprehension

About Toxemia of Pregnancy

Toxemia is a disorder of pregnant women that is characterized by elevated blood pressure, swelling of the feet and hands, and loss of protein in the urine. It occurs in the third trimester, usually after the 20th week of gestation. The cause of toxemia is not known. It is more common in women who are carrying twins, who have high blood pressure before pregnancy, and who are pregnant for the first time. Toxemia is also more common in women 35 years of age and older. If severe, toxemia of pregnancy may progress to serious problems for both mother and child—including MISCARRIAGE. Toxemia of pregnancy is also known as pre-eclampsia or eclampsia, depending on its severity.

Blood Group Links

There is an association with blood group O women and the risk of toxemia of pregnancy and subsequent loss of the fetus. Whether this is the result of blood group incompatibility between the mother and fetus is still open to debate[1].

Therapies, Toxemia of Pregnancy

ALL BLOOD GROUPS:

Preventive measures that can be taken prior to pregnancy include the following:

- Dietary changes in line with Blood Type Diet recommendations
- Weight loss (if OBESE)
- Exercise, according to blood type recommendations, to build cardiovascular strength and keep blood pressure normal

BLOOD GROUP A:

1. Liver Support Protocol
2. Detoxification Protocol

BLOOD GROUP B:

1. Liver Support Protocol
2. Detoxification Protocol

BLOOD GROUP AB:

1. Liver Support Protocol
2. Detoxification Protocol

BLOOD GROUP O:

1. Liver Support Protocol
2. Detoxification Protocol

Related Topics

Cardiovascular disease

Infertility

Insulin resistance

Obesity

REFERENCES

1. Lauritsen JG, Grunnet N, Jensen OM. Materno-fetal ABO incompatibility as a cause of spontaneous abortion. *Clin Genet.* 1975;7:308–316.

TOXICITY, BOWEL (INDICANURIA)–

Intestinal putrefaction measured by a high urine indican level, typically the result of microbial overgrowth.

Bowel toxicity, indicanuria	RISK		
	LOW	AVERAGE	HIGH
GROUP A			
GROUP B			
GROUP AB			
GROUP O			

Symptoms

- Detectable with indican urine test

About Indicanuria

Normally, the liver and kidneys are able to efficiently cleanse the blood and digestive tracts on a daily basis. Bowel toxicity arises when the capabilities of these organs are overwhelmed, or they are otherwise prevented from performing their functions.

One simple way of measuring bowel toxicity is the Obermayer test of urinary indican. The test measures the amount of indican in a sample of first morning urine. Indican is a conversion product of another chemical, indole, which is a marker for incomplete protein breakdown.

High urinary indican levels, a condition called indicanuria, result from the absorption of indoles and indicans by the gut, and their elimination through the kidneys. Indoles are produced by bac-

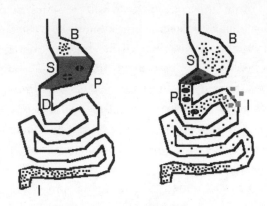

CAUSES OF INDICANURIA

Elevated levels of indican in the urine usually result from inappropriate conversion of tryptophan into indole by bacteria in the upper intestines. LEFT: In a healthy system, the residual levels of acid in the stomach (S) act as a barrier to bacteria (B) entering the upper intestines (D). The high stomach acid also helps protein digestion (P). Some bacteria may enter the lower intestines (I) from the colon, but they do not inhabit the upper intestines. RIGHT: In a sick system, low stomach acid (S) does not serve as an effective barrier to bacteria (B), which can pass through and colonize the upper intestine. The low stomach acid also does not completely break down the proteins (P), which serve as a food source for the bacteria and attracts more bacteria from the lower intestines The putrefaction of these undigested protein residues produces by-products called indoles, which then are absorbed through the blood stream and eliminated as indican by the kidneys through the urine.

terial putrefaction of excess tryptophan from the diet that is not absorbed in the intestinal tract. Though examination of the urine is the preferred method of testing, indican is not made in the blood, but rather in the intestines. It is absorbed through the colon wall into the blood, and is then excreted by the kidneys.

Indican has been shown to be a co-carcinogen; that is, a substance that is not carcinogenic in itself, but rather promotes the carcinogenicity of other cancer-causing chemicals. High levels of urinary indican also signal that large amounts of protein are being lost in the intestinal tract instead of being absorbed as nutrients.

More important, indican is a reflection of sickness and putrefaction in the bowel. A toxic bowel problem can result in a plethora of symptoms, and contribute to a variety of diseases. Some of the most common signs of bowel toxicity are INDIGESTION, BAD BREATH, yeast overgrowth, lack of energy, HEADACHES and irritability, joint problems, AUTOIMMUNE DISORDERS, and PREMENSTRUAL SYNDROME.

General Risk Factors and Causes

- *Old age:* Up to half of elderly hospitalized patients excrete an abnormally high concentration of indican, compared to younger individuals. This may be due to age-related changes in the effectiveness of digestion, such as a lack of sufficient enzymes or stomach acid.

- *Lack of stomach acid:* The acid pool in the stomach is a potent barrier to microbes entering the small intestine. Low stomach acid production is a very common occurrence in the elderly, especially elderly women. Since one of the prime functions of stomach acid is to facilitate the breakdown of proteins, low stomach acid may prevent the complete breakdown of proteins, preventing them from being fully assimilated. These leftovers may then serve as food for bacteria, which can pass through the stomach or migrate upward from the lower small intestine.

- *Use of antibiotics:* Antibiotics, especially the use of two or more antibiotics in tandem, can predispose individuals to the putrefaction of tryptophan and the production of indican. These drugs include kanamycin, the antifungal metronidazole, cefotaxime, and Bactrim (trimethoprim and sulfamethoxazole).

- *Improper diet:* Dietary lectins can cause malabsorption of proteins, leading to elevated indican levels. This is believed to result from the interference of lectins with the function of the protein-splitting enzyme trypsin. Chronic constipation has been associated with bacterial overgrowth of the upper intestines, and consequent putrefaction of tryptophan into indole.

- *Liver or kidney dysfunction:* Individuals with chronic, active HEPATITIS without CIRRHOSIS have been shown to have high urinary indican levels. In 34 patients with complete recovery, a follow-up study 10 years later revealed that, with the normalization of liver function, general liver tests, and detoxification parameters, the production of indican also normalized. Kidney patients with uremia (a condition produced by toxins from protein breakdown) also show high indican levels.

- *Saccharin:* The artificial sweetener saccharin produces phenomenal increases in levels of urinary indican. Many artificial sweeteners are linked to BLADDER CANCER in animals. Bladder cancer is also linked to high indican levels.

- CELIAC *and* INFLAMMATORY BOWEL DISEASE: Increased indican has been observed in most inflammatory conditions of the bowel, including CELIAC DISEASE, ULCERATIVE COLITIS, and CROHN'S DISEASE.

- *High intake of dietary methionine:* High dietary levels of the sulfur-containing amino acid methionine have been shown to increase levels of indican in the urine. Methionine also increases levels of another class of toxins called polyamines as well. High dietary sources of methionine include milk, casein, egg whites, dried cod fish, sesame meal, wheat gluten, and wheat germ. Intestinal dysbiosis and pathogenic bacterial overgrowth leading to production of indican is a by-product.

Blood Group Links

All blood groups are susceptible to indicanuria if they fail to follow their specific dietary guidelines. However, it should be noted that blood groups A and AB have low stomach acid, which can be a precipitating factor.

Therapies, Indicanuria

BLOOD GROUP A:

1. Detoxification Protocol
2. Intestinal Health Protocol
3. Liver Support Protocol

BLOOD GROUP B:

1. Detoxification Protocol
2. Intestinal Health Protocol
3. Liver Support Protocol

BLOOD GROUP AB:

1. Detoxification Protocol
2. Intestinal Health Protocol
3. Liver Support Protocol

BLOOD GROUP O:

1. Detoxification Protocol

2. Intestinal Health Protocol
3. Liver Support Protocol

Related Topics

Bacterial disease (general)

Digestion

TOXICITY, BOWEL (POLYAMINES)—*Excessive production or intake of a class of biologic amines called polyamines.*

Bowel toxicity, polyamines	RISK		
	LOW	AVERAGE	HIGH
GROUP A	▓	▓	
GROUP B	▓		
GROUP AB	▓	▓	
GROUP O	▓		

Symptoms

- Cramping or flatulence
- Difficulty losing weight
- Fatigue
- Skin rashes and itching
- Headache
- Low blood sugar
- Cold hands and feet
- Lack of libido

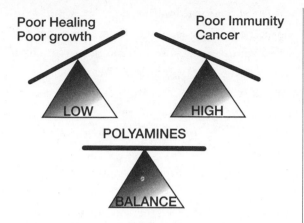

MODULATION OF POLYAMINE LEVELS IN THE BODY

In health, polyamine levels are balanced between the amounts sufficent to sustain cell repair functions (usually present in the diet), and the over production which can depress the immune response and support the growth of many cancers.

About Polyamines

Polyamines are part of a class of proteins called biogenic amines, and are present in low concentrations in all human, animal, and plant cells. Polyamines are essential for the maintenance of high metabolic activity in a normally functioning and healthy body. Not only the intestine, but all of the other organs of the body require polyamines for their growth, renewal, and metabolism. All cell growth requires certain amounts of polyamines. They are also critical to the healthy function of the nervous system, and the growth of young children.

Many biochemistry textbooks refer to the polyamines as "dead flesh proteins." This image is employed because, when living tissue is shocked or dies, its protein structure cracks open. Bacteria or enzymes contained in the food itself subsequently convert many of the protein fragments into polyamines. This is why polyamines are found in very high amounts in the tissues of severely injured trauma patients, and in foods that have been morphologically shocked by excessive processing, such as rapid freezing. Though many advocates of vegetarianism use polyamines as a justification for an all-vegetarian lifestyle, polyamines are found just as abundantly in meats and seafood as they are in vegetables, grains, fruits, and sprouts.

Problems arise when polyamine levels increase to levels that compromise growth and metabolism. The concentration of polyamines inside the cell is tightly regulated. The range of cellular polyamine concentration is determined at the lower limit by their absolute requirement for cell growth, and at the upper limit by their potential toxicity.

Polyamines are both synthesized in the body, and are also derived from the diet, either in the form of foods that are in themselves high in polyamines, or by the action of the bacteria in the gut, synthesizing polyamines from dietary amino acids. These two methods are referred to as exogenous (outside manufacture by gut bacteria) and endogenous (inside manufacture by the liver and other organs). Bacteria can produce polyamines by metabolizing amino acids found in food. Many strains of bacteria are capable of manufacturing polyamines, including *Bacillus*, *Clostridium*, *Enterobacteriaceae*, *Enterococcus*, *Klebsiella*, *Morganella*, and *Proteus*. Often, the process of producing polyamines by bacteria begins long before the

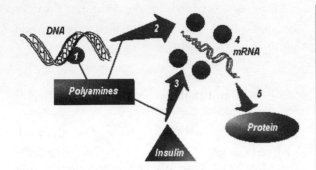

Inside the cell, polyamines work to increase growth by two separate mechanisms. The first (1) involves having a direct influence on specific growth-promoting genes. The second mechanism involves the enhancement of the production of the various cell proteins needed for growth. By this mechanism polyamines amplify the effects of DNA (2) and insulin (3) by acting to stabilize messenger RNA (4). This results in the synthesis of larger amounts of protein (5).

food is eaten. Frozen, canned, preserved, and otherwise tainted foods are loaded with polyamines.

When manufactured by the body, polyamines are derived from the amino acid ornithine, through the actions of the enzyme ornithine decarboxylase (ODC). Almost all tissues can manufacture polyamines, but the liver makes the vast majority of them. In humans, the starting point of polyamine synthesis is the amino acid ornithine. Ornithine is a nonessential amino acid, in the sense that the body can make ornithine from other amino acids through what is called the ornithine cycle. This pathway converts either of two other amino acids, arginine or citrulline, into ornithine.

Arginine, also a nonessential amino acid, may not be quite so nonessential after all. Recent evidence has placed into question the widely held belief that adult mammals, including human beings, can meet all of their arginine needs by synthesis from other amino acids. Arginine is one of the most versatile amino acids in animal cells, serving as a precursor for the synthesis not only of polyamines, but also of proteins, NITRIC OXIDE, urea, proline, and glutamate. Arginine is critical for the synthesis of creatine, a major source of high-energy phosphate for regeneration of energy production in muscle, and a favorite of bodybuilders everywhere.

The first polyamine to be produced is putrescine. Putrescine is made from ornithine by the action of ODC. Putrescine can then be converted to two other polyamines, spermine and spermidine, each of which has slightly different effects in the body. Because both spermidine and spermine are made from putrescine, and putrescine is made from the amino acid ornithine by the enzyme ODC, blocking ODC is usually sufficient to block the synthesis of all three polyamines.

ODC is the first enzyme in the biosynthesis of polyamines in all mammal cells. It is also called the rate-limiting enzyme, because it lies at a choke point at which you can control the production of other polyamines by controlling ODC.

The control over ODC (and consequently over polyamines) is a very exquisite and precise process. Cell growth and differentiation depend on precise control of the levels of polyamines inside the cell. ODC is one of those ephemeral enzymes that doesn't last very long in the cell: Protein-splitting enzymes degrade it very rapidly. This is known as a half-life, which is just the amount of time for the original amount of a chemical in the body to drop by half. The half-life of ODC is one of the shortest known for any enzyme in any species of mammal, and provides the cell a way to rapidly change polyamine synthesis.

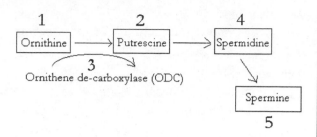

POLYAMINE SYNTHESIS

The amino acid ornithine (1) serves as the starting point for polyamine synthesis. It is converted to putrescine (2) by the actions of the enzyme ornithine decarboxylase (3). From putrescine, the other polyamines spermidine (4) and spermine (5) can also be synthesized.

Inhibition of ODC results in a drop in polyamine synthesis, and an arrest of cell growth; this can sometimes be reversed by the use of external polyamines from the diet. Not surprisingly, human cells are equipped with a very efficient transport system for snaring these extracellular polyamines and putting them to work.

Polyamines are essential to cellular proliferation and differentiation. Children have high levels of polyamines, and bodybuilders certainly feel that they also need high levels. It was believed that most of the polyamines needed for growth were synthesized in the gut. However, recent studies have shown that polyamines accumulated in the small bowel are largely obtained from the food consumed in our diet.

How polyamines stimulate growth is far from clear. What we do know is that they have a profound stabilizing effect on a cell's genetic material (DNA). One mechanism for their involvement in growth processes may be via their influence on the activity of growth-promoting genes. The size and electrical charge of the polyamines permit them to interact with huge molecules such as DNA and RNA, and pass through phospholipid membranes and compartments with ease.

Polyamines and Cell Growth

There appears to be an intimate relationship between polyamines, RNA, and the hormone insulin. Insulin, whose primary effect once inside the cell is to activate growth, does this by providing stimulation to the protein-synthesizing factory of the cell, the ribosomes. Ribosomes act on instructions from messenger RNA, which carries the blueprint for which particular type of protein is coded in the DNA. Polyamines seem to stabilize and amplify the information contained in messenger RNA, which serves to increase the protein produced from it.

Human milk is very high in polyamines, particularly spermine; they are thought to account for the protective effect of human milk against allergies. The data indicate that human milk provides substantial amounts of spermine and spermidine to newborns and infants, which could potentially modulate the maturation of the infant's intestines. In one study, the polyamine concentration of human milk was measured from 60 women during a period extending from the first week to the sixth month of lactation, and compared with the polyamine content of 18 infant formulas. The spermine and spermidine content of these formulas was lower that that of the human milk.

During the first week after birth, putrescine levels in human milk remain very low and vary little, while spermidine and spermine concentrations rise markedly during the first 3 days, reaching levels that are 12 times higher than the values measured on the first day. In artificial powdered formulas, the polyamine concentration is approximately 10 times lower than that found in human milk.

Low maternal protein intake decreases the activity of ODC, which consequently lowers the levels of polyamines in the placenta. This has been shown to result in reduced fetal growth. Perhaps this is part of the reason that the offspring of strictly vegetarian parents are typically smaller than average.

In sufficient amounts, polyamines, particularly putrescine, are important in maintaining the healthy structure and function of the intestinal mucosa, which seems to require vitamin D as well as putrescine. Long-term feeding of polyamine-deficient diets to animals results in shrinking of the intestinal lining in both the small intestine and the colon.

In infants, polyamines are very important growth factors. Their high concentration in human milk probably helps explain why breast-fed babies are on average a bit larger than those fed formula, and have a lower incidence of FOOD ALLERGIES later in life.

Polyamines and Cancer

Cancer cells are voracious consumers of polyamines. In fact, the strategy of polyamine deprivation shows great promise as a new cancer treatment, especially against cancers that are themselves hormonally sensitive, such as prostate and breast cancer. Many new anti-cancer drugs are being prepared that block the ability of cancer cells to benefit from polyamines. By and large, these drugs work by inhibiting ODC, the enzyme that synthesizes polyamines. One of these drugs, alpha-difluoromethylornithine (DFMO), shows great promise in treating prostate cancer.

In addition to stimulating cell growth, high polyamine levels inhibit the anti-cancer response of the body through specialized anti-tumor cells, called natural killer (NK) cells. By blocking the manufacture and uptake from the intestines, deprivation and lowering of polyamines increases NK cell activity.

It is believed that certain vitamins should be avoided by cancer patients, such as folic acid in patients receiving certain forms of chemotherapy. Widespread use of vitamin B_6 (pyridoxal) is fairly common, abetted by misguided proponents who advocate its use for just about anything. There is ample evidence that vitamin B_6 has a profoundly stimulating effect on ODC, and consequently on polyamine synthesis. As such, it should have no place in the nutritional treatment of patients with active cancer, or in the supplementation regimen for patients who are predisposed to cancer.

Changes in ODC activity and polyamine synthesis, and changes in the expression of the blood group antigens are considered two of the most important biological markers of a precancerous colon. This has led researchers to hypothesize that the monitoring of both blood type alterations and polyamine levels may eventually become an important screening tool in the early detection and prevention of colon cancer.

Polyamines made by gut bacteria, or present in food itself, are an important stimulus to tumor growth. Studies have shown that when polyamines were systematically blocked by the use of drugs that inhibit ODC, and all external sources were eliminated by a polyamine-free diet and decontamination of the gastrointestinal tract, the number of METASTASES (tumor spread) was significantly reduced.

Perhaps the higher levels of polyamines typical in growing children may help explain why certain types of cancers, particularly LEUKEMIAS and LYMPHOMAS, tend to be so much more aggressive in them. There is some evidence that high polyamine levels act as promoters of other tumors.

Polyamines in Food

The concentration of polyamines in spoiled food can be toxic. Fish tissue, which is more perishable than animal tissue, is very susceptible to microorganism invasion. This is why freshly caught fish stored at moderate temperature (60°F, 15.5°C) will remain unspoiled for only 1 day or less. A condition called scombroid poisoning is associated with polyamine toxicity. This seafood poisoning got its name from its source, the widespread consumption of the *Scombroidea* species (mackerel, tuna, bluefish, and skipjack). These fish, and other rapidly moving fish such as mahimahi (yellow-fin dolphin), sardines, anchovies, and herring, are subject to rapid microbial decomposition.

All of these fish have a relatively high content of the amino acid histidine in their tissues. Bacterial decomposition of the fish converts the histidine to histamine. Histamine can reach fairly high concentrations without the development of any off-flavors that would cause these fish to be

rejected as spoiled and thus inedible. Some individuals claim to have detected a sharp, peppery taste in conjunction with this type of seafood poisoning.

Histamine has a relatively low oral toxicity, and in most cases, the histamine will not produce the observed toxicity. However, putrescine is also encountered in fish. Putrescine actually enhances the effects of histamine, and causes a violent allergic reaction. Histamine and putrescine are chemically stable, and will not be reduced by cooking, freezing, or other processing.

The symptoms of scombroid poisoning can begin in less than 10 minutes or up to 2 hours after consumption of the tainted fish. Most of the acute symptoms vanish within 16 to 24 hours. The symptoms resemble a severe allergic reaction, and may include a facial flush, tightness of the chest, sweating, nausea, vomiting, tingling, body rash (hives or itching wheals), severe headache, shortness of breath, dizziness, throbbing, thirst, and diarrhea.

Paraquat, the herbicide sprayed by the government on marijuana plants in the 1970s, is a substantial lung carcinogen. Its cancer-causing abilities have in part been shown to be the result of huge increases of polyamines in the lungs.

Most dietary lectins have been shown to be potent inducers of polyamine production in the gut. This is probably the result of the intestinal cells synthesizing large amounts of polyamines in an effort to repair the damage caused by the lectins. Lectins typically damage the delicate finger-like projections of the mucosa called microvilli.

Many lectins cause growth increases in several organs, including the liver, pancreas, and spleen.

Enlargements of these organs are the result of a huge influx of polyamines into the organs.

Wheat germ lectin induces significant polyamine production. Incorporating wheat germ lectin into the diet of lab animals reduced the digestibility and utilization of dietary proteins, and significantly interfered with the growth of the animals. As a result of its binding and uptake by the cells of the small intestine, wheat germ lectin induced extensive polyamine-dependent growth of the small bowel tissue by increasing its content of proteins, RNA, and DNA. An appreciable portion of the absorbed wheat germ lectin was transported across the gut wall into the systemic circulation, where it was deposited in the walls of the blood and lymphatic vessels. Wheat germ lectin also induced growth of the pancreas. These same effects have been shown to occur with several bean and legume lectins as well.

Therapies, Polyamines

ALL BLOOD GROUPS:

1. Avoid guar gum, carrageenan, and large amounts of pectin.

2. Avoid canned or flash-frozen vegetables: The shock to the tissues of many foods processed in this manner allows for the release of many polyamines, either prior to pasteurization or upon thawing.

3. Avoid the amino acids ornithine, cysteine, and methionine. Ornithine and methionine are precursors of polyamines. Ornithine is the direct precursor to putrescine; methionine

and cysteine are intermediates in the synthesis of polyamines.

BLOOD GROUP A:

1. Detoxification Protocol
2. Intestinal Health Protocol
3. Liver Support Protocol
4. Antibacterial Protocol

BLOOD GROUP B:

1. Detoxification Protocol
2. Intestinal Health Protocol
3. Liver Support Protocol
4. Antibacterial Protocol

BLOOD GROUP AB:

1. Detoxification Protocol
2. Intestinal Health Protocol
3. Liver Support Protocol
4. Antibacterial Protocol

BLOOD GROUP O:

1. Detoxification Protocol
2. Intestinal Health Protocol
3. Liver Support Protocol
4. Antibacterial Protocol

Related Topics

Bacterial disease (general)

Digestion

Immunity

Liver disease

TOXIC SHOCK SYNDROME–*See Bacterial disease, pneumonia*

TRIGLYCERIDES–*See Hypertriglyceridernia*

TUBERCULOSIS–*See Bacterial disease, tuberculosis*

TYPHOID–*See Bacterial disease, typhoid*

ULCER, DUODENAL–*A type of ulcer in the upper gastrointestinal tract that occurs in mucosa that has contact with acid and pepsin.*

Duodenal ulcer	RISK		
	LOW	AVERAGE	HIGH
GROUP A			
GROUP B			
GROUP AB			
GROUP O			
NON-SECRETORS			

Symptoms

- Epigastric pain (often burning, gnawing, or vague; somewhat relieved by food or antacids)

- Epigastric tenderness with palpation, especially in the midline section of the abdomen

About Duodenal Ulcers

Duodenal ulcers occur when the effects of acid and pepsin overwhelm the body's natural ability to defend itself with mucus production. Most duodenal ulcers occur in the first part of the duodenum. They are typically round or oval, less than 1 centimeter in diameter, and are chronic and recurrent (60% of healed ulcers will recur within 1 year, and 80% to 90% will recur within 2 years).

General Causes and Risk Factors

Predisposing factors for ulcer development include family history, cigarette smoking, and mental or emotional stress, anger, or anxiety. Recent estimates indicate that up to 10% of the population will experience a duodenal ulcer at some time during their life. The condition is more common in males, and is more common than gastric ulcers.

Additional causes and aggravating factors include the following:

- Abnormal bacterial flora, producing urease. This converts urea present in the stomach, producing localized ammonia and bicarbonate. It migrates into the mucosa, where it inhibits mucus-secreting cells. It also produces protease and lipase, which digest the mucus layer.

- Poor nutritional status, especially inadequate levels of zinc, vitamin A, glutamine, and vitamin E

- Smoking, decreasing bicarbonate and decreasing gastric emptying time

- Aspirin, irritating membranes and increasing their permeability

- Caffeine and alcohol, both stimulating acid secretion

Blood Group Links

The association between blood group O and duodenal ulcers was one of the first made by researchers, dating back to 1936[1]. An investigation of the relationship of ABO blood groups and stomach cancer, duodenal ulcer, and stomach ulcer revealed that a statistically higher level of free hydrochloric acid was found in blood group O than in blood group A[2]. In addition, non-secretors have a higher level of duodenal ulcers[3].

Therapies, Duodenal Ulcer

BLOOD GROUP A:

1. Antibacterial Protocol
2. Stomach Health Protocol
3. Intestinal Health Protocol

BLOOD GROUP B:

1. Antibacterial Protocol
2. Stomach Health Protocol
3. Intestinal Health Protocol

BLOOD GROUP AB:

1. Antibacterial Protocol
2. Stomach Health Protocol
3. Intestinal Health Protocol

BLOOD GROUP O:

1. Antibacterial Protocol
2. Stomach Health Protocol
3. Intestinal Health Protocol

Related Topics

Bacterial disease (general)

Cancer, stomach

Digestion

Ulcer, *H. pylori*

Ulcer, peptic

REFERENCES

1. Shahid A, Zuberi SJ, Siddiqui AA, Waqar MA. Genetic markers and duodenal ulcer. *JPMA J Pak Med Assoc.* 1997; 47:135–137.
2. Pals G, Defize J, Pronk JC, et al. Relations between serum pepsinogen levels, pepsinogen phenotypes, ABO blood groups, age and sex in blood donors. *Ann Hum Biol.* 1985; 12:403–411.
3. Kolster J, Castro D, Kolster C, Quintero M, Callegari C. [HLA, blood group, secretory factor, pepsinogen I, and *Helicobacter pylori* in duodenal ulcer patients.] *G E N.* 1993; 47:247–256.

ULCER, *HELICOBACTER PYLORI*–*A bacterial infection increasingly implicated as the primary cause of nonerosive gastritis.*

H. pylori ulcer	RISK		
	LOW	AVERAGE	HIGH
GROUP A			
GROUP B			
GROUP AB			
GROUP O			
NON-SECRETORS			

Symptoms

Most patients with *H. pylori*–associated gastritis are asymptomatic.

About *H. pylori* Ulcer

There is currently a consensus in medical science that most gastric ulcers are caused by infection with *H. pylori*. There is strong evidence linking *H. pylori* infection with the subsequent development of stomach cancer, although as yet the mechanism is not fully understood. Apparently, *H. pylori* infection and its attendant inflammation increase the proliferation of stomach cells, and incite early precancerous changes. Type A individuals seem most prone to developing stomach cancer.

In 1994, the World Health Organization declared *H. pylori* to be a grade I carcinogen for gastric adenocarcinoma and mucosa-associated lymphoid tissue tumors of the stomach. Although the exact mode of transmission is unclear, the organism has been cultured from stool, saliva, and dental plaque, which implicates oral–oral or fecal–oral transmission. Infections tend to cluster in families, and in residents of custodial institutions. Nurses and gastroenterologists appear to be at high risk, and bacteria have been transmitted by improperly disinfected endoscopes.

Blood Group Links

In the early 1950s, it was discovered that blood group O predominated in the development of all types of stomach ulcers at a rate of approximately two to one over the other blood groups. These findings have been reproduced so frequently— over 25 studies in the last 20 years—with the same consistent result that the conclusions are not questioned[1,2].

In several studies, non-secretors of ABO substances have been found to have a significantly higher rate of gastric and duodenal ulcers. Some researchers have suggested that secretor status might influence bacterial colonization density, or the ability of *H. pylori* to attach to gastroduodenal cells. Because non-secretors are limited in their ability to secrete blood group antigens into the mucus secretions of their digestive tract, they have trouble preventing the attachment of *H. pylori* bacteria. The lack of antigens contributes to colonization by *H. pylori*.

When specific antigens are free-floating in the mucus, it acts to bind up some of the *H. pylori* before it can contact and attach to tissues. Secretors have the ability to put some biological decoys or metabolic false targets into secretions to deter the *H. pylori* from attaching. Non-secretors are unable to mount an aggressive immune response against this organism[3–10].

Therapies, *H. pylori* Ulcer

BLOOD GROUP A:

1. Antibacterial Protocol

2. Stomach Health Protocol

3. Cancer Prevention Protocol

BLOOD GROUP B:

1. Antibacterial Protocol

2. Stomach Health Protocol

3. Intestinal Health Protocol

BLOOD GROUP AB:

1. Antibacterial Protocol

2. Stomach Health Protocol

3. Cancer Prevention Protocol

BLOOD GROUP O:

1. Antibacterial Protocol

2. Stomach Health Protocol

3. Intestinal Health Protocol

Related Topics

Bacterial disease (general)

Cancer, stomach

Digestion

Ulcer, duodenal

Ulcer, peptic

REFERENCES

1. Mentis A, Blackwell CC, Weir DM, Spiliadis C, Dailianas A, Skandalis N. ABO blood group, secretor status and detection of *Helicobacter pylori* among patients with gastric or duodenal ulcers. *Epidemiol Infect.* 1991;106:221–229.

2. Alkout AM, Blackwell CC, Weir DM. Increased inflammatory responses of persons of blood group O to *Helicobacter pylori. J Infect Dis.* 2000;181:1364–1369.

3. Suadicani P, Hein HO, Gyntelberg F. Genetic and lifestyle determinants of peptic ulcer. A study of 3,387 men aged 54 to 74 years: The Copenhagen Male Study. *Scand J Gastroenterol.* 1999;34:12–17.

4. Hein HO, Suadicani P, Gyntelberg F. Genetic markers for stomach ulcer. A study of 3,387 men aged 54 to 74 years from The Copenhagen Male Study. *Ugeskr Laeger.* 1998; 160:5045–5046.

5. Dickey W, Collins JS, Watson RG, Sloan JM, Porter KG. Secretor status and *Helicobacter pylori* infection are independent risk factors for gastroduodenal disease. *Gut.* 1993; 34:351–353.

6. Sumii K, Inbe A, Uemura N, et al. Multiplicative effect of hyperpepsinogenemia I and non-secretor status on the risk of duodenal ulcer in siblings. *Gastroenterol Jpn.* 1990;25: 157–161.

7. Oberhuber G, Kranz A, Dejaco C, et al. Blood groups Lewis(b) and ABH expression in gastric mucosa: lack of inter-relation with *Helicobacter pylori* colonisation and occurrence of gastric MALT lymphoma. *Gut.* 1997;41:37–42.

8. Su B, Hellstrom PM, Rubio C, et al. Type I *Helicobacter pylori* shows Lewis(b)-independent adherence to gastric cells requiring de novo protein synthesis in both host and bacteria. *J Infect Dis.* 1998;178:1379–1390.

9. Alkout AM, Blackwell CC, Weir DM, et al. Isolation of a cell surface component of *Helicobacter pylori* that binds H type 2, Lewis(a), and Lewis(b) antigens. *Gastroenterology.* 1997;112:1179–1187.

10. Klaamas K, Kurtenkov O, Ellamaa M, Wadstrom T. The *Helicobacter pylori* seroprevalence in blood donors related to Lewis (a,b) histo-blood group phenotype. *Eur J Gastroenterol Hepatol.* 1997;9:367–370.

ULCER, PEPTIC–_A type of ulcer in the upper gastrointestinal tract that occurs in mucosa that has contact with acid and pepsin._

Peptic ulcer	RISK		
	LOW	AVERAGE	HIGH
GROUP A	░	░	
GROUP B	░	░	
GROUP AB	░	░	
GROUP O	░	░	░
NON-SECRETORS	░	░	░

Symptoms

- Epigastric pain (often made worse from food and not helped by antacids)
- Hemorrhage (25% of people)
- Anorexia
- Nausea and vomiting

About Peptic Ulcers

Peptic ulcers are typically seen in individuals age 50 or older, and occur equally in men and women. Almost all peptic ulcers are located in the antrum, the hollow of the stomach. Benign ulcers almost always occur with gastritis. Unlike duodenal ulcers, which appear to follow high acid–pepsin secretion, gastric ulcers are more often due to the lack of protection from the mucosal cells, as patients with gastric ulcers tend to have normal or even reduced amounts of hydrochloric acid secretion. There is a strong association with con-

sumption of aspirin, steroids, and nonsteroidal anti-inflammatory drugs (NSAIDs).

General Causes and Risk Factors

- Decreased production of protective substances lining the stomach
- Abnormal bacterial flora
- Poor nutritional status, especially inadequate levels of zinc, vitamin A, and glutamine
- Smoking, decreasing bicarbonate and decreasing gastric emptying time

Blood Group Links

The characteristics of peptic ulcer and non-ulcer dyspepsia in young men were studied in 202 consecutive military conscripts admitted to the Central Military Hospital in Helsinki because of long-standing upper abdominal complaints. Active peptic ulceration was found in 48 individuals, inactive peptic ulcer disease was diagnosed in 77 patients, non-ulcer dyspepsia was diagnosed in 52 patients. (In 25 cases, the reason for symptoms was another disease, and these individuals were excluded from the study.) A control series was established with 30 healthy young male volunteers without symptoms. In conclusion, the status of gastroduodenal mucosa, gastric secretion pattern, and distribution of some genetic markers among the patients indicated that young onset peptic ulcer and non-ulcer dyspepsia were two separate entities. The researchers concluded that _Helicobacter_-positive antrum gastritis is the best determinant of ulcer risk, but also Lewis (a+) phenotype, non-secretor status, and group O blood were indicators of an increased risk of peptic ulcer[1].

In another study, the concentrations of gastrin were measured by radioimmune assay in the sera (blood) of 121 healthy Greek volunteers of both sexes and of different ABO blood groups, aged 20 to 70 years. Samples were obtained after fasting from all the participants, then at 10 minutes and 40 minutes after a test meal for 42 of the volunteers. An increase was found in the mean concentrations of gastrin in all of the groups after the meal. Blood groups O and B showed an increase within 10 minutes after the meal, while groups A and AB did not show it for 40 minutes[2].

Therapies, Peptic Ulcer

BLOOD GROUP A:

1. Antibacterial Protocol
2. Stomach Health Protocol

BLOOD GROUP B:

1. Antibacterial Protocol
2. Stomach Health Protocol

BLOOD GROUP AB:

1. Antibacterial Protocol
2. Stomach Health Protocol

BLOOD GROUP O:

1. Antibacterial Protocol
2. Stomach Health Protocol

Related Topics

Bacterial disease (general)

Cancer, stomach

Digestion

Ulcer, duodenal

Ulcer, peptic

REFERENCES

1. Cederberg A, Varis K, Salmi HA, Sipponen P, Harkonen M, Sarna S. Young onset peptic ulcer disease and non-ulcer dyspepsia are separate entities. *Scand J Gastroenterol Suppl.* 1991;186:33–44.

2. Melissinos K, Alegakis G, Archimandritis AJ, Theodoropoulos G. Serum gastrin concentrations in healthy people of the various ABO blood groups. *Acta Hepatogastroenterol (Stuttg).* 1978;25:482–486.

ULCERATIVE COLITIS–*See Colitis, ulcerative*

UNIPOLAR DEPRESSION–*See Depression, unipolar*

URINARY TRACT INFECTION–*See Cystitis*

UTERINE CANCER–*See Cancer, uterine*

UTERINE FIBROIDS–*See Fibroids, uterine*

V

VAGINAL CANCER–_See Cancer, gynecological tumors_

VAGINITIS–_See Fungal disease, candidiasis (vaginal)_

VENOUS THROMBOEMBOLISM–_See Blood clotting disorders_

VIRAL DISEASE, ACQUIRED IMMUNE DEFICIENCY SYNDROME (AIDS)–_A breakdown of the body's immune system, resulting from infection with the human immunodeficiency virus (HIV)._

AIDS	RISK		
	LOW	AVERAGE	HIGH
GROUP A			
GROUP B			
GROUP AB			
GROUP O			
NON-SECRETOR			

Symptoms

- Pneumocystic pneumonia
- _Candida_ infection (thrush)
- Kaposi's sarcoma
- Cryptococcal meningitis

About AIDS

The human immunodeficiency virus (HIV) is transmitted through blood and bodily fluids. The most common risk factors include:

- Sexual contact with an infected person
- Sharing a hypodermic needle (injection drug use) with an infected person
- Being born to an infected mother
- Blood-to-blood contact with infected blood

Once infected with HIV, the body will try to fight the infection by creating antibodies. It is the presence of these antibodies in blood that causes an individual to test HIV positive.

Being HIV positive won't necessarily cause illness, but once a person has the virus it continues to weaken the immune system. Full-blown AIDS is usually diagnosed in the presence of an opportunistic infection, such as pneumonia or thrush. However, the progression of the disease can be tracked through blood tests, which determine the number of T-helper cells. AIDS attacks these T cells, gradually destroying them and leaving the body open to infection.

The Role of T-Lymphocyte Cells

T lymphocytes (T cells) enable the immune system to recognize and destroy foreign substances (such as bacteria, virus, and fungi). T cells comprise 80% to 90% of circulating lymphocytes, and may survive up to 30 years. T cells can be categorized as helper/inducer (CD4) cells and as suppressor/cytotoxic (CD8) cells.

There are two types of T-helper cells:

- T_H1 (inflammatory helper cells) produce cytokines that promote cellular immune responses. These cytokines include interleukin 2 (IL-2), immune interferon gamma (IFN-γ), and tumor necrosis factor-beta (TNF-β).

- T_H2 (helper cells) produce interleukins 2, 4, 6, and 10, all of which prompt the production of antibodies.

Cytotoxic or cytolytic T cells kill cells that produce foreign antigens, such as tumor cells, virus-infected cells, and foreign tissue grafts. Cytoxic T cells are identified by the presence of the CD8 marker. These cells can suppress the immune response, and are sometimes referred to as suppressor T cells.

Blood Group Links

Blood group antigens play a critical role in the activity of T cells. Therefore, although people of every blood group are susceptible to infection with HIV after exposure, they will vary in their susceptibility to the opportunistic infections that result from a weakened immune system.

There is some evidence that HIV-infected blood group A and AB individuals may produce anti-A antibodies, thus weakening their ability to fight infections[1].

It is also known that stress plays a significant role in the weakening of the immune system. In particular, stress affects the body's ability to produce immunoglobulin A (IgA), one of the primary defenses against infection which is found in the mucosal secretions of the digestive system, mouth, lungs, urinary tract, and other body cavities. IgA is the first line of defense against bacterial and viral infections. Blood group A and to some degree blood group B are particularly vulnerable to stress-related conditions, due to their naturally higher levels of cortisol.

Therapies, AIDS

ALL BLOOD GROUPS:

Since many of the opportunistic infections cause nausea, diarrhea, and mouth sores, AIDS is often a wasting disease. Adherence to the blood type diet is especially critical.

BLOOD GROUP A:

1. Antiviral Protocol

2. Yeast/Fungus Resistance Protocol

3. Chemotherapy Adjunct Protocol

4. Immune-Enhancing Protocol

BLOOD GROUP B:

1. Antiviral Protocol

2. Yeast/Fungus Resistance Protocol

3. Chemotherapy Adjunct Protocol

4. Immune-Enhancing Protocol

BLOOD GROUP AB:

1. Antiviral Protocol

2. Yeast/Fungus Resistance Protocol

3. Chemotherapy Adjunct Protocol

4. Immune-Enhancing Protocol

BLOOD GROUP O:

1. Antiviral Protocol

2. Yeast/Fungus Resistance Protocol

3. Chemotherapy Adjunct Protocol

4. Immune-Enhancing Protocol

Related Topics

Bacterial disease (general)

Blood transfusion

Fungal disease, candidiasis

Immunity

Infectious disease

Viral disease, hepatitis B and C

REFERENCES

1. Friedli F, et al. *Clin Immunopathology*. 1996;80:96–100.

VIRAL DISEASE, HEPATITIS B AND C–

Diffuse liver inflammation caused by specific hepatotropic viruses.

Hepatitis B and C	RISK		
	LOW	AVERAGE	HIGH
GROUP A			
GROUP B			
GROUP AB			
GROUP O			

Symptoms

- Profound anorexia

- Distaste for cigarettes (an early manifestation for smokers)

- Malaise

- Nausea and vomiting

- Fever

- Darkened urine (in 3 to 10 days)

- Jaundice

About Hepatitis B and C

Hepatitis is a disorder in which viruses or other mechanisms produce inflammation in liver cells, resulting in their injury or destruction. In most cases, this inflammatory process is triggered when the immune system fights off infections caused by viruses. It can also be caused, however, by an overactive immune system that attacks its own liver cells. Inflammation of the liver can also occur from medical problems, drugs, alcoholism, chemicals, and environmental toxins. Hepatitis varies in severity from a self-limited condition with total recovery, to a life-threatening or life-long disease.

The hepatitis B virus (HBV) is the most thoroughly characterized and complex agent. It is transmitted through blood transfusions, contaminated needles, and sexual contact.

Hepatitis C

Until blood screening began in 1990, the primary mode of known transmission was through transfusions. It is also transmitted through contaminated needles, and possibly via sexual transmission. In 40% of cases, the cause of transmission remains unknown. Most cases of hepatitis C (HVC) infection are subclinical, even in the acute stage. The infection has a much higher rate of remaining in a chronic state (about 75%) than does hepatitis B. Hepatitis C is often uncovered in routine blood work by the serendipitous detection of anti-HCV in apparently healthy persons. It may not be found for many years after infection.

Blood Group Links

The ABO blood groups and their relationship with the hepatitis B antigen (HBsAg) were studied in 500 blood donors and 76 patients. Most of the blood donors belonged to blood group B, but HBsAg was found to be most prevalent in blood group A. In a second study, 76 patients clinically diagnosed with viral hepatitis showed a similar trend, with the highest percentage of HBsAg-

positive individuals found in group A. In both studies, this trend was found to be statistically significant. None of the individuals with the AB blood group showed HBsAg. The absence of HbsAg made group AB especially susceptible to a more virulent form of hepatitis B[1]. Another study, which screened 330 blood donors for HBsAg to study its relationship to blood groups, found that blood group O donors had the highest HBsAg prevalence rate, 4.3%, as opposed to none for group AB donors[2].

Therapies, Hepatitis B and C

ALL BLOOD GROUPS:

Post-transfusion infections with hepatitis are minimized by avoiding unnecessary transfusions, using volunteers rather than paid donors, and screening all donors for HBsAg and anti-HCV. Screening is almost universally available, and it has dramatically decreased, but not eliminated, hepatitis B and C infections acquired through medical care. There is no vaccine against HCV. Vaccination against HBV gives an almost universal anti-HBsAg response in normal recipients, and has resulted in a dramatic reduction (about 90%) in the incidence of HBV infection. Dialysis patients, cirrhotic patients, and other immunocompromised recipients respond less well. The few healthy persons who fail to mount an anti-HBsAg response have no obvious immunologic defect.

BLOOD GROUP A:

1. Antiviral Protocol

2. Immune-Enhancing Protocol

BLOOD GROUP B:

1. Antiviral Protocol

2. Immune-Enhancing Protocol

BLOOD GROUP AB:

1. Antiviral Protocol

2. Immune-Enhancing Protocol

BLOOD GROUP O:

1. Antiviral Protocol

2. Immune-Enhancing Protocol

Related Topics

Bacterial disease (general)

Blood transfusion

Fungal disease, candidiasis

Immunity

Infectious disease

Viral disease, AIDS

REFERENCES

1. Lenka MR, Ghosh E, Bhattacharyya PK. ABO blood groups in relation to hepatitis-B surface antigen (Australia antigen). *Trans R Soc Trop Med Hyg.* 1981;75:688–690.

2. Gupta, HL, Tandon, SK, Pandit, N, Sinha, VP, Gajendra-gadkar, S. Incidence of viral hepatitis in relation to ABO blood groups. *J Commun Dis.* 1988;20:159–160.

VIRAL DISEASE, INFLUENZA–*A viral infection, sometimes called "the flu," which is actually caused by a very specific and devastating viral agent.*

Influenza	RISK		
	LOW	AVERAGE	HIGH
GROUP A	▨		
GROUP B (A-strain only)	▨	▨	
GROUP AB	▨	▨	▨
GROUP O	▨		
SECRETORS			
MN BLOOD GROUP			

Symptoms

- Fever
- Cough
- Sore throat
- Runny nose
- Headache
- Chills and muscle ache
- Deep fatigue

About Influenza

Influenza is a perennial killer, appearing every winter like clockwork. On several occasions in the 20th century, influenza has reached epidemic proportions. The Spanish Flu of 1918 to 1919 killed 500,000 people in the United States, and 20 million worldwide. The Asian Flu of 1957 to 1958 caused 70,000 deaths in America alone. The Hong

Kong Flu of 1968 to 1969 took 34,000 lives. In the 21st century, the flu remains just as deadly. As many as 20,000 people in the United States still die from it every year—the victims are mostly the elderly, the immunosuppressed, and those with preexisting conditions such as DIABETES, ASTHMA, or HEART DISEASE.

Although people often use the term "flu" to describe a wide range of symptoms that include anything from a fever to a cough, the influenza virus is a very specific pathogen. Influenza causes a fever; respiratory symptoms such as COUGHING, a sore throat, and a runny nose; and HEADACHE, muscle ache, and deep FATIGUE. Influenza is usually designated as a type *A* or a type *B*. This delineation has no relation to blood group; rather, it describes particular strains. To differentiate influenza strain A or B from blood group A or B, the influenza strain *A* or *B* will be italicized in this section.

Blood Group Links

Blood group A demonstrates an ability to generate a quick and substantial antibody response against influenza type *A* (H1N1), and even more so against type *A* (H3N2). The response against the influenza *B* virus is less strong. Overall, blood group A tends to acquire only the less virulent forms of the virus. If they become ill, they do so less severely than others.

Blood group B has the weakest defense against *A* (H3N2), and a slightly better defense against *A* (H1N1). The type *A* (H3N2) antigen can still be found in healthy group B individuals as long as 5 months after their recovery from the flu. There

may be no symptoms, but the virus has nevertheless been given a safe harbor. Blood group B, however, has an extremely strong advantage against influenza *B* strains over any of the other blood types. The immune response happens much more quickly and persists far longer than that of the other blood groups[1].

Blood group AB has a relatively poor ability to generate antibodies against any of the influenza viruses. The flu is problematic every year for group AB individuals. Immunological investigations of the time course of serum anti-HA and anti-NA antibodies against influenza *A* and *B* viruses in the female and male population with ABO blood groups were carried out for several months. The persons with the blood group AB were shown to be most sensitive to influenza *A* and *B*. They were affected by the epidemic virus earlier and more severely than those with the other blood groups[2].

Blood group O has an overall lower risk for influenza.

Secretors are more susceptible to influenza than non-secretors. ABO secretors are significantly over-represented among patients with influenza viruses *A* and *B*, rhinoviruses, respiratory syncytial viruses, and echoviruses[3]. MN blood group individuals have more protection against influenza[4].

Therapies, Influenza

BLOOD GROUP A:

1. Antiviral Protocol

2. Immune-Enhancing Protocol

BLOOD GROUP B:

1. Antiviral Protocol

2. Immune-Enhancing Protocol

BLOOD GROUP AB:

1. Antiviral Protocol

2. Immune-Enhancing Protocol

BLOOD GROUP O:

1. Antiviral Protocol

2. Immune-Enhancing Protocol

Related Topics

Bacterial disease (general)

Immunity

Infectious disease

Viral disease, AIDS

REFERENCES

1. Naikhin AN, Katorgina LG, Tsantsyna IM, et al. [Indicators of collective immunity to influenza depending on the blood group and sex of the population]. *Vopr Virusol.* 1989;34: 419–423.

2. The relationship between epidemic influenza (A(H1N1) and ABO blood group. *J Hyg (Lond).* 1981;87:139–146.

3. Vojvodie S. [Inhibitory activity of blood group antigens M and N in inhibition of virus hemagglutination reactions of influenza viruses]. *Med Pregl.* 2000;53:7–14.

4. Raza MW, Blackwell CC, Molyneaux P, et al. Association between secretor status and respiratory viral illness. *BMJ.* 1991;303(6806):815–818.

VIRAL DISEASE, MONONUCLEOSIS—*Infection with the Epstein-Barr virus.*

Mononucleosis	RISK		
	LOW	AVERAGE	HIGH
GROUP A			
GROUP B			
GROUP AB			
GROUP O			
RH-NEGATIVE			

Symptoms

- Fatigue
- Weakness
- Sore throat
- Fever
- Swollen lymph nodes in neck and armpits
- Swollen tonsils
- Headache
- Skin rash
- Loss of appetite
- Nausea
- Vomiting
- Weight loss

About Mononucleosis

Mononucleosis (commonly referred to as "mono") is caused by the Epstein-Barr virus and it is spread by intimate contact—the reason it's often called the "kissing disease." Mono infections usually arc not very serious; some people with mono have such minimal symptoms that the infection goes unrecognized. Most people have been exposed to the Epstein-Barr virus by the time they are 35 years old and have built up antibodies which make them immune to future infection. Full-blown mono is common among people aged 7 to 35; and the highest incidence is found among people aged 15 and 24.

Blood Group Links

Mononucleosis shows a somewhat higher incidence in blood group B and in all Rh-negative individuals.

Therapies, Mononucleosis

BLOOD GROUP A:
1. Antiviral Protocol
2. Immune-Enhancing Protocol

BLOOD GROUP B:
1. Antiviral Protocol
2. Immune-Enhancing Protocol

BLOOD GROUP AB:
1. Antiviral Protocol
2. Immune-Enhancing Protocol

BLOOD GROUP O:
1. Antiviral Protocol
2. Immune-Enhancing Protocol

Related Topics

Bacterial disease (general)

Immunity

Infectious disease

VIRAL DISEASE, MUMPS–*A viral infection that attacks the parotid salivary glands.*

Mumps	RISK		
	LOW	AVERAGE	HIGH
GROUP A	░		
GROUP B	░		
GROUP AB	░	░	
GROUP O	░		
RH-NEGATIVE	░	░	░

Symptoms

- Swollen, painful salivary glands on one or both sides of the face
- Fever
- Weakness and fatigue
- Orchitis (tenderness and swelling of a testicle)

About Mumps

Mumps is a viral infection of the parotid glands—salivary glands located below and in front of the ears. The disease spreads through close contact with someone who has mumps. Mumps is usually not very serious, and cases have dropped off significantly since the appearance of the mumps vaccine in the 1960s. Mumps is more serious when it is contracted by adults, among whom rare cases result in encephalitis, pancreatitis, and swelling of the testicles.

Blood Group Links

Rh-negative individuals appear to be more susceptible to mumps than others.

Therapies, Mumps

BLOOD GROUP A:

1. Antiviral Protocol

2. Immune-Enhancing Protocol

BLOOD GROUP B:

1. Antiviral Protocol

2. Immune-Enhancing Protocol

BLOOD GROUP AB:

1. Antiviral Protocol

2. Immune-Enhancing Protocol

BLOOD GROUP O:

1. Antiviral Protocol

2. Immune-Enhancing Protocol

Related Topics

Immunity

Infectious disease

VITILIGO–*A congenital or acquired decrease in melanin production.*

Vitiligo	RISK		
	LOW	AVERAGE	HIGH
GROUP A	▒		
GROUP B	▒	▒	
GROUP AB	▒		
GROUP O	▒	▒	
RH-NEGATIVE	▒	▒	▒

Symptoms

- White patches (depigmentation) on sun-exposed areas of the skin

- White patches in the armpits and groin and around the mouth, eyes, nostrils, navel, and genitals

- Premature graying of hair

About Vitiligo

Vitiligo generally appears in one of three patterns. In the focal pattern, the depigmentation is limited to one or two areas. In the segmental pattern, people develop depigmented patches on only one side of their bodies. However, most people who have vitiligo experience the generalized pattern, in which depigmentation occurs on different parts of the body. In addition to white patches on the skin, people with vitiligo may have premature graying of the scalp hair, eyelashes, eyebrows, and beard. People with dark skin may notice a loss of color inside their mouths.

The cause of vitiligo is not known, but doctors and researchers have several different theories. One theory is that people develop antibodies that destroy the melanocytes in their own bodies. Another theory is that melanocytes destroy themselves.

Vitiligo seems to be more common in people with certain autoimmune diseases, including HYPERTHYROIDISM, adrenal disorders, and PERNICIOUS ANEMIA.

Blood Group Links

Blood group B has been shown to have an increased incidence of vitiligo.

Therapies, Vitiligo

ALL BLOOD GROUPS:

Treatment for vitiligo is primarily for the cosmetic disfigurement. Topical corticosteroids occasionally help. Oral and topical psoralens with ultraviolet A (PUVA) have been used, but treatment is protracted and results vary. Khellin, a furanochromone, can be used in combination with PUVA. However, 100 to 200 treatments are required to achieve a satisfactory result.

BLOOD GROUP A:

1. Skin Health Protocol
2. Yeast/Fungus Resistance Protocol

BLOOD GROUP B:

1. Skin Health Protocol
2. Yeast/Fungus Resistance Protocol

BLOOD GROUP AB:

1. Skin Health Protocol
2. Yeast/Fungus Resistance Protocol

BLOOD GROUP O:

1. Skin Health Protocol
2. Yeast/Fungus Resistance Protocol

Related Topics

Autoimmune disease (general)

VOMITING–*See Nausea*

VON WILLEBRAND FACTOR–*See Blood clotting disorders*

VULVAR CANCER–*See Cancer, gynecological tumors*

W

WEIGHT LOSS–*See Obesity*

WHEEZING–*See Asthma*

Y

YELLOWING OF THE SKIN–_See Liver_
disease

YERSINIA–_See Bacterial disease,_ Yersinia
(Plague)

PART THREE

Blood Group Protocols

1. BLOOD GROUP MEDICAL AND HEALTH PROTOCOLS

2. BLOOD GROUP FOOD BASE

3. BLOOD GROUP SUPPLEMENT BASE

ONE

Blood Group Medical and Health Protocols

The following 30 blood group–specific protocols are the functional health strategies to be used in addition to diet, exercise, and general medical recommendations. You will find suggestions for their use in the Therapies portions of part 2, A–Z Blood Group Guide to Health and Medical Conditions. You may also use them individually as needed for general health and well-being.

Note: These protocols are not meant as substitutes for the medical advice of physicians and other health care professionals. Rather, they are intended to enhance medical treatments and provide overall health benefits.

The Protocols

1. Allergy Control Protocols
2. Antibacterial Protocols
3. Antibiotic Support Protocols
4. Anti-Inflammation Protocols
5. Antistress Protocols
6. Antiviral Protocols

7. Arthritis Protocols

8. Blood-Building Protocols

9. Cancer Prevention Protocols

10. Cardiovascular Protocols

11. Chemotherapy Adjunct Protocols

12. Chronic Illness Recovery Protocols

13. Cognitive Improvement Protocols

14. Detoxification Protocols

15. Fatigue-Fighting Protocols

16. Female Balancing Protocols

17. Immune-Enhancing Protocols

18. Intestinal Health Protocols

19. Liver Support Protocols

20. Male Health Protocols

21. Menopause Support Protocols

22. Metabolic Enhancement Protocols

23. Nerve Health Protocols

24. Pulmonary Support Protocols

25. Sinus Health Protocols

26. Skin Health Protocols

27. Stomach Health Protocols

28. Surgery Recovery Protocols

29. Urinary Tract Health Protocols

30. Yeast/Fungus Resistance Protocols

1. ALLERGY CONTROL PROTOCOLS

Use this protocol for 4 weeks.

BLOOD GROUP A

☐ Hawthorn (*Crataegus* sp), standardized extract, 100 mg: 1–2 capsules, twice daily

☐ Vitamin C (preferably from Rose Hips or Acerola Cherry), 250 mg: 1 capsule daily

☐ Quercetin, 500 mg: 1 capsule with meals, 2–3× daily

☐ Stinging Nettle leaf (*Urtica dioica*), 500 mg: 1–2 capsules, twice daily away from food

BLOOD GROUP B

☐ Potassium citrate, 99 mg: 1–2 capsules, twice daily

☐ MSM (methylsulfonylmethane), 500 mg: 1–2 capsules, twice daily

☐ Magnesium, 650 mg: 1 capsule, twice daily

☐ Pantothenic acid (vitamin B_5), 500 mg: twice daily

BLOOD GROUP AB

☐ Frankincense (*Boswellia serrata*), 400 mg (standardized to contain 37.5% boswellic acids): 2 capsules, twice daily

☐ Magnolia flower (*Magnolia lilflora*), 50 mg: 1–2 capsules, twice daily

☐ Quercetin, 500 mg: 1 capsule with meals, 2–3× daily

BLOOD GROUP O

☐ Frankincense (*Boswellia serrata*), 400 mg (standardized to contain 37.5% boswellic acids): 2 capsules, twice daily

☐ Yerba maté tea (*Ilex paraguariensis*): 1–3 cups, daily

☐ Stinging Nettle leaf (*Urtica dioica*), 500 mg: 1–2 capsules, twice daily away from food

☐ Pantothenic acid (vitamin B$_5$), 500 mg: twice daily

NON-SECRETORS
Add:

☐ Schisandra/Wu-Wei-Zi berry (*Schizandra chinensis*), 450 mg: 1 capsule, twice daily

☐ Vitamin C (preferably from acerola cherry or rose hips), 250 mg: 1 capsule daily

GENERAL RECOMMENDATIONS USABLE BY ALL GROUPS

☐ Bromelain (Pineapple enzyme), 500 mg: 1–3 tablets four times daily between meals, gradually decreasing

2. ANTIBACTERIAL PROTOCOLS
Use this protocol for 3 weeks.

BLOOD GROUP A

☐ Oregon Grape (*Berberis aquifolium*), 250–500 mg: 1–2 capsules, twice daily

☐ Old Man's Beard (*Usnea barbata*) tincture: 7–10 drops in warm water before meals

☐ Baptisia tinctorialis (homeopathic remedy) 6c–30c: 3–5 pellets, daily away from food

BLOOD GROUP B

☐ *Coriolus versicolor* mushroom, 300 mg: 1–2 capsules, daily

☐ Schisandra/Wu-Wei-Zi (*Schisandra chinensis*), 250–500 mg: 1–2 capsules, daily

☐ Siberian ginseng (*Eleutherococcus senticosus*), 500 mg: 1–2 capsules, daily

BLOOD GROUP AB

☐ Astragalus (*Astragalus membranaceus*), 500 mg: 1–2 capsules, twice daily

☐ Ligustrum (*Ligustrum lucidum*), 250–500 mg: 1–2 capsules, daily away from food

BLOOD GROUP O

☐ Astragalus (*Astragalus membranaceus*), 500 mg: 1–2 capsules, twice daily

☐ Kutki (*Picrorhiza kurroa*), 400 mg: 1–2 capsules daily

NON-SECRETORS
Add:

☐ Vitamin A, 10,000 IU: 1 capsule, daily

☐ Zinc, 15 mg: daily

GENERAL RECOMMENDATIONS USABLE BY ALL GROUPS

☐ Vitamin C (from acerola cherry or rose hips), 250 mg: 1 capsule, twice daily

☐ Larch arabinogalactan (*Larix officinalis*) "ARA6"*: 1 tbsp, twice daily in juice or water

☐ Probiotic supplement, preferably ABO specific

3. ANTIBIOTIC SUPPORT PROTOCOLS
Use this protocol for 4 weeks.[1]

BLOOD GROUP A

☐ Bromelain (pineapple enzyme), 500 mg: 1–2 capsules with each dose of antibiotic

☐ Echinacea/Purple Coneflower (*Echinacea purpura*) tincture: 15 drops, twice daily

BLOOD GROUP B

☐ Alpha lipoic acid, 100 mg: 2 capsules daily

☐ Baptisia tinctoris (homeopathic remedy) (6c): 2–3 pellets, twice daily

BLOOD GROUP AB

☐ Bromelain (pineapple enzyme), 500 mg: 1–2 capsules with each dose of antibiotic

☐ Huang Lian (Rhizoma Coptidis), 200 mg: 1 capsule, daily[2]

*Entries that appear in quotation marks are available through North American Pharmacal. See back page for details.

BLOOD GROUP O

☐ Proteolytic enzymes (pancreatin 4x): 1 capsule with each dose of antibiotic

☐ Bladderwrack (*Fucus vesiculosus*), 150 mg: 1 capsule, daily

NON-SECRETORS
Add:

☐ Glutathione, 100 mg: 1 capsule, twice daily

☐ Caprylic acid, 250 mg: 1 capsule, with meals

GENERAL RECOMMENDATIONS USABLE BY ALL GROUPS

☐ Probiotic supplement, preferably ABO specific

☐ Larch arabinogalactan (ARA6): 1 tbsp daily

☐ Multivitamin, preferably ABO specific

NOTES:

1. Avoid calcium supplementation if using antibiotics in the tetracycline and quinolone families.

2. Regular use of Huang Lian (Rhizoma Coptidis) in large dosage (greater than 3 grams daily) may cause diarrhea.

4. ANTI-INFLAMMATION PROTOCOLS
Use this protocol for 4–8 weeks.

BLOOD GROUP A

☐ Kava Kava (*Piper mysticum*) standardized extract (30% kavalactones), 250 mg: 1 capsule, twice daily

☐ Fish oil capsules (3 grams of EPA plus DHA): 1 capsule, daily[1]

☐ White Willow bark (*Salix alba*), 300 mg, standardized extract, 14% salicin: 1 capsule, once or twice daily

☐ Frankincense (*Boswellia serrata*), 400 mg (standardized to contain 37.5% boswellic acids): 2 capsules, twice daily

☐ Holy Basil (*Ocimum sanctum*) leaf extract, 50 mg: 1–2 capsules, twice daily

BLOOD GROUP B

☐ MSM (methylsulfonylmethane), 500 mg: 1–2 capsules, twice daily

☐ Cat's Claw (*Uncaria tomentosa*), 500 mg: 1–2 capsules, twice daily

☐ OPCs (oligomeric proanthocyanidins), 100 mg: 1 capsule, daily

☐ Curcumin (Turmeric: *Curcuma longa*), 95% curcuminoids, 300–500 mg: 1 capsule, once or twice daily

☐ Jiaogulan (*Gynostemma pentaphyllum*), 60 mg, gynostemma whole glucosides: 1–2 capsules, twice daily

BLOOD GROUP AB

☐ Frankincense (*Boswellia serrata*), 400 mg (standardized to contain 37.5% boswellic acids): 2 capsules, twice daily

☐ Curcumin (Turmeric: *Curcuma longa*), 95% curcuminoids, 300–500 mg: 1 capsule, once or twice daily

☐ Bilberry extract (Vaccinium), 25 mg anthocyanosides calculated as anthocyanidins: 1–2 capsules, twice daily

☐ Jiaogulan (*Gynostemma pentaphyllum*), 60 mg, gynostemma whole glucosides: 1–2 capsules, twice daily

BLOOD GROUP O

☐ Glucosamine sulphate, 500 mg: 1–2 capsules away from food, twice daily

☐ Joshua Tree (*Yucca brevifolia*), concentrated yucca saponins, 400–500 mg: 1–2 capsules, twice daily

☐ Ginger root (Rhizoma Zingiberis: *Zingiber officinalis*)

☐ Cayenne pepper (*Capsicum* sp), 300 mg: 1–2 capsules with meals

NON-SECRETORS
Add:

☐ 5-HTP (5-Hydroxytryptophan), 150 mg: 1 capsule, twice daily (non-secretors)

☐ Lectin-blocking formula ("Deflect") specific for ABO group: 2 capsules with meals (non-secretors)

GENERAL RECOMMENDATIONS USABLE BY ALL GROUPS

☐ Bromelain (Pineapple enzyme), 500 mg: 1–3 tablets, four times daily between meals, gradually decreasing dose and frequency as symptoms improve

NOTES:

1. Fish oil should not be taken by women who are or could become pregnant. Consult your doctor first.

5. ANTISTRESS PROTOCOLS
Use this protocol for 8 weeks.

BLOOD GROUP A

☐ Chamomile (*Matricaria chamomilla*) herbal tincture: 25 drops in warm water, two or three times daily

☐ Spreading Hogweed (*Boerhaavia diffusa*), 250 mg: 1–2 capsules, twice daily

☐ Brahmi (*Bacopa monnieri*), 200 mg: 1–2 capsules, twice daily

☐ Yoga or Tai Chi: 25–30 minutes, five times weekly

☐ Oatstraw (*Avena sativa*), 750 mg: 1–2 capsules, twice daily

☐ Holy Basil (*Ocimum sanctum*) leaf extract, 50 mg: 1–2 capsules, twice daily

BLOOD GROUP B

☐ Cordyceps (*Cordyceps sinensis*), 500 mg: 1–2 capsules, twice daily

☐ GABA (gamma amino butyric acid), 500 mg: 1 capsule, twice daily

☐ Inositol, 500 mg: 1–2 capsules, twice daily

☐ Schisandra/Wu-Wei-Zi (*Schizandra chinensis*) herbal tincture: 15–25 drops, twice daily

☐ Meditation, visualization, chanting, singing: 25 minutes daily

BLOOD GROUP AB

☐ Cordyceps (*Cordyceps sinensis*), 500 mg: 1–2 capsules, twice daily

☐ Brahmi (*Bacopa monnieri*), 200 mg: 1–2 capsules, twice daily

☐ Wild Hops (*Humulus* sp) freeze dried, 250 mg: 1–2 capsules, before bed

☐ Astragalus (*Astragalus membranaceus*), 500 mg: 1–2 capsules, twice daily

☐ Meditation, visualization, yoga, or Tai Chi: 25–30 minutes, five times weekly

BLOOD GROUP O

☐ Russian Rhodiola (*Rhodiola rosea*), 250 mg: 1–2 capsules, three times daily

☐ L-Tyrosine, 500 mg: 1 capsule, twice daily[1]

☐ Valerian (*Valeriana officinalis*), 0.5% essential oils, 500 mg: 1–2 capsules, before bed

☐ Aerobics, swimming, cycling: 25 minutes, four times weekly

NON-SECRETORS
Add:

☐ Maitake extract (*Grifola frondosa*), 500 mg: 2–3 capsules, twice daily (non-secretors)

☐ 5-HTP (5-hydroxytryptophan), 150 mg: 1 capsule, twice daily (non-secretors)

GENERAL RECOMMENDATIONS USABLE BY ALL GROUPS

☐ Calcium, 1000 mg (preferably from sea plants)

☐ Multivitamin (preferably blood group specific)

NOTES:

1. Do not take L-Tyrosine supplement if you are on a MAO inhibitor–type drug.

6. ANTIVIRAL PROTOCOLS
Use this protocol for 2 weeks.

BLOOD GROUP A

☐ Asian Ginseng (*Panax ginseng*), 250 mg: 1–2 capsules, daily

☐ Linden (*Tilia* sp) tea: 1–3 cups, daily

☐ Fo-Ti (*Polygonum multiflorum*), 250 mg: 1–2 capsules, daily

☐ Noni (*Morinda citrifolia*) fruit extract, 250 mg: 1–2 capsules, daily

BLOOD GROUP B

☐ *Coriolus versicolor* mushroom, 300 mg: 1–2 capsules, daily

☐ Siberian ginseng (*Eleutherococcus senticosus*), 500 mg: 1–2 capsules, daily

☐ Gokharu/Caltrop (*Tribulus terrestris*) fruit extract (20% furanosterols), 50 mg: 1–2 capsules, daily

☐ Chlorella (*Chlorella regularis*), 200 mg: 1–2 capsules, daily

BLOOD GROUP AB

☐ Linden (*Tilia* sp) tea: 1–3 cups, daily

☐ L-arginine, 500 mg: 1–2 capsules, daily

☐ Chlorella (*Chlorella regularis*), 200 mg: 1–2 capsules, daily

☐ Siberian ginseng (*Eleutherococcus senticosus*), 500 mg: 1–2 capsules, daily

BLOOD GROUP O

☐ Astragalus (*Astragalus membranaceus*), 500 mg: 1–2 capsules, twice daily

☐ Kutki (*Picrorhiza kurroa*), 400 mg: 1–2 capsules, daily

☐ L-glutamine, 500 mg: 1–2 capsules, daily

NON-SECRETORS
Add:

☐ Vitamin A 10,000 IU: 1 capsule, daily

☐ Zinc, 15 mg: daily

GENERAL RECOMMENDATIONS USABLE BY ALL GROUPS

☐ Vitamin C (from acerola cherry or rose hips) 250 mg: 1 capsule, twice daily

☐ Larch arabinogalactan (*Larix officinalis*) "ARA6": 1 tbsp, twice daily in juice or water

☐ Elderberry extract ("Proberry Capsules"): 1–2 capsules, twice daily

7. ARTHRITIS PROTOCOLS
Use this protocol for 12 weeks.

BLOOD GROUP A

☐ Chondroitin sulfate, 600 mg: 2 capsules, daily, away from food

☐ Glucosamine sulfate, 500 mg: 2–3 capsules, daily, away from food

☐ Betaine HCl, 250 mg: 1 capsule with large meals

☐ Fish oil capsules (3 grams of EPA plus DHA): 1 capsule, daily[1]

BLOOD GROUP B

☐ Glucosamine sulfate, 500 mg: 3–4 capsules daily away from food

☐ S-adenosyl-methionine (SAMe), 400 mg: 1–2 capsules, daily[2]

☐ Niacinamide (vitamin B₃), 50 mg: 2 capsules, daily[3]

BLOOD GROUP AB

☐ Chondroitin sulfate, 600 mg: 2 capsules daily away from food

☐ Niacinamide (vitamin B₃), 50 mg: 2 capsules, daily[3]

BLOOD GROUP O

☐ N-acetyl glucosamine, 250–500 mg: 3–4 capsules, daily, away from food

☐ Frankincense (*Boswellia serrata*), 500 mg: 1–2 capsules with meals

☐ L-Phenylalanine, 250 mg: 1–2 capsules between meals[4]

☐ Rhus tox (homeopathic medicine), 6c–30c: 3–5 pellets, away from food, daily

NON-SECRETORS
Add:

☐ Lectin-blocking formula ("Deflect") specific for ABO group: 2 capsules with meals

☐ Boron, 1 mg: 1 capsule, daily

GENERAL RECOMMENDATIONS USABLE BY ALL GROUPS

☐ Vitamin C (from acerola cherry or rose hips), 250 mg: 1 capsule, twice daily

NOTES:

1. Fish oil should not be taken by women who are or could become pregnant. Consult your physician first.

2. SAMe may be detrimental in people with Parkinson's disease.

3. Niacinamide is almost always safe to take, though rare liver problems have occurred at amounts in excess of 1,000 mg per day.

4. People with phenylketonuria must not supplement with phenylalanine. Some research suggests that tardive dyskinesia patients may process phenylalanine abnormally. Until more is known, it makes sense for people with this condition to avoid phenylalanine supplementation.

8. BLOOD-BUILDING PROTOCOLS
Use this protocol for 4 weeks.

BLOOD GROUP A

☐ Floradix "Liquid Iron and Herbs": 1–2 teaspoons, daily

☐ Methylcobalamin ("active B_{12}"), 500 mcg: 2 capsules, daily, away from food

☐ Folic acid, 400 mcg: 1 tablet, daily

☐ Betaine HCl, 250 mg: 1 capsule with large meals

☐ Noni (*Morinda citrifolia*) fruit extract, 250 mg: 1–2 capsules, daily

BLOOD GROUP B

☐ Iron citrate, 50 mg: 1–2 capsules, twice daily

☐ Liquid chlorophyll: 1 tbsp, daily

☐ Folic acid, 400 mcg: 1 tablet, daily

BLOOD GROUP AB

☐ Iron citrate, 50 mg: 1–2 capsules, twice daily

☐ Yellow dock (*Rumex crispus*), 250 mg: 1–2 capsules, daily

☐ Methylcobalamin ("active B_{12}"), 500 mcg: 2 capsules daily away from food

BLOOD GROUP O

☐ Liver extract (aqueous extract best), 500 mg: 1–2 capsules, twice daily away from food

☐ Copper citrate, 3 mg: 1 capsule, daily (for 2–3 weeks)

☐ Stinging Nettle leaves (*Urtica dioica*), 500 mg: 1 capsule, twice daily

☐ Pyridoxine (vitamin B_6), 50–200 mg: daily

GENERAL RECOMMENDATIONS USABLE BY ALL GROUPS

☐ Vitamin C (from Acerola Cherry or rose hips), 250 mg: 1 capsule, twice daily

9. CANCER PREVENTION PROTOCOLS
Use this protocol for 4 weeks, discontinue for 4 weeks, then restart.

BLOOD GROUP A

☐ Quercetin, 500 mg: 1 capsule, twice daily

☐ Maitake extract (*Grifola frondosa*), 500 mg: 2–3 capsules, twice daily

☐ Curcumin (Turmeric: *Curcuma longa*), 95% curcuminoids, 300–500 mg: 1 capsule, once or twice daily

☐ Tarragon (*Artemisia dracunculus*), 100 mg, daily

☐ Burdock root (*Arctium* sp) tea: 1–3 cups, daily

☐ Noni (*Morinda citrifolia*) fruit extract, 250 mg: 1–2 capsules, daily

☐ Escargot/Roman Snail (*Helix pomatia*), "Helix plus": 1–2 capsules, daily

BLOOD GROUP B

☐ *Coriolus versicolor* mushroom, 300 mg: 1–2 capsules, daily

☐ Astragalus (*Astragalus membranaceus*), 500 mg: 1–2 capsules, twice daily

☐ Selenium, 50 mcg: 1–2 capsules, twice daily

☐ Sweet Fennel (*Foeniculum vulgare*), 250 mg: 1–2 capsules, daily

BLOOD GROUP AB

☐ Quercetin, 500 mg: 1 capsule, twice daily

☐ Selenium, 50 mcg: 1–2 capsules, twice daily

☐ Curcumin (Turmeric: *Curcuma longa*), 95% curcuminoids, 300–500 mg: 1 capsule, once or twice daily

☐ Sweet Basil (*Ocimum basilium*), 100–250 mg: 1 capsule, daily

☐ Roman Snail (*Helix pomatia*), "Helix plus": 1–2 capsules, daily

BLOOD GROUP O

☐ Maitake extract (*Grifola frondosa*), 500 mg: 2–3 capsules, twice daily

☐ Astragalus (*Astragalus membranaceus*), 500 mg: 1–2 capsules, twice daily

☐ Rosemary (*Romarinus* sp) extract 5:1 concentrate, 50 mg: 1 capsule, daily

☐ Tarragon (*Artemisia dracunculus*), 100 mg: daily

NON-SECRETORS
Add:

☐ Probiotic supplement, preferably ABO specific

GENERAL RECOMMENDATIONS USABLE BY ALL GROUPS

☐ Co Enzyme Q10, 30 mg: 2 capsules, daily

☐ Green tea: 1–3 cups, daily

☐ Typhoid vaccine (injectable, not oral): repeat every 3–5 years

☐ Larch arabinogalactan (*Larix officinalis*) "ARA6": 1 tbsp, twice daily, in juice or water

10. CARDIOVASCULAR PROTOCOLS
Use this protocol for 4–8 weeks.

BLOOD GROUP A

☐ Hawthorn (*Crataegus* sp) standardized extract, 100 mg: 1–2 capsules, twice daily

☐ Ginger (*Zingiber* sp), 1.5% essential oils: 1–2 capsules, twice daily

☐ Pantethine, 500 mg: 1 capsule, twice daily

☐ Gingko (*Gingko biloba*), 24% standardized extract, 60 mg: 1–2 capsules, daily[1]

☐ Artichoke leaf (*Cynara scolymnus*), 500 mg: 2 capsules, twice daily[2]

BLOOD GROUP B

☐ OPCs (oligomeric proanthocyanidins), 100 mg: 1 capsule, daily

☐ Alpha lipoic acid, 50 mg: 1 capsule, daily

☐ Curcumin (Turmeric: *Curcuma longa*), 95% curcuminoids, 300–500 mg: 1 capsule, once or twice daily

☐ Fenugreek (*Trigonella foenum-graecum*), 500 mg, defatted seeds: 1–2 capsules, twice daily

BLOOD GROUP AB

☐ Hawthorn (*Crataegus* sp), standardized extract, 100 mg: 1–2 capsules, twice daily

☐ OPCs (oligomeric proanthocyanidins), 100 mg: 1 capsule, daily

☐ Standardized Chinese Garlic Extract (*Allium sativum*), 400 mg: 1 capsule, twice daily

☐ Pantethine, 500 mg: 1 capsule, twice daily

BLOOD GROUP O

☐ Arjuna Myrobalan (*Terminalia arjuna*), 2% Arjunolic acid, 250 mg: twice daily

☐ Coleus (*Coleus forskohlii*), standardized extract, 125 mg: 1 capsule, twice daily

☐ L-Carnitine, 50 mg: 1–2 capsules, twice daily

☐ Guggul Gum (*Commiphora mukul*), standardized for 25 mg guggulsterones of types E and Z: 1 capsule, once or twice daily

☐ Artichoke leaf (*Cynara scolymnus*), 500 mg: 2 capsules, twice daily[2]

NON-SECRETORS
Add:

☐ Co Enzyme Q10, 30 mg: 1 capsule, twice daily with a fatty meal (non-secretors)

☐ He-Shou-Wu, Fo-Ti (*Polygonum multiflorum*) 250 mg: 1 capsule, twice daily (non-secretors)

☐ *N*-acetyl glucosamine, 250 mg: 1 capsule with meals (NN blood group), 2–3× daily

☐ Dandelion (*Taraxacum officinale*), 250 mg: 1 capsule, twice daily (MN blood group)

GENERAL RECOMMENDATIONS USABLE BY ALL GROUPS

☐ Folic acid, 400 mcg: 2 tablets, daily

☐ Probiotic supplement, preferably ABO specific

NOTES:

1. Gingko is not appropriate for persons with blood clotting disorders.

2. Individuals with gall bladder disease should use artichoke only under medical supervision.

11. CHEMOTHERAPY ADJUNCT PROTOCOLS

Use this protocol for 3 weeks, discontinue for 1 week, then restart.

BLOOD GROUP A

☐ Astragalus (*Astragalus membranaceus*), 500 mg: 1–2 capsules, twice daily

☐ *Coriolus versicolor* mushroom, 300 mg: 1–2 capsules, daily

BLOOD GROUP B

☐ Thoroughwax/Bei-Chai-Hu (*Bupleurum chinense*), 500 mg: 1 capsule, twice daily

☐ Maitake extract (*Grifola frondosa*), 500 mg: 2–3 capsules, twice daily (non-secretors)

BLOOD GROUP AB

☐ Astragalus (*Astragalus membranaceus*), 500 mg: 1–2 capsules, twice daily

☐ *Coriolus versicolor* mushroom, 300 mg: 1–2 capsules, daily

BLOOD GROUP O

☐ Standardized Chinese Garlic Extract (*Allium sativum*), 400 mg: 1 capsule, twice daily

☐ Schisandra/Wu-Wei-Zi (*Schizandra chinensis*) herbal tincture: 15–25 drops, twice daily

NON-SECRETORS
Add:

☐ Vitamin A 10,000 IU: 1 capsule, daily

GENERAL RECOMMENDATIONS USABLE BY ALL GROUPS

☐ Probiotic supplement, preferably ABO specific

☐ Larch arabinogalactan (*Larix officinalis*) "ARA6": 1 tbsp, twice daily in juice or water

☐ Green tea: 1–3 cups, daily

12. CHRONIC ILLNESS RECOVERY PROTOCOLS

Use this protocol for 6 weeks.

BLOOD GROUP A

☐ Ashwaganda (*Withania somnifera*), 250 mg: 1 capsule, twice daily

☐ Pantothenic acid, 250 mg: 1–2 capsules, twice daily

☐ Potassium citrate, 99 mg: twice daily

BLOOD GROUP B

☐ Phosphatidyl choline, 1 gram: 2 capsules, daily

☐ Siberian ginseng (*Eleutherococcus senticosus*), 250 mg: 1 capsule, twice daily

☐ Magnesium, 350 mg: 1 capsule, twice daily

BLOOD GROUP AB

☐ L-arginine, 500 mg: 1–2 capsules, daily

☐ Pantothenic acid, 250 mg: 1–2 capsules, twice daily

☐ Zinc, 25 mg: 1 capsule, daily

BLOOD GROUP O

☐ Gotu Kola leaf (*Hydrocotyle asiatica*), 250 mg, standardized extract: 1 capsule, twice daily[1]

☐ L-Carnitine, 50 mg: 1–2 capsules, twice daily

☐ Sarsaparilla (*Smilax* sp), standardized extract, 150 mg: 1 capsule, twice daily

NON-SECRETORS
Add:

☐ Dandelion (*Taraxacum officinale*), 250 mg: 1 capsule, twice daily (MN blood group)

GENERAL RECOMMENDATIONS USABLE BY ALL GROUPS

☐ General multivitamin, preferably ABO specific

☐ Vitamin C (from Acerola Cherry or rose hips), 250 mg: 1 capsule, twice daily

NOTES:

1. Do not use Gotu Kola leaf if you are pregnant.

---

13. COGNITIVE IMPROVEMENT PROTOCOLS
Use this protocol for 4 weeks.

BLOOD GROUP A

☐ Brahmi (*Bacopa monnieri*), 200 mg: 1–2 capsules, twice daily

☐ OPCs (oligomeric proanthocyanidins), 100 mg: 1 capsule, daily

☐ Methylcobalamin ("active B_{12}"), 400 mcg: 1 capsule before bed

☐ Spreading Hogweed (*Boerhaavia diffusa*), 250 mg: 1–2 capsules, twice daily

BLOOD GROUP B

☐ Siberian ginseng (*Eleutherococcus senticosus*), 250 mg: 1 capsule, twice daily

☐ Inositol, 500 mg: 1–2 capsules, twice daily

☐ Gokharu/Caltrop (*Tribulus terrestris*), 150 mg: 1 capsule, daily

☐ Gingko (*Gingko biloba*), 24% standardized extract, 60 mg: 1–2 capsules, daily[1]

BLOOD GROUP AB

☐ Brahmi (*Bacopa monnieri*), 200 mg: 1–2 capsules, twice daily

☐ Siberian ginseng (*Eleutherococcus senticosus*), 250 mg: 1 capsule, twice daily

☐ OPCs (oligomeric proanthocyanidins), 100 mg: 1 capsule, daily

☐ Thiamine hydrochloride (vitamin B_1), 50 mg: 1 capsule, twice daily

BLOOD GROUP O

☐ Russian Rhodiola (*Rhodiola rosea*), 250 mg: 1–2 capsules, twice daily

☐ Thiamine hydrochloride (vitamin B_1), 50 mg: 1 capsule, twice daily

☐ Amla/Indian Gooseberry (*Phyllanthus emblica*), 250 mg: 1–2 capsules, daily

☐ Folic acid, 400 mcg: 2 tablets, daily

GENERAL RECOMMENDATIONS USABLE BY ALL GROUPS

☐ Multivitamin supplement, preferably ABO specific

NOTES:

1. Gingko is not appropriate for persons with blood clotting disorders.

14. DETOXIFICATION PROTOCOLS
Use this protocol for 1 week.

BLOOD GROUP A

☐ Cleavers (*Galium aparine*) tea: 2–3 teaspoons of the herb in a cup of hot water, steep for 10 to 15 minutes. Drink 1 to 2 cups per day.

☐ Dandelion (*Taraxacum officinale*), 250 mg: 1 capsule, twice daily (MN blood group)

☐ Fig powder: 1 tbsp before bed with a large glass of water

☐ Dry skin brushing: Immediately before showering or bathing, start with the feet and gently brush up toward the heart. Brush from the extremities toward the center. Brush gently in a circular motion around your abdomen and breasts/chest area. The proper dry skin brush is made of vegetable bristles that are neither too stiff nor too soft. It shouldn't scratch, but you should feel some friction against the skin.

BLOOD GROUP B

☐ Thoroughwax/Bei-Chai-Hu (*Bupleurum chinense*), 500 mg: 1 capsule, twice daily

☐ Flaxseeds (*Linum usitatissimum*): 1 tbsp added to 8 oz water, allow to soak overnight, drink in morning

☐ L-glutathione, 100 mg: 1 capsule, twice daily

☐ Epsom Salt Baths: Take a shower first, then start with a very clean tub; fill the tub with the hottest water you can stand. Begin with ¼ cup of Epsom salts, work up gradually to 4 cups, and soak as long as ½ hour. If you experience light-headedness, drain the tub, and wait until you feel steady enough to leave the tub.

BLOOD GROUP AB

☐ Burdock root (*Arctium* sp) tea: 1–3 cups, daily

☐ Yarrow (*Achillea millefolium*), 250 mg: 1–2 capsules, daily

☐ Flaxseeds (*Linum usitatissimum*): 1 tbsp added to 8 oz water, allow to soak overnight, drink in morning

☐ Dry skin brushing: Immediately before showering or bathing, start with the feet and gently brush up toward the heart. Brush from the extremities toward the center. Brush gently in a circular motion around your abdomen and breasts/chest area. The proper dry skin brush is made of vegetable bristles that are neither too stiff nor too soft. It shouldn't scratch, but you should feel some friction against the skin.

BLOOD GROUP O

☐ Bladderwrack (*Fucus vesiculosus*), 100 mg: 1–2 capsules, with meals 2–3× daily

☐ Standardized Chinese Garlic Extract (*Allium sativum*), 400 mg: 1 capsule, twice daily

☐ Prune powder: 1 tbsp before bed with a large glass of water

☐ Saunas and steam treatments as appropriate to your constitution and physical strength

NON-SECRETORS

Add:

☐ Lectin-blocking formula ("Deflect") specific for ABO group: 2 capsules with meals 2–3× daily

GENERAL RECOMMENDATIONS USABLE BY ALL GROUPS

☐ Probiotic supplement, preferably ABO specific

☐ Triphala—a combination of Amla (*Phyllanthus emblica*), Beleric Myrobalan (*Terminalia belerica*), and Chebulic Myrobalan (*Terminalia chebula*), 650–1000 mg: 1 capsule, twice daily

15. FATIGUE-FIGHTING PROTOCOLS

Use this protocol for 4 weeks.

BLOOD GROUP A

☐ Methylcobalamin (active B_{12}), 400 mcg: 1 capsule before bed

☐ Ashwaganda (*Withania somnifera*), 250 mg: 1 capsule, twice daily

☐ Nicotinamide adenine dinucleotide (NADH), 10–20 mg: 1 capsule in morning

☐ Pantothenic acid, 250 mg: 1–2 capsules, twice daily

☐ Vitamin C (from acerola cherry or rose hips), 250 mg: 1 capsule, twice daily

BLOOD GROUP B

☐ Siberian ginseng (*Eleutherococcus senticosus*), 250 mg: 1 capsule, twice daily

☐ Magnesium, 350 mg: 2 capsules, twice daily

☐ Melatonin, 3 mg: 1 capsule at bedtime

☐ Licorice (*Glycyrrhiza* sp): 1 cup of tea, twice daily[1]

☐ Potassium, 99 mg, twice daily

BLOOD GROUP AB

☐ Ginseng (*Panax* sp), 250 mg: 1 capsule, twice daily

☐ Nicotinamide adenine dinucleotide (NADH): 10–20 mg in morning

☐ Licorice (*Glycyrrhiza* sp): 1 cup of tea, twice daily[1]

☐ Potassium, 99 mg: 1 capsule, twice daily

☐ Vitamin C (from Acerola Cherry or rose hips), 250 mg: 1 capsule, twice daily

BLOOD GROUP O

☐ Methylcobalamin (active B_{12}), 400 mcg: 1 capsule before bed

☐ Russian Rhodiola (*Rhodiola rosea*), 250 mg: 1–2 capsules, twice daily

☐ L-Tyrosine, 250 mg: 1 capsule, twice daily

☐ Coleus (*Coleus forskohlii*), 150 mg: 1 capsule, twice daily

☐ Sarsaparilla (*Smilax* sp) standardized extract, 150 mg: 1 capsule, twice daily

NON-SECRETORS
Add:

☐ Co Enzyme Q10, 30 mg: 1 capsule, twice daily with a fatty meal (non-secretors)

GENERAL RECOMMENDATIONS USABLE BY ALL GROUPS

☐ General multivitamin, preferably ABO specific

☐ Probiotic supplement, preferably ABO specific

NOTES:

1. Licorice can cause sodium and water retention. It should be used with a potassium supplement or in combination with a high-potassium diet.

16. FEMALE BALANCING PROTOCOLS
Use this protocol for 4 weeks.

BLOOD GROUP A

☐ Chamomile (*Matricaria chamomilla*)

☐ Black Cohosh (*Cimicifuga racemosa*), standardized to 2.5% triterpene glycosides: 1–2 capsules, twice daily[1]

☐ Parsley leaf (*Petroselinum* sp), 400 mg: 1–2 capsules, twice daily

☐ Blessed Thistle (*Cnicus benedictus*) tincture: 5–10 drops in warm water, twice daily

☐ Black Currant seed oil capsules, 500 mg: 2–3 capsules, daily

BLOOD GROUP B

☐ Chaste Berry (*Vitex agnus-castus*), 400 mg, standardized: 1 capsule, twice daily

☐ Raspberry leaf (*Rubus* sp) tincture: 15–20 drops, twice daily

☐ Motherwort (*Leonurus cardiaca*) tincture: 10–15 drops, daily

☐ Black Currant seed oil capsules, 500 mg: 2–3 capsules, daily

BLOOD GROUP AB

☐ Dong Quai (*Angelica sinensis*), 500 mg: 1 capsule, twice daily

☐ Celery seed extract, 450 mg: 1 capsule, twice daily

☐ Parsley leaf (*Petroselinum* sp), 400 mg: 1–2 capsules, twice daily

☐ Motherwort (*Leonurus cardiaca*) tincture: 10–15 drops in warm water, daily

BLOOD GROUP O

☐ Squaw Vine (*Mitchella repens*) tincture: 10 drops in warm water, twice daily

☐ Vitamin B_6 (pyridoxal 5 phosphate), 50 mg: 1–3 capsules, daily

☐ Gotu Kola leaf (*Hydrocotyle asiatica*), 250 mg standardized extract: 1 capsule, twice daily[2]

☐ Bladderwrack (*Fucus vesiculosus*), 200 mg: 1 capsule, twice daily

☐ Blessed Thistle (*Cnicus benedictus*) tincture: 5–10 drops in warm water, twice daily

NON-SECRETORS
Add:

☐ Probiotic supplement, preferably ABO specific

GENERAL RECOMMENDATIONS USABLE BY ALL GROUPS

☐ Coriander extract (*Coriandrum sativum*), tincture: 7–10 drops, twice daily

☐ Magnesium, 650 mg: 1 capsule, twice daily (reduce if stools loosen)

☐ Hibiscus tea: 1–2 cups, daily

NOTES:

1. Do not take Black Cohosh if you have high blood pressure or heart disease.

2. Do not use Gotu Kola leaf if you are pregnant.

---

17. IMMUNE-ENHANCING PROTOCOLS
Use this protocol for 4 weeks.

BLOOD GROUP A

☐ Zinc, 25 mg: 1 capsule, daily

☐ Vitamin A, 10,000 IU: 1 capsule, daily

☐ Astragalus (*Astragalus membranaceus*), 500 mg: 1–2 capsules, twice daily

☐ Vitamin C (preferably from acerola cherry or rose hips), 250 mg: 1 capsule, daily

BLOOD GROUP B

☐ Maitake extract (*Grifola frondosa*), 500 mg: 2–3 capsules, twice daily

☐ Cordyceps (*Cordyceps sinensis*), 500 mg: 1–2 capsules, twice daily

☐ Job's Tears (*Coix lacryma-jobi*), 250 mg: 1–2 capsules, twice daily

☐ L-Arginine, 250 mg: 1–2 capsules, twice daily

☐ Sage (*Salvia officinalis*) tincture: 7–15 drops, twice daily

BLOOD GROUP AB

☐ Zinc, 25 mg: 1 capsule, daily

☐ Astragalus (*Astragalus membranaceus*), 500 mg: 1–2 capsules, twice daily

☐ Reishi mushroom (*Ganoderma senensis*), 500 mg: 1 capsule, twice daily

☐ Vitamin C (preferably from acerola cherry or rose hips), 250 mg: 1 capsule, daily

BLOOD GROUP O

☐ Woad root (*Isatis tinctoris*), 400 mg or tea: 1 capsule, twice daily (alternately, 1 cup tea, twice daily)

☐ Reishi mushroom (*Ganoderma senensis*), 500 mg: 1 capsule, twice daily

☐ Chuanxinlian (*Andrographis paniculata*), 350 mg: 1 capsule two or three times daily[1]

☐ Osha root (*Ligusticum porteri*), 250 mg: 1 capsule, twice daily[2]

NON-SECRETORS
Add:

☐ Elderberry concentrate "Proberry": 1 tsp, twice daily

☐ Codonopsis (*Codonopsitis lanceolate*), 400 mg: 1 capsule, twice daily

GENERAL RECOMMENDATIONS USABLE BY ALL GROUPS

☐ Larch arabinogalactan (*Larix officinalis*) "ARA6": 1 tbsp, twice daily in juice or water

☐ Probiotic supplement, preferably ABO specific

☐ Multivitamin supplement, preferably ABO specific

NOTES:

1. Chuanxinlian should not be used for longer than 3 weeks.

2. Osha is an endangered species.

---

18. INTESTINAL HEALTH PROTOCOLS
Use this protocol for 4 weeks.

BLOOD GROUP A

☐ Quercetin, 500 mg: 1 capsule with meals

☐ Black Currant seed oil capsules, 500 mg: 2–3 capsules, daily

☐ *Aloe vera*, 200 mg: 1 capsule with meals

☐ Jerusalem artichoke powder (*Helianthus tuberosus*), 750 mg: 1 capsule, twice daily

☐ Chicory powder (*Cichorium intybus*), 400 mg: 1 capsule, twice daily

☐ Burdock root (*Arctium* sp) tea: 1–3 cups, daily

BLOOD GROUP B

☐ Magnesium, 350 mg: 1 capsule, twice daily

☐ Rice-derived tocotrienols, 50 mg: 1–2 capsules, daily

☐ Elecampane (*Inula helenium*), 500 mg: 1 capsule with meals

☐ Chlorophyll liquid: 1 tsp, twice daily

BLOOD GROUP AB

☐ Bovine colostrums, 500 mg: 1–2 capsules, twice daily

☐ Dandelion (*Taraxacum officinale*), 300 mg: twice daily

☐ Standardized Chinese Garlic Extract (*Allium sativum*), 400 mg: 1 capsule, twice daily

☐ Quercetin, 500 mg: 1 capsule with meals

BLOOD GROUP O

☐ L-Glutamine, 200 mg: 1–2 capsules, twice daily

☐ Bovine colostrums, 500 mg: 1–2 capsules, twice daily

☐ NAG (*N*-acetyl-glucosamine), 200 mg: 1 capsule, twice daily

☐ Chicory powder (*Cichorium intybus*), 400 mg: 1 capsule, twice daily

NON-SECRETORS
Add:

☐ Caprylic acid, 350 mg: 1–2 capsules, twice daily away from food

GENERAL RECOMMENDATIONS USABLE BY ALL GROUPS

☐ Ghee (clarified butter) 1 tsp, twice daily

☐ ABO specific lectin blocking formula "Deflect": 1 capsule with meals 2–3× daily

☐ Larch arabinogalactan (*Larix officinalis*) "ARA6": 1 tbsp, twice daily in juice or water

☐ Probiotic supplement, preferably ABO specific

19. LIVER SUPPORT PROTOCOLS
Use this protocol for 4 weeks.

BLOOD GROUP A

☐ False Daisy (*Eclipta alba*), 300 mg: 1–2 capsules, daily

☐ Artichoke extract (*Cynara scolymnus*), 160 mg standardized to contain 13%–18% caffeylquinic acids calculated as chlorogenic acid: 1 capsule, twice daily

☐ L-Glutathione, 500 mg: 1 capsule, twice daily

☐ Alpha lipoic acid, 100 mg: 1 capsule, twice daily

BLOOD GROUP B

☐ Beet leaf and root, 100 mg: 2 capsules, twice daily

☐ Licorice root tea (*Glycyrrhiza* sp): 1 cup, once or twice daily[1]

☐ Potassium citrate, 99 mg: 1 capsule, daily

☐ Curcumin (Turmeric: *Curcuma longa*), 95% curcuminoids, 300–500 mg: 1 capsule, once or twice daily

☐ Fenugreek (*Trigonella foenum-graecum*), 500 mg, defatted seeds: 1–2 capsules, twice daily

BLOOD GROUP AB

☐ Beet leaf and root, 100 mg: 2 capsules, twice daily

☐ Milk Thistle extract (*Silybum marianum*), 175 mg: 2–3 capsules, daily

☐ Alpha lipoic acid, 100 mg: 1 capsule, twice daily

☐ Curcumin (Turmeric: *Curcuma longa*), 95% curcuminoids, 300–500 mg: 1 capsule, once or twice daily

☐ Thoroughwax/Bei-Chai-Hu (*Bupleurum chinense*), 500 mg: 1 capsule, twice daily

BLOOD GROUP O

☐ Milk Thistle extract (*Silybum marianum*), 175 mg: 2–3 capsules, daily

☐ Artichoke extract (*Cynara scolymnus*), 160 mg standardized to contain 13%–18% caffeylquinic acids calculated as chlorogenic acid: 1–2 capsules, daily

☐ Phyllanthus (*Phyllanthus amarus*), 500 mg: 1–2 capsules, daily

NON-SECRETORS
Add:

☐ Dandelion root (*Taraxacum officinale*), 200 mg: 1–2 capsules, twice daily

GENERAL RECOMMENDATIONS USABLE BY ALL GROUPS

☐ L-Glutathione, 500 mg: 1 capsule, twice daily

NOTES:

1. Licorice can cause sodium and water retention. It should be used with a potassium supplement or in combination with a high-potassium diet.

20. MALE HEALTH PROTOCOLS
Use this protocol for 4 weeks.

BLOOD GROUP A

☐ Stinging Nettle root (*Urtica dioica*), "UDA Plus," 200 mg: 1–2 capsules, twice daily

☐ Saw Palmetto extract (*Serenoa* sp), 50–100 mg of saw palmetto berry extract, standardized to contain 85–95% fatty acids and sterols: 1–2 capsules, twice daily

☐ False Unicorn Root (*Chaemelirium luteum, helonias*) tincture: 10–15 drops, twice daily in warm water

☐ Pumpkin seeds (*Cucurbita pepo*): 1–3 handfuls, daily

BLOOD GROUP B

☐ Saw Palmetto extract (*Serenoa* sp), 50–100 mg of saw palmetto berry extract, standardized to contain 85–95% fatty acids and sterols: 1–2 capsules, twice daily

☐ L-Arginine, 250 mg: 1–2 capsules, twice daily

☐ Peruvian Balsam bark (*Myroxylon pereira*), 50 mg: 1–2 capsules, daily

BLOOD GROUP AB

☐ Saw Palmetto extract (*Serenoa* sp), 50–100 mg of saw palmetto berry extract, standardized to contain 85–95% fatty acids and sterols: 1–2 capsules, twice daily

☐ L-Arginine, 250 mg: 1–2 capsules, twice daily

☐ Lycopene extract, 3 mg: 1–2 capsules, daily

BLOOD GROUP O

☐ Stinging Nettle root (*Urtica dioica*), "UDA Plus," 200 mg: 1–2 capsules, twice daily

☐ Pygeum (*Pygeum africanum*) extract, 50 mg: 1–2 capsules, daily

☐ False Daisy (*Eclipta alba*), 100 mg: 1 capsule, twice daily

☐ Man Vine (*Agonandra racemosa*) tincture: 6–15 drops, once or twice daily

☐ Pumpkin seeds (*Cucurbita pepo*): 1–3 handfuls, daily

GENERAL RECOMMENDATIONS USABLE BY ALL GROUPS

☐ Zinc, 25 mg: 1 capsule, daily

☐ L-Alanine, 250 mg: 1 capsule, twice daily

☐ L-Glycine, 250 mg: 1 capsule, twice daily

21. MENOPAUSE SUPPORT PROTOCOLS
Use this protocol for 6 weeks.

BLOOD GROUP A

☐ Black Cohosh (*Cimicifuga racemosa*), standardized to 2.5% triterpene glycosides: 1–2 capsules, twice daily[1]

☐ Squaw Vine (*Mitchella repens*) tincture: 10 drops in warm water, twice daily

☐ Soy isoflavones, 50 mg: 1 capsule, daily

☐ Vitamin B_6 (pyridoxine), 50 mg: daily

☐ Chamomile tea (*Matricaria chamomilla*): 1–3 cups, daily

BLOOD GROUP B

☐ Motherwort (*Leonurus cardiaca*) tincture: 10–15 drops, daily

☐ Magnesium, 350 mg: 2 capsules, twice daily

☐ Methylcobalamine ("active B_{12}"), 400 mcg: 1 capsule before bed

☐ Dong Quai (*Angelica sinensis*), 250 mg: 1–2 capsules, daily

BLOOD GROUP AB

☐ Black Cohosh (*Cimicifuga racemosa*), standardized to 2.5% triterpene glycosides: 1–2 capsules, twice daily[1]

☐ Vitamin B_6 (pyridoxine), 50 mg: daily

☐ Methylcobalamin ("active B_{12}"), 400 mcg: 1 capsule before bed

☐ Sage tea (*Salvia officinalis*): 1–2 cups, daily

BLOOD GROUP O

☐ Chaste Berry (*Vitex agnus-castus*), 400 mg standardized: 1 capsule, twice daily

☐ Horsetail (*Equisetum arvense*) 500 mg: 1 capsule, twice daily

☐ Manganese 10 mg: 1 capsule, daily

☐ Vervain (*Verbena officinalis*) tea: 1–2 cups, daily

NON-SECRETORS AND OTHER SUBTYPES
Add:

☐ Vitamin A 10,000 IU: 1 capsule, daily

☐ Boron, 1 mg: 1 capsule, daily

GENERAL RECOMMENDATIONS USABLE BY ALL GROUPS

☐ Calcium, 1000 mg (preferably from sea plants, such as "Phytocal")

☐ Vitamin D, 400 IU: daily (800 IU daily for non-secretors)

☐ General multivitamin, preferably ABO specific

NOTES:

1. Do not take Black Cohosh if you have high blood pressure or heart disease.

22. METABOLIC ENHANCEMENT PROTOCOLS
Use this protocol for 4 weeks.

BLOOD GROUP A

☐ Gotu Kola (*Centella asiatica*), 100 mg: 1–2 capsules, twice daily[1]

☐ Triphala—a combination of Amla (*Phyllanthus emblica*), Beleric Myrobalan (*Terminalia belerica*), and Chebulic Myrobalan (*Terminalia chebula*), 500 mg: 1 capsule, twice daily

☐ L-Tyrosine, 250 mg: 1–2 capsules, twice daily

BLOOD GROUP B

☐ Watermelon seed, 300 mg: 1–2 capsules, twice daily

☐ Ginger root (Rhizoma Zingiberis: *Zingiber officinalis*), 500 mg: 1–2 capsules with meals

☐ Fenugreek (*Trigonella foenum-graecum*), 500 mg, defatted seeds: 1–2 capsules, twice daily

BLOOD GROUP AB

☐ L-Cysteine, 500 mg: 1 capsule, twice daily

☐ Triphala—a combination of Amla (*Phyllanthus emblica*), Beleric Myrobalan (*Terminalia belerica*), and Chebulic Myrobalan (*Terminalia chebula*) 500 mg: 1 capsule, twice daily

BLOOD GROUP O

☐ Bladderwrack (*Fucus vesiculosus*), 200 mg: 1 capsule, twice daily

☐ Dandelion (*Taraxacum officinale*), 250 mg: 1 capsule, twice daily

☐ Guggul Gum (*Commiphora mukul*), standardized for 25 mg guggulsterones of types E and Z: 1 capsule, once or twice daily

GENERAL RECOMMENDATIONS USABLE BY ALL GROUPS

☐ Lectin-blocking formula ("Deflect") specific for ABO group: 2 capsules with meals

☐ Green tea: 1–3 cups, daily

NOTES:

1. Do not use Gotu Kola leaf if you are pregnant.

---

23. NERVE HEALTH PROTOCOLS
Use this protocol for 4 weeks.

BLOOD GROUP A

☐ Methylcobalamine ("active B_{12}"), 400 mcg: 1 capsule before bed

☐ Choline bitartrate, 500 mg: 1–2 capsules, daily

☐ DHA (docosahexaenoic acid), 100 mg: 1 capsule, twice daily

☐ Vinpocetin, 25 mg: 1 capsule, twice daily

BLOOD GROUP B

☐ NADH (Nicotinamide adenine dinucleotide), 50 mg: 1 tablet, twice daily

☐ DHA (docosahexaenoic acid), 100 mg: 1 capsule, twice daily

☐ Inositol, 250 mg: 1–2 capsules, daily

☐ Blessed Thistle (*Cnicus benedictus*), 250 mg: 1–2 capsules, daily

BLOOD GROUP AB

☐ DHA (docosahexaenoic acid), 100 mg: 1 capsule, twice daily

☐ Choline bitartrate, 500 mg: 1–2 capsules, daily

☐ Vinpocetin, 25 mg: 1 capsule, twice daily

☐ L-glutamine, 250 mg: 1 capsule, twice daily

BLOOD GROUP O

☐ Methylcobalamine ("active B_{12}"), 400 mcg: 1 capsule before bed

☐ Blessed Thistle (*Cnicus benedictus*), 250 mg: 1–2 capsules, daily

☐ NADH (Nicotinamide adenine dinucleotide), 50 mg: 1 tablet, twice daily

☐ Phosphatidylserine, 100 mg: 2 capsules, daily

GENERAL RECOMMENDATIONS USABLE BY ALL GROUPS

☐ Wild Oat extract (*Avene sativa*) 250 mg: 1–2 capsules, daily

---

24. PULMONARY SUPPORT PROTOCOLS
Use this protocol for 6 weeks.

BLOOD GROUP A

☐ Quercetin, 500 mg: 1 capsule with meals

☐ Horseradish (*Cochlearia armoracia*), fresh: ½ to 1 tsp, twice daily

☐ Gokharu/Caltrop (*Tribulus terrestris*), 150 mg: 1 capsule, daily

☐ MSM (methylsulfonylmethane), 500 mg: 1–2 capsules, twice daily

BLOOD GROUP B

☐ *N*-acetyl-cysteine, 500 mg: 1 capsule, twice daily

☐ Thyme (*Thymus vulgaris*) tincture: 5–10 drops, twice daily

☐ Ginger (*Zingiber* sp), 1.5% essential oils: 1–2 capsules, twice daily

BLOOD GROUP AB

☐ Quercetin, 500 mg: 1 capsule with meals 2–3× daily

☐ Ginger (*Zingiber* sp), 1.5% essential oils: 1–2 capsules, twice daily

☐ Horehound (*Marrubium vulgare*) tincture: 7–10 drops, daily

☐ MSM (methylsulfonylmethane), 500 mg: 1–2 capsules, twice daily

BLOOD GROUP O

☐ *N*-acetyl-cysteine 500 mg 1 capsule, twice daily

☐ Noni (*Morinda citrifolia*) fruit extract 250 mg: 1–2 capsules, daily

☐ Mullein (*Verbascum thapsus*) tea: 1–2 cups, daily

NON-SECRETORS
Add:

☐ Vitamin A, 10,000 IU: 1 capsule, daily

☐ Co Enzyme Q10: 3 mg, twice daily with meals 1–2× daily

GENERAL RECOMMENDATIONS USABLE BY ALL GROUPS

☐ Larch arabinogalactan (*Larix officinalis*) "ARA6": 1 tbsp, twice daily in juice or water

☐ Zinc, 15 mg: daily

☐ Vitamin C (from Acerola Cherry or rose hips), 250 mg: 1 capsule, twice daily

25. SINUS HEALTH PROTOCOLS
Use this protocol for 4 weeks.

BLOOD GROUP A

☐ Stone Root (*Collinsonia canadensis*), 200 mg: 1–2 capsules, twice daily

☐ Stinging Nettle leaf (*Urtica dioica*), 500 mg: 1–2 capsules, twice daily away from food

BLOOD GROUP B

☐ Magnolia flower (*Magnolia lilflora*), 50 mg: 1–2 capsules, twice daily

☐ Wild Indigo (*Baptisia tinctoria*) tincture: 3–7 drops, twice daily

BLOOD GROUP AB

☐ Stone Root (*Collinsonia canadensis*), 200 mg: 1–2 capsules, twice daily

☐ Stinging Nettle leaf (*Urtica dioica*), 500 mg: 1–2 capsules, twice daily away from food

BLOOD GROUP O

☐ Stinging Nettle leaf (*Urtica dioica*), 500 mg: 1–2 capsules, twice daily away from food

☐ MSM (methylsulfonylmethane), 500 mg: 1–2 capsules, twice daily

NON-SECRETORS
Add:

☐ Vitamin A, 10,000 IU: 1 capsule, daily

☐ Elderberry concentrate, "Proberry": 1 tsp, twice daily

GENERAL RECOMMENDATIONS USABLE BY ALL GROUPS

☐ Vitamin C (from Acerola Cherry or rose hips), 250 mg: 1 capsule, twice daily

☐ Neti Pots the natural way to keep your sinus passages clear and healthy.

☐ Yerba Santa (*Eriodictyon californicum*) tincture: 10–15 drops, twice daily in warm water

☐ Anise essential oil (*Pimpinella anisum*): added to nebulizer or vaporizer

26. SKIN HEALTH PROTOCOLS
Use this protocol for 4 weeks.

BLOOD GROUP A

☐ Pantethine, 500 mg: 1 capsule, twice daily

☐ Burdock root (*Arctium* sp) tea: 1–3 cups, daily

☐ Vitamin A, 10,000 IU: 1 capsule, daily

☐ Holy Basil (*Ocimum sanctum*) leaf extract, 50 mg: 1–2 capsules, twice daily

BLOOD GROUP B

☐ OPCs (oligomeric proanthocyanidins), 100 mg: 1 capsule, daily

☐ Pantothenic acid (vitamin B_5), 500 mg: twice daily

☐ Sarsaparilla (*Smilax officinalis*), 250 mg: 1–2 capsules, daily

BLOOD GROUP AB

☐ OPCs (oligomeric proanthocyanidins), 100 mg: 1 capsule, daily

☐ Vitamin A, 10,000 IU: 1 capsule, daily

☐ Red Clover (*Trifolium pratense*) tincture: 5 drops, once or twice daily

BLOOD GROUP O

☐ Pantothenic acid (vitamin B_5), 500 mg: twice daily

☐ Vitamin A, 10,000 IU: 1 capsule, daily

☐ Biotin, 2 mg: 2 capsules, daily

NON-SECRETORS
Add:

☐ Probiotic supplement, preferably ABO specific

☐ Tea Tree (*Leptospermum* sp) oil lotion (5%): apply topically, twice daily

GENERAL RECOMMENDATIONS USABLE BY ALL GROUPS

☐ Topical treatment with Witch-hazel (*Hammamelis virginiana*) as needed

☐ Topical treatment with Marigold juice (*Calendula officinales*) as needed

☐ Zinc, 15 mg: 1 capsule, twice daily

☐ Niacinamide creme (4%): apply topically, twice daily

27. STOMACH HEALTH PROTOCOLS

Use this protocol for 4 weeks.

BLOOD GROUP A

☐ Old Man's Beard (*Usnea barbata*) tincture: 7–10 drops in warm water before meals

☐ Gentian (*Gentiana lutea*) tincture: 5 drops in warm water before meals

☐ Natrum carbonicum 6c (homeopathic cell salt): 2–3 tablets between meals

BLOOD GROUP B

☐ Marshmallow (*Althea officinalis*), 250 mg: 1 capsule with meals 1–2X daily

☐ Cabbage powder, 400 mg: 1 capsule with meals, 1–2X daily

☐ Fenugreek (*Trigonella foenum-graecum*), 500 mg defatted seeds: 1 capsule, twice daily

☐ L-Glycine, 250 mg: 1 capsule, twice daily

BLOOD GROUP AB

☐ Slippery Elm (*Ulmus rubra*), 250 mg: 1 capsule, twice daily

☐ Parsley leaf (Petroselinum sp), 400 mg: 1–2 capsules, twice daily

☐ DGL Licorice (*Glycyrrhiza* sp), 150 mg, capsules or chewable tablets: 1 before meals[1]

BLOOD GROUP O

☐ Bladderwrack (*Fucus vesiculosus*), 100 mg: 1–2 capsules with meals, 2–3X daily

☐ DGL Licorice (*Glycyrrhiza* sp), 150 mg capsules or chewable tablets: 1 before meals[1]

☐ American Cranesbill (*Geranium maculatum*), 250 mg: 1 capsule with meals, 1–2X daily

☐ L-Glycine, 250 mg: 1 capsule, twice daily

NON-SECRETORS
Add:

☐ ABO specific lectin-blocking formula ("Deflect"): 1 capsule with meals, 2–3X daily

☐ Probiotic supplement, preferably ABO specific

GENERAL RECOMMENDATIONS USABLE BY ALL GROUPS

☐ Ginger root (Rhizoma Zingiberis: *Zingiber officinalis*), 200 mg: 1 capsule before meals

NOTES:

1. De-glycyrrhizinated (DGL) licorice has no side effects. Anyone with an ulcer should be treated by a physician.

28. SURGERY RECOVERY PROTOCOLS

Start this protocol 2 weeks before surgery and discontinue 2 weeks after surgery.

BLOOD GROUP A

☐ Gotu Kola (*Centella asiatica*), 100 mg: 1–2 capsules, twice daily[1]

☐ Vitamin E, 400 IU: 1 capsule, daily

☐ Horse Chestnut (*Aesculus hippocastanum*), 90 mg: 1 capsule, daily

☐ Chamomile (*Matricaria chamomilla*) herbal tincture: 25 drops in warm water 2–3 times, daily

BLOOD GROUP B

☐ Rehmannia root (*Rehmannia glutinosa*), 200 mg: 1 capsule, daily

☐ White Atractylodes (*Atractylodis macrocephalae*), 250 mg: 1 capsule, daily

☐ L-Arginine, 250 mg: 1–2 capsules, twice daily

☐ Plantain (*Plantaginis lanceolatae*), 250 mg: 1 capsule, daily

BLOOD GROUP AB

☐ Astragalus (*Astragalus membranaceus*), 500 mg: 1–2 capsules, twice daily

☐ Gotu Kola (*Centella asiatica*), 100 mg: 1–2 capsules, twice daily[1]

☐ Chamomile (*Matricaria chamomilla*) herbal tincture: 25 drops in warm water, two or three times daily

☐ Horsetail (*Equisetum arvense*), 500 mg: 1 capsule, twice daily

BLOOD GROUP O

☐ Horse Chestnut (*Aesculus hippocastanum*), 90 mg: 1 capsule, daily

☐ Rehmannia root (*Rehmannia glutinosa*), 200 mg: 1 capsule, daily

☐ Copper, 2 mg: 1 capsule, daily

☐ Horsetail (*Equisetum arvense*), 500 mg: 1 capsule, twice daily

GENERAL RECOMMENDATIONS USABLE BY ALL GROUPS

☐ Vitamin C (from Acerola Cherry or rose hips), 250 mg: 1 capsule, twice daily

☐ Zinc, 25 mg: 1 capsule, daily

☐ Bromelain (Pineapple enzyme), 500 mg: 1 capsule, twice daily after surgery

NOTES:

1. Do not use Gotu Kola leaf if you are pregnant.

29. URINARY TRACT HEALTH PROTOCOLS

Use this protocol for 4 weeks.

BLOOD GROUP A

☐ Cranberry capsules, 500 mg: 1–2 capsules, twice daily

☐ Bearberry (*Arctostaphylos uva-ursi*), 150–250 mg: 1–2 capsules, twice daily

☐ Corn Silk, 150 mg: 1 capsule, daily

☐ Old Man's Beard (*Usnea barbata*) tincture: 7–10 drops in warm water before meals

BLOOD GROUP B

☐ Cranberry capsules, 500 mg: 1–2 capsules, twice daily

☐ Buchu herb concentrate (*Barosma betulina*): 250 mg: 1–2 capsules, twice daily

☐ Bearberry (*Arctostaphylos uva-ursi*), 150–250 mg: 1–2 capsules, twice daily

BLOOD GROUP AB

☐ Cranberry capsules, 500 mg: 1–2 capsules, twice daily

☐ Chickweed (*Stellaria media*) tea: 1–2 cups, daily

☐ Parsley leaf (*Petroselinum* sp), 400 mg: 1–2 capsules, twice daily

BLOOD GROUP O

☐ Bromelain (Pineapple enzyme), 500 mg: 1–2 capsules, twice daily

☐ Bearberry (*Arctostaphylos uva-ursi*), 150–250 mg: 1–2 capsules, twice daily

☐ Horsetail (*Equisetum arvense*) 500 mg: 1 capsule, twice daily

NON-SECRETORS
Add:

☐ Vitamin A, 10,000 IU: 1 capsule, daily

☐ ABO specific lectin-blocking formula ("Deflect"): 1 capsule with meals 2–3× daily

GENERAL RECOMMENDATIONS USABLE BY ALL GROUPS

☐ Vitamin C (from Acerola Cherry or rose hips), 250 mg: 1 capsule, twice daily

☐ Probiotic supplement, preferably ABO specific

30. YEAST/FUNGUS RESISTANCE PROTOCOLS

Use this protocol for 6 weeks.

BLOOD GROUP A

☐ Stinging Nettle root (*Urtica dioica*), "UDA Plus": 1–2 capsules, twice daily

☐ Elecampane (*Inula helenium*), 500 mg: 1 capsule with meals 1–2× daily

☐ Caprylic acid, 350 mg: 1–2 capsules, twice daily away from food

□ Betaine HCl, 250 mg: 1 capsule with large meals

□ Oregon Grape (*Berberis aquifolium*), 250–500 mg: 1–2 capsules, twice daily

BLOOD GROUP B

□ Oregano (*Origanum vulgare*) tincture: 4–7 drops, twice daily

□ Thyme (*Thymus vulgaris*) tincture: 5–10 drops, twice daily

□ Coriander seeds (*Coriandrum sativum*) tincture: 2–3 drops, twice daily

□ Rosemary (*Rosmarinus officinalis*)

□ Olive oil: 1 tbsp, twice daily between meals

BLOOD GROUP AB

□ Thyme (*Thymus vulgaris*) tincture: 5–10 drops, twice daily

□ Elecampane (*Inula helenium*), 500 mg: 1 capsule with meals 1–2× daily

□ Slippery Elm (*Ulmus rubra*), 400 mg: 2–3 capsules with meals 1–2× daily

□ Olive oil: 1 tbsp, twice daily between meals

□ Betaine HCl, 250 mg: 1 capsule with large meals

BLOOD GROUP O

□ Caprylic acid, 350 mg: 1–2 capsules, twice daily away from food

□ Clove fruit (*Eugenia* sp), 50 mg: 1 capsule, daily

□ Standardized Chinese Garlic Extract (*Allium sativum*), 400 mg: 1 capsule, twice daily

□ Stinging Nettle root (*Urtica dioica*), "UDA Plus": 1–2 capsules, twice daily

□ Bladderwrack (*Fucus vesiculosus*), "Fucus Plus": 1 capsule with meals, 2–3× daily

NON-SECRETORS
Add:

□ Zinc, 15 mg: daily

GENERAL RECOMMENDATIONS USABLE BY ALL GROUPS

□ Larch arabinogalactan (*Larix officinalis*) "ARA6": 1 tbsp, twice daily in juice or water

□ Probiotic supplement, preferably ABO specific

Blood Group Food Base

This is the most detailed blood group–related food analysis to date. It not only provides values for ABO blood groups, non-secretors, and minor blood groups, but also offers an explanation for why each food is considered beneficial, neutral, or to be avoided.

Note: The basic values for each blood group are for secretors. Non-secretor variants are listed where appropriate.

▪ MEAT

Food item	BLOOD GROUP A	BLOOD GROUP B	BLOOD GROUP AB	BLOOD GROUP O
Bacon/Ham/Pork	AVOID: Provokes abnormal blood reaction; inhibits proper gastric function or blocks assimilation.	AVOID: Provokes abnormal blood reaction.	AVOID: Contains component that can modify known disease susceptibility.	AVOID: Provokes abnormal blood reaction; contains component that can modify known disease susceptibility.

MEAT, CONTINUED

Food Item	BLOOD GROUP A	BLOOD GROUP B	BLOOD GROUP AB	BLOOD GROUP O
Beef	AVOID: Secretory insufficiency; increases intestinal imbalance; increases polyamine or indican levels; inhibits proper gastric function or blocks assimilation.	NEUTRAL	AVOID: Contains component that can modify known disease susceptibility.	BENEFICIAL: Provides high-quality protein; increases lean muscle mass.
Buffalo	AVOID: Secretory insufficiency; increases intestinal imbalance; increases polyamine or indican levels; inhibits proper gastric function or blocks assimilation.	NEUTRAL	AVOID: Contains component that can modify known disease susceptibility.	BENEFICIAL: Provides high-quality protein; increases lean muscle mass.
Chicken	NEUTRAL	AVOID: Contains lectin or other agglutinin.	AVOID: Contains lectin or other agglutinin.	NEUTRAL
Cornish Hen	NEUTRAL	AVOID: Contains lectin or other agglutinin.	AVOID: Contains lectin or other agglutinin.	NEUTRAL
Duck	AVOID: Secretory insufficiency; increases polyamine or indican levels; inhibits proper gastric function or blocks assimilation. Non-secretor variant: NEUTRAL	AVOID: Provokes abnormal blood reaction.	AVOID: Contains component that can modify known disease susceptibility.	NEUTRAL
Goat	AVOID: Secretory insufficiency; induces intestinal imbalance; increases polyamine or indican levels; inhibits proper gastric function or blocks assimilation. Non-secretor variant: NEUTRAL	BENEFICIAL: Nutrient-dense food.	NEUTRAL	NEUTRAL

◼ MEAT, CONTINUED

Food Item	BLOOD GROUP A	BLOOD GROUP B	BLOOD GROUP AB	BLOOD GROUP O
Goose	AVOID: Secretory insufficiency. Increases polyamine or indican levels; inhibits proper gastric function or blocks assimilation. Non-secretor variant: NEUTRAL	AVOID: Contains lectin or other agglutinin; increases polyamine or indican levels.	AVOID: Secretory insufficiency; induces intestinal imbalance.	NEUTRAL
Grouse	NEUTRAL	AVOID: Provokes abnormal blood reaction.	AVOID: Provokes abnormal blood reaction.	NEUTRAL
Guinea Hen	NEUTRAL	AVOID: Contains lectin or other agglutinin.	AVOID: Contains lectin or other agglutinin.	NEUTRAL
Heart (Beef)	AVOID: Secretory insufficiency; induces intestinal imbalance; increases polyamine or indican levels; inhibits proper gastric function or blocks assimilation.	AVOID: Increases polyamine or indican levels. Non-secretor variant: NEUTRAL	AVOID: Contains component that can modify known disease susceptibility.	BENEFICIAL: Provides high-quality protein; increases lean muscle mass.
Horse	AVOID: Secretory insufficiency; induces intestinal imbalance; increases polyamine or indican levels; inhibits proper gastric function or blocks assimilation.	AVOID: Increases polyamine or indican levels. Non-secretor variant: NEUTRAL	AVOID: Secretory insufficiency; induces intestinal imbalance.	NEUTRAL
Lamb	AVOID: Secretory insufficiency; induces intestinal imbalance; increases polyamine or indican levels; inhibits proper gastric function or blocks assimilation.	BENEFICIAL: Nutrient-dense food.	NEUTRAL Non-secretor variant: BENEFICIAL	BENEFICIAL: Provides high-quality protein; increases lean muscle mass. Non-secretor variant: NEUTRAL
Liver (Calf)	AVOID: Secretory insufficiency; induces intestinal imbalance; increases polyamine levels; inhibits proper gastric function or blocks assimilation.	NEUTRAL Non-secretor variant: BENEFICIAL	NEUTRAL	BENEFICIAL: Provides high-quality protein; increases lean muscle mass. Non-secretor variant: NEUTRAL

■ MEAT, CONTINUED

Food Item	BLOOD GROUP A	BLOOD GROUP B	BLOOD GROUP AB	BLOOD GROUP O
Mutton	AVOID: Secretory insufficiency; induces intestinal imbalance; increases polyamine levels; inhibits proper gastric function or blocks assimilation. Non-secretor variant: NEUTRAL	BENEFICIAL: High density nutrient.	NEUTRAL Non-secretor variant: BENEFICIAL	BENEFICIAL: Provides high-quality protein; increases lean muscle mass.
Ostrich	NEUTRAL	NEUTRAL	NEUTRAL	NEUTRAL Non-secretor variant: BENEFICIAL
Partridge	AVOID: Secretory insufficiency; increases polyamine or indican levels; inhibits proper gastric function or blocks assimilation. Non-secretor variant: NEUTRAL	AVOID: Contains lectin or other agglutinin; increases polyamine or indican levels.	AVOID: Contains lectin or other agglutinin.	NEUTRAL Non-secretor variant: BENEFICIAL
Pheasant	AVOID: Secretory insufficiency; increases polyamine or indican levels; inhibits proper gastric function or blocks assimilation; Non-secretor variant: NEUTRAL	NEUTRAL	NEUTRAL	NEUTRAL; Non-secretor variant: BENEFICIAL
Quail	AVOID: Secretory insufficiency; induces intestinal imbalance; increases polyamine or indican levels; inhibits proper gastric function or blocks assimilation. Non-secretor variant: NEUTRAL	AVOID: Increases polyamine or indican levels.	AVOID Non-secretor variant: NEUTRAL	AVOID Non-secretor variant: NEUTRAL

■ MEAT, CONTINUED

Food Item	BLOOD GROUP A	BLOOD GROUP B	BLOOD GROUP AB	BLOOD GROUP O
Rabbit	AVOID: Secretory insufficiency; induces intestinal imbalance; inhibits proper gastric function or blocks assimilation. Non-secretor variant: NEUTRAL	BENEFICIAL: High-density nutrient.	NEUTRAL Non-secretor variant: BENEFICIAL	NEUTRAL Non-secretor variant: BENEFICIAL
Squab	NEUTRAL	AVOID: Increases polyamine or indican levels. Non-secretor variant: NEUTRAL	AVOID: Contains lectin or other agglutinin; provokes reaction in blood (non-lectin).	NEUTRAL Non-secretor variant: BENEFICIAL
Squirrel	AVOID: Secretory insufficiency; induces intestinal imbalance; increases polyamine or indican levels; inhibits proper gastric function or blocks assimilation.	AVOID: Provokes abnormal blood reaction; increases polyamine or indican levels.	AVOID: Contains lectin or other agglutinin; provokes abnormal blood reaction.	NEUTRAL
Sweetbreads	AVOID: Secretory insufficiency; induces intestinal imbalance; increases polyamine or indican levels; inhibits proper gastric function or blocks assimilation.	AVOID: Increases polyamine or indican levels. Non-secretor variant: NEUTRAL	AVOID: Increases polyamine or indican levels.	BENEFICIAL: Provides high-quality protein; increases lean muscle mass.
Turkey	NEUTRAL Non-secretor variant: BENEFICIAL	NEUTRAL	BENEFICIAL: Healthy alternative to more common variety of foods that are classed as avoids.	NEUTRAL
Turtle	AVOID: Provokes abnormal blood reaction. Non-secretor variant: NEUTRAL	AVOID: Provokes abnormal blood reaction.	AVOID: Provokes abnormal blood reaction.	AVOID Non-secretor variant: NEUTRAL
Veal	AVOID: Secretory insufficiency; increases polyamine or indican levels; inhibits proper gastric function or blocks assimilation.	NEUTRAL	AVOID: Secretory insufficiency; increases polyamine or indican levels; inhibits proper gastric function or blocks assimilation.	BENEFICIAL: Provides high-quality protein; increases lean muscle mass.

▪ MEAT, CONTINUED

Food Item	BLOOD GROUP A	BLOOD GROUP B	BLOOD GROUP AB	BLOOD GROUP O
Venison	AVOID: Secretory insufficiency; increases polyamine or indican levels; inhibits proper gastric function or blocks assimilation.	BENEFICIAL: Nutrient-dense food.	AVOID: Contains component that can modify known disease susceptibility. Non-secretor variant: NEUTRAL	BENEFICIAL: Provides high-quality protein; increases lean muscle mass.

▪ FISH

Food Item	BLOOD GROUP A	BLOOD GROUP B	BLOOD GROUP AB	BLOOD GROUP O
Abalone	NEUTRAL	NEUTRAL	NEUTRAL	AVOID: Induces intestinal imbalance.
Anchovy	AVOID: Provokes abnormal blood reaction; inhibits proper gastric function or blocks assimilation. Non-secretor variant: NEUTRAL	AVOID: Provokes abnormal blood reaction; contains lectin or other agglutinin.	AVOID: Provokes abnormal blood reaction; contains lectin or other agglutinin.	NEUTRAL Non-secretor variant: AVOID
Barracuda	AVOID: Contains lectin or other agglutinin; metabolic inhibitor; inhibits proper gastric function or blocks assimilation.	AVOID: Provokes abnormal blood reaction. Non-secretor variant: NEUTRAL	AVOID: Contains lectin or other agglutinin.	AVOID: Increases intestinal imbalance.
Bass (Bluegill)	AVOID: Contains lectin or other agglutinin; metabolic inhibitor; inhibits proper gastric function or blocks assimilation.	AVOID: Provokes abnormal blood reaction.	AVOID: Provokes abnormal blood reaction.	BENEFICIAL: Nutrient-dense food; increases lean muscle mass.
Bass (Sea)	NEUTRAL	AVOID: Contains lectin or other agglutinin.	AVOID: Provokes abnormal blood reaction.	BENEFICIAL Non-secretor variant: NEUTRAL
Bass (Striped)	AVOID: Contains lectin or other agglutinin; metabolic inhibitor; inhibits proper gastric function or blocks assimilation.	AVOID: Provokes abnormal blood reaction.	AVOID: Provokes abnormal blood reaction.	BENEFICIAL Non-secretor variant: NEUTRAL

■ FISH, CONTINUED

Food Item	BLOOD GROUP A	BLOOD GROUP B	BLOOD GROUP AB	BLOOD GROUP O
Beluga	AVOID: Contains lectin or other agglutinin; metabolic inhibitor; inhibits proper gastric function or blocks assimilation. Non-secretor variant: NEUTRAL	AVOID: Increases polyamine or indican levels.	AVOID: Increases polyamine or indican levels.	NEUTRAL
Bluefish	AVOID: Provokes abnormal blood reaction; inhibits proper gastric function or blocks assimilation. Non-secretor variant: NEUTRAL	NEUTRAL	NEUTRAL	NEUTRAL
Bullhead	NEUTRAL	NEUTRAL	NEUTRAL	NEUTRAL
Butterfish	NEUTRAL	AVOID: Increases polyamine or indican levels. Non-secretor variant: NEUTRAL	NEUTRAL	NEUTRAL
Carp	BENEFICIAL: Contains component that positively influences known disease susceptibility.	NEUTRAL Non-secretor variant: BENEFICIAL	NEUTRAL	NEUTRAL
Catfish	AVOID: Provokes abnormal blood reaction; inhibits proper gastric function or blocks assimilation.	NEUTRAL	NEUTRAL	AVOID Non-secretor variant: NEUTRAL
Caviar	AVOID: Provokes abnormal blood reaction; inhibits proper gastric function or blocks assimilation. Non-secretor variant: NEUTRAL	BENEFICIAL Non-secretor variant: NEUTRAL	NEUTRAL	NEUTRAL
Chub	NEUTRAL	NEUTRAL	NEUTRAL	NEUTRAL

▪ FISH, CONTINUED

Food Item	BLOOD GROUP A	BLOOD GROUP B	BLOOD GROUP AB	BLOOD GROUP O
Clam	AVOID: Provokes abnormal blood reaction; inhibits proper gastric function or blocks assimilation.	AVOID: Contains lectin or other agglutinin.	AVOID: Contains lectin or other agglutinin.	NEUTRAL
Cod	BENEFICIAL: Nutrient-dense food; contains component that positively influences known disease susceptibility.	BENEFICIAL: Nutrient-dense food.	BENEFICIAL: Nutrient-dense food; contains component that positively influences known disease susceptibility.	BENEFICIAL: Nutrient-dense food; increases lean muscle mass.
Conch	AVOID: Provokes abnormal blood reaction; inhibits proper gastric function or blocks assimilation; increases polyamine or indican levels.	AVOID: Increases polyamine or indican levels.	AVOID: Provokes abnormal blood reaction; inhibits proper gastric function or blocks assimilation; increases polyamine or indican levels.	AVOID: Increases intestinal imbalance.
Crab	AVOID: Secretory insufficiency; provokes abnormal blood reaction; inhibits proper gastric function or blocks assimilation.	AVOID: Provokes abnormal blood reaction.	AVOID: Contains component that can modify known disease susceptibility.	NEUTRAL Non-secretor variant: AVOID
Croaker	NEUTRAL	BENEFICIAL: Nutrient-dense food.	NEUTRAL	NEUTRAL
Cusk	NEUTRAL: Non-secretor variant: BENEFICIAL	NEUTRAL	NEUTRAL	NEUTRAL
Drum	NEUTRAL Non-secretor variant: BENEFICIAL	NEUTRAL	NEUTRAL	NEUTRAL
Eel/Japanese Eel	AVOID: Provokes abnormal blood reaction; contains lectin or other agglutinin; metabolic inhibitor; inhibits proper gastric function or blocks assimilation.	AVOID: Contains lectin or other agglutinin.	AVOID: Contains lectin or other agglutinin.	NEUTRAL

▪ FISH, CONTINUED

Food Item	BLOOD GROUP A	BLOOD GROUP B	BLOOD GROUP AB	BLOOD GROUP O
Flounder	AVOID: Contains lectin or other agglutinin; metabolic inhibitor; provokes abnormal blood reaction; inhibits proper gastric function or blocks assimilation. Non-secretor variant: NEUTRAL	BENEFICIAL: Nutrient-dense food. Non-secretor variant: NEUTRAL	AVOID: Contains lectin or other agglutinin.	NEUTRAL
Frog	AVOID: Provokes abnormal blood reaction; increases polyamine or indican levels; inhibits proper gastric function or blocks assimilation. Non-secretor variant: NEUTRAL	AVOID: Provokes abnormal blood reaction.	AVOID: Contains lectin or other agglutinin.	AVOID: Increases intestinal imbalance.
Gray Sole	AVOID: Contains lectin or other agglutinin; metabolic inhibitor; provokes reaction in blood (non-lectin); inhibits proper gastric function or blocks assimilation. Non-secretor variant: NEUTRAL	NEUTRAL	AVOID: Contains lectin or other agglutinin.	NEUTRAL
Grouper	AVOID: Contains lectin or other agglutinin; metabolic inhibitor; provokes reaction in blood (non-lectin); inhibits proper gastric function or blocks assimilation. Non-secretor variant: NEUTRAL	BENEFICIAL: Nutrient-dense food.	BENEFICIAL: Nutrient-dense food; contains component that positively influences known disease susceptibility.	NEUTRAL
Haddock	AVOID: Contains lectin or other agglutinin; metabolic inhibitor; provokes abnormal blood reaction; inhibits proper gastric function or blocks assimilation. Non-secretor variant: NEUTRAL	BENEFICIAL: Nutrient-dense food.	AVOID: Contains lectin or other agglutinin.	NEUTRAL

■ FISH, CONTINUED

Food Item	BLOOD GROUP A	BLOOD GROUP B	BLOOD GROUP AB	BLOOD GROUP O
Hake	AVOID: Contains lectin or other agglutinin; metabolic inhibitor; inhibits proper gastric function or blocks assimilation. Non-secretor variant: NEUTRAL	BENEFICIAL: Nutrient-dense food.	AVOID: Contains lectin or other agglutinin.	NEUTRAL Non-secretor variant: BENEFICIAL
Halfmoon Fish	NEUTRAL Non-secretor variant: BENEFICIAL	NEUTRAL	NEUTRAL	NEUTRAL
Halibut	AVOID: Contains lectin or other agglutinin; metabolic inhibitor; inhibits proper gastric function or blocks assimilation. Non-secretor variant: NEUTRAL	BENEFICIAL: Nutrient-dense food. Non-secretor variant: NEUTRAL	AVOID: Contains lectin or other agglutinin.	BENEFICIAL: Contains an agglutinin that modifies disease susceptibility. Non-secretor variant: NEUTRAL
Harvest Fish	AVOID: Inhibits proper gastric function or blocks assimilation. Non-secretor variant: BENEFICIAL	BENEFICIAL: Nutrient-dense food.	NEUTRAL	NEUTRAL
Herring	AVOID: Increases polyamine or indican levels; provokes abnormal blood reaction; inhibits proper gastric function or blocks assimilation. Non-secretor variant: NEUTRAL	NEUTRAL	NEUTRAL Non-secretor variant: BENEFICIAL	NEUTRAL Non-secretor variant: BENEFICIAL
Lobster	AVOID: Secretory insufficiency; provokes abnormal blood reaction; inhibits proper gastric function or blocks assimilation.	AVOID: Provokes abnormal blood reaction; increases polyamine or indican levels.	AVOID: Provokes abnormal blood reaction.	NEUTRAL

■ **FISH, CONTINUED**

Food Item	BLOOD GROUP A	BLOOD GROUP B	BLOOD GROUP AB	BLOOD GROUP O
Mackerel	BENEFICIAL: Contains component that positively influences known disease susceptibility.	BENEFICIAL: Nutrient-dense food.	BENEFICIAL: Nutrient-dense food; contains component that positively influences known disease susceptibility.	NEUTRAL Non-secretor variant: BENEFICIAL
Mahi-mahi	NEUTRAL	BENEFICIAL: Nutrient-dense food.	BENEFICIAL: Nutrient-dense food.	NEUTRAL
Monkfish	BENEFICIAL: Contains component that positively influences known disease susceptibility.	BENEFICIAL: Contains component that positively influences known disease susceptibility.	BENEFICIAL: Contains component that positively influences known disease susceptibility.	NEUTRAL
Mullet	NEUTRAL Non-secretor variant: BENEFICIAL	NEUTRAL	NEUTRAL	NEUTRAL
Muskellunge	NEUTRAL Non-secretor variant: BENEFICIAL	NEUTRAL	NEUTRAL	AVOID: Increases intestinal imbalance; increases polyamine or indican levels.
Mussels	AVOID: Contains lectin or other agglutinin; metabolic inhibitor; inhibits proper gastric function or blocks assimilation. Non-secretor variant: NEUTRAL	AVOID: Provokes reaction in blood (non-lectin); inhibits proper gastric function or blocks assimilation.	NEUTRAL	NEUTRAL Non-secretor variant: AVOID
Octopus	AVOID: Provokes reaction in blood (non-lectin); inhibits proper gastric function or blocks assimilation. Non-secretor variant: NEUTRAL	AVOID: Provokes reaction in blood (non-lectin).	AVOID: Provokes reaction in blood (non-lectin).	AVOID: Gastric irritant; inhibits proper digestive function.
Opaleye Fish	AVOID: Provokes abnormal blood reaction; inhibits proper gastric function or blocks assimilation. Non-secretor variant: NEUTRAL	NEUTRAL	NEUTRAL	NEUTRAL

■ FISH, CONTINUED

Food Item	BLOOD GROUP A	BLOOD GROUP B	BLOOD GROUP AB	BLOOD GROUP O
Orange Roughy	NEUTRAL	NEUTRAL	NEUTRAL	NEUTRAL
Oyster	AVOID: Provokes abnormal blood reaction; inhibits proper gastric function or blocks assimilation.	AVOID: Provokes abnormal blood reaction.	AVOID: Contains component that can modify known disease susceptibility.	NEUTRAL
Parrotfish	NEUTRAL	NEUTRAL	NEUTRAL	NEUTRAL
Perch (Ocean)	NEUTRAL	BENEFICIAL: Nutrient-dense food.	NEUTRAL	BENEFICIAL: Nutrient-dense food; increases lean muscle mass.
Perch (Silver)	BENEFICIAL: Contains component that positively influences known disease susceptibility.	NEUTRAL	NEUTRAL	BENEFICIAL: Nutrient-dense food; increases lean muscle mass.
Perch (White)	NEUTRAL	NEUTRAL	NEUTRAL	BENEFICIAL: Nutrient-dense food; increases lean muscle mass.
Perch (Yellow)	BENEFICIAL: Contains component that positively influences known disease susceptibility.	NEUTRAL	NEUTRAL	BENEFICIAL: Provides high-quality protein; increases lean muscle mass.
Pickerel	BENEFICIAL: Contains component that positively influences known disease susceptibility.	BENEFICIAL: Nutrient-dense food.	BENEFICIAL: Contains component that positively influences known disease susceptibility.	NEUTRAL
Pike	NEUTRAL	BENEFICIAL: Nutrient-dense food. Non-secretor variant: NEUTRAL	BENEFICIAL: Nutrient-dense food; contains component that positively influences known disease susceptibility.	BENEFICIAL: Nutrient-dense food; increases lean muscle mass.
Pollack	BENEFICIAL: Contains component that positively influences known disease susceptibility.	AVOID: Provokes abnormal blood reaction.	NEUTRAL	AVOID: Contains lectin or other agglutinin.
Pompano	NEUTRAL	NEUTRAL	NEUTRAL	NEUTRAL

FISH, CONTINUED

Food Item	BLOOD GROUP A	BLOOD GROUP B	BLOOD GROUP AB	BLOOD GROUP O
Porgy	NEUTRAL	BENEFICIAL: Nutrient-dense food.	BENEFICIAL: Nutrient-dense food.	NEUTRAL
Red Snapper	BENEFICIAL: Contains component that positively influences known disease susceptibility.	NEUTRAL	BENEFICIAL: Contains component that positively influences known disease susceptibility.	BENEFICIAL: Metabolic enhancer. Non-secretor variant: NEUTRAL
Rosefish	NEUTRAL Non-secretor variant: BENEFICIAL	NEUTRAL	NEUTRAL	NEUTRAL
Sailfish	NEUTRAL	NEUTRAL	BENEFICIAL: Nutrient-dense food; contains component that positively influences known disease susceptibility.	NEUTRAL
Salmon	BENEFICIAL: Nutrient-dense food; contains component that positively influences known disease susceptibility.	BENEFICIAL: Nutrient-dense food. Non-secretor variant: NEUTRAL	BENEFICIAL: Nutrient-dense food; contains component that positively influences known disease susceptibility.	NEUTRAL
Salmon Roe	NEUTRAL	AVOID: Contains lectin or other agglutinin.	AVOID: Contains lectin or other agglutinin.	AVOID Non-secretor variant: NEUTRAL
Sardine	BENEFICIAL: Contains component that positively influences known disease susceptibility.	BENEFICIAL: Nutrient-dense food.	BENEFICIAL: Nutrient-dense food; contains component that positively influences known disease susceptibility.	NEUTRAL Non-secretor variant: BENEFICIAL
Scallop	AVOID: Provokes abnormal blood reaction; inhibits proper gastric function or blocks assimilation. Non-secretor variant: NEUTRAL	NEUTRAL Non-secretor variant: AVOID	NEUTRAL	NEUTRAL
Scrod	NEUTRAL	NEUTRAL	NEUTRAL	NEUTRAL

■ FISH, CONTINUED

Food Item	BLOOD GROUP A	BLOOD GROUP B	BLOOD GROUP AB	BLOOD GROUP O
Scup	AVOID: Contains lectin or other agglutinin; metabolic inhibitor; inhibits proper gastric function or blocks assimilation. Non-secretor variant: NEUTRAL	NEUTRAL	NEUTRAL	NEUTRAL
Shad	AVOID: Contains lectin or other agglutinin; metabolic inhibitor; inhibits proper gastric function or blocks assimilation. Non-secretor variant: NEUTRAL	BENEFICIAL: Nutrient-dense food.	BENEFICIAL: Nutrient-dense food; contains component that positively influences known disease susceptibility.	BENEFICIAL: Nutrient-dense food; increases lean muscle mass.
Shark	NEUTRAL	NEUTRAL	NEUTRAL	NEUTRAL
Shrimp	AVOID: Secretory insufficiency; inhibits cardiovascular function; inhibits proper gastric function or blocks assimilation.	AVOID: Provokes abnormal blood reaction.	AVOID: Enhances effect of other food toxins; increases polyamine or indican levels; contains component that can modify known disease susceptibility.	NEUTRAL
Smelt	NEUTRAL	NEUTRAL	NEUTRAL	NEUTRAL
Snail (Escargot/*Helix pomatia***)**	BENEFICIAL: Contains an agglutinin that modifies disease susceptibility.	AVOID: Contains lectin or other agglutinin. Non-secretor variant: NEUTRAL	BENEFICIAL: Contains an agglutinin that modifies disease susceptibility.	NEUTRAL
Sole	AVOID: Contains lectin or other agglutinin; metabolic inhibitor; inhibits proper gastric function or blocks assimilation.	BENEFICIAL Non-secretor variant: NEUTRAL	AVOID: Contains lectin or other agglutinin.	BENEFICIAL: Nutrient-dense food; increases lean muscle mass.
Squid (Calamari)	AVOID: Contains lectin or other agglutinin; metabolic inhibitor; inhibits proper gastric function or blocks assimilation.	NEUTRAL	NEUTRAL	AVOID: Contains lectin or other agglutinin.

FISH, CONTINUED

Food Item	BLOOD GROUP A	BLOOD GROUP B	BLOOD GROUP AB	BLOOD GROUP O
Sturgeon	NEUTRAL	BENEFICIAL: Nutrient-dense food.	BENEFICIAL: Nutrient-dense food; contains component that positively influences known disease susceptibility.	BENEFICIAL: Nutrient-dense food; increases lean muscle mass.
Sucker	NEUTRAL Non-secretor variant: BENEFICIAL	NEUTRAL	NEUTRAL	NEUTRAL
Sunfish	NEUTRAL	NEUTRAL	NEUTRAL	NEUTRAL
Swordfish	NEUTRAL Non-secretor variant: BENEFICIAL	NEUTRAL	NEUTRAL	BENEFICIAL: Provides high-quality protein; increases lean muscle mass.
Tilapia	NEUTRAL	NEUTRAL	NEUTRAL	NEUTRAL
Tilefish	AVOID: Contains lectin or other agglutinin; metabolic inhibitor; inhibits proper gastric function or blocks assimilation. Non-secretor variant: NEUTRAL	NEUTRAL	NEUTRAL	BENEFICIAL: Provides high-quality protein; increases lean muscle mass.
Trout (Brook)	NEUTRAL Non-secretor variant: BENEFICIAL	AVOID: Contains lectin or other agglutinin.	AVOID: Contains lectin or other agglutinin. Non-secretor variant: NEUTRAL	NEUTRAL
Trout (Rainbow)	BENEFICIAL: Contains component that positively influences known disease susceptibility.	AVOID: Contains lectin or other agglutinin.	AVOID: Contains lectin or other agglutinin. Non-secretor variant: NEUTRAL	BENEFICIAL: Provides high-quality protein; increases lean muscle mass.
Trout (Sea)	BENEFICIAL: Contains component that positively influences known disease susceptibility.	AVOID: Contains lectin or other agglutinin.	AVOID: Contains lectin or other agglutinin. Non-secretor variant: NEUTRAL	NEUTRAL

FISH, CONTINUED

Food Item	BLOOD GROUP A	BLOOD GROUP B	BLOOD GROUP AB	BLOOD GROUP O
Tuna	NEUTRAL	NEUTRAL	BENEFICIAL: Contains component that positively influences known disease susceptibility.	NEUTRAL
Weakfish	NEUTRAL	NEUTRAL	NEUTRAL	NEUTRAL
Whitefish	BENEFICIAL: Contains component that positively influences known disease susceptibility.	NEUTRAL	NEUTRAL	NEUTRAL
Whiting	BENEFICIAL: Contains component that positively influences known disease susceptibility.	NEUTRAL	AVOID: Contains lectin or other agglutinin.	NEUTRAL
Yellowtail	NEUTRAL	AVOID: Provokes abnormal blood reaction. Non-secretor variant: NEUTRAL	AVOID: Contains lectin or other agglutinin.	BENEFICIAL: Provides high-quality protein; increases lean muscle mass.

DAIRY

Food Item	BLOOD GROUP A	BLOOD GROUP B	BLOOD GROUP AB	BLOOD GROUP O
American Cheese	AVOID: Provokes abnormal blood reaction; increases polyamine or indican levels.	AVOID: Provokes reaction in blood (non-lectin); increases polyamine or indican levels.	AVOID: Provokes abnormal blood reaction.	AVOID: Provokes reaction in blood (non-lectin); contains component that can modify known disease susceptibility.
Blue Cheese	AVOID: Provokes reaction in blood (non-lectin); increases polyamine or indican levels; inhibits proper gastric function or blocks assimilation.	AVOID: Increases polyamine or indican levels.	AVOID: Increases polyamine or indican levels.	AVOID: Provokes reaction in blood (non-lectin); contains component that can modify known disease susceptibility.
Brie Cheese	AVOID: Increases polyamine or indican levels; inhibits proper gastric function or blocks assimilation.	NEUTRAL	AVOID: Increases polyamine or indican levels.	AVOID: Provokes reaction in blood (non-lectin).

■ **DAIRY, CONTINUED**

Food Item	BLOOD GROUP A	BLOOD GROUP B	BLOOD GROUP AB	BLOOD GROUP O
Butter	AVOID: Secretory insufficiency; provokes reaction in blood (non-lectin).	NEUTRAL	AVOID: Contains component that can modify known disease susceptibility.	NEUTRAL
Buttermilk	AVOID: Inhibits proper gastric function or blocks assimilation.	NEUTRAL	AVOID: Increases polyamine or indican levels.	AVOID: Provokes reaction in blood (non-lectin).
Camembert Cheese	AVOID: Increases polyamine or indican levels; inhibits proper gastric function or blocks assimilation.	NEUTRAL Non-secretor variant: AVOID	AVOID: Increases polyamine or indican levels.	AVOID: Provokes reaction in blood (non-lectin).
Casein	AVOID: Provokes abnormal blood reaction.	NEUTRAL	NEUTRAL	AVOID: Provokes abnormal blood reaction.
Cheddar Cheese	AVOID: Provokes abnormal blood reaction.	NEUTRAL Non-secretor variant: AVOID	NEUTRAL	AVOID: Provokes abnormal blood reaction.
Colby Cheese	AVOID: Inhibits proper gastric function or blocks assimilation.	NEUTRAL	NEUTRAL	AVOID: Metabolic inhibitor.
Cottage Cheese	AVOID: Inhibits proper gastric function or blocks assimilation. Non-secretor variant: NEUTRAL	BENEFICIAL: Provides optimal amino acid (lysine/arginine) ratio. Non-secretor variant: NEUTRAL	BENEFICIAL: Provides optimal amino acid (lysine/arginine) ratio.	AVOID: Metabolic inhibitor.
Cream Cheese	AVOID: Inhibits proper gastric function or blocks assimilation.	NEUTRAL	NEUTRAL	AVOID: Provokes abnormal blood reaction.
Edam Cheese	AVOID: Provokes abnormal blood reaction; inhibits proper gastric function or blocks assimilation.	NEUTRAL	NEUTRAL	AVOID: Provokes abnormal blood reaction.
Emmenthal Cheese	AVOID: Provokes abnormal blood reaction; increases polyamine or indican levels; inhibits proper gastric function or blocks assimilation.	NEUTRAL Non-secretor variant: AVOID	NEUTRAL Non-secretor variant: AVOID	AVOID: Provokes abnormal blood reaction.

▪ DAIRY, CONTINUED

Food Item	BLOOD GROUP A	BLOOD GROUP B	BLOOD GROUP AB	BLOOD GROUP O
Farmer Cheese	NEUTRAL	BENEFICIAL: Provides optimal amino acid (lysine/arginine) ratio.	BENEFICIAL: Provides optimal amino acid (lysine/arginine) ratio.	NEUTRAL Non-secretor variant: AVOID
Feta Cheese	NEUTRAL	BENEFICIAL: Provides optimal amino acid (lysine/arginine) ratio.	BENEFICIAL: Provides optimal amino acid (lysine/arginine) ratio.	NEUTRAL Non-secretor variant: AVOID
Ghee (clarified butter)	NEUTRAL	NEUTRAL Non-secretor variant: BENEFICIAL	NEUTRAL Non-secretor variant: BENEFICIAL	NEUTRAL
Goat Cheese	NEUTRAL	BENEFICIAL: Provides optimal amino acid (lysine/arginine) ratio.	BENEFICIAL Non-secretor variant: NEUTRAL	NEUTRAL Non-secretor variant: AVOID
Gouda Cheese	AVOID: Provokes abnormal blood reaction; inhibits proper gastric function or blocks assimilation.	NEUTRAL	NEUTRAL	AVOID: Provokes abnormal blood reaction; increases intestinal imbalance; increases polyamine or indican levels.
Gruyère Cheese	AVOID: Provokes abnormal blood reaction; inhibits proper gastric function or blocks assimilation.	NEUTRAL	NEUTRAL	AVOID: Provokes abnormal blood reaction; contains component that can modify known disease susceptibility.
Half & Half	AVOID: Provokes abnormal blood reaction; inhibits proper gastric function or blocks assimilation.	NEUTRAL	AVOID: Increases polyamine or indican levels.	AVOID: Provokes abnormal blood reaction; increases intestinal imbalance; increases polyamine or indican levels.
Ice Cream	AVOID: Provokes abnormal blood reaction; inhibits proper gastric function or blocks assimilation.	AVOID: Provokes abnormal blood reaction.	AVOID: Provokes abnormal blood reaction.	AVOID: Provokes abnormal blood reaction; increases intestinal imbalance; increases polyamine or indican levels.
Jarlsberg Cheese	AVOID: Inhibits proper gastric function or blocks assimilation.	NEUTRAL Non-secretor variant: AVOID	NEUTRAL	AVOID: Increases intestinal imbalance; increases polyamine or indican levels.

■ DAIRY, CONTINUED

Food Item	BLOOD GROUP A	BLOOD GROUP B	BLOOD GROUP AB	BLOOD GROUP O
Kefir	NEUTRAL	BENEFICIAL: Provides optimal amino acid (lysine/arginine) ratio; cultured food.	BENEFICIAL: Provides optimal amino acid (lysine/arginine) ratio; cultured food.	AVOID: Metabolic inhibitor.
Milk (Cow: Skim or 2%)	AVOID: Provokes abnormal blood reaction; inhibits proper gastric function or blocks assimilation.	BENEFICIAL: Provides optimal amino acid (lysine/arginine) ratio. Non-secretor variant: NEUTRAL	NEUTRAL	AVOID: Provokes abnormal blood reaction; metabolic inhibitor.
Milk (Cow: Whole)	AVOID: Provokes abnormal blood reaction; inhibits proper gastric function or blocks assimilation.	BENEFICIAL: Provides optimal amino acid (lysine/arginine) ratio. Non-secretor variant: NEUTRAL	AVOID: Contains component that can modify known disease susceptibility.	AVOID: Provokes abnormal blood reaction; contains component that can modify known disease susceptibility.
Milk (Goat)	NEUTRAL Non-secretor variant: AVOID	BENEFICIAL: Provides optimal amino acid (lysine/arginine) ratio.	BENEFICIAL: Provides optimal amino acid (lysine/arginine) ratio.	AVOID: Provokes abnormal blood reaction.
Monterey Jack Cheese	AVOID: Provokes abnormal blood reaction; inhibits proper gastric function or blocks assimilation.	NEUTRAL Non-secretor variant: AVOID	NEUTRAL	AVOID: Increases polyamine or indican levels.
Mozzarella Cheese	NEUTRAL	BENEFICIAL: Provides optimal amino acid (lysine/arginine) ratio.	BENEFICIAL: Provides optimal amino acid (lysine/arginine) ratio.	NEUTRAL Non-secretor variant: AVOID
Muenster Cheese	AVOID: Provokes abnormal blood reaction; inhibits proper gastric function or blocks assimilation.	NEUTRAL Non-secretor variant: AVOID	NEUTRAL	AVOID: Provokes abnormal blood reaction; contains component that can modify known disease susceptibility.
Neufchatel Cheese	AVOID: Provokes abnormal blood reaction.	NEUTRAL	NEUTRAL	AVOID: Provokes abnormal blood reaction; contains component that can modify known disease susceptibility.

■ **DAIRY, CONTINUED**

Food Item	BLOOD GROUP A	BLOOD GROUP B	BLOOD GROUP AB	BLOOD GROUP O
Paneer	NEUTRAL	BENEFICIAL: Provides optimal amino acid (lysine/arginine) ratio; cultured food.	NEUTRAL	AVOID: Provokes abnormal blood reaction; metabolic inhibitor.
Parmesan Cheese	AVOID: Increases polyamine or indican levels; inhibits proper gastric function or blocks assimilation.	NEUTRAL Non-secretor variant: AVOID	AVOID: Increases polyamine or indican levels.	AVOID: Increases polyamine or indican levels.
Provolone Cheese	AVOID: Increases polyamine or indican levels; inhibits proper gastric function or blocks assimilation.	NEUTRAL Non-secretor variant: AVOID	AVOID: Increases polyamine or indican levels.	AVOID: Increases polyamine or indican levels.
Quark Cheese	NEUTRAL	NEUTRAL	NEUTRAL	AVOID: Contains component that can modify known disease susceptibility.
Ricotta Cheese	NEUTRAL	BENEFICIAL: Provides optimal amino acid (lysine/arginine) ratio.	BENEFICIAL: Provides optimal amino acid (lysine/arginine) ratio.	AVOID: Provokes abnormal blood response.
Sour Cream (low-/nonfat)	NEUTRAL Non-secretor variant: AVOID	NEUTRAL	BENEFICIAL: Provides optimal amino acid (lysine/arginine) ratio; cultured food.	AVOID: Contains component that can modify known disease susceptibility.
String Cheese	AVOID: Provokes abnormal blood reaction; inhibits proper gastric function or blocks assimilation.	AVOID: Provokes abnormal blood reaction.	NEUTRAL	AVOID: Provokes abnormal blood reaction; increases intestinal imbalance; increases polyamine or indican levels.
Swiss Cheese	AVOID: Provokes abnormal blood reaction; increases polyamine or indican levels; inhibits proper gastric function or blocks assimilation.	NEUTRAL Non-secretor variant: AVOID	NEUTRAL Non-secretor variant: AVOID	AVOID: Increases polyamine or indican levels.

DAIRY, CONTINUED

Food Item	BLOOD GROUP A	BLOOD GROUP B	BLOOD GROUP AB	BLOOD GROUP O
Whey	AVOID: Provokes abnormal blood reaction; inhibits proper gastric function or blocks assimilation. Non-secretor variant: NEUTRAL	NEUTRAL Non-secretor variant: BENEFICIAL	NEUTRAL	AVOID: Provokes abnormal blood reaction.
Yogurt	NEUTRAL	BENEFICIAL: Provides optimal amino acid (lysine/arginine) ratio; cultured food.	BENEFICIAL Non-secretor variant: NEUTRAL	AVOID: Provokes abnormal blood reaction.

EGG

Food Item	BLOOD GROUP A	BLOOD GROUP B	BLOOD GROUP AB	BLOOD GROUP O
Chicken Egg	NEUTRAL	NEUTRAL	NEUTRAL Non-secretor variant: BENEFICIAL	NEUTRAL
Chicken: Egg White	NEUTRAL	NEUTRAL	BENEFICIAL: Nutrient-dense food.	NEUTRAL
Chicken: Egg Yolk	NEUTRAL	NEUTRAL	NEUTRAL Non-secretor variant: BENEFICIAL	NEUTRAL
Duck Egg	NEUTRAL	AVOID: Provokes abnormal blood reaction.	AVOID: Contains lectin or other agglutinin.	NEUTRAL
Goose Egg	NEUTRAL	AVOID: Provokes abnormal blood reaction.	NEUTRAL	AVOID Non-secretor variant: NEUTRAL
Quail Egg	NEUTRAL	AVOID: Provokes abnormal blood reaction.	NEUTRAL	AVOID Non-secretor variant: NEUTRAL

▪ BEAN/LEGUME

Food Item	BLOOD GROUP A	BLOOD GROUP B	BLOOD GROUP AB	BLOOD GROUP O
Adzuki Bean	BENEFICIAL: Contains component that either blocks polyamine synthesis or lowers indican levels. Non-secretor variant: NEUTRAL	AVOID: Contains lectin or other agglutinin.	AVOID: Contains lectin or other agglutinin.	BENEFICIAL: Contains an agglutinin that modifies disease susceptibility. Non-secretor variant: NEUTRAL
Black Bean	BENEFICIAL: Contains component that either blocks polyamine synthesis or lowers indican levels. Non-secretor variant: NEUTRAL	AVOID: Contains lectin or other agglutinin.	AVOID: Contains lectin or other agglutinin.	NEUTRAL
Black-eyed Pea	BENEFICIAL: Contains component that either blocks polyamine synthesis or lowers indican levels. Non-secretor variant: NEUTRAL	AVOID: Contains lectin or other agglutinin.	AVOID: Contains lectin or other agglutinin.	BENEFICIAL: Contains an agglutinin that modifies disease susceptibility. Non-secretor variant: NEUTRAL
Cannellini Bean	NEUTRAL	NEUTRAL	NEUTRAL	NEUTRAL
Copper Bean	AVOID: Contains lectin or other agglutinin; metabolic inhibitor. Non-secretor variant: NEUTRAL	NEUTRAL	NEUTRAL	AVOID: Contains lectin or other agglutinin.
Fava (Broad) Bean	BENEFICIAL: Contains component that either blocks polyamine synthesis or lowers indican levels. Non-secretor variant: NEUTRAL	NEUTRAL	AVOID: Contains lectin or other agglutinin. Non-secretor variant: NEUTRAL	NEUTRAL Non-secretor variant: AVOID
Garbanzo Bean (Chickpea)	AVOID: Contains lectin or other agglutinin; metabolic inhibitor.	AVOID: Contains lectin or other agglutinin.	AVOID: Contains lectin or other agglutinin; metabolic inhibitor.	NEUTRAL Non-secretor variant: AVOID

▪ BEAN/LEGUME, CONTINUED

Food Item	BLOOD GROUP A	BLOOD GROUP B	BLOOD GROUP AB	BLOOD GROUP O
Green/Snap/String Bean	BENEFICIAL: Contains component which either blocks polyamine synthesis or lowers indican levels.	NEUTRAL	NEUTRAL	NEUTRAL
Jicama	NEUTRAL	NEUTRAL	NEUTRAL Non-secretor variant: AVOID	NEUTRAL
Kidney Bean	AVOID: Contains lectin or other agglutinin; metabolic inhibitor. Non-secretor variant: NEUTRAL	BENEFICIAL: Contains component which either blocks polyamine synthesis or lowers indican levels. Non-secretor variant: NEUTRAL	AVOID: Contains lectin or other agglutinin.	AVOID: Contains lectin or other agglutinin; metabolic inhibitor.
Lentil (Domestic)	BENEFICIAL: Contains an agglutinin that modifies disease susceptibility.	AVOID: Contains lectin or other agglutinin.	NEUTRAL	AVOID Non-secretor variant: NEUTRAL
Lentil (Green)	BENEFICIAL: Contains an agglutinin that modifies disease susceptibility.	AVOID: Flocculates serum or precipitates serum proteins; contains lectin or other agglutinin.	BENEFICIAL: Contains an agglutinin that modifies disease susceptibility.	AVOID Non-secretor variant: NEUTRAL
Lentil (Red)	BENEFICIAL: Contains an agglutinin which modifies disease susceptibility.	AVOID: Contains lectin or other agglutinin.	NEUTRAL	AVOID Non-secretor variant: NEUTRAL
Lima Bean	AVOID: Contains lectin or other agglutinin; metabolic inhibitor.	BENEFICIAL: Contains component which either blocks polyamine synthesis or lowers indican levels. Non-secretor variant: NEUTRAL	AVOID: Contains lectin or other agglutinin.	NEUTRAL
Mung Bean/Sprouts	NEUTRAL	AVOID: Contains lectin or other agglutinin.	AVOID: Contains lectin or other agglutinin.	NEUTRAL

■ BEAN/LEGUME, CONTINUED

Food Item	BLOOD GROUP A	BLOOD GROUP B	BLOOD GROUP AB	BLOOD GROUP O
Navy Bean	AVOID: Contains lectin or other agglutinin; metabolic inhibitor. Non-secretor variant: NEUTRAL	BENEFICIAL: Contains component that either blocks polyamine synthesis or lowers indican levels. Non-secretor variant: NEUTRAL	BENEFICIAL Non-secretor variant: NEUTRAL	AVOID: Contains lectin or other agglutinin.
Northern Bean	NEUTRAL	NEUTRAL	NEUTRAL	NEUTRAL
Pinto Bean	BENEFICIAL: Contains component that either blocks polyamine synthesis or lowers indican levels.	AVOID: Provokes abnormal blood reaction.	BENEFICIAL: Contains an agglutinin that modifies disease susceptibility.	AVOID Non-secretor variant: NEUTRAL
Snap Bean	NEUTRAL	NEUTRAL	NEUTRAL	NEUTRAL
Soybean	BENEFICIAL: Contains an agglutinin that modifies disease susceptibility. Non-secretor variant: NEUTRAL	NEUTRAL Non-secretor variant: AVOID	BENEFICIAL Non-secretor variant: NEUTRAL	NEUTRAL Non-secretor variant: AVOID
Soy Cheese	BENEFICIAL: Contains an agglutinin that modifies disease susceptibility. Non-secretor variant: NEUTRAL	AVOID: Contains lectin or other agglutinin; metabolic inhibitor.	NEUTRAL Non-secretor variant: AVOID	NEUTRAL Non-secretor variant: AVOID
Soy Flakes	BENEFICIAL: Contains an agglutinin that modifies disease susceptibility. Non-secretor variant: NEUTRAL	AVOID: Contains lectin or other agglutinin; metabolic inhibitor.	NEUTRAL	NEUTRAL Non-secretor variant: AVOID
Soy Granules (Lecithin)	BENEFICIAL: Contains an agglutinin that modifies disease susceptibility. Non-secretor variant: NEUTRAL	AVOID: Contains lectin or other agglutinin; metabolic inhibitor.	NEUTRAL	NEUTRAL Non-secretor variant: AVOID

▪ BEAN/LEGUME, CONTINUED

Food Item	BLOOD GROUP A	BLOOD GROUP B	BLOOD GROUP AB	BLOOD GROUP O
Soy Milk	BENEFICIAL: Contains an agglutinin that modifies disease susceptibility. Non-secretor variant: NEUTRAL	AVOID: Contains lectin or other agglutinin; metabolic inhibitor. Non-secretor variant: NEUTRAL	NEUTRAL Non-secretor variant: AVOID	NEUTRAL Non-secretor variant: AVOID
Tamarind Bean	AVOID: Provokes abnormal blood reaction.	NEUTRAL	NEUTRAL	AVOID: Gastric irritant; inhibits proper digestive function; increases intestinal imbalance; increases polyamine or indican levels.
Tempeh (fermented soy)	BENEFICIAL: Contains an agglutinin that modifies disease susceptibility. Non-secretor variant: NEUTRAL	AVOID: Contains lectin or other agglutinin; metabolic inhibitor.	BENEFICIAL Non-secretor variant: NEUTRAL	NEUTRAL Non-secretor variant: AVOID
Tofu (soy cake)	BENEFICIAL: Contains an agglutinin that modifies disease susceptibility. Non-secretor variant: NEUTRAL	AVOID: Contains lectin or other agglutinin; metabolic inhibitor.	BENEFICIAL Non-secretor variant: NEUTRAL	NEUTRAL Non-secretor variant: AVOID
White Bean	NEUTRAL	NEUTRAL	NEUTRAL	NEUTRAL

▪ NUT/SEED

Food Item	BLOOD GROUP A	BLOOD GROUP B	BLOOD GROUP AB	BLOOD GROUP O
Almond/Almond Butter	NEUTRAL	NEUTRAL	NEUTRAL	NEUTRAL
Almond Cheese	NEUTRAL	NEUTRAL	NEUTRAL	NEUTRAL Non-secretor variant: AVOID
Almond Milk	NEUTRAL	NEUTRAL	NEUTRAL	NEUTRAL Non-secretor variant: AVOID

■ NUT/SEED, CONTINUED

Food Item	BLOOD GROUP A	BLOOD GROUP B	BLOOD GROUP AB	BLOOD GROUP O
Beechnut	NEUTRAL	NEUTRAL	NEUTRAL	AVOID: Provokes abnormal blood reaction.
Brazil Nut	AVOID: Provokes abnormal blood reaction; inhibits proper gastric function or blocks assimilation.	NEUTRAL	NEUTRAL Non-secretor variant: AVOID	AVOID: Provokes abnormal blood reaction.
Butternut	NEUTRAL	NEUTRAL	NEUTRAL	NEUTRAL
Cashew/Cashew Butter	AVOID: Provokes abnormal blood reaction; contains lectin or other agglutinin; metabolic inhibitor; inhibits proper gastric function or blocks assimilation.	AVOID: Provokes abnormal blood reaction.	NEUTRAL Non-secretor variant: AVOID	AVOID: Contains component that can modify known disease susceptibility.
Chestnut	NEUTRAL	NEUTRAL	BENEFICIAL: Contains component that either blocks polyamine synthesis or lowers indican levels.	AVOID: Provokes abnormal blood reaction.
Filbert (Hazelnut)	NEUTRAL	AVOID: Provokes abnormal blood reaction.	AVOID: Provokes abnormal blood reaction.	NEUTRAL
Flaxseed (Linseed)	BENEFICIAL: Contains component that positively influences known disease susceptibility.	NEUTRAL	NEUTRAL	BENEFICIAL: Contains component that positively influences known disease susceptibility. Non-secretor variant: NEUTRAL
Hickory	NEUTRAL	NEUTRAL	NEUTRAL	NEUTRAL
Litchi	NEUTRAL	NEUTRAL	NEUTRAL	AVOID: Increases intestinal imbalance; increases polyamine or indican levels.
Macadamia	NEUTRAL	NEUTRAL	NEUTRAL	NEUTRAL
Peanut/Peanut Butter	BENEFICIAL: Contains an agglutinin that modifies disease susceptibility.	AVOID: Contains lectin or other agglutinin.	BENEFICIAL Non-secretor variant: NEUTRAL	AVOID: Contains lectin or other agglutinin.

■ **NUT/SEED, CONTINUED**

Food Item	BLOOD GROUP A	BLOOD GROUP B	BLOOD GROUP AB	BLOOD GROUP O
Pecan/Pecan Butter	NEUTRAL	NEUTRAL	NEUTRAL	NEUTRAL
Pine Nut (Pignola)	NEUTRAL	AVOID: Provokes abnormal blood reaction.	NEUTRAL	NEUTRAL
Pistachio	AVOID: Provokes abnormal blood reaction; inhibits proper gastric function or blocks assimilation.	AVOID: Provokes abnormal blood reaction.	NEUTRAL Non-secretor variant: AVOID	AVOID: Increases polyamine or indican levels; inhibits proper gastric function or blocks assimilation.
Poppy Seed	NEUTRAL	AVOID: Contains lectin or other agglutinin.	AVOID: Contains lectin or other agglutinin.	AVOID: Enhances effect of other food toxins; contains component that can modify known disease susceptibility.
Pumpkin Seed/Pumpkin Seed Butter	BENEFICIAL: Contains an agglutinin that modifies disease susceptibility.	AVOID: Provokes abnormal blood reaction. Non-secretor variant: NEUTRAL	AVOID: Contains lectin or other agglutinin.	BENEFICIAL: Contains component that positively influences known disease susceptibility.
Safflower Seed	NEUTRAL Non-secretor variant: AVOID	AVOID: Contains lectin or other agglutinin; provokes abnormal blood reaction.	NEUTRAL	NEUTRAL Non-secretor variant: AVOID
Sesame Butter/Tahini	NEUTRAL	AVOID: Contains lectin or other agglutinin.	AVOID: Contains lectin or other agglutinin.	NEUTRAL
Sesame Seed	NEUTRAL	AVOID: Contains lectin or other agglutinin. Provokes abnormal blood reaction.	AVOID: Contains lectin or other agglutinin.	NEUTRAL
Sunflower Seed/Sunflower Seed Butter	NEUTRAL: Non-secretor variant: AVOID	AVOID: Contains lectin or other agglutinin; provokes abnormal blood reaction.	AVOID: Contains lectin or other agglutinin.	AVOID: Contains lectin or other agglutinin.
Walnut (Black)	BENEFICIAL: Contains component that either blocks polyamine synthesis or lowers indican levels.	BENEFICIAL: Contains component that either blocks polyamine synthesis or lowers indican levels.	BENEFICIAL: Contains component that either blocks polyamine synthesis or lowers indican levels.	BENEFICIAL: Contains component that either blocks polyamine synthesis or lowers indican levels.

NUT/SEED, CONTINUED

Food Item	BLOOD GROUP A	BLOOD GROUP B	BLOOD GROUP AB	BLOOD GROUP O
Walnut (English)	BENEFICIAL: Contains component that either blocks polyamine synthesis or lowers indican levels.	NEUTRAL Non-secretor variant: BENEFICIAL	BENEFICIAL: Contains component that either blocks polyamine synthesis or lowers indican levels.	BENEFICIAL: Contains component that either blocks polyamine synthesis or lowers indican levels.

GRAIN

Food Item	BLOOD GROUP A	BLOOD GROUP B	BLOOD GROUP AB	BLOOD GROUP O
Amaranth	BENEFICIAL: Contains an agglutinin that modifies disease susceptibility.	AVOID: Contains lectin or other agglutinin. Non-secretor variant: NEUTRAL	BENEFICIAL: Contains an agglutinin that modifies disease susceptibility.	NEUTRAL
Artichoke Flour/Pasta	BENEFICIAL: Healthy alternative to more common variety of foods which are classed as avoids; contains component that positively influences known disease susceptibility.	AVOID: Contains lectin or other agglutinin. Non-secretor variant: NEUTRAL	AVOID: Contains lectin or other agglutinin.	NEUTRAL Non-secretor variant: AVOID
Barley	NEUTRAL	NEUTRAL	NEUTRAL	AVOID: Metabolic inhibitor.
Buckwheat/Kasha	BENEFICIAL: Healthy alternative to more common variety of foods which are classed as avoids. Non-secretor variant: NEUTRAL	AVOID: Contains lectin or other agglutinin.	AVOID: Contains lectin or other agglutinin.	NEUTRAL Non-secretor variant: AVOID
Corn (all)	NEUTRAL Non-secretor variant: AVOID	AVOID: Contains lectin or other agglutinin.	AVOID: Contains lectin or other agglutinin.	AVOID: Contains lectin or other agglutinin; metabolic inhibitor; contains component that can modify known disease susceptibility.
Cornmeal	NEUTRAL Non-secretor variant: AVOID	AVOID: Contains lectin or other agglutinin.	AVOID: Contains lectin or other agglutinin.	AVOID: Contains lectin or other agglutinin; metabolic inhibitor; contains component that can modify known disease susceptibility.

■ GRAIN, CONTINUED

Food Item	BLOOD GROUP A	BLOOD GROUP B	BLOOD GROUP AB	BLOOD GROUP O
Couscous (Cracked Wheat)	NEUTRAL Non-secretor variant: AVOID	AVOID: Provokes abnormal blood reaction.	NEUTRAL	AVOID: Contains lectin or other agglutinin; metabolic inhibitor; contains component that can modify known disease susceptibility.
Essene Bread (Manna Bread)	BENEFICIAL: Healthy alternative to more common variety of foods which are classed as avoids Non-secretor variant: NEUTRAL	BENEFICIAL: Healthy alternative to more common variety of foods which are classed as avoids.	BENEFICIAL: Healthy alternative to more common variety of foods which are classed as avoids.	BENEFICIAL: Healthy alternative to more common variety of foods which are classed as avoids.
Ezekiel Bread	BENEFICIAL: Healthy alternative to more common variety of foods which are classed as avoids. Non-secretor variant: NEUTRAL	BENEFICIAL: Healthy alternative to more common variety of foods which are classed as avoids. Non-secretor variant: NEUTRAL	BENEFICIAL: Healthy alternative to more common variety of foods which are classed as avoids.	NEUTRAL
Gluten Flour	NEUTRAL Non-secretor variant: AVOID	AVOID: Provokes abnormal blood reaction.	NEUTRAL	AVOID: Contains lectin or other agglutinin; metabolic inhibitor; contains component that can modify known disease susceptibility.
Gluten-Free Bread	NEUTRAL	NEUTRAL	NEUTRAL	NEUTRAL Non-secretor variant: AVOID
Kamut	NEUTRAL	AVOID: Provokes abnormal blood reaction.	AVOID: Increases polyamine or indican levels.	NEUTRAL
Millet	NEUTRAL	BENEFICIAL: Healthy alternative to more common variety of foods which are classed as avoids.	BENEFICIAL: Healthy alternative to more common variety of foods which are classed as avoids.	NEUTRAL

■ **GRAIN, CONTINUED**

Food Item	BLOOD GROUP A	BLOOD GROUP B	BLOOD GROUP AB	BLOOD GROUP O
Oat Flour	BENEFICIAL: Contains component that positively influences known disease susceptibility. Non-secretor variant: NEUTRAL	BENEFICIAL: Contains component that either blocks polyamine synthesis or lowers indican levels. Non-secretor variant: NEUTRAL	BENEFICIAL: Contains component that positively influences known disease susceptibility.	NEUTRAL Non-secretor variant: AVOID
Oat/Oat Bran/Oatmeal	BENEFICIAL: Contains component that positively influences known disease susceptibility. Non-secretor variant: NEUTRAL	BENEFICIAL: Contains component that either blocks polyamine synthesis or lowers indican levels. Non-secretor variant: NEUTRAL	BENEFICIAL: Contains component that positively influences known disease susceptibility.	NEUTRAL Non-secretor variant: AVOID
Popcorn	NEUTRAL Non-secretor variant: AVOID	AVOID: Contains lectin or other agglutinin.	AVOID: Contains lectin or other agglutinin.	AVOID: Contains lectin or other agglutinin; metabolic inhibitor; contains component which can modify known disease susceptibility.
Quinoa	NEUTRAL	NEUTRAL	NEUTRAL	NEUTRAL
Rice (Cream of)	NEUTRAL	NEUTRAL	NEUTRAL	NEUTRAL
Rice (Puffed)	NEUTRAL	BENEFICIAL: Contains an agglutinin that modifies disease susceptibility.	BENEFICIAL: Contains an agglutinin that modifies disease susceptibility.	NEUTRAL
Rice (White/Brown/Basmati) Bread	NEUTRAL	NEUTRAL	BENEFICIAL: Contains an agglutinin that modifies disease susceptibility.	NEUTRAL
Rice (Wild)	NEUTRAL	AVOID Non-secretor variant: NEUTRAL	BENEFICIAL: Contains an agglutinin that modifies disease susceptibility.	NEUTRAL
Rice Bran	NEUTRAL	BENEFICIAL: Contains an agglutinin that modifies disease susceptibility.	BENEFICIAL: Contains an agglutinin that modifies disease susceptibility.	NEUTRAL

■ **GRAIN, CONTINUED**

Food Item	BLOOD GROUP A	BLOOD GROUP B	BLOOD GROUP AB	BLOOD GROUP O
Rice Cake/Flour	NEUTRAL	BENEFICIAL: Contains an agglutinin that modifies disease susceptibility.	BENEFICIAL: Contains an agglutinin that modifies disease susceptibility.	NEUTRAL
Rice Milk	NEUTRAL	BENEFICIAL: Contains an agglutinin that modifies disease susceptibility.	BENEFICIAL: Contains an agglutinin that modifies disease susceptibility.	NEUTRAL
Rye Flour (Whole Rye)	BENEFICIAL: Healthy alternative to more common variety of foods which are classed as avoids.	AVOID: Contains lectin or other agglutinin.	BENEFICIAL: Healthy alternative to more common variety of foods which are classed as avoids.	NEUTRAL
Rye/100% Rye Bread	BENEFICIAL: Healthy alternative to more common variety of foods which are classed as avoids.	AVOID: Contains lectin or other agglutinin.	BENEFICIAL: Healthy alternative to more common variety of foods which are classed as avoids.	NEUTRAL
Soba Noodles (100% Buckwheat)	BENEFICIAL: Healthy alternative to more common variety of foods which are classed as avoids. Non-secretor variant: NEUTRAL	AVOID: Contains lectin or other agglutinin.	AVOID: Contains lectin or other agglutinin.	NEUTRAL Non-secretor variant: AVOID
Sorghum	NEUTRAL	AVOID: Contains lectin or other agglutinin. Non-secretor variant: NEUTRAL	AVOID: Increases polyamine or indican levels.	AVOID: Increases polyamine or indican levels.
Soy Flour/Bread	BENEFICIAL: Contains an agglutinin that modifies disease susceptibility. Non-secretor variant: NEUTRAL	NEUTRAL Non-secretor variant: AVOID	BENEFICIAL Non-secretor variant: AVOID	NEUTRAL Non-secretor variant: AVOID
Spelt (whole)	NEUTRAL	BENEFICIAL Non-secretor variant: NEUTRAL	BENEFICIAL Non-secretor variant: NEUTRAL	NEUTRAL Non-secretor variant: AVOID

GRAIN, CONTINUED

Food Item	BLOOD GROUP A	BLOOD GROUP B	BLOOD GROUP AB	BLOOD GROUP O
Spelt Flour/Products	NEUTRAL	NEUTRAL	NEUTRAL	NEUTRAL Non-secretor variant: AVOID
Tapioca	NEUTRAL	AVOID Non-secretor variant: NEUTRAL	AVOID: Increases polyamine or indican levels.	NEUTRAL Non-secretor variant: AVOID
Teff	AVOID: Provokes abnormal blood reaction. Non-secretor variant: NEUTRAL	AVOID: Contains lectin or other agglutinin.	AVOID: Contains lectin or other agglutinin; provokes abnormal blood reaction.	NEUTRAL
Wheat (Bran)	AVOID: Contains lectin or other agglutinin; metabolic inhibitor.	AVOID: Contains lectin or other agglutinin; metabolic inhibitor.	NEUTRAL	AVOID: Contains lectin or other agglutinin; metabolic inhibitor; contains component that can modify known disease susceptibility.
Wheat (Germ)	AVOID: Provokes abnormal blood reaction; contains lectin or other agglutinin; metabolic inhibitor.	AVOID: Provokes abnormal blood reaction.	NEUTRAL Non-secretor variant: AVOID	AVOID: Contains lectin or other agglutinin; metabolic inhibitor; contains component that can modify known disease susceptibility.
Wheat (Gluten Flour Products)	NEUTRAL Non-secretor variant: AVOID	AVOID: Provokes abnormal blood reaction; contains lectin or other agglutinin; metabolic inhibitor.	NEUTRAL Non-secretor variant: AVOID	AVOID: Contains lectin or other agglutinin; metabolic inhibitor; contains component that can modify known disease susceptibility.
Wheat (Refined Unbleached)	NEUTRAL Non-secretor variant: AVOID	NEUTRAL Non-secretor variant: AVOID	AVOID: Contains lectin or other agglutinin.	AVOID: Contains lectin or other agglutinin; metabolic inhibitor; contains component that can modify known disease susceptibility.

▪ GRAIN, CONTINUED

Food Item	BLOOD GROUP A	BLOOD GROUP B	BLOOD GROUP AB	BLOOD GROUP O
Wheat (Semolina Flour Products)	NEUTRAL Non-secretor variant: AVOID	NEUTRAL Non-secretor variant: AVOID	NEUTRAL Non-secretor variant: AVOID	AVOID: Contains lectin or other agglutinin; metabolic inhibitor; contains component that can modify known disease susceptibility.
Wheat (White Flour Products)	NEUTRAL Non-secretor variant: AVOID	NEUTRAL Non-secretor variant: AVOID	NEUTRAL Non-secretor variant: AVOID	AVOID: Contains lectin or other agglutinin; metabolic inhibitor; contains component that can modify known disease susceptibility.
Wheat (Whole Wheat Products)	AVOID: Provokes abnormal blood reaction; contains lectin or other agglutinin; metabolic inhibitor.	AVOID: Provokes abnormal blood reaction.	NEUTRAL Non-secretor variant: AVOID	AVOID: Contains lectin or other agglutinin; metabolic inhibitor; contains component that can modify known disease susceptibility.
Wheat Bread (Sprouted Commercial, Except Essene and Ezekiel)	NEUTRAL	NEUTRAL Non-secretor variant: AVOID	NEUTRAL	AVOID: Contains lectin or other agglutinin; metabolic inhibitor; contains component that can modify known disease susceptibility.

▪ VEGETABLE/VEG JUICE

Food Item	BLOOD GROUP A	BLOOD GROUP B	BLOOD GROUP AB	BLOOD GROUP O
Agar	NEUTRAL Non-secretor variant: AVOID	NEUTRAL Non-secretor variant: AVOID	NEUTRAL Non-secretor variant: AVOID	NEUTRAL Non-secretor variant: AVOID
Alfalfa Sprouts	BENEFICIAL: Contains component that positively influences known disease susceptibility. Non-secretor variant: NEUTRAL	NEUTRAL	BENEFICIAL: Contains component that positively influences known disease susceptibility.	AVOID: Contains component that can modify known disease susceptibility.

■ VEGETABLE/VEG JUICE, CONTINUED

Food Item	BLOOD GROUP A	BLOOD GROUP B	BLOOD GROUP AB	BLOOD GROUP O
Aloe/Aloe Tea/Aloe Juice	BENEFICIAL: Contains an agglutinin that modifies disease susceptibility. Non-secretor variant: NEUTRAL	AVOID: Contains lectin or other agglutinin.	AVOID: Contains component that can modify known disease susceptibility.	AVOID: Contains lectin or other agglutinin; contains component that can modify known disease susceptibility.
Artichoke (Globe/Jerusalem)	BENEFICIAL: Contains component that positively influences known disease susceptibility.	AVOID Non-secretor variant: NEUTRAL	AVOID: Contains lectin or other agglutinin.	BENEFICIAL: Contains component that positively influences known disease susceptibility.
Arugula	NEUTRAL	NEUTRAL	NEUTRAL	NEUTRAL
Asparagus	NEUTRAL	NEUTRAL	NEUTRAL	NEUTRAL
Asparagus Pea	NEUTRAL	NEUTRAL	NEUTRAL	NEUTRAL
Bamboo Shoot	NEUTRAL	NEUTRAL	NEUTRAL	NEUTRAL
Beet	NEUTRAL	BENEFICIAL: Contains component that positively influences known disease susceptibility.	BENEFICIAL Non-secretor variant: NEUTRAL	NEUTRAL
Beet Greens	BENEFICIAL: Contains component that positively influences known disease susceptibility.	BENEFICIAL: Contains component that positively influences known disease susceptibility.	BENEFICIAL: Contains component that positively influences known disease susceptibility.	BENEFICIAL: Contains component that positively influences known disease susceptibility.
Bok Choy	NEUTRAL	NEUTRAL	NEUTRAL	NEUTRAL
Broccoli	BENEFICIAL: Contains component that positively influences known disease susceptibility.	BENEFICIAL: Contains component that positively influences known disease susceptibility.	BENEFICIAL: Contains component that positively influences known disease susceptibility.	BENEFICIAL: Contains component that positively influences known disease susceptibility.
Brussels Sprouts	NEUTRAL	BENEFICIAL: Contains component that positively influences known disease susceptibility.	NEUTRAL	NEUTRAL Non-secretor variant: AVOID

■ VEGETABLE/VEG JUICE, CONTINUED

Food Item	BLOOD GROUP A	BLOOD GROUP B	BLOOD GROUP AB	BLOOD GROUP O
Cabbage (Chinese/ Red/White)	AVOID: Provokes abnormal blood reaction; secretory insufficiency; increases intestinal imbalance.	BENEFICIAL: Contains component that positively influences known disease susceptibility. Non-secretor variant: NEUTRAL	NEUTRAL	NEUTRAL Non-secretor variant: AVOID
Cabbage Juice	NEUTRAL	BENEFICIAL: Contains component that positively influences known disease susceptibility. Non-secretor variant: NEUTRAL	BENEFICIAL: Contains component that positively influences known disease susceptibility.	NEUTRAL Non-secretor variant: AVOID
Caper	AVOID: Flocculates serum or precipitates serum proteins.	NEUTRAL	AVOID: Flocculates serum or precipitates serum proteins.	AVOID: Metabolic inhibitor.
Carrot	BENEFICIAL: Contains an agglutinin that modifies disease susceptibility. Non-secretor variant: NEUTRAL	BENEFICIAL: Contains component that positively influences known disease susceptibility.	NEUTRAL	NEUTRAL Non-secretor variant: BENEFICIAL
Carrot Juice	BENEFICIAL: Contains an agglutinin that modifies disease susceptibility. Non-secretor variant: NEUTRAL	NEUTRAL	BENEFICIAL: Contains an agglutinin that modifies disease susceptibility.	NEUTRAL
Cauliflower	NEUTRAL	BENEFICIAL: Contains component that positively influences known disease susceptibility.	BENEFICIAL: Contains component that positively influences known disease susceptibility.	AVOID: Metabolic inhibitor.
Celeriac	NEUTRAL	NEUTRAL	NEUTRAL	NEUTRAL
Celery/Celery Juice	BENEFICIAL: Contains component that positively influences known disease susceptibility. Non-secretor variant: NEUTRAL	NEUTRAL	BENEFICIAL: Contains component that positively influences known disease susceptibility.	NEUTRAL

■ **VEGETABLE/VEG JUICE, CONTINUED**

Food Item	BLOOD GROUP A	BLOOD GROUP B	BLOOD GROUP AB	BLOOD GROUP O
Chicory	BENEFICIAL: Contains component that positively influences known disease susceptibility.	NEUTRAL	NEUTRAL	BENEFICIAL: Contains component that either blocks polyamine synthesis or lowers indican levels.
Chili Pepper	AVOID: Flocculates serum or precipitates serum proteins. Non-secretor variant: NEUTRAL	NEUTRAL	AVOID: Gastric irritant; inhibits proper digestive function.	NEUTRAL
Collard Greens	BENEFICIAL: Contains component that positively influences known disease susceptibility.	BENEFICIAL: Contains component that positively influences known disease susceptibility.	BENEFICIAL: Contains component that either blocks polyamine synthesis or lowers indican levels.	BENEFICIAL: Contains component that positively influences known disease susceptibility.
Cucumber	NEUTRAL	NEUTRAL	BENEFICIAL: Contains an agglutinin that modifies disease susceptibility.	AVOID: Contains lectin or other agglutinin.
Cucumber Juice	NEUTRAL	NEUTRAL	NEUTRAL	AVOID: Contains lectin or other agglutinin.
Daikon Radish	NEUTRAL	NEUTRAL	NEUTRAL	NEUTRAL
Dandelion	BENEFICIAL: Contains component that positively influences known disease susceptibility.	NEUTRAL	BENEFICIAL: Contains component that either blocks polyamine synthesis or lowers indican levels.	BENEFICIAL: Contains component that either blocks polyamine synthesis or lowers indican levels.
Eggplant	AVOID: Contains lectin or other agglutinin; metabolic inhibitor. Non-secretor variant: NEUTRAL	BENEFICIAL: Contains an agglutinin that modifies disease susceptibility. Non-secretor variant: NEUTRAL	BENEFICIAL: Contains an agglutinin that modifies disease susceptibility.	NEUTRAL Non-secretor variant: AVOID
Endive	NEUTRAL	NEUTRAL	NEUTRAL	NEUTRAL
Escarole	BENEFICIAL: Contains component that positively influences known disease susceptibility.	NEUTRAL	NEUTRAL	BENEFICIAL: Contains component that positively influences known disease susceptibility.

■ **VEGETABLE/VEG JUICE, CONTINUED**

Food Item	BLOOD GROUP A	BLOOD GROUP B	BLOOD GROUP AB	BLOOD GROUP O
Fennel	BENEFICIAL: Contains component that either blocks polyamine synthesis or lowers indican levels. Non-secretor variant: NEUTRAL	NEUTRAL	NEUTRAL	NEUTRAL
Fiddlehead Fern	NEUTRAL	NEUTRAL	NEUTRAL	NEUTRAL Non-secretor variant: BENEFICIAL
Garlic	BENEFICIAL: Contains an agglutinin that modifies disease susceptibility. Non-secretor variant: NEUTRAL	NEUTRAL Non-secretor variant: BENEFICIAL	BENEFICIAL: Contains an agglutinin that modifies disease susceptibility.	NEUTRAL Non-secretor variant: BENEFICIAL
Ginger	BENEFICIAL: Contains component that either blocks polyamine synthesis or lowers indican levels.	BENEFICIAL: Contains componcnt that positively influences known disease susceptibility.	NEUTRAL Non-secretor variant: BENEFICIAL	BENEFICIAL: Contains component that positively influences known disease susceptibility.
Horseradish	BENEFICIAL: Contains component that either blocks polyamine synthesis or lowers indican levels. Non-secretor variant: NEUTRAL	NEUTRAL	NEUTRAL	BENEFICIAL: Contains component that positively influences known disease susceptibility.
Juniper	AVOID: Secretory insufficiency; induces intestinal imbalance.	AVOID: Provokes abnormal blood reaction.	NEUTRAL Non-secretor variant: AVOID	AVOID: Gastric irritant; inhibits proper digestive function.
Kale	BENEFICIAL: Contains component that positively influences known disease susceptibility.	BENEFICIAL	BENEFICIAL: Contains component that positively influences known disease susceptibility.	BENEFICIAL: Contains component that positively influences known disease susceptibility.
Kelp	NEUTRAL	NEUTRAL	NEUTRAL	BENEFICIAL: metabolic enhancer.

■ **VEGETABLE/VEG JUICE, CONTINUED**

Food Item	BLOOD GROUP A	BLOOD GROUP B	BLOOD GROUP AB	BLOOD GROUP O
Kohlrabi	BENEFICIAL: Contains component that positively influences known disease susceptibility.	NEUTRAL	NEUTRAL	BENEFICIAL: Contains component that positively influences known disease susceptibility.
Leek	BENEFICIAL: Contains an agglutinin that modifies disease susceptibility.	NEUTRAL	NEUTRAL	AVOID: Contains lectin or other agglutinin; metabolic inhibitor.
Lettuce (except Romaine)	NEUTRAL	NEUTRAL	NEUTRAL	NEUTRAL
Lettuce (Romaine)	BENEFICIAL: Contains component that positively influences known disease susceptibility.	NEUTRAL	NEUTRAL	BENEFICIAL: Contains component that positively influences known disease susceptibility. Non-secretor variant: NEUTRAL
Mushroom (Abalone)	NEUTRAL	NEUTRAL	AVOID: Provokes abnormal blood reaction.	NEUTRAL
Mushroom (Domestic white "Button," "Silver Dollar")	BENEFICIAL: Contains an agglutinin that modifies disease susceptibility. Non-secretor variant: AVOID	NEUTRAL	NEUTRAL	AVOID Non-secretor variant: NEUTRAL
Mushroom (Enoki)	NEUTRAL	NEUTRAL	NEUTRAL	NEUTRAL
Mushroom (Maitake)	BENEFICIAL: Contains an agglutinin that modifies disease susceptibility.	NEUTRAL	BENEFICIAL: Contains an agglutinin that modifies disease susceptibility.	NEUTRAL
Mushroom (Oyster)	NEUTRAL	NEUTRAL	NEUTRAL	NEUTRAL
Mushroom (Portobello)	NEUTRAL	NEUTRAL	NEUTRAL	NEUTRAL
Mushroom (Shiitake)	AVOID: Provokes abnormal blood reaction.	BENEFICIAL: Contains component that positively influences known disease susceptibility.	AVOID: Provokes abnormal blood reaction.	AVOID: Contains component that can modify known disease susceptibility.

■ **VEGETABLE/VEG JUICE, CONTINUED**

Food Item	BLOOD GROUP A	BLOOD GROUP B	BLOOD GROUP AB	BLOOD GROUP O
Mushroom (Straw)	NEUTRAL	NEUTRAL	NEUTRAL	NEUTRAL
Mustard Greens	NEUTRAL	BENEFICIAL: Contains component that positively influences known disease susceptibility.	BENEFICIAL: Contains component that positively influences known disease susceptibility.	AVOID Non-secretor variant: NEUTRAL
Okra	BENEFICIAL: Contains an agglutinin that modifies disease susceptibility.	NEUTRAL Non-secretor variant: BENEFICIAL	NEUTRAL	BENEFICIAL: Contains component that positively influences known disease susceptibility.
Olive (Black)	AVOID: Secretory insufficiency; induces intestinal imbalance; provokes abnormal blood reaction; inhibits proper gastric function or blocks assimilation.	AVOID: Provokes abnormal blood reaction.	AVOID: Increases polyamine or indican levels.	AVOID: Contains component that can modify known disease susceptibility.
Olive (Greek/Spanish)	AVOID: Provokes abnormal blood reaction.	AVOID: Provokes abnormal blood reaction.	NEUTRAL	NEUTRAL Non-secretor variant: AVOID
Olive (Green)	NEUTRAL Non-secretor variant: AVOID	AVOID: Provokes abnormal blood reaction.	NEUTRAL	NEUTRAL Non-secretor variant: AVOID
Onion (Red/ Spanish/ Yellow/ White/Green)	BENEFICIAL: Contains component that positively influences known disease susceptibility.	NEUTRAL Non-secretor variant: BENEFICIAL	NEUTRAL	BENEFICIAL: Contains component that positively influences known disease susceptibility.
Oyster Plant	NEUTRAL	NEUTRAL	NEUTRAL	NEUTRAL
Parsnip	BENEFICIAL: Contains an agglutinin that modifies disease susceptibility.	BENEFICIAL: Contains an agglutinin that modifies disease susceptibility.	BENEFICIAL: Contains an agglutinin that modifies disease susceptibility.	BENEFICIAL: Contains an agglutinin that modifies disease susceptibility. Non-secretor variant: NEUTRAL
Pea (Green/Pod/Snow)	NEUTRAL	NEUTRAL	NEUTRAL	NEUTRAL

■ **VEGETABLE/VEG JUICE, CONTINUED**

Food Item	BLOOD GROUP A	BLOOD GROUP B	BLOOD GROUP AB	BLOOD GROUP O
Pepper (Green/ Yellow/Jalapeño)	AVOID: Provokes abnormal blood reaction. Non-secretor variant: NEU-TRAL	BENEFICIAL Non-secretor variant: NEU-TRAL	AVOID: Provokes abnormal blood reaction.	NEUTRAL
Pepper (Red/Cayenne)	AVOID	BENEFICIAL: Contains component that positively influences known disease susceptibility. Non-secretor variant: NEU-TRAL	AVOID: Provokes abnormal blood reaction.	BENEFICIAL: Contains component that positively influences known disease susceptibility.
Pickle (in brine)	NEUTRAL Non-secretor variant: AVOID	NEUTRAL	AVOID: Gastric irritant; inhibits proper digestive function.	AVOID: Contains component that can modify known disease susceptibility.
Pickle (in vinegar)	AVOID: Provokes abnormal blood reaction.	NEUTRAL	AVOID: Provokes abnormal blood reaction.	AVOID: Contains component that can modify known disease susceptibility.
Pimento	NEUTRAL	NEUTRAL	NEUTRAL	NEUTRAL
Poi	NEUTRAL	NEUTRAL	NEUTRAL Non-secretor variant: AVOID	NEUTRAL Non-secretor variant: AVOID
Potato (Sweet)	AVOID: Secretory insufficiency; induces intestinal imbalance; inhibits proper gastric function or blocks assimilation.	BENEFICIAL: Contains component that positively influences known disease susceptibility.	BENEFICIAL: Contains component that positively influences known disease susceptibility.	BENEFICIAL: Contains component that positively influences known disease susceptibility. Non-secretor variant: NEU-TRAL
Potato (White/ Red/Blue/Yellow)	AVOID: Contains lectin or other agglutinin; metabolic inhibitor; provokes abnormal blood reaction.	NEUTRAL Non-secretor variant: AVOID	NEUTRAL	AVOID: Contains lectin or other agglutinin; contains component that can modify known disease susceptibility; metabolic inhibitor.

▨ VEGETABLE/VEG JUICE, CONTINUED

Food Item	BLOOD GROUP A	BLOOD GROUP B	BLOOD GROUP AB	BLOOD GROUP O
Pumpkin	BENEFICIAL: Contains component that positively influences known disease susceptibility.	AVOID Non-secretor variant: NEUTRAL	NEUTRAL	BENEFICIAL: Contains component that positively influences known disease susceptibility.
Radicchio	NEUTRAL	NEUTRAL	NEUTRAL	NEUTRAL
Radish	NEUTRAL	AVOID: Provokes abnormal blood reaction.	AVOID: Provokes abnormal blood reaction.	NEUTRAL
Radish Sprouts	NEUTRAL	AVOID: Provokes abnormal blood reaction.	AVOID: Provokes abnormal blood reaction.	NEUTRAL
Rappini	BENEFICIAL: Contains component that positively influences known disease susceptibility. Non-secretor variant: NEUTRAL	NEUTRAL	NEUTRAL	NEUTRAL
Rhubarb	AVOID: Secretory insufficiency.	AVOID: Provokes abnormal blood reaction.	AVOID: Contains component that can modify known disease susceptibility.	AVOID: Gastric irritant; inhibits proper digestive function; contains component that can modify known disease susceptibility.
Rutabaga	NEUTRAL	NEUTRAL	NEUTRAL	NEUTRAL
Sauerkraut	AVOID: Provokes abnormal blood reaction.	NEUTRAL	NEUTRAL	NEUTRAL Non-secretor variant: AVOID
Scallion	NEUTRAL	NEUTRAL	NEUTRAL	NEUTRAL
Seaweed	NEUTRAL	NEUTRAL	NEUTRAL	BENEFICIAL: Metabolic enhancer.
Shallot	NEUTRAL	NEUTRAL	NEUTRAL	NEUTRAL
Spinach/Spinach Juice	BENEFICIAL: Contains component that positively influences known disease susceptibility.	NEUTRAL	NEUTRAL	BENEFICIAL: Contains component that positively influences known disease susceptibility.

▪ VEGETABLE/VEG JUICE, CONTINUED

Food Item	BLOOD GROUP A	BLOOD GROUP B	BLOOD GROUP AB	BLOOD GROUP O
Squash (Summer/Winter)	NEUTRAL	NEUTRAL	NEUTRAL	NEUTRAL
Swiss Chard	BENEFICIAL: Contains an agglutinin that modifies disease susceptibility.	NEUTRAL	NEUTRAL	BENEFICIAL: Contains component that positively influences known disease susceptibility.
Taro	NEUTRAL	NEUTRAL	NEUTRAL Non-secretor variant: AVOID	AVOID: Metabolic inhibitor.
Tomato/Tomato Juice	AVOID: Contains lectin or other agglutinin; metabolic inhibitor; provokes abnormal blood reaction. Non-secretor variant: NEUTRAL	AVOID: Provokes abnormal blood reaction. Non-secretor variant: NEUTRAL	NEUTRAL Non-secretor variant: BENEFICIAL	NEUTRAL
Turnip	BENEFICIAL: Contains an agglutinin that modifies disease susceptibility.	NEUTRAL	NEUTRAL	BENEFICIAL: Contains component that either blocks polyamine synthesis or lowers indican levels. Non-secretor variant: NEUTRAL
Water Chestnut	NEUTRAL	NEUTRAL	NEUTRAL	NEUTRAL
Watercress	NEUTRAL	NEUTRAL	NEUTRAL	NEUTRAL
Yam	AVOID: Secretory insufficiency; induces intestinal imbalance.	BENEFICIAL: Contains component that positively influences known disease susceptibility.	BENEFICIAL: Contains component that positively influences known disease susceptibility.	NEUTRAL
Yucca	AVOID: Provokes abnormal blood reaction.	NEUTRAL	NEUTRAL	AVOID: Metabolic inhibitor.
Zucchini	NEUTRAL	NEUTRAL	NEUTRAL	NEUTRAL

▪ FRUIT/FRUIT JUICE

Food Item	BLOOD GROUP A	BLOOD GROUP B	BLOOD GROUP AB	BLOOD GROUP O
Apple/Apple Juice/Cider	NEUTRAL	NEUTRAL	NEUTRAL	NEUTRAL Non-secretor variant: AVOID
Apricot/Apricot Juice	BENEFICIAL: Contains component that positively influences known disease susceptibility.	NEUTRAL	NEUTRAL	NEUTRAL Non-secretor variant: AVOID
Asian Pear	NEUTRAL	NEUTRAL	NEUTRAL	AVOID: Contains lectin or other agglutinin.
Avocado	NEUTRAL	AVOID: Contains lectin or other agglutinin.	AVOID: Contains lectin or other agglutinin.	AVOID Non-secretor variant: BENEFICIAL
Banana	AVOID: Contains lectin or other agglutinin; metabolic inhibitor; provokes abnormal blood reaction. Non-secretor variant: NEUTRAL	BENEFICIAL: Contains an agglutinin that modifies disease susceptibility. Non-secretor variant: NEUTRAL	AVOID: Contains lectin or other agglutinin.	BENEFICIAL: Contains an agglutinin that modifies disease susceptibility.
Bitter Melon	AVOID: Contains lectin or other agglutinin.	AVOID: Contains lectin or other agglutinin.	AVOID: Contains lectin or other agglutinin.	AVOID: Contains lectin or other agglutinin; contains component that can modify known disease susceptibility.
Blackberry/Blackberry Juice	BENEFICIAL: Contains component that either blocks polyamine synthesis or lowers indican levels.	NEUTRAL Non-secretor variant: BENEFICIAL	NEUTRAL Non-secretor variant: BENEFICIAL	AVOID: Contains lectin or other agglutinin.
Blueberry	BENEFICIAL: Contains component that either blocks polyamine synthesis or lowers indican levels.	NEUTRAL Non-secretor variant: BENEFICIAL	NEUTRAL Non-secretor variant: BENEFICIAL	BENEFICIAL: Contains component that either blocks polyamine synthesis or lowers indican levels.
Boysenberry	BENEFICIAL: Contains component that either blocks polyamine synthesis or lowers indican levels.	NEUTRAL Non-secretor variant: BENEFICIAL	NEUTRAL	NEUTRAL

■ **FRUIT/FRUIT JUICE, CONTINUED**

Food Item	BLOOD GROUP A	BLOOD GROUP B	BLOOD GROUP AB	BLOOD GROUP O
Breadfruit	NEUTRAL	NEUTRAL	NEUTRAL	NEUTRAL
Canang Melon	NEUTRAL	NEUTRAL	NEUTRAL	NEUTRAL
Cantaloupe	NEUTRAL Non-secretor variant: AVOID	NEUTRAL Non-secretor variant: AVOID	NEUTRAL Non-secretor variant: AVOID	AVOID: Increases intestinal imbalance.
Casaba Melon	NEUTRAL Non-secretor variant: AVOID	NEUTRAL	NEUTRAL	NEUTRAL
Cherry (all)	BENEFICIAL: Contains component that either blocks polyamine synthesis or lowers indican levels.	NEUTRAL Non-secretor variant: BENEFICIAL	BENEFICIAL: Contains component that either blocks polyamine synthesis or lowers indican levels.	BENEFICIAL: Contains component that either blocks polyamine synthesis or lowers indican levels.
Cherry Juice (Black)	BENEFICIAL: Contains component that either blocks polyamine synthesis or lowers indican levels.	NEUTRAL Non-secretor variant: BENEFICIAL	BENEFICIAL: Contains component that either blocks polyamine synthesis or lowers indican levels.	BENEFICIAL: Contains component that either blocks polyamine synthesis or lowers indican levels.
Christmas Melon	NEUTRAL	NEUTRAL	NEUTRAL	NEUTRAL
Coconut	AVOID: Provokes abnormal blood reaction. Non-secretor variant: NEUTRAL	AVOID: Provokes abnormal blood reaction.	AVOID: Enhances effect of other food toxins.	AVOID: Enhances effect of other food toxins; provokes abnormal blood reaction.
Coconut Milk	AVOID: Provokes abnormal blood reaction. Non-secretor variant: NEUTRAL	AVOID: Provokes abnormal blood reaction.	AVOID: Provokes abnormal blood reaction.	AVOID: Enhances effect of other food toxins; contains component that can modify known disease susceptibility.
Cranberry	BENEFICIAL: Contains component that either blocks polyamine synthesis or lowers indican levels.	BENEFICIAL: Contains component that either blocks polyamine synthesis or lowers indican levels.	BENEFICIAL: Contains component that either blocks polyamine synthesis or lowers indican levels.	NEUTRAL
Cranberry Juice	NEUTRAL Non-secretor variant: BENEFICIAL	BENEFICIAL: Contains component that positively influences known disease susceptibility.	BENEFICIAL: Contains component that either blocks polyamine synthesis or lowers indican levels.	NEUTRAL

■ **FRUIT/FRUIT JUICE, CONTINUED**

Food Item	BLOOD GROUP A	BLOOD GROUP B	BLOOD GROUP AB	BLOOD GROUP O
Crenshaw Melon	NEUTRAL	NEUTRAL	NEUTRAL	NEUTRAL
Currants (Black/Red)	NEUTRAL	NEUTRAL Non-secretor variant: BENEFICIAL	NEUTRAL	NEUTRAL
Date (all)	NEUTRAL	NEUTRAL	NEUTRAL	NEUTRAL Non-secretor variant: AVOID
Dewberry	NEUTRAL	NEUTRAL	AVOID: Provokes abnormal blood reaction.	NEUTRAL
Elderberry (Dark Blue/Purple)	NEUTRAL Non-secretor variant: BENEFICIAL	NEUTRAL Non-secretor variant: BENEFICIAL	NEUTRAL Non-secretor variant: BENEFICIAL	NEUTRAL
Fig (Fresh/Dried)	BENEFICIAL: Contains component that positively influences known disease susceptibility.	NEUTRAL Non-secretor variant: BENEFICIAL	BENEFICIAL: Contains component that either blocks polyamine synthesis or lowers indican levels.	BENEFICIAL: Contains component that either blocks polyamine synthesis or lowers indican levels.
Gooseberry	NEUTRAL	NEUTRAL	BENEFICIAL: Contains component that either blocks polyamine synthesis or lowers indican levels.	NEUTRAL
Grape (all)	NEUTRAL	BENEFICIAL: Contains component that either blocks polyamine synthesis or lowers indican levels.	BENEFICIAL: Contains component that either blocks polyamine synthesis or lowers indican levels.	NEUTRAL
Grapefruit	BENEFICIAL: Contains component that positively influences known disease susceptibility.	NEUTRAL	BENEFICIAL: Contains component that positively influences known disease susceptibility.	NEUTRAL
Grapefruit Juice	BENEFICIAL: Contains component that positively influences known disease susceptibility.	NEUTRAL	NEUTRAL	NEUTRAL

■ FRUIT/FRUIT JUICE, CONTINUED

Food Item	BLOOD GROUP A	BLOOD GROUP B	BLOOD GROUP AB	BLOOD GROUP O
Guava/Guava Juice	NEUTRAL	NEUTRAL Non-secretor variant: BENEFICIAL	AVOID: Provokes abnormal blood reaction.	BENEFICIAL: Healthy alternative to more common variety of foods which are classed as avoids.
Honeydew	AVOID: Provokes abnormal blood reaction.	NEUTRAL Non-secretor variant: AVOID	NEUTRAL Non-secretor variant: AVOID	AVOID: Enhances effect of other food toxins.
Kiwi	NEUTRAL	NEUTRAL	BENEFICIAL: Contains component that either blocks polyamine synthesis or lowers indican levels.	AVOID: Metabolic inhibitor.
Kumquat	NEUTRAL	NEUTRAL	NEUTRAL	NEUTRAL
Lemon/Lemon Juice	BENEFICIAL: Contains component that positively influences known disease susceptibility.	NEUTRAL	BENEFICIAL: Contains component that positively influences known disease susceptibility.	NEUTRAL
Lime/Lime Juice	BENEFICIAL: Contains component that positively influences known disease susceptibility. Non-secretor variant: NEUTRAL	NEUTRAL	NEUTRAL Non-secretor variant: BENEFICIAL	NEUTRAL
Loganberry	NEUTRAL	NEUTRAL	BENEFICIAL: Contains component that either blocks polyamine synthesis or lowers indican levels.	NEUTRAL
Mango/Mango Juice	AVOID: Provokes abnormal blood reaction; increases polyamine or indican levels. Non-secretor variant: NEUTRAL	NEUTRAL	AVOID: Increases polyamine or indican levels.	BENEFICIAL: Contains component that positively influences known disease susceptibility.
Mulberry	NEUTRAL	NEUTRAL	NEUTRAL	NEUTRAL
Muskmelon	NEUTRAL	NEUTRAL	NEUTRAL	NEUTRAL

■ **FRUIT/FRUIT JUICE, CONTINUED**

Food Item	BLOOD GROUP A	BLOOD GROUP B	BLOOD GROUP AB	BLOOD GROUP O
Nectarine/ Nectarine Juice	NEUTRAL	NEUTRAL	NEUTRAL	NEUTRAL
Orange/Orange Juice	AVOID: Increases polyamine or indican levels; inhibits proper gastric function or blocks assimilation.	NEUTRAL	AVOID: Increases polyamine or indican levels.	AVOID: Increases polyamine or indican levels; metabolic inhibitor.
Papaya/Papaya Juice	AVOID: Provokes abnormal blood reaction.	BENEFICIAL: Contains component that either blocks polyamine synthesis or lowers indican levels.	NEUTRAL	NEUTRAL
Peach	NEUTRAL	NEUTRAL	NEUTRAL	NEUTRAL
Pear/Pear Juice	NEUTRAL	NEUTRAL	NEUTRAL	NEUTRAL
Persian Melon	NEUTRAL	NEUTRAL	NEUTRAL	NEUTRAL
Persimmon	NEUTRAL	AVOID: Contains lectin or other agglutinin.	AVOID: Contains lectin or other agglutinin.	NEUTRAL
Pineapple	BENEFICIAL: Contains component that positively influences known disease susceptibility.	BENEFICIAL: Contains component that positively influences known disease susceptibility.	BENEFICIAL: Contains component that positively influences known disease susceptibility.	NEUTRAL
Pineapple Juice	BENEFICIAL: Contains component that positively influences known disease susceptibility.	BENEFICIAL: Contains component that positively influences known disease susceptibility.	NEUTRAL	BENEFICIAL: Contains component that positively influences known disease susceptibility.
Plantain	AVOID: Provokes abnormal blood reaction.	NEUTRAL	NEUTRAL	AVOID: Contains lectin or other agglutinin.
Plum (Dark/Green/Red)	BENEFICIAL: Contains component that either blocks polyamine synthesis or lowers indican levels.	BENEFICIAL: Contains component that either blocks polyamine synthesis or lowers indican levels.	BENEFICIAL: Contains component that either blocks polyamine synthesis or lowers indican levels.	BENEFICIAL: Contains component that either blocks polyamine synthesis or lowers indican levels.
Pomegranate	NEUTRAL	AVOID: Contains lectin or other agglutinin.	AVOID: Contains lectin or other agglutinin.	NEUTRAL Non-secretor variant: BENEFICIAL

▪ FRUIT/FRUIT JUICE, CONTINUED

Food Item	BLOOD GROUP A	BLOOD GROUP B	BLOOD GROUP AB	BLOOD GROUP O
Prickly Pear	NEUTRAL	AVOID: Provokes abnormal blood reaction.	AVOID: Provokes abnormal blood reaction.	NEUTRAL Non-secretor variant: BENEFICIAL
Prune	BENEFICIAL: Contains component that either blocks polyamine synthesis or lowers indican levels.	NEUTRAL	NEUTRAL Non-secretor variant: AVOID	BENEFICIAL: Contains component that either blocks polyamine synthesis or lowers indican levels.
Quince	NEUTRAL	NEUTRAL	AVOID: Contains lectin or other agglutinin.	NEUTRAL
Raisin	NEUTRAL	NEUTRAL	NEUTRAL	NEUTRAL
Raspberry	NEUTRAL	NEUTRAL Non-secretor variant: BENEFICIAL	NEUTRAL	NEUTRAL
Sago Palm	NEUTRAL	NEUTRAL	AVOID: Metabolic inhibitor.	NEUTRAL
Spanish Melon	NEUTRAL	NEUTRAL	NEUTRAL	NEUTRAL
Starfruit (Carambola)	NEUTRAL	AVOID: Contains lectin or other agglutinin.	AVOID: Provokes abnormal blood reaction.	NEUTRAL
Strawberry	NEUTRAL	NEUTRAL	NEUTRAL	NEUTRAL Non-secretor variant: AVOID
Tangerine	AVOID: Provokes abnormal blood reaction; increases polyamine or indican levels. Non-secretor variant: NEUTRAL	NEUTRAL	NEUTRAL Non-secretor variant: AVOID	AVOID: Increases polyamine or indican levels; metabolic inhibitor.
Water & Lemon	BENEFICIAL: Contains component that positively influences known disease susceptibility.	NEUTRAL	NEUTRAL	NEUTRAL

■ FRUIT/FRUIT JUICE, CONTINUED

Food Item	BLOOD GROUP A	BLOOD GROUP B	BLOOD GROUP AB	BLOOD GROUP O
Watermelon	NEUTRAL Non-secretor variant: BEN-EFICIAL	BENEFICIAL: Contains component that positively influences known disease susceptibility.	BENEFICIAL: Contains component that positively influences known disease susceptibility.	NEUTRAL
Youngberry	NEUTRAL	NEUTRAL	NEUTRAL	NEUTRAL

■ OIL

Food Item	BLOOD GROUP A	BLOOD GROUP B	BLOOD GROUP AB	BLOOD GROUP O
Almond Oil	NEUTRAL	NEUTRAL	NEUTRAL	NEUTRAL Non-secretor variant: BEN-EFICIAL
Black Currant Seed Oil	BENEFICIAL: Contains component that positively influences known disease susceptibility.	NEUTRAL Non-secretor variant: BEN-EFICIAL	NEUTRAL	NEUTRAL
Borage Seed Oil	NEUTRAL	AVOID: Provokes abnormal blood reaction.	NEUTRAL	NEUTRAL Non-secretor variant: AVOID
Canola Oil	NEUTRAL	AVOID: Provokes abnormal blood reaction.	NEUTRAL	NEUTRAL Non-secretor variant: AVOID
Castor Oil	AVOID: Secretory insufficiency.	AVOID: Provokes abnormal blood reaction.	NEUTRAL	AVOID: Contains lectin or other agglutinin.
Coconut Oil	AVOID: Provokes abnormal blood reaction.	AVOID: Provokes abnormal blood reaction.	AVOID: Enhances effect of other food toxins.	AVOID Non-secretor variant: NEU-TRAL
Cod Liver Oil	NEUTRAL Non-secretor variant: BEN-EFICIAL	NEUTRAL	NEUTRAL	NEUTRAL Non-secretor variant: AVOID

■ **OIL, CONTINUED**

Food Item	BLOOD GROUP A	BLOOD GROUP B	BLOOD GROUP AB	BLOOD GROUP O
Corn Oil	AVOID: Secretory insufficiency; interferes with cardiovascular activity.	AVOID: Contains lectin or other agglutinin.	AVOID: Contains lectin or other agglutinin.	AVOID: Contains lectin or other agglutinin.
Cottonseed Oil	AVOID: Secretory insufficiency; interferes with cardiovascular activity.	AVOID: Provokes abnormal blood reaction.	AVOID: Contains component that can modify known disease susceptibility.	AVOID: Enhances effect of other food toxins; metabolic inhibitor.
Evening Primrose Oil	NEUTRAL	NEUTRAL	NEUTRAL	AVOID: Enhances effect of other food toxins.
Flax Seed (Linseed) Oil	BENEFICIAL: Contains component that positively influences known disease susceptibility.	NEUTRAL Non-secretor variant: BENEFICIAL	NEUTRAL	BENEFICIAL Non-secretor variant: NEUTRAL
Olive Oil	BENEFICIAL: Contains component that positively influences known disease susceptibility.	BENEFICIAL: Contains component that positively influences known disease susceptibility.	BENEFICIAL: Contains component that positively influences known disease susceptibility.	BENEFICIAL: Contains component that positively influences known disease susceptibility.
Peanut Oil	AVOID: Secretory insufficiency; interferes with cardiovascular activity. Non-secretor variant: NEUTRAL	AVOID: Provokes abnormal blood reaction.	NEUTRAL	AVOID: Enhances effect of other food toxins; provokes abnormal blood reaction; metabolic inhibitor.
Safflower Oil	NEUTRAL Non-secretor variant: AVOID	AVOID: Provokes abnormal blood reaction.	AVOID: Contains component that can modify known disease susceptibility.	AVOID: Increases polyamine or indican levels; inhibits proper gastric function or blocks assimilation.
Sesame Oil	NEUTRAL Non-secretor variant: BENEFICIAL	AVOID: Contains lectin or other agglutinin.	AVOID: Contains lectin or other agglutinin.	NEUTRAL
Soy Oil	NEUTRAL	AVOID: Contains lectin or other agglutinin.	NEUTRAL	AVOID: Provokes abnormal blood reaction.
Sunflower Oil	NEUTRAL	AVOID: Contains lectin or other agglutinin.	AVOID: Contains lectin or other agglutinin.	AVOID: Provokes abnormal blood reaction.

OIL, CONTINUED

Food Item	BLOOD GROUP A	BLOOD GROUP B	BLOOD GROUP AB	BLOOD GROUP O
Walnut Oil	BENEFICIAL: Contains component that either blocks polyamine synthesis or lowers indican levels.	NEUTRAL Non-secretor variant: BENEFICIAL	BENEFICIAL: Contains component that either blocks polyamine synthesis or lowers indican levels.	NEUTRAL Non-secretor variant: BENEFICIAL
Wheat Germ Oil	NEUTRAL	NEUTRAL	NEUTRAL	AVOID: Provokes abnormal blood reaction; increases intestinal imbalance; increases polyamine or indican levels.

HERB/SPICE

Food Item	BLOOD GROUP A	BLOOD GROUP B	BLOOD GROUP AB	BLOOD GROUP O
Acacia (Arabic Gum)	AVOID: Provokes abnormal blood reaction; contains lectin or other agglutinin; metabolic inhibitor; increases lectin activity and binding.	AVOID: Provokes abnormal blood reaction.	AVOID: Provokes abnormal blood reaction.	AVOID: Provokes abnormal blood reaction.
Allspice	NEUTRAL	AVOID: Provokes abnormal blood reaction.	AVOID: Provokes abnormal blood reaction.	NEUTRAL
Anise	NEUTRAL	NEUTRAL	AVOID: Provokes abnormal blood reaction.	NEUTRAL
Arrowroot	NEUTRAL	NEUTRAL	NEUTRAL	NEUTRAL
Basil	NEUTRAL	NEUTRAL	NEUTRAL	NEUTRAL Non-secretor variant: BENEFICIAL
Bay Leaf	NEUTRAL	NEUTRAL	NEUTRAL Non-secretor variant: BENEFICIAL	NEUTRAL Non-secretor variant: BENEFICIAL
Bergamot	NEUTRAL	NEUTRAL	NEUTRAL	NEUTRAL
Caraway	NEUTRAL	NEUTRAL	NEUTRAL	NEUTRAL

▪ HERB/SPICE, CONTINUED

Food Item	BLOOD GROUP A	BLOOD GROUP B	BLOOD GROUP AB	BLOOD GROUP O
Cardamom	NEUTRAL	NEUTRAL	NEUTRAL	NEUTRAL
Carob	NEUTRAL	NEUTRAL	NEUTRAL	BENEFICIAL: Healthy alternative to more common variety of foods which are classed as avoids. Non-secretor variant: NEUTRAL
Chervil	NEUTRAL	NEUTRAL	NEUTRAL	NEUTRAL
Chili Powder	AVOID: Provokes abnormal blood reaction. Non-secretor variant: NEUTRAL	NEUTRAL	NEUTRAL	NEUTRAL
Chives	NEUTRAL	NEUTRAL	NEUTRAL	NEUTRAL
Chocolate	NEUTRAL	NEUTRAL	NEUTRAL	NEUTRAL
Cilantro	NEUTRAL Non-secretor variant: BENEFICIAL	NEUTRAL	NEUTRAL	NEUTRAL
Cinnamon	NEUTRAL	AVOID: Provokes abnormal blood reaction.	NEUTRAL	NEUTRAL Non-secretor variant: AVOID
Clove	NEUTRAL	NEUTRAL	NEUTRAL	NEUTRAL
Coriander	NEUTRAL	NEUTRAL	NEUTRAL	NEUTRAL
Cornstarch	NEUTRAL Non-secretor variant: AVOID	AVOID: Contains lectin or other agglutinin.	AVOID: Contains lectin or other agglutinin.	AVOID: Contains lectin or other agglutinin; metabolic inhibitor; contains component that can modify known disease susceptibility.
Cream of Tartar	NEUTRAL	NEUTRAL	NEUTRAL	NEUTRAL

■ **HERB/SPICE, CONTINUED**

Food Item	BLOOD GROUP A	BLOOD GROUP B	BLOOD GROUP AB	BLOOD GROUP O
Cumin	NEUTRAL	NEUTRAL	NEUTRAL	NEUTRAL
Curry	NEUTRAL	BENEFICIAL: Contains component that either blocks polyamine synthesis or lowers indican levels.	BENEFICIAL: Contains component that either blocks polyamine synthesis or lowers indican levels.	BENEFICIAL: Contains component that either blocks polyamine synthesis or lowers indican levels.
Dill	NEUTRAL	NEUTRAL	NEUTRAL	NEUTRAL
Dulse	NEUTRAL	NEUTRAL	NEUTRAL	BENEFICIAL: Metabolic enhancer.
Guarana	NEUTRAL	AVOID: Increases polyamine or indican levels; inhibits proper gastric function or blocks assimilation.	AVOID: Increases polyamine or indican levels; inhibits proper gastric function or blocks assimilation.	AVOID: Enhances effect of other food toxins.
Licorice Root	NEUTRAL	BENEFICIAL: Contains component that positively influences known disease susceptibility.	NEUTRAL	NEUTRAL Non-secretor variant: BENEFICIAL
Mace	NEUTRAL	NEUTRAL	NEUTRAL	AVOID: Provokes abnormal blood reaction.
Marjoram	NEUTRAL	NEUTRAL	NEUTRAL	NEUTRAL
Mustard, Dry	BENEFICIAL: Contains component that either blocks polyamine synthesis or lowers indican levels.	NEUTRAL	NEUTRAL	NEUTRAL
Nutmeg	NEUTRAL	NEUTRAL	NEUTRAL	AVOID Non-secretor variant: NEUTRAL
Oregano	NEUTRAL	NEUTRAL Non-secretor variant: BENEFICIAL	BENEFICIAL: Contains component that either blocks polyamine synthesis or lowers indican levels.	NEUTRAL Non-secretor variant: BENEFICIAL
Paprika	NEUTRAL	NEUTRAL	NEUTRAL	NEUTRAL

◼ HERB/SPICE, CONTINUED

Food Item	BLOOD GROUP A	BLOOD GROUP B	BLOOD GROUP AB	BLOOD GROUP O
Parsley	BENEFICIAL: Contains component that either blocks polyamine synthesis or lowers indican levels. Non-secretor variant: NEUTRAL	BENEFICIAL: Contains component that either blocks polyamine synthesis or lowers indican levels.	BENEFICIAL: Contains component that either blocks polyamine synthesis or lowers indican levels.	BENEFICIAL: Contains component that positively influences known disease susceptibility.
Pepper (Black/White)	AVOID: Provokes abnormal blood reaction.	AVOID: Provokes abnormal blood reaction; increases polyamine or indican levels.	AVOID: Gastric irritant; inhibits proper digestive function.	AVOID: Gastric irritant; inhibits proper digestive function; contains component that can modify known disease susceptibility.
Pepper (Peppercorn/ Red Flakes)	AVOID: Provokes abnormal blood reaction.	NEUTRAL	AVOID: Gastric irritant; inhibits proper digestive function.	NEUTRAL
Peppermint	NEUTRAL	NEUTRAL	NEUTRAL	NEUTRAL
Rosemary	NEUTRAL	NEUTRAL	NEUTRAL	NEUTRAL
Saffron	NEUTRAL	NEUTRAL	NEUTRAL	NEUTRAL Non-secretor variant: BENEFICIAL
Sage	NEUTRAL	NEUTRAL	NEUTRAL	NEUTRAL
Savory	NEUTRAL	NEUTRAL	NEUTRAL	NEUTRAL
Senna	NEUTRAL Non-secretor variant: AVOID	NEUTRAL	NEUTRAL	NEUTRAL
Spearmint	NEUTRAL	NEUTRAL	NEUTRAL	NEUTRAL
Tamarind	NEUTRAL	NEUTRAL	NEUTRAL	NEUTRAL
Tarragon	NEUTRAL	NEUTRAL	NEUTRAL	NEUTRAL Non-secretor variant: BENEFICIAL
Thyme	NEUTRAL	NEUTRAL	NEUTRAL	NEUTRAL

■ HERB/SPICE, CONTINUED

Food Item	BLOOD GROUP A	BLOOD GROUP B	BLOOD GROUP AB	BLOOD GROUP O
Turmeric	BENEFICIAL: Contains component that either blocks polyamine synthesis or lowers indican levels. Non-secretor variant: NEUTRAL	NEUTRAL	NEUTRAL Non-secretor variant: BENEFICIAL	BENEFICIAL: Contains component that either blocks polyamine synthesis or lowers indican levels. Non-secretor variant: NEUTRAL
Vanilla	NEUTRAL	NEUTRAL	NEUTRAL	NEUTRAL Non-secretor variant: AVOID
Wintergreen	AVOID: Provokes abnormal blood reaction. Non-secretor variant: NEUTRAL	NEUTRAL	NEUTRAL	NEUTRAL

■ CONDIMENT

Food Item	BLOOD GROUP A	BLOOD GROUP B	BLOOD GROUP AB	BLOOD GROUP O
Apple Pectin	NEUTRAL	NEUTRAL	NEUTRAL	NEUTRAL
Carrageenan	AVOID: Contains lectin or other agglutinin; metabolic inhibitor.	AVOID: Provokes abnormal blood reaction; metabolic inhibitor.	AVOID: Increases polyamine or indican levels.	AVOID: Contains component that can modify known disease susceptibility.
Gelatin, Plain	AVOID: Contains lectin or other agglutinin; metabolic inhibitor.	AVOID: Increases polyamine or indican levels; metabolic inhibitor; inhibits proper gastric function or blocks assimilation.	AVOID: Metabolic inhibitor.	NEUTRAL
Guar Gum	AVOID: Contains lectin or other agglutinin; metabolic inhibitor.	AVOID: Increases polyamine or indican levels; metabolic inhibitor; inhibits proper gastric function or blocks assimilation.	AVOID: Metabolic inhibitor.	AVOID: Provokes abnormal blood reaction.
Jam/Jelly (OK ingredients)	NEUTRAL	NEUTRAL	NEUTRAL	NEUTRAL

CONDIMENT, CONTINUED

Food Item	BLOOD GROUP A	BLOOD GROUP B	BLOOD GROUP AB	BLOOD GROUP O
Ketchup	AVOID: Provokes abnormal blood reaction; contains lectin or other agglutinin; metabolic inhibitor.	AVOID: Contains lectin or other agglutinin.	AVOID: Enhances effect of other food toxins.	AVOID: Contains lectin or other agglutinin.
Mayonnaise	AVOID: Provokes abnormal blood reaction.	NEUTRAL	NEUTRAL	NEUTRAL Non-secretor variant: AVOID
Miso	BENEFICIAL: Contains an agglutinin that modifies disease susceptibility.	AVOID: Contains lectin or other agglutinin.	BENEFICIAL Non-secretor variant: NEUTRAL	NEUTRAL Non-secretor variant: AVOID
MSG	AVOID: Increases polyamine or indican levels.	AVOID: Increases polyamine or indican levels; metabolic inhibitor.	AVOID: Enhances effect of other food toxins.	AVOID Non-secretor variant: NEUTRAL
Mustard (with vinegar and wheat)	AVOID	NEUTRAL Non-secretor variant: AVOID	AVOID: Gastric irritant; inhibits proper digestive function.	AVOID: Gastric irritant; inhibits proper digestive function.
Mustard (with vinegar, wheat-free).	NEUTRAL	NEUTRAL	AVOID: Gastric irritant; inhibits proper digestive function.	AVOID: Gastric irritant; inhibits proper digestive function.
Mustard (with wheat, vinegar-free)	BENEFICIAL: Contains component that either blocks polyamine synthesis or lowers indican levels.	NEUTRAL Non-secretor variant: AVOID	NEUTRAL Non-secretor variant: AVOID	AVOID: Gastric irritant; inhibits proper digestive function.
Mustard (wheat-free, vinegar-free)	BENEFICIAL: Contains component that either blocks polyamine synthesis or lowers indican levels.	NEUTRAL	NEUTRAL	NEUTRAL
Pickle Relish	AVOID: Provokes abnormal blood reaction.	NEUTRAL Non-secretor variant: AVOID	AVOID: Gastric irritant; inhibits proper digestive function.	AVOID: Gastric irritant; inhibits proper digestive function.
Salad Dressing (OK ingredients)	NEUTRAL	NEUTRAL	NEUTRAL	NEUTRAL

■ **CONDIMENT, CONTINUED**

Food Item	BLOOD GROUP A	BLOOD GROUP B	BLOOD GROUP AB	BLOOD GROUP O
Sea Salt	NEUTRAL	NEUTRAL	NEUTRAL	NEUTRAL
Soy Sauce	BENEFICIAL: Contains an agglutinin that modifies disease susceptibility. Non-secretor variant: NEUTRAL	AVOID: Contains lectin or other agglutinin.	NEUTRAL	NEUTRAL Non-secretor variant: AVOID
Tamari (wheat-free)	BENEFICIAL: Contains an agglutinin that modifies disease susceptibility. Non-secretor variant: NEUTRAL	NEUTRAL	NEUTRAL	NEUTRAL Non-secretor variant: AVOID
Vinegar (Apple Cider)	AVOID: Provokes abnormal blood reaction.	NEUTRAL	AVOID: Gastric irritant; inhibits proper digestive function.	NEUTRAL Non-secretor variant: AVOID
Vinegar (Balsamic/ White/Red/Rice)	AVOID: Provokes abnormal blood reaction.	NEUTRAL	AVOID: Gastric irritant; inhibits proper digestive function.	AVOID: Gastric irritant; inhibits proper digestive function.
Worcestershire Sauce	AVOID: Increases polyamine or indican levels.	AVOID: Increases polyamine or indican levels.	AVOID: Increases polyamine or indican levels.	AVOID: Increases polyamine or indican levels.
Yeast (Baker's)	NEUTRAL	NEUTRAL	NEUTRAL	NEUTRAL
Yeast (Brewer's)	NEUTRAL Non-secretor variant: BENEFICIAL	NEUTRAL Non-secretor variant: BENEFICIAL	NEUTRAL Non-secretor variant: BENEFICIAL	NEUTRAL Non-secretor variant: BENEFICIAL

■ **SWEETENER**

Food Item	BLOOD GROUP A	BLOOD GROUP B	BLOOD GROUP AB	BLOOD GROUP O
Almond Extract	NEUTRAL	AVOID: Increases polyamine or indican levels.	AVOID: Increases polyamine or indican levels; flocculates serum or precipitates serum proteins.	NEUTRAL

◾ SWEETNER, CONTINUED

Food Item	BLOOD GROUP A	BLOOD GROUP B	BLOOD GROUP AB	BLOOD GROUP O
Aspartame	AVOID: Provokes abnormal blood reaction; inhibits proper gastric function or blocks assimilation.	AVOID: Inhibits proper gastric function or blocks assimilation; metabolic inhibitor.	AVOID: Metabolic inhibitor.	AVOID: Metabolic inhibitor.
Barley Malt	BENEFICIAL: Healthy alternative to more common variety of foods which are classed as avoids. Non-secretor variant: NEUTRAL	AVOID: Provokes abnormal blood reaction.	AVOID: Increases polyamine or indican level.	NEUTRAL Non-secretor variant: AVOID
Corn Syrup	NEUTRAL Non-secretor variant: AVOID	AVOID: Contains lectin or other agglutinin.	AVOID: Contains lectin or other agglutinin.	AVOID: Metabolic inhibitor; contains lectin or other agglutinin.
Dextrose	NEUTRAL Non-secretor variant: AVOID	AVOID: Provokes abnormal blood reaction.	AVOID: Enhances effect of other food toxins.	AVOID: Metabolic inhibitor.
Fructose	NEUTRAL	NEUTRAL Non-secretor variant: AVOID	AVOID: Metabolic inhibitor.	AVOID: Metabolic inhibitor.
Honey	NEUTRAL	NEUTRAL	NEUTRAL Non-secretor variant: AVOID	NEUTRAL Non-secretor variant: AVOID
Invert Sugar	NEUTRAL Non-secretor variant: AVOID	AVOID: Provokes abnormal blood reaction.	AVOID: Metabolic inhibitor.	AVOID: Metabolic inhibitor.
Maltodextrin	NEUTRAL Non-secretor variant: AVOID	AVOID: Contains lectin or other agglutinin; increases polyamine or indican levels.	AVOID: Metabolic inhibitor.	AVOID: Metabolic inhibitor.
Maple Syrup	NEUTRAL	NEUTRAL	NEUTRAL Non-secretor variant: AVOID	NEUTRAL Non-secretor variant: AVOID

■ SWEETNER, CONTINUED

Food Item	BLOOD GROUP A	BLOOD GROUP B	BLOOD GROUP AB	BLOOD GROUP O
Molasses	NEUTRAL	NEUTRAL	NEUTRAL	NEUTRAL
Molasses (Blackstrap)	BENEFICIAL: Contains component which positively influences known disease susceptibility. Non-secretor variant: NEUTRAL	BENEFICIAL: Contains component that positively influences known disease susceptibility.	BENEFICIAL: Contains component that positively influences known disease susceptibility.	NEUTRAL
Rice Syrup	NEUTRAL	NEUTRAL	NEUTRAL Non-secretor variant: AVOID	NEUTRAL Non-secretor variant: AVOID
Stevia	NEUTRAL	AVOID Non-secretor variant: NEUTRAL	NEUTRAL	NEUTRAL Non-secretor variant: AVOID
Sucanat	AVOID: Provokes abnormal blood reaction.	AVOID: Provokes abnormal blood reaction.	AVOID: Metabolic inhibitor.	NEUTRAL Non-secretor variant: AVOID
Sugar (Brown/White)	NEUTRAL	NEUTRAL Non-secretor variant: AVOID	NEUTRAL Non-secretor variant: AVOID	NEUTRAL Non-secretor variant: AVOID

■ BEVERAGE

Food Item	BLOOD GROUP A	BLOOD GROUP B	BLOOD GROUP AB	BLOOD GROUP O
Beer	AVOID: Provokes abnormal blood reaction. Non-secretor variant: NEUTRAL	NEUTRAL	NEUTRAL Non-secretor variant: AVOID	AVOID: Contains component that can modify known disease susceptibility.
Coffee (Regular/Decaf)	BENEFICIAL: Contains an agglutinin that modifies disease susceptibility.	NEUTRAL Non-secretor variant: AVOID	AVOID: Provokes abnormal blood reaction.	AVOID: Contains component that can modify known disease susceptibility.

▪ BEVERAGE, CONTINUED

Food Item	BLOOD GROUP A	BLOOD GROUP B	BLOOD GROUP AB	BLOOD GROUP O
Green Tea	BENEFICIAL: Contains component that either blocks polyamine synthesis or lowers indican levels.	BENEFICIAL: Contains component that positively influences known disease susceptibility.	BENEFICIAL: Contains component that either blocks polyamine synthesis or lowers indican levels.	BENEFICIAL: Contains component that either blocks polyamine synthesis or lowers indican levels.
Liquor (Distilled)	AVOID: Secretory insufficiency.	AVOID: Inhibits proper gastric function or blocks assimilation. Non-secretor variant: NEUTRAL	AVOID Non-secretor variant: NEUTRAL	AVOID: Contains component that can modify known disease susceptibility.
Seltzer Water	AVOID: Secretory insufficiency; inhibits proper gastric function or blocks assimilation. Non-secretor variant: NEUTRAL	AVOID: Inhibits proper gastric function or blocks assimilation; metabolic inhibitor. Non-secretor variant: NEUTRAL	NEUTRAL	BENEFICIAL: Contains component that positively influences known disease susceptibility.
Soda (Club)	AVOID: Secretory insufficiency.	AVOID: Inhibits proper gastric function or blocks assimilation. Non-secretor variant: NEUTRAL	NEUTRAL	BENEFICIAL: Contains component which positively influences known disease susceptibility.
Soda (Misc./Diet/Cola)	AVOID: Secretory insufficiency; inhibits proper gastric function or blocks assimilation.	AVOID: Inhibits proper gastric function or blocks assimilation.	AVOID: Metabolic inhibitor.	AVOID: Inhibits proper digestive function.
Tea (Black Regular/Decaf)	AVOID: Secretory insufficiency. Non-secretor variant: NEUTRAL	NEUTRAL Non-secretor variant: AVOID	AVOID: Contains component that can modify known disease susceptibility.	AVOID: Contains component that can modify known disease susceptibility.
Wine (Red)	BENEFICIAL: Contains component that either blocks polyamine synthesis or lowers indican levels.	NEUTRAL Non-secretor variant: BENEFICIAL	NEUTRAL Non-secretor variant: BENEFICIAL	NEUTRAL Non-secretor variant: BENEFICIAL
Wine (White)	NEUTRAL Non-secretor variant: BENEFICIAL	NEUTRAL Non-secretor variant: BENEFICIAL	NEUTRAL	AVOID: Contains component that can modify known disease susceptibility.

═══

THREE

Blood Group Supplement Base

Use this supplement database as a cross-reference for the blood group protocols, and to gain additional information about the specific supplements recommended in each protocol. Listed here are the individualized blood group–specific beneficial effects of each supplement. This list is not intended as a comprehensive description of all supplements and their benefits, but as a targeted reference to help each blood group gain their maximum health benefits.

COMMON NAME	BLOOD GROUP–SPECIFIC BENE-FICIAL EFFECT	PRIMARY ACTION
Aloe	➤ GROUP A Intestinal Health	Used to treat minor cuts and burns. Also useful as a laxative.
American Cranesbill	➤ GROUP O Stomach Health	Used as an astringent and to treat gastrointestinal bleeding.

COMMON NAME	BLOOD GROUP–SPECIFIC BENEFICIAL EFFECT	PRIMARY ACTION
Arabinogalactan	➤ ALL BLOOD GROUPS Antibacterial Antibiotic Support Antiviral Cancer Prevention Chemotherapy Adjunct Immune-Enhancing Pulmonary Support Yeast/Fungus Resistance	An immune modulator and adaptogenic agent. Also used as a source of dietary fiber and to treat digestive ailments.
Arginine	➤ GROUP B Immune-Enhancing Male Health Surgery Recovery ➤ GROUP AB Antiviral Chronic Illness Recovery	Facilitates immune function. Increases nitric oxide and assists in wound healing.
Artichoke leaf	➤ GROUP A Cardiovascular Liver Support ➤ GROUP O Cardiovascular Liver Support	Digestive tonic that enhances liver function and promotes detoxification.
Ascorbic acid **[see vitamin C/rose hips]**		
Ashwaghanda	➤ GROUP A Chronic Illness Recovery Fatigue-Fighting	Adaptogenic herb that promotes healthy stress response.
Astragalus	➤ GROUP A Chemotherapy Adjunct Immune-Enhancing ➤ GROUP B Cancer Prevention ➤ GROUP AB Antibacterial Antistress Chemotherapy Adjunct Immune-Enhancing Surgery Recovery	Immune modulator. Increases natural killer (NK) cell activity. Helps in the treatment of Alzheimer's disease. Aids in boosting chemotherapy support and immune function. Fights common cold/sore throat, infection.

COMMON NAME	BLOOD GROUP–SPECIFIC BENEFICIAL EFFECT	PRIMARY ACTION
Astragalus, (cont.)	➤ GROUP O Antibacterial Antiviral Cancer Prevention	
Bearberry	➤ GROUP B Urinary Tract Health	Supports proper bladder function.
Brahmi (*Bacopa monniera*)	➤ GROUP A Anti-Stress Cognitive Improvement ➤ GROUP AB Anti-Stress Cognitive Improvement	Antioxidant support for brain and nervous system. Also used to promote longevity, and to combat nervous system deficit due to injury and stroke.
Balsam bark	➤ GROUP B Male Health	Used to treat asthma, bronchitis, colic, cough, eczema, gout, itch, ringworm, skin troubles, stomachache, and hormonal dysfunction.
Baptisia tinctorialls (home remedy)	➤ GROUP A Antibacterial ➤ GROUP B Antibiotic Support	Used as a circulatory stimulant, antiseptic, laxative, and tonic. Has antimicrobial properties.
Beet leaf/root	➤ GROUP B Liver Support ➤ GROUP AB Liver Support	Acts as a laxative and also helps to promote liver health.
Beta carotene [see Vitamin A]		
Betaine HCl	➤ GROUP A Arthritis Blood-Building Yeast/Fungus Resistance ➤ GROUP AB Yeast/Fungus Resistance	Increases stomach acidity. Helps break down proteins for further digestion in the small intestine.
Bilberry	➤ GROUP AB Anti-Inflammation	Inhibits platelet aggregation. Increases membrane protection, which protects the stomach. Lowers blood glucose levels. Prevents free radical damage.

COMMON NAME	BLOOD GROUP–SPECIFIC BENE-FICIAL EFFECT	PRIMARY ACTION
Biotin	➤ **GROUP O** Skin Health	Antifungal in large doses.
Black cohosh	➤ **GROUP A** Female Balancing Menopause Support ➤ **GROUP AB** Menopause Support	Smooth muscle relaxant. Used to treat hot flashes and the symptoms of premenstrual syndrome.
Black currant seed oil	➤ **GROUP A** Female Balancing Intestinal Health	Source of omega-6 oils. Anti-inflammatory. Used to treat rheumatoid arthritis and infections. Also useful for kidney and blood health.
Bladderwrack (kelp)	➤ **GROUP O** Antibiotic Support Detoxification Stomach Health Yeast/Fungus Resistance	Metabolic aid. Traditional herbal medicine for weight loss. Kelp is a source of iodine, assisting in thyroid hormone production.
Spreading hogweed (*Boerhaavia diffusa*)	➤ **GROUP A** Antistress Cognitive Improvement	A stress modifier and liver protector.
Boron	➤ **NON-SECRETORS** Arthritis Menopause Support	Helps maintain healthy bones. Enhances metabolism of calcium, magnesium, copper, phosphorus, and vitamin D.
Bupleurem	➤ **GROUP B** Chemotherapy Adjunct Detoxification ➤ **GROUP AB** Liver Support	A Chinese herb with anti-inflammatory, adaptogenic, and sedative properties.
Burdock root	➤ **GROUP A** Cancer Prevention Intestinal Health Skin Health ➤ **GROUP AB** Detoxification	An immune modulator and blood purifier.
Calcium, citrate	➤ **ALL BLOOD GROUPS** Antistress Menopause Support	Needed to form bones and teeth and also required for blood clotting, transmission of signals in nerve cells, and muscle contraction.

COMMON NAME	BLOOD GROUP–SPECIFIC BENEFICIAL EFFECT	PRIMARY ACTION
Caprylic acid	➤ **GROUP A** Yeast/Fungus Resistance ➤ **GROUP O** Yeast/Fungus Resistance ➤ **NON-SECRETORS** Antibiotic Support Intestinal Health	Antifungal, antiseptic. Produced in the body in small amounts, antifungal in human sweat and sebum. Natural component of coconut oil, palm nut oil, butter fat, and other vegetable and animal sources, synthesized from caprylic alcohol (octanol) found in coconut oil.
Cat's claw	➤ **GROUP B** Anti-Inflammation	Immune modulator. Used to treat inflammation, rheumatism, gastric ulcers, tumors, and dysentery.
Cayenne pepper	➤ **GROUP O** Anti-Inflammation	Digestive stimulant. Used to treat diseases of the circulatory system, and as a remedy for rheumatic pains and arthritis.
Celery seed extract	➤ **GROUP AB** Female Balancing	Used to treat rheumatoid arthritis and urinary tract infections. Contains a component that has an anti-inflammatory effect on the tissues of the body.
Chamomile	➤ **GROUP A** Antistress Female Balancing Menopause Support Surgery Recovery ➤ **GROUP AB** Surgery Recovery	Nerve tonic. Calming and soothing; folk remedy for colic.
Chaste berry	➤ **GROUP O** Menopause Support	Female tonic. Acts upon the pituitary gland—specifically on the production of luteinizing hormone—to increase progesterone production and help regulate a woman's cycle.
Chickweed	➤ **GROUP AB** Urinary Tract Health	Bile stimulant. Used to treat asthma, indigestion, and skin diseases. Soothes and protects abraded mucus membranes.
Chlorella	➤ **GROUP B** Antiviral ➤ **GROUP AB** Antiviral	Immune modulator.
Chondroitin sulfate	➤ **GROUP A** Arthritis ➤ **GROUP AB** Arthritis	May have some benefits in regenerating joint cartilage. Chondroitin sulfate is a major constituent of cartilage, providing structure, holding water and nutrients, and allowing other molecules to move through cartilage.

COMMON NAME	BLOOD GROUP–SPECIFIC BENEFICIAL EFFECT	PRIMARY ACTION
Clove	➤ GROUP O Yeast/Fungus Resistance	An anti-inflammatory and anti-ulcer compound. Promotes resistance against *Candida albicans.*
Codonopsis	➤ NON-SECRETORS Immune-Enhancing	Used to treat diabetes, chronic cough and shortness of breath, prolapsed (fallen) uterus, lack of appetite, fatigue and tired limbs, and diarrhea and vomiting.
Coleus	➤ GROUP O Cardiovascular Fatigue-Fighting	Enhances intracellular energy production. Can lower blood pressure by relaxing arteriolar smooth muscle. Has a positive effect on the heart muscle, and is an inhibitor of platelet aggregation.
Colostrum, bovine	➤ GROUP AB Intestinal Health	Immune modulator. A highly concentrated source of powerful immune and growth factors produced from the mammary glands within the first 24–72 hours after giving birth. Generally contains immuniglobulins such as IgG, IgA, IgE, IgD, and IgM.
Copper citrate	➤ GROUP O Blood-Building Surgery Recovery	Maintains healthy blood cells, and is needed to absorb and use iron. Also part of the antioxidant enzyme superoxide dismutase (SOD).
Co enzyme Q10	➤ ALL BLOOD GROUPS Cancer Prevention ➤ NON-SECRETORS Cardiovascular Fatigue-Fighting Pulmonary Support	Increases intracellular energy. Protects against angina and congestive heart failure. A powerful antioxidant that protects the body from free radicals.
Cordyceps	➤ GROUP B Antistress Immune-Enhancing ➤ GROUP AB Anti-Stress	An antimicrobial agent, used to treat cough, night sweats, and bacterial infections. Useful as a treatment in recovering from a long illness.
Coriander	➤ ALL BLOOD GROUPS Female Balancing ➤ GROUP B Yeast/Fungus Resistance	Antispasmodic, appetizer, calmative. Also used topically for infections and joint pain.
Coriolus versicolor	➤ GROUP A Chemotherapy Adjunct ➤ GROUP B Antibacterial Antiviral Cancer Prevention	Extract is one of the most thoroughly researched all-natural products with proven benefit in cancer. Significant immune system benefit clearly demonstrated in dozens of published clinical studies.

COMMON NAME	BLOOD GROUP–SPECIFIC BENE-FICIAL EFFECT	PRIMARY ACTION
Coriolus versicolor (*cont.*)	➤ **GROUP AB** Chemotherapy Adjunct	
Corn silk	➤ **GROUP A** Urinary Tract Health	Urinary tract tonic.
Cranberry capsules	➤ **GROUP A** Urinary Tract Health ➤ **GROUP B** Urinary Tract Health ➤ **GROUP AB** Urinary Tract Health	Used to treat cystitis for both bacterial (*Escherichia coli*) and yeast-related cystitis.
Curcumin (turmeric)	➤ **GROUP A** Cancer Prevention ➤ **GROUP B** Cardiovascular Liver Support ➤ **GROUP AB** Cancer Prevention Liver Support	Used to treat many conditions, including poor vision, rheumatic pains, and coughs. Protects the liver and improves cardiovascular health.
Cysteine, *N*-acetyl (NAC)	➤ **GROUP AB** Metabolic Enhancement	Helps break down mucus.
Dandelion	➤ **GROUP A** Detoxification ➤ **GROUP AB** Intestinal Health ➤ **GROUP O** Metabolic Enhancement ➤ **NON-SECRETORS** Cardiovascular Liver Support	Leaves are a diuretic, used to treat constipation, edema (water retention), indigestion, and heartburn. Provides pregnancy and postpartum support. Roots used to treat alcohol withdrawal, constipation, indigestion, heartburn, and liver ailments, also to provide pregnancy and postpartum support.
Deflect	➤ **ALL BLOOD GROUPS** Intestinal Health Metabolic Enhancement	Acts as sacrificial molecules to preferentially bind to dietary lectins in the gastrointestinal tract before they can cross into the bloodstream.

COMMON NAME	BLOOD GROUP–SPECIFIC BENE-FICIAL EFFECT	PRIMARY ACTION
Deflect (*cont.*)	➤ NON-SECRETORS Anti-Inflammation Arthritis Detoxification Stomach Health Urinary Tract Health	
DHEA	➤ GROUP A Antistress	Blunts hormonal effects of stress and aging.
Dong quai	➤ GROUP B Menopause Support ➤ GROUP AB Female Balancing	Female tonic. Used to treat abnormal menstruation, suppressed menstrual flow, painful or difficult menstruation, and uterine bleeding. Dong quai traditionally used for hot flashes associated with perimenopause. Also used for both men and women with cardiovascular disease, including high blood pressure, and problems with peripheral circulation.
Echinacea	➤ GROUP A Antibiotic Support	Immune modulator. Increases the production and activity of white blood cells. Used to treat common cold/sore throat (for symptoms), infection, and influenza.
Elderberry (concentrate—"Proberry")	➤ ALL BLOOD GROUPS Antiviral ➤ NON-SECRETORS Immune-Enhancing Sinus Health	Antiviral; anti-oxidant. Used to treat bronchitis, common cold/sore throat, infection, and influenza.
Elecampane	➤ GROUP A Yeast/Fungus Resistance ➤ GROUP B Intestinal Health ➤ GROUP AB Yeast/Fungus Resistance	Promotes insulin sensitivity, lowers cortisol, provides fiber substrate needed to promote growth of friendly bacteria.
Escargot (Roman snail)	➤ GROUP A Cancer Prevention ➤ GROUP AB Cancer Prevention	Immune modulator.
Essential fatty acids	➤ GROUP A Cardiovascular Nerve Health	Used to treat Crohn's disease, high blood pressure, high triglycerides, rheumatoid arthritis, and ulcerative colitis. Also associated with treatments for memory loss, dementia, and visual problems.

COMMON NAME	BLOOD GROUP–SPECIFIC BENE-FICIAL EFFECT	PRIMARY ACTION
Essential fatty acids (*cont.*)	➤ GROUP B Nerve Health ➤ GROUP AB Cardiovascular Nerve Health ➤ GROUP O Anti-Inflammation Intestinal Health	
False daisy	➤ GROUP A Liver Support ➤ GROUP O Male Health	Liver protectant.
False unicorn root	➤ GROUP A Male Health	Supports reproductive health, for both men and women.
Fennel	➤ GROUP B Cancer Prevention	Used to treat colic, indigestion, and heartburn. Seeds are a common cooking spice, particularly for use with fish. After meals, they are used in several cultures to prevent gas and upset stomach. The seeds are also used in Latin America to increase the flow of breast milk. Fennel has also been used as a remedy for cough and colic in infants.
Fenugreek	➤ GROUP B Cardiovascular Immune-Enhancing Liver Support Metabolic Enhancement	Used to treat digestive distress, atherosclerosis, diabetes, and high triglycerides. Chinese herbalists use it for kidney problems and conditions affecting the male reproductive tract.
Feverfew	➤ ALL BLOOD GROUPS Metabolic Enhancement	Migraine remedy.
Fish oils	➤ GROUP A Anti-Inflammation Arthritis	Blood thinner, anti-inflammatory. Used to treat Crohn's disease, high blood pressure, high triglycerides, and rheumatoid arthritis.
Flaxseed husks	➤ GROUP A Intestinal Health	A source of fiber, used to treat constipation. Also thins the blood, protects arteries from damage, inhibits blood clots, reduces triglycerides, lowers LDL blood cholesterol, lowers blood pressure, and reduces risk of heart attack and stroke.
Floradix (liquid iron and herbs)	➤ GROUP A Blood-Building	Useful for anemic conditions or when there is a general need for blood building.

COMMON NAME	BLOOD GROUP–SPECIFIC BENEFICIAL EFFECT	PRIMARY ACTION
Folic acid [see Vitamin B]		
Frankincense (*Boswellia serrata*)	➤ GROUP A Anti-Inflammation ➤ GROUP AB Allergy Control Anti-Inflammation ➤ GROUP O Arthritis	Used to treat arthritis and inflammation.
GABA	➤ GROUP B Anti-Stress	Mild tranquilizer.
Garlic (standardized Chinese extract)	➤ GROUP AB Cardiovascular ➤ GROUP O Chemotherapy Adjunct Detoxification Yeast/Fungus Resistance	Antimicrobial. Used to treat high blood pressure and high triglycerides.
Garlic (standardized extract)	➤ GROUP AB Intestinal Health	Antimicrobial and also acts as a blood thinner.
Genistein (soy extract)	➤ GROUP A Cancer Prevention ➤ GROUP AB Cancer Prevention	Phytoestrogen. Isoflavones in soy, primarily genistein and daidzein, have been well researched for antioxidant and phytoestrogenic properties, and shown in studies to be potent aromatase inhibitors. Saponins enhance immune function and bind to cholesterol to limit its absorption in the intestine. Phytosterols and other components of soy have been reported to lower cholesterol levels.
Gentian	➤ GROUP A Stomach Health	Stomach tonic. Promotes appetite; improves digestion.
Ginger root	➤ ALL BLOOD GROUPS Stomach Health ➤ GROUP A Cardiovascular ➤ GROUP B Metabolic Enhancement Pulmonary Support	Stomach tonic. Used to treat anorexia, flatulence, gastric and intestinal spasms, acute colds, and painful menstruation.

COMMON NAME	BLOOD GROUP–SPECIFIC BENE-FICIAL EFFECT	PRIMARY ACTION
Ginger root (*cont.*)	➤ GROUP AB Pulmonary Support ➤ GROUP O Anti-Inflammation	
Gingko	➤ GROUP A Cardiovascular ➤ GROUP B Cognitive Improvement	Increases cerebral circulation. Used to treat Alzheimer's disease, atherosclerosis, cerebrovascular insufficiency, congestive heart failure, depression, diabetes, and impotence/infertility.
Ginseng, Chinese	➤ GROUP A Antiviral ➤ GROUP AB Fatigue-Fighting	Adaptogen; promotes healthy stress response. Used to treat heart disease, stress, diabetes mellitus, poor digestion, weakness after long illness/injury/surgery, and the effects of aging.
Ginseng, Siberian	➤ GROUP B Antibacterial Antiviral Chronic Illness Recovery Cognitive Improvement Fatigue-Fighting ➤ GROUP AB Antiviral Cognitive Improvement	Adaptogen; promotes healthy stress response, increases stamina and endurance, encourages normal adrenal gland function, enhances mental acuity, and combats harmful toxins.
Glucosamine sulfate	➤ GROUP O Anti-Inflammation	Supports connective tissue. Used to treat kidney stones and osteoarthritis, and for wound healing.
Glucosamine, *N*-acetyl (NAG)	➤ GROUP A Arthritis ➤ GROUP B Arthritis	Binds lectins, breaks down mucus, and protects the liver.
Glutamine	➤ GROUP O Antiviral Intestinal Health ➤ GROUP AB Nerve Health	An amino acid that is transformed into the GABA class of neurotransmitters. Helps with nerve transmission; can be soothing to the gut, serves as a source of fuel for cells lining the intestines. Alcohol withdrawal support, HIV support, peptic ulcer, ulcerative colitis, inflammatory bowel disease.

COMMON NAME	BLOOD GROUP–SPECIFIC BENEFICIAL EFFECT	PRIMARY ACTION
Gokharu	➤ GROUP A Pulmonary Support ➤ GROUP B Cognitive Improvement	Can raise testosterone levels by increasing luteinizing hormone. Balances stress hormones.
Goldenseal	➤ ALL BLOOD GROUPS Immune-Enhancing	Antibacterial. Used to treat mucous membrane infections and inflammations, upper respiratory ailments, influenza, gastroenteritis, infectious diarrhea, giardiasis, peptic ulcers, and uterine hemorrhage.
Gotu kola	➤ GROUP A Metabolic Enhancement Surgery Recovery ➤ GROUP AB Surgery Recovery ➤ GROUP O Female Balancing Metabolic Enhancement	Aids in rapid wound healing, chronic venous insufficiency, mental function, minor burns, scars, skin ulcers, varicose veins, and wound healing.
Green tea	➤ ALL BLOOD GROUPS Cancer Prevention Chemotherapy Adjunct Metabolic Enhancement	Antioxidant. Reduces cancer risk, gingivitis (periodontal disease), high cholesterol, high blood pressure, and high triglycerides. Improves immune function and guards against cardiovascular disease.
Gum, guggul	➤ GROUP O Cardiovascular Metabolic Enhancement	Lowers cholesterol. Gugulipid offers considerable benefit in preventing and treating atherosclerotic vascular disease (heart disease). Most effective in lowering LDL cholesterol and triglycerides. Also raises the level of good cholesterol (HDL). Guggul exhibits a cholesterol lowering ability unlike any other natural substance. In human trials of gugulipid, cholesterol levels dropped 14% to 27% in a 4- to 12-week period, while triglyceride levels dropped from 22% to 30%.
Hawthorn	➤ GROUP A Allergy Control Cardiovascular ➤ GROUP AB Cardiovascular	Promotes improved heart function. Used to treat angina, atherosclerosis, congestive heart failure, and high blood pressure. Improves coronary artery blood flow and the contractions of the heart muscle.
Helix pomatia	➤ GROUP A Cancer Prevention ➤ GROUP AB Cancer Prevention	Lectin in *Helix pomatia*, through its ability to recognize the altered products on metastatic cells, appears to act by turning off a cancer cell's "cloaking device" and allowing it to be more visible to the immune system.

COMMON NAME	BLOOD GROUP–SPECIFIC BENE-FICIAL EFFECT	PRIMARY ACTION
He shou wu ("Fo-Ti")	➤ GROUP A Antiviral ➤ NON-SECRETORS Cardiovascular	Eastern and Western herbalists recommend Fo-Ti as supplement to maintain youthful vigor, increase energy, tone the kidneys and liver, and purify the blood. Also employed as a remedy for insomnia, stomach upset, and diabetes; contains a number of glycosides that account for the herbs use as a remedy for stomach disorders and constipation. He shou wu roots may contain compounds with mild cardiovascular and anti-inflammatory effects.
Hibiscus	➤ ALL BLOOD GROUPS Female Balancing	Acts as an adaptogen for the female reproductive system.
Holy basil	➤ GROUP A Anti-Inflammation Antistress Skin Health	Lowers cortisol; prevents stress-related breakdown.
Hops	➤ GROUP AB Antistress	Nerve tonic. Soothes the stomach and promotes healthy digestion.
Horehound	➤ GROUP AB Pulmonary Support	Expectorant, bitter tonic, and antiseptic. Normalizes irregular heartbeat in small amounts. Vasodilator.
Horse chestnut	➤ GROUP A Surgery Recovery ➤ GROUP O Surgery Recovery	Used to treat varicose veins, bruising, chronic venous insufficiency, edema (water retention), hemorrhoids, and minor injuries.
Horseradish root	➤ GROUP A Pulmonary Support	Used to treat sinus conditions, bronchitis, chronic obstructive sinusitis, pulmonary disease, common cold/sore throat, indigestion, and heartburn.
Horsetail	➤ GROUP AB Surgery Recovery ➤ GROUP O Menopause Support Surgery Recovery Urinary Tract Health	Used to treat brittle nails, edema (water retention) as a diuretic, osteoarthritis, osteoporosis, and rheumatoid arthritis.
Huang lian	➤ GROUP AB Antibiotic Support	Shown to block the adherence of harmful bacteria.
Indol-3-carbinol	➤ GROUP A Cancer Prevention Chemotherapy Adjunct	Compounds found in cruciferous vegetables like cabbage, Brussels sprouts, cauliflower, collards, and broccoli help to transform dangerous estrogen into more benign forms. Shown to stop the growth of breast-cancer cells.

COMMON NAME	BLOOD GROUP–SPECIFIC BENE-FICIAL EFFECT	PRIMARY ACTION
Indol-3-carbinol (*cont.*)	➤ GROUP AB Cancer Prevention Chemotherapy Adjunct	
Inositol	➤ GROUP B Anti-Stress Cognitive Improvement Nerve Health	Component of cell membrane important in restoring cell fluidity and function.
Inula	➤ GROUP A Yeast/Fungus resistance ➤ GROUP B Intestinal Health ➤ GROUP AB Yeast/Fungus Resistance	Promotes insulin sensitivity, lowers cortisol, provides fiber substrate needed to promote growth of friendly bacteria.
Iron citrate	➤ GROUP B Blood-Building ➤ GROUP AB Blood-Building	Blood health.
Isatis	➤ GROUP O Immune-Enhancing	Immune modulator.
Jiaogulan	➤ GROUP B Anti-Inflammation ➤ GROUP AB Anti-Inflammation	Acts as an anti-inflammatory agent.
Job's tears	➤ GROUP B Immune-Enhancing	Antioxidant.
Kava kava	➤ GROUP A Anti-Inflammation	Sedative, hypnotic, also noted for initiating a state of contentment, a greater sense of well-being, and enhanced mental acuity, memory, and sensory perception. Used traditionally to treat pain. Kava-lactones may have anti-anxiety, analgesic (pain-relieving), muscle-relaxing, and anti-convulsant effects.
Kelp	➤ GROUP O Metabolic Enhancement Female Balancing	Known for its properties of metabolic enhancement. Concentrated source of minerals, including iodine, potassium, magnesium, calcium, and iron. As a source of iodine, assists in making thyroid hormones.

COMMON NAME	BLOOD GROUP–SPECIFIC BENE-FICIAL EFFECT	PRIMARY ACTION
L-carnitine	➤ GROUP O Cardiovascular Chronic Illness Recovery	Enhances intracellular energy processes; helpful in some types of muscular dystrophy.
L-glutathione	➤ ALL BLOOD GROUPS Liver Support ➤ GROUP B Detoxification ➤ NON-SECRETORS/SUBTYPES Antibiotic Support	One of the body's most powerful antioxidants.
L-phenylalanine	➤ GROUP O Arthritis relief	Used to treat osteoarthritis, Parkinson's disease, and rheumatoid arthritis. Also thought to be effective in treating depression and alcohol withdrawal. L-phenylalanine can be converted to L-tyrosine (another amino acid) and subsequently to L-dopa, norepinephrine, and epinephrine.
L-tryptophan (5HT)	➤ NON-SECRETORS Antistress Anti-Inflammation	Helps balance neurotransmitters.
Kutki (Picrorhiza)	➤ O Antibacterial Antiviral	Liver protectant. Also used to treat asthma, acute and chronic infections, immune conditions, and autoimmune disease.
Licorice (DGL) (De-glycyrrhizinated)	➤ GROUP B Fatigue-Fighting Liver Support ➤ GROUP AB Fatigue-Fighting Stomach Health ➤ GROUP O Stomach Health	Used to treat stomach ulcers, canker sores (mouth ulcers), indigestion, and heartburn.
Linden	➤ GROUP A Antiviral ➤ GROUP B Antiviral ➤ GROUP AB Antiviral	Anti-inflammatory and nerve health agent.

COMMON NAME	BLOOD GROUP–SPECIFIC BENE-FICIAL EFFECT	PRIMARY ACTION
Lipoic acid	➤ **GROUP A** Liver Support ➤ **GROUP B** Antibiotic Support Cardiovascular ➤ **GROUP AB** Liver Support	Lipoic acid, a vitamin-like substance that contains sulfur, is important to the body in the production of energy. Also effective against water- and fat-soluble free radical damage. Helps catecholamine elimination. Enhances sensitivity to insulin.
Liver extract	➤ **GROUP O** Blood-Building	Used to treat anemia.
Lysine	➤ **GROUP B** Anti-Stress ➤ **GROUP AB** Antistress	Essential amino acid needed for growth, and to help maintain nitrogen balance in the body. Appears to help the body absorb and conserve calcium.
Ma huang	➤ **GROUP B** Allergy Control	Decongestant. Used to treat asthma, congestion, cough, chronic obstructive pulmonary disease, weight loss, and obesity.
Magnesium	➤ **ALL BLOOD GROUPS** Female Balancing ➤ **GROUP B** Allergy Control Chronic Illness Recovery Fatigue-Fighting Intestinal Health Menopausal Support	Nerve and digestive health. Needed for bone, protein, and fatty acid formation, making new cells, activating B vitamins, relaxing muscles, and clotting blood.
Magnolia flower	➤ **GROUP B** Sinus Health ➤ **GROUP AB** Allergy Control	Sinus and allergy remedy.
Maitake mushroom extract	➤ **GROUP A** Cancer Prevention ➤ **GROUP B** Chemotherapy Adjunct Immune-Enhancing	Immune modulator. Used to treat diabetes, high cholesterol, HIV-related conditions, high blood pressure, high triglycerides, and infection. Useful as a chemotherapy support.

COMMON NAME	BLOOD GROUP–SPECIFIC BENEFICIAL EFFECT	PRIMARY ACTION
Maitake mushroom extract (*cont.*)	➤ GROUP O Cancer Prevention ➤ NON-SECRETORS Antistress	
Man root	➤ GROUP O Male Health	Immune tonic. Used to treat infections, gastrointestinal disturbances, kidney ailments, and liver ailments.
Manganese	➤ GROUP O Menopause Support	Needed for healthy skin, bone, and cartilage formation, as well as glucose tolerance. Useful in hypoglycemia and osteoporosis.
Marigold	➤ ALL BLOOD GROUPS Skin Health	Used to treat inflammation, eczema, and various skin conditions.
Marshmallow	➤ GROUP B Stomach Health	Excellent demulcent, soothing to mucus membranes, such as those in the gastrointestinal tract.
Melatonin	➤ GROUP B Fatigue-Fighting	Aid to sleep. Shortens the time needed to go to sleep, reduces the number of night awakenings, and improves sleep quality. May help down-regulate FGF receptors.
Methionine	➤ GROUP B Arthritis	Essential amino acid. Helpful for aiding liver detoxification.
Methylcobalamin [see vitamin B_{12}]		
Milk thistle	➤ GROUP AB Liver Support ➤ GROUP O Liver Support	Functions as a liver protectant and antioxidant.
Moducare (plant sterols and sterolins)	➤ ALL BLOOD GROUPS Immune-Enhancing	Enhances immunity by acting as an immune adaptogen. The plant sterols and sterolins help support a normal, balanced T-helper 1 to T-helper 2 response, which is essential for proper immune functioning. Guards against a hyperactive immune system.
Motherwort	➤ GROUP B Female Balancing Menopause Support ➤ GROUP AB Female Balancing	Tonic and laxative used to treat menstrual difficulties and menopausal symptoms.

COMMON NAME	BLOOD GROUP–SPECIFIC BENEFICIAL EFFECT	PRIMARY ACTION
MSM (methylsulfonylmethane)	➤ **GROUP A** Pulmonary Support ➤ **GROUP B** Allergy Control Anti-Inflammation ➤ **GROUP AB** Pulmonary Support ➤ **GROUP O** Sinus Health	Promotes joint and pulmonary health.
Mullein	➤ **GROUP O** Pulmonary Support	Used to treat asthma, bronchitis, chronic obstructive pulmonary disease, common cold/sore throat, cough, and recurrent ear infection.
NAG	➤ **GROUP B** Pulmonary Support ➤ **GROUP O** Arthritis Intestinal Health ➤ **NON-SECRETORS** Cardiovascular	Used to treat obesity by binding onto certain lectins that promote insulin resistance.
Niacinamide [see Vitamin B₃]		
Noni	➤ **GROUP A** Blood-Building Cancer Prevention ➤ **GROUP O** Pulmonary Support	An anti-inflammatory agent and an antioxidant.
Old man's beard	➤ **GROUP A** Antibacterial Stomach Health Urinary Tract Health	Antibiotic; inhibits growth of bacteria.

COMMON NAME	BLOOD GROUP–SPECIFIC BENE-FICIAL EFFECT	PRIMARY ACTION
OPCs (oligomeric proanthocyanidins)	➤ **GROUP A** Cognitive Improvement ➤ **GROUP B** Anti-Inflammation Cardiovascular Skin Health ➤ **GROUP AB** Cognitive Improvement Skin Health	A class of nutrients belonging to the flavinoid family. Two of the main functions of OPCs are as antioxidants and in the stabilization of collagen and maintenance of elastin, which are components of connective tissue.
Oregano	➤ **GROUP B** Yeast/Fungus Resistance	Common herb used in cooking. Antifungal and anti-inflammatory.
Oregon grape	➤ **GROUP A** Antibacterial Yeast/Fungus Resistance	Berberine inhibits the ability of bacteria to attach to human cells, which helps prevent infections, particularly in the throat and urinary tract, and enhances immune cell function. Used to treat infection, parasites, poor digestion, psoriasis, and urinary tract infections.
Osha root	➤ **GROUP O** Immune-Enhancing	Antiviral agent, used to treat herpes, sore throats, colds, flu, and as a bronchial expectorant. Has immune stimulating properties as well.
Pancreatic enzymes	➤ **GROUP O** Antibiotic Support	Digestive aid.
Pantethine (active B$_5$) [see also Vitamin B$_5$]	➤ **GROUP A** Cardiovascular Skin Support ➤ **GROUP AB** Cardiovascular	Lowers cholesterol.
Pantothenic acid [see Vitamin B$_5$]		
Parsley leaf	➤ **GROUP A** Female Balancing ➤ **GROUP B** Female Balancing ➤ **GROUP AB** Female Balancing Stomach Health Urinary Tract Health	Used as a stomach tonic, antioxidant, and a diuretic. Encourages uric acid elimination. Increases milk in lactating women. Inhibits histamine release. Tones uterine muscles.

COMMON NAME	BLOOD GROUP–SPECIFIC BENEFICIAL EFFECT	PRIMARY ACTION
Phosphatidyl choline (lecithin)	➤ **GROUP B** Chronic Illness Recovery ➤ **GROUP AB** Nerve Health	Nerve and circulatory remedy. Used to treat anxiety, eczema, gallbladder attacks, hepatitis, manic depression, and liver ailments.
Picrorhiza	➤ **GROUP O** Antibacterial Antiviral	Liver protectant. Also used to treat asthma, acute and chronic infections, immune conditions, and autoimmune disease.
Pineapple enzyme (Bromelain)	➤ **ALL BLOOD GROUPS** Allergy Control Anti-Inflammation Surgery Recovery ➤ **GROUP A** Antibiotic Support ➤ **GROUP O** Urinary Tract Health	Inflammation modulator. Bromelain is an anti-inflammatory agent. Used to treat minor injuries, particularly sprains and strains, muscle injuries, and the pain, swelling, and tenderness that accompany sports injuries. Also good for angina, asthma, minor injuries, and urinary tract infection.
Potassium citrate	➤ **GROUP A** Chronic Illness Recovery ➤ **GROUP B** Allergy Control Fatigue-Fighting Liver Support ➤ **GROUP AB** Fatigue-Fighting	Supports proper nerve function. Needed to regulate water balance, levels of acidity, blood pressure, and neuromuscular function. Required for carbohydrate and protein metabolism.
Primrose oil	➤ **ALL BLOOD GROUPS** Female Balancing	Anti-inflammatory, blood thinner, and blood vessel dilator. Evening primrose oil (EPO) contains gamma linolenic acid (GLA), a fatty acid that the body converts to a hormone-like substance called prostaglandin E1 (PGE1), helpful to the female cycle.
Probiotics	➤ **ALL BLOOD GROUPS** Antibiotic Support Cardiovascular Chemotherapy Adjunct Detoxification Fatigue-Fighting Immune-Enhancing Intestinal Health Stomach Health Urinary Tract Health Yeast/Fungus Resistance	Beneficial bacteria, such as *Lactobacillus acidophilus* and *Bifidobacterium bifidum*, are called probiotics. Probiotic bacteria favorably alter the intestinal microflora balance, inhibit the growth of harmful bacteria, promote good digestion, boost immune function, and increase resistance to infection. Individuals with flourishing intestinal colonies of beneficial bacteria are better equipped to fight the growth of disease-causing bacteria.

COMMON NAME	BLOOD GROUP–SPECIFIC BENE-FICIAL EFFECT	PRIMARY ACTION
Probiotics (*cont.*)	➤ NON-SECRETORS Cancer Prevention Skin Health	
Pygeum extract	➤ GROUP O Male Health	Supports prostate health.
Pyridoxal [see Vitamin B₆]		
Quercetin	➤ GROUP A Cancer Prevention Intestinal Health Pulmonary Support ➤ GROUP AB Cancer Prevention Intestinal Health	Antioxidant. Acts as an antihistamine and has anti-inflammatory activity. Inhibits the enzyme aldose reductase, which can decrease the buildup of sorbitol. Sorbitol has been linked to nerve, kidney, and eye damage in diabetics.
Raspberry leaf	➤ GROUP B Female Balancing	Female tonic. Used for pregnancy and postpartum support.
Red clover	➤ GROUP AB Skin Health	Blood clot inhibitor and blood purifier.
Rehmannia root	➤ GROUP B Surgery Recovery ➤ GROUP O Surgery Recovery	Promotes healing of injured bones and blood clotting. Commonly used in clinics in the orient and is called di-huang, or "yellow earth." Used to treat diabetes, constipation, urinary tract problems, anemia, dizziness, and irregular menstrual flow.
Reishi mushroom	➤ GROUP AB Immune-Enhancing ➤ GROUP O Immune-Enhancing	Promotes long-term antiviral resistance. Helps lower blood pressure as well as decrease low-density lipoprotein (LDL) and triglyceride levels. Also helps to reduce blood clotting.
Rhodiola	➤ GROUP O Antistress Fatigue-Fighting Cognitive Improvement	Anti-stress remedy. Prevents stress-induced catecholamine activity in the heart, and promotes stable heart contractility.
Rhus tox	➤ GROUP O Arthritis	Homeopathic remedy made from poison ivy. Used to treat skin ailments, achy joints, and rheumatic pains.

COMMON NAME	BLOOD GROUP–SPECIFIC BENEFICIAL EFFECT	PRIMARY ACTION
Rose hips **[see Vitamin C/rose hips]**		
Rosemary	➤ **GROUP B** Yeast/Fungus Resistance ➤ **GROUP O** Cancer Prevention	Has potent antibacterial effects, and can relax smooth muscles in the lungs. May inhibit cancer formation.
Sage	➤ **GROUP B** Immune-Enhancing ➤ **GROUP AB** Menopause Support	Antibacterial, especially against *Staphylococcus aureus*. Also has antiseptic and antispasmodic properties. Stimulates muscles of the uterus.
Saint John's wort	➤ **GROUP A** Antistress	Antidepressant. Promotes neurotransmitter balance. Used to treat anxiety, depression, herpes simplex/cold sores, HIV-related conditions, and recurrent ear infections.
Sarsaparilla	➤ **GROUP B** Skin Health ➤ **GROUP O** Fatigue-Fighting Chronic Illness Recovery	General tonic. Used to treat arthritis, cancer, skin diseases, and psoriasis.
Saw palmetto	➤ **GROUP A** Male Health ➤ **GROUP B** Male Health ➤ **GROUP AB** Male Health	Prostate remedy.
Schisandra	➤ **GROUP B** Antibacterial Anti-Stress	Supports proper nerve health. Used to treat common cold/sore throat, fatigue, hepatitis, and stress.
Slippery elm	➤ **GROUP AB** Stomach Health Yeast/Fungus Resistance	Digestive protectant. Used to treat common cold/sore throat, cough, Crohn's disease, and gastritis.

COMMON NAME	BLOOD GROUP–SPECIFIC BENEFICIAL EFFECT	PRIMARY ACTION
Squaw vine	➤ **GROUP A** Menopause Support ➤ **GROUP O** Female Balancing	Used to treat menstrual problems and menopausal symptoms.
Stinging Nettle leaf	➤ **GROUP A** Allergy Control Sinus Health ➤ **GROUP AB** Sinus Health ➤ **GROUP O** Allergy Control Blood-Building Sinus Health	Anti-inflammatory. Used to treat hay fever, sinusitis, and prostate enlargement.
Stinging Nettle, root	➤ **GROUP A** Male Health Yeast/Fungus Resistance ➤ **GROUP O** Male Health Yeast/Fungus Resistance	Supports healthy immune function. The root has effects on hormones and proteins that carry sex hormones (such as testosterone or estrogen) in the human body. It also contains a "super lectin" called UDA, which inhibits viruses.
Stone root	➤ **GROUP A** Sinus Health ➤ **GROUP AB** Sinus Health	Helps support healthy sinus function. Stimulates and tones the alimentary mucous membranes. Strengthen structure and function of veins.
Sweet basil	➤ **GROUP AB** Cancer Prevention	Tonic to stimulate entire system. Can be used to relax smooth muscles of the gastrointestinal tract and has anti-cancer properties.
Tarragon	➤ **GROUP A** Cancer Prevention ➤ **GROUP O** Cancer Prevention	Primarily a cooking spice. Known to contain over 50 anti-cancer compounds.
Tea tree oil	➤ **NON-SECRETORS** Skin Health	Oil from tree acts as fungicide. Also useful topically for the treatment of eczema of the hands.

COMMON NAME	BLOOD GROUP–SPECIFIC BENE-FICIAL EFFECT	PRIMARY ACTION
Thiamine [see Vitamin B,]		
Thistle, blessed	➤ GROUP A Female Balancing ➤ GROUP O Female Balancing	Reduces fever. Used to treat digestive problems, including gas, constipation, stomach upset, and liver and gallbladder diseases.
Thyme	➤ GROUP B Pulmonary Support Yeast/Fungus Resistance ➤ GROUP AB Yeast/Fungus Resistance	Antibacterial and antifungal agent.
Tribulus	➤ GROUP B Antibacterial	Adaptogen. Promotes healthy stress response.
Triphala	➤ ALL BLOOD GROUPS Detoxification ➤ GROUP A Metabolic Enhancement ➤ GROUP AB Metabolic Enhancement	Acts to detoxify and help enhance metabolic efficiency.
Turmeric	➤ GROUP B Anti-Inflammation ➤ GROUP AB Anti-Inflammation	Used to treat many conditions, including poor vision, rheumatic pains, and coughs. Increases milk production. Protects against free radical damage. Reduces inflammation by lowering histamine levels, and possibly by increasing production of natural cortisone by the adrenal glands. Protects the liver from a number of toxic compounds. Shown to reduce platelets from clumping together, which in turn improves circulation and helps protect against atherosclerosis.
Tyrosine	➤ GROUP A Metabolic Enhancement ➤ GROUP O Antistress Fatigue-Fighting	Nonessential amino acid that acts as a precursor to thyroid hormone.
Uva Ursi	➤ GROUP B Urinary Tract Health	Supports proper bladder function.

COMMON NAME	BLOOD GROUP–SPECIFIC BENE-FICIAL EFFECT	PRIMARY ACTION
Valerian	➤ **GROUP O** Antistress	Used to treat anxiety and insomnia.
Vervain	➤ **GROUP O** Menopause Support	Nerve tonic, sedative, antispasmodic, and hypotensive agent.
Vitamin A	➤ **GROUP A** Immune-Enhancing Skin Health ➤ **GROUP AB** Skin Health ➤ **GROUP O** Skin Health ➤ **NON-SECRETORS** Antibacterial Antiviral Chemotherapy Adjunct Menopause Support Pulmonary Support Sinus Health Urinary Tract Health	Antioxidant and immune enhancer. Necessary for formation of bone, protein, and growth hormone. Also essential for normal reproduction and lactation.
Vitamin B **(Folic Acid)**	➤ **ALL BLOOD GROUPS** Cardiovascular ➤ **GROUP A** Blood-Building ➤ **GROUP B** Blood-Building ➤ **GROUP O** Cognitive Improvement	Necessary for the proper functioning of antidepressant agents like Zoloft and Prozac. Lowers homocysteine, builds blood. Used to treat celiac disease, Crohn's disease, depression, and gingivitis. Useful for pregnancy and postpartum support.
Vitamin B$_1$ **(Thiamine)**	➤ **GROUP AB** Cognitive Improvement ➤ **GROUP O** Cognitive Improvement	Nerve health. Needed to process carbohydrates, fat, and protein. Every cell of the body requires vitamin B$_1$. Used to treat fibromyalgia, canker sores, and minor injuries. Helpful in HIV support, and pregnancy and postpartum support.

COMMON NAME	BLOOD GROUP–SPECIFIC BENE-FICIAL EFFECT	PRIMARY ACTION
Vitamin B_3 (Niacin)	➤ ALL BLOOD GROUPS Skin Health ➤ GROUP B Arthritis Nerve Health ➤ GROUP AB Arthritis	The body uses vitamin B_3 in the process of releasing energy from carbohydrates. Needed to form fat from carbohydrates and to process alcohol. Niacin form of vitamin B_3 also regulates cholesterol.
Vitamin B_5 (Pantothenic acid)	➤ GROUP A Chronic Illness Recovery Fatigue-Fighting ➤ GROUP B Allergy Control Skin Health ➤ GROUP AB Chronic Illness Recovery ➤ GROUP O Allergy Control Skin Health	Helps blunt effects of stress, activates the adrenal glands.
Vitamin B_6	➤ GROUP A Menopause Support ➤ GROUP AB Menopause Support ➤ GROUP O Female Balancing Blood-Building	Helps protein metabolism. Helps to make and take apart many amino acids, and also needed to make serotonin, melatonin, and dopamine. Aids in the formation of several neurotransmitters, and thus an essential nutrient in regulation of mental processes and possibly mood.
Vitamin B_{12} Methylcobalamin	➤ GROUP A Blood-Building Cognitive Improvement Fatigue-Fighting Nerve Health ➤ GROUP B Menopause Support ➤ GROUP AB Blood-Building Menopause Support Nerve Health	Methylcobalamin is a specific form of B_{12} needed for nervous system health.

COMMON NAME	BLOOD GROUP–SPECIFIC BENE-FICIAL EFFECT	PRIMARY ACTION
Vitamin B$_{12}$ Methylcobalamin (*cont.*)	➤ **GROUP O** Fatigue-Fighting	
Vitamin C (preferably rose hips)	➤ **ALL BLOOD GROUPS** Arthritis Blood-Building Chronic Illness Recovery Pulmonary Support Sinus Health Surgical Recovery Urinary Tract Health ➤ **GROUP A** Allergy Fatigue Fighting Immune Enhancing ➤ **GROUP AB** Fatigue-Fighting Immune-Enhancing ➤ **NON-SECRETOR/ SUBTYPES** Allergy	
Vitamin D	➤ **ALL BLOOD GROUPS** Menopause Support	Most important role is maintaining blood levels of calcium, which it accomplishes by increasing absorption of calcium from food and reducing urinary calcium loss. Plays a role in immunity and blood cell formation.
Vitamin E	➤ **ALL BLOOD GROUPS** Surgical Recovery	Powerful antioxidant that protects cell membranes and other fat-soluble parts of the body, such as LDL cholesterol. Helps in wound healing and decreases the amount of adhesions that may form after certain surgeries.
Vitamin K	➤ **GROUP O** Surgery Recovery	Needed for proper bone formation and blood clotting, in both cases by helping the body transport calcium.
Vitex	➤ **GROUP B** Female Balancing	Used to treat fibrocystic breast disease, infertility (female), menopause, menstrual difficulties, and premenstrual syndrome.
Watermelon seed	➤ **GROUP B** Metabolic Enhancement	Acts as a diuretic and to balance metabolism.
White atractylodes	➤ **GROUP B** Surgical Recovery	Protects the liver and increases the secretion of bile and gastric juice.

COMMON NAME	BLOOD GROUP–SPECIFIC BENE-FICIAL EFFECT	PRIMARY ACTION
Wild indigo	➤ GROUP B Sinus Health	Immune modulator. Used to treat common cold/sore throat, Crohn's disease, influenza, and sinusitis.
Wild oat	➤ ALL BLOOD GROUPS Nerve Health ➤ GROUP A Anti-Stress	Nerve tonic. Used to treat anxiety, eczema, high cholesterol, high triglycerides, insomnia, and nicotine withdrawal.
Wild yam	➤ GROUP O Menopause Support	Source of progesterone. Used to treat abdominal cramps, high cholesterol, high triglycerides, menopausal symptoms, muscle pain, and spasms.
Willow bark	➤ GROUP A Anti-Inflammation	Anti-inflammatory. Used to treat bursitis, fever, headache (tension), osteoarthritis, and rheumatoid arthritis.
Witchhazel	➤ ALL BLOOD GROUPS Skin Health	Astringent. Used to treat hemorrhoids, wounds, painful tumors, insect bites, and ulcers.
Woad root	➤ GROUP O Immune-Enhancing	Immune modulator.
Yarrow	➤ GROUP AB Detoxification	Supports intestinal health.
Yellow dock	➤ GROUP AB Blood-Building	Blood tonic. Used to treat skin conditions that are attributed to toxic metabolites from maldigestion and poor liver function.
Yerba Santa	➤ ALL BLOOD GROUPS Sinus Health ➤ GROUP O Allergy Control	Mild decongestant and expectorant.
Yucca	➤ GROUP O Anti-Inflammation	Anti-inflammatory agent.

COMMON NAME	BLOOD GROUP–SPECIFIC BENE-FICIAL EFFECT	PRIMARY ACTION
Zinc	➤ **ALL BLOOD GROUPS** Male Health Pulmonary Support Skin Health Surgical Recovery ➤ **GROUP A** Immune-Enhancing ➤ **GROUP AB** Chronic Illness Recovery Immune-Enhancing ➤ **NON-SECRETORS** Antibacterial Antiviral Yeast/Fungus resistance	Maintains proper immune function. Component of more than 300 enzymes that are needed to repair wounds, maintain fertility, synthesize protein, help cells reproduce, preserve vision, boost immunity, and protect against free radicals.

Self Testing

HOME BLOOD TYPING KITS

North American Pharmacal, Inc., is the official distributor of Home Blood Type Testing Kits. Each kit costs $7.95 and is a single-use disposable educational device capable of determining one individual's ABO and rhesus blood type. Results are obtained within about 4 to 5 minutes. If you have several friends or family members who need to learn their blood type, you will need to order a separate home blood-typing kit for each individual.

All U.S. orders are shipped via UPS ground (shipping and handling cost is $5.25 per order irrespective of the number of kits ordered). Expedited shipping methods (UPS second day or next day) are available but cost more. Please contact the customer service department to inquire about rates for expedited shipping to your area.

If you are ordering a kit to be shipped outside of the U.S., shipping rates can vary dramatically and can be quite expensive. Please contact our customer service department prior to placing your order for an estimate of shipping charges for non-U.S. orders.

To order a single Home Blood Typing Kit, please enclose $7.95 plus $5.25 for shipping and handling and send to:

North American Pharmacal, Inc.
5 Brook Street
Norwalk, CT 06851
Telephone: 203-866-7664
Fax: 203-838-4066
Toll Free: 1-877-ABO-TYPE (1-877-226-8973)
www.4yourtype.com

To contact Dr. Peter D'Adamo or to get more information on the Blood Type Diet, you can go to his website www.dadamo.com. The website has an interactive message board and archives of past posts and questions to the board. This is currently the only vehicle available for additional information regarding Dr. D'Adamo's ongoing research on blood type and individuality.

Blood Type Specialty Products

North American Pharmacal, Inc., is the official distributor of the Blood Type Diet Specialty Products.

The product line includes a home blood type kit, the secretor test, books, educational materials, supplements, meal replacement bars, teas and support materials that have been specifically crafted to address the unique requirements of each blood type.

North American Pharmacal, Inc.
5 Brook Street
Norwalk, CT 06851
Telephone: 203-866-7664
Fax: 203-838-4066
Toll Free: 1-877-ABO-TYPE (1-877-226-8973)
www.4yourtype.com